TECHNIQUES AND PROCEDURES
OF
ANESTHESIA

Third Edition, Third Printing

Techniques and Procedures of

ANESTHESIA

By

JOHN ADRIANI, M.D.

Director, Department of Anesthesiology, Charity Hospital
Professor of Surgery, School of Medicine
Tulane University of Louisiana
and
Clinical Professor of Surgery and Pharmacology
School of Medicine, Louisiana State University
New Orleans, Louisiana

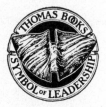

CHARLES C THOMAS · PUBLISHER

Springfield · Illinois · U.S.A.

Published and Distributed Throughout the World by
CHARLES C THOMAS • PUBLISHER
Bannerstone House
301-327 East Lawrence Avenue, Springfield, Illinois, U.S.A.

© 1947, 1956, and 1964, by CHARLES C THOMAS • PUBLISHER
ISBN 0-398-00015-8
Library of Congress Catalog Card Number: 63-12294

First Edition, First Printing, 1947
First Edition, Second Printing, 1949
First Edition, Third Printing, 1950
First Edition, Fourth Printing, 1952
First Edition, Fifth Printing, 1953
First Edition, Sixth Printing, 1954
Second Edition, First Printing, 1956
Second Edition, Second Printing, 1960
Third Edition, First Printing, 1964
Third Edition, Second Printing, 1969
Third Edition, Third Printing, 1972

Printed in the United States of America
B-7

INTRODUCTION

The technique of anesthesia cannot be learned from books. For the most part, the instruction must be practical and can only be taught in the operating room. However, this practical instruction should be supplemented by organized lectures or classroom work.

The author has found that an outline of procedures based upon the fundamentals of anesthesia simplifies and expedites the process of teaching and learning for both instructor and pupil. This outline of procedures and techniques has been employed by the author as a guide for beginners in anesthesia.

It is obvious that an author cannot assemble a book of procedures which would please and satisfy every anesthetist who is engaged in teaching anesthesia. *The material which must be compressed into an outline of this sort is vast.* Adequate condensation is not possible without slighting topics and details which, to some teachers, may appear more important than the topics and details outlined.

Each anesthetist ultimately develops his own technique and manner of performing his duties. It would appear, then, that almost as many individual techniques exist for a given procedure as there are anesthetists. However, closer scrutiny will reveal that these seemingly varied techniques are all based upon the same fundamental principles and that they differ from one another only in minor details.

The techniques described in this book are those which illustrate fundamental principles and which the author has found adaptable for student personnel and suitable in his management of the Department of Anesthesia at Charity Hospital of Louisiana at New Orleans.

The author lays no claim to originality of any of the techniques outlined. Many have been employed for so long a period of time that they are now accepted medical practice. Others have been introduced recently and are described with modifications. Reference is made to the original description of a technique or procedure and its author, whenever this is possible, and particularly in the case of newer techniques. The methods of regional anesthesia are based upon the approaches advocated by Labat and his teachers and pupils.

The author wishes to stress the fact that there is no such thing as a "routine" in the administration of anesthetics. Each situation and each patient which the student encounters presents a different problem. No two situations are identical. Each step in the performance of one's duties has an underlying reason behind its execution. The reason may be a physiologic, pharmacologic or other equally important fact. An attempt has been made in this outline not only *to enumerate the technical details* of anesthesia but *the associated reasons for executing them* in the manner described.

The conduct of anesthesia is influenced by such variable factors as the disease with which the patient is afflicted, the type of operation to be performed, the skill and dexterity of the surgeon, or the pharmacologic effect of the drug upon the patient. In order to be a skillful technician, the anesthetist must possess a knowledge of the fundamental sciences, diagnostic acumen, and that faculty which, in medicine, is known as judgment. The student will do well, if he wishes to balance his training, to pursue parallel reading in the fundamental sciences of anatomy, chemistry, physiology, pharmacology, pathology, and in clinical subjects related to the field of anesthesiology.

The author wishes to acknowledge the assistance, suggestions and criticisms of Dr. Ralph Sappenfield, Anesthetist, Miami, Florida; Dr. Keith Stratford, Salt Lake City, formerly assistant resident in surgery, Tulane Unit, Charity Hospital of Louisiana at New Orleans; and of Dr. Douglass Batten, Anesthetist, San Diego, California in the preparation of this volume.

J. A.

New Orleans

PREFACE TO THIRD EDITION

Anesthesiology continues to change. The changes since this volume was last revised have been gradual and have been neither remarkable nor astounding. New drugs have been introduced while certain of the older ones have been relegated to the background. The search for a non-flamable inhalation anesthetic has continued. The fluorine containing hydrocarbons and thers are now with us.

In spite of the addition of new drugs, innovations and a number of renements in techniques, the basic principles of anesthesiology have changed little if at all. The general plan of this edition, therefore, remains the same as that of two previous editions. Older techniques and the use of some agent which now have been supplanted are still retained in this volume for both the sake of completeness or for those who perchance might have the occasion to use them. This edition has been brought up-to-date to include new techniques, drugs or methods now in general use.

JOHN ADRIANI, M D.

PREFACE TO SECOND EDITION

A dozen years have elapsed since the material for the first edition of this book was assembled. During that time there have been numerous refinements and innovations in anesthesia. New drugs have been introduced requiring new techniques or modification of old techniques. Some of these did not stand the test of even a few years time and are no longer used. Others have proved useful and are with us yet. The more important of these advances and uses of new drugs have been included in this edition. It is hoped that this edition will continue to be as useful as the first has proved to be as evidenced by the continued demand for the volume during the past decade.

The writer is grateful to Dr. Meyer Saklad, to Dr. C. R. Stephen, and to Dr. Robert Hosler for the use of illustrations from their respective books, *Inhalation Therapy, Elements of Pediatric Anesthesia,* and *Cardiac Resuscitation,* and to Dr. Donovan Campbell and Dr. Roger Witt for assistance in proofreading.

JOHN ADRIANI, M.D.

CONTENTS

TECHNIQUES AND PROCEDURES
OF
ANESTHESIA

PART I

GENERAL CONSIDERATIONS

TYPES OF ANESTHESIA

The types of anesthesia may be classified according to the routes of administration of drugs employed.

The following types are available:

1. *Inhalation:* Narcosis is produced by inhalation of gases or vapors of highly volatile liquids.
2. *Regional:* Anesthesia is obtained by applying a drug along the course of a nerve. Sensation is abolished by one of the following methods:
   a. Spinal anesthesia: The drug is applied to the anterior and posterior roots and sympathetic fibers of the nerve as it passes from the spinal cord through the subarachnoid space.
   b. Epidural anesthesia: The drug is applied to the nerve as it passes from the dura but while it is still in the canal of the vertebral column.
   c. Nerve block: The drug is applied at some point along the course of the nerve before it divides into its terminal branches.
   d. Topical, field block, and infiltration: The drug is applied at the nerve endings. (Physical agents such as pressure and cold may be applied to nerve endings to produce anesthesia also.)
3. *Intravascular:* Narcosis is obtained by injecting an aqueous solution of a drug directly into the blood stream as follows:
   a. By intravenous injection.
   b. By intra-arterial injection.
   c. By intramedullary injection (marrow puncture).
4. *Rectal:* Narcosis is obtained by administering an aqueous or oily solution of a drug as an enema. Provides basal narcosis.
5. *Intraperitoneal:* Narcosis is obtained by injecting an aqueous solution of a drug into the peritoneal cavity. The drug is absorbed into the systemic circulation from the serous surface. This technique is limited chiefly to animals.
6. *Oral:* Narcosis is obtained by ingestion of solutions of drugs or the pure drugs so that they are absorbed through the upper portion of the gastro-intestinal tract. No suitable oral preparation available for anesthesia.
7. *Subcutaneous and Intramuscular:* Narcosis is obtained by injecting aqueous or oily solutions of soluble drugs into these tissues. No suitable preparation available for anesthesia.

3

AVAILABLE DRUGS

Drugs used for anesthesia are central nervous system depressants. Two types are recognized—the volatile and non-volatile.

Volatile drugs are gases or liquids with low boiling points. The currently used gases are nitrous oxide, ethylene and cyclopropane. The currently used liquids are *ether, vinethene, chloroform, ethyl chloride halothane, methoxyflurane* and *trichlorethylene*.

The non-volatile drugs are solids or liquids with vapor pressures too low to be effective at room temperature. Currently used drugs are *avertin, chloral, paraldehyde, pentothal, evipal, surital, the narcotics, morphine, dilaudid demerol, methadon, nisentil* and *dromoran*.

The local anesthetics are non-volatile substances also. The currently used drugs are described in Part VI.

COMBINATIONS OF DRUGS AND ROUTES

In present day anesthesia practice, combinations of drugs and routes are used. Some of the currently employed combinations are as follows:

1. Inhalation plus basal narcosis induced by injecting a non-volatile drug intravenously, intramuscularly or rectally. Example: nitrous oxide oxygen plus pentothal intravenously.
2. Inhalation plus basal narcosis plus a muscle relaxant. Example: nitrous oxide oxygen plus pentothal plus curare.
3. Regional plus inhalation. Example: spinal block plus cyclopropane.
4. Regional plus basal narcosis induced by injecting a non-volatile drug intravenously, intramuscularly or rectally. Example: spinal block plus pentothal.

GENERAL DUTIES OF THE ANESTHETIST

Duties

Reasons

1. The anesthetist should visit the patient in advance of operation in order to evaluate the patient as an operative risk and to decide upon premedication, type, and techniques of administration of anesthesia.

Familiarity with the patient's abnormalities is necessary in order to avoid the many pitfalls of anesthesia.

2. The anesthetist should assemble all the necessary equipment and be prepared to induce anesthesia at least 15 minutes before the scheduled time of operation.

Induction of anesthesia may be prolonged as a result of technical difficulties, slow action of drugs or other allowable delays, thus interfering with the progress of the surgical team.

3. The anesthetist should verify the

In large institutions confusion may

TABLE I

General Properties and Characteristics of Currently Employed Inhalational Anesthetic Drugs

Name	Chemical Name	Formula	Description	B.P. or M.P.	S.G.	Stability	Preservative	Packaged	Accepted	Remarks
Ether Vinyl ether	Diethyl oxide	C_2H_6	Colorless mobile inflammable liquid with pungent odor.	B.P. 36-37° C.	Liq. .718 at 15° C. Vap. 2.6	Oxidized by air or oxygen light or heat to peroxides.	Copper or iron.	Dark bottles, cans.	U.S.P.	Contains up to 4% alcohol from manufacturing process.
Vinethene	Vinyl oxide	C_2H_3 C_2H_3	Colorless inflammable liquid with garlic like odor.	B.P. 28-29° C.	Liq. .77 at 20° C. Vap. 2.2	Polymerizes to resins. Decomposed by acids.	Basic substances, amines or other.	Dark bottles.	U.S.P.	Contains 4% added alcohol to elevate boiling point.
Chloroform	Trichlormethane	$CHCl_3$	Sweet pungent liquid yielding heavy vapor.	B.P. 60-61° C.	Vap. 4.12	Oxidized by air, oxygen, light or heat.	Ethyl alcohol.	Dark bottles.	U.S.P.	Contains added alcohol to act as a preservative.
Ethyl chloride	Monochlorethane	C_2H_5Cl	Colorless mobile highly volatile liquid.	B.P. 12.5-15° C.	Liq. .921 at 20° C. Vap. 2.28	Hydrolized to alcohol and hydrochloric acid.	None added.	Dark glass or metal amplon.	U.S.P.	Contains alcohol from manufacturing process.
Trilene	Trichlorethylene	C_2HCl_3	Sweet pungent mobile liquid	B.P. 87° C.		Oxidized by air, oxygen, light, heat and soda lime	Thymol	Dark bottles	U.S.P.	
Halothane (Fluothane)	1 Trifluro 2 Bromo 2 Chlorethane	F Br $\vert$ $\vert$ F—C—C—Cl $\vert$ $\vert$ F H	Sweet smelling somewhat pungent liquid yielding heavy vapor	B.P. 51° C.		Stable. Decomposed to acids by light			N.N.D.	Non-flammable
Ethylene	Ethene	C_2H_4	Colorless gas with an etheral odor.	B.P. 103° C.	Vap. .97	Stable at ordinary conditions.	None added, keep in a cool place.	Compressed into a liquid and stored in steel cylinders.	U.S.P.	Carbon monoxide a possible impurity.
Cyclopropane	Trimethylene	C_3H_6	Colorless, sweet smelling gas.	B.P. -34° C.	Vap. 1.46	Stable at ordinary temperatures and pressures.	None added, keep in cool place.	Compressed into a liquid and stored in light metal cylinders.	U.S.P.	A polymer of propylene in presence of iron at 100° C. may be converted to propylene.
Nitrous oxide	Nitrogen monoxide	N_2O	Colorless, sweet smelling gas.	B.P. -89° C.	Vap. 1.54	Stable.	None added, keep in cool place	Compressed into a liquid and stored in heavy metal cylinders	U.S.P.	Noninflammable, but supports combustion.

nature of the contemplated operation and name of the patient with the patient himself before anesthesia is induced.

occur and the wrong patient may be operated upon or the wrong operation may be attempted.

4. The anesthetist should verify the patient's age and note whether or not permission for operation on the patient's chart has been signed.

Minor females and males (under 21 years) may not sign for consent for operation. (In most states married males and females may sign consent even though not of age.)

5. **The anesthetist should have the patient under continued surveillance from the moment of induction of anesthesia until he is returned to bed.**

The anesthetist is responsible for the patient so long as it is dangerous to entrust him to less experienced individuals who may care for him in the post anesthetic period.

6. The anesthetist should maintain an accurate and complete record of the entire procedure and note all events as they occur.

Records are essential for many reasons: (1) As future references in the event of complications, (2) for case analysis, (3) as an aid to prognostication during surgery, (4) for a source of statistical data (punch card), and (5) for medicolegal purposes.

SELECTION OF ANESTHESIA

Anesthesia cannot be selected on an empiric basis. *No rule can be formulated regarding selection of a nesthesia.* Each case must be considered on its own merits.

The following variable factors should be considered in each individual case:

1. The type and duration of operation to be performed, and the depth of anesthesia required to complete it.
2. The physical state of the patient.
3. The skill and dexterity of the surgeon and the degree of muscle relaxation demanded by the surgeon.
4. The skill of the anesthetist.
5. The pharmacological action of drugs in question and their relationship to the underlying disease.

Comment: Often any one of several techniques may be employed. The choice rests upon individual preference, availability of apparatus and drugs and the wishes of the anesthetist to accommodate, the surgeon all other factors being equal.

TABLE II

SELECTION OF ANESTHESIA IN THE ORDER ON THEIR GREATEST DESIRABILITY, MOST
USEFULNESS OR LEAST OBJECTIONABLE FEATURES

Problems Encountered	Choices	Remarks

HEAD

1. Skull—Intracranial Operations—Craniotomy, Lobotomy, Plastics on Cranium

Problems Encountered	Choices	Remarks
Clinical 1. May be comatose, irrational psychotic, uncooperative, dehydrated, emaciated. 2. May have respiratory failure requiring artificial respiration throughout operation. 3. May have expanding lesions, infections, hemorrhage, trauma all leading to increased intracranial pressure. *Surgical* 1. May be unusually long. 2. Use high frequency current (explosion hazard). 3. Excessive bleeding may be encountered (neoplasms). 4. Are done in prone or other awkward positions. Requires endotracheal tube. 5. Scalp highly vascular (add epinephrine with local). 6. No relaxation necessary. 7. May need to be awake in certain operations (for stimulation of cortical areas). 8. Bone difficult to anesthetize with local anesthesia. *Anesthetic* 1. Coughing or straining, raises intracranial pressure. 2. Projectile vomiting may occur increasing possibility of aspiration. 3. CO_2 excess or anoxia to be avoided. Raise intracranial pressure. 4. Anesthetist must be away from operative field. Intratracheal tube required. 5. Reflex changes may cause circulatory and respiratory disturbance.	1. Local. 2. Nitrous oxide-halothane 3. Pentothal or avertin basal, nitrous oxide intratracheally with topical. 4. Nitrous oxide—ether oxygen sequence. 5. Nitrous oxide-trilene *Less Desirable or Contra-indicated* 4. Ethylene or cyclopropane. 5. Pentothal alone. 6. Avertin alone or with local.	Most suitable for most operations. Non-flammable. Most desirable from standpoint of flammability in noncooperative patients. Most suitable, but flammable Use justified only when others are contraindicated. Not flammable. Flammable. Airway not under control. Excessive quantity required. Airway not under control. Operation outlasts narcosis.

2. Skull—Ventriculogram

Problems Encountered	Choices	Remarks
Clinical 1. May be comatose, irrational psychotic, uncooperative, dehydrated, emaciated. 2. May have respiratory failure requiring constant artificial respiration. *Surgical* 1. Short duration. 2. No relaxation needed. 3. Done in semi-upright or sitting position. 4. Respiratory failure may be present or may occur. *Anesthetic* 1. Must remain anesthetized until x-rays are taken.	1. Local. 2. Nitrous oxide-halothane 3. Nitrous oxide intratracheally with topical and basal of pentothal. 4. Nitrous oxide—ether-oxygen sequence intratracheally. 5. Cyclopropane and oxygen. *Not Desirable or Contraindicated* Any of the above without an intratracheal airway. *Children* 1. 1 or 2. 2. Local.	Suitable when rational. Non-flammable Suitable when electro-surgical unit is used. Flammable. Used when nonvolatile drugs are not desired. CO_2 retention may raise intracranial pressure. Flammable. Suitable if cooperative.

TABLE II—(continued)

Problems Encountered	Choices	Remarks

3. Skull—Encephalogram

Problems Encountered	Choices	Remarks
Clinical 1. May be comatose, irrational psychotic, uncooperative, dehydrated, emaciated. *Surgical* 1. Usually performed in sitting position. 2. Usually brief. 3. May cause shock or respiratory failure. *Anesthetic* 1. Airway not easily maintained. 2. Must remain narcotized until X-Rays are taken. 3. Fire hazard present due to X-Ray unit. 4. Respiratory failure secondary to neurological disease may occur.	1. Local with sedation. 2. Pentothal basal intravenously and nitrous oxide. 3. Pentothal basal alone. 4. Nitrous oxide-halothane 5. Open drop ether. 6. Avertin alone. 7. Trilene analgesia	Suitable for cooperative subjects who are not comatose. Non-flammable, most practical. Large amounts of barbiturate often required. Non-flammable. Suitable for children. Respond to pain induced by air injection and struggle. Reflexes not abolished.

4. Skull—Extracranial Operations—Plastic-Operation, Removal of Cyst, etc.

Problems Encountered	Choices	Remarks
Clinical 1. Patients usually in good condition. 2. Intracranial pressure rarely affected. *Surgical* 1. May be minor and brief. 2. Scalp highly vascular (add epinephrine with local). 3. Relaxation not needed. *Anesthetic* 1. Anesthetist must be out of operative field. 2. May be done in prone position. 3. Bone difficult to anesthetize with local anesthesia.	1. Local. 2. Cyclopropane intratracheally. 3. Nitrous oxide or ethylene with ether intratracheally. 4. Nitrous oxide intratracheally, topical and pentothal basal. 5. Halothane-nitrous oxide *Less Desirable or Contraindicated* 5. Anesthetics listed above with no intratracheal airway. 6. Pentothal alone. 7. Avertin alone. *Children* 1. Cyclopropane intratracheally. 2. Ether intratracheally. 3. Nitrous oxide intratracheally with basal of avertin or pentothal.	Most suitable. Labile, rapid acting. When 1 and 2 are not desired When fire hazard exists. Non-flammable Airway not under control. Excess drug needed. Airway not under control. Same as 6.

5. Eye—Evisceration, Plastic on Lids, Retinal Operations, Removal of Tumors, Muscle Transplants, Removal of Cataracts, Lens Transplants, Relief of Glaucoma, etc.

Problems Encountered	Choices	Remarks
Clinical 1. Many are very young or in upper age groups. 2. Glaucoma may be present—Avoid atropine. *Surgical* 1. Eyeball must be fixed—deeper anesthesia required. 2. Nausea, vomiting in postoperative period must be avoided. *Anesthetic* 1. Anesthetist must be away from operative field. Endotracheal tube required to control airway. 2. Coughing and sneezing impair surgical result. 3. Head and face covered by drapes.	1. Local. 2. Cyclopropane intratracheally and muscle relaxant. 3. Pentothal, nitrous oxide intratracheally, muscle relaxant. 4. Halothane-nitrous oxide *Less Desirable* 4. Ether intratracheally. 5. Local and muscle relaxant. 6. Ether insufflation. *Children* 1. Cyclopropane or ether intratracheally. 2. Insufflation ether. 3. Halothane-nitrous oxide	Best suited for adults. Nausea may occur. Prolonged depression postoperatively—nausea minimal. Non-flammable Nausea and vomiting frequent. Airway not under control. Not advised. Airway not under control. Ordinarily used. Not advised. Airway not under control. Non-flammable.

TABLE II—(*continued*)

Problems Encountered	Choices	Remarks

6. Face—Plastic Surgery, Reduction of Fractures, Excisions of Moles or Scars, Incisions and Drainage

Problems Encountered	Choices	Remarks
Surgical	1. Block of branches of 5th Nerve.	Not always satisfactory and of sufficient duration.
1. Areas may be highly vascular.		
2. Relaxation not needed.	2. Cyclopropane intratrache- ally.	Most desirable.
3. May be lengthy.		
4. Electrosurgical unit may be used.	3. Pentothal basal, nitrous ox- ide intratracheally with topical.	Suitable for short procedures or when electrical equipment is used.
Anesthetic	4. Ether intratracheally pre- ceded by nitrous oxide or ethylene.	Used when 1 and 2 are contra- indicated.
1. Anesthetist must be away from opera- tive field. Intratracheal tube needed.	5. Halothane-nitrous oxide.	Non-flammable.
	6. Local infiltration.	In simple brief procedures.
	Children	
	1. Cyclopropane intratrache- ally.	Most desirable because of la- bility and rapidity of action.
	2. Ether intratracheally.	
	3. Pentothal basal-nitrous ox- ide intratracheally.	

7. Ear—Mastoidectomy

Problems Encountered	Choices	Remarks
Clinical	1. Cyclopropane intratrache- ally.	Labile—rapid recovery.
1. May have acute infection.		
2. Sepsis fever, etc. may be present.	2. Nitrous oxide and pento- thal basal.	Used when fire hazard is pres- ent.
3. May have signs of meningeal irritation or increased intracranial pressure.	3. Nitrous oxide or ethylene followed by ether.	When 1 and 2 cannot be used.
4. Acute in children most often—chronic in adults.	4. Halothane-nitrous oxide.	Non-flammable.
5. In children more often than adults.	*Less Desirable or Not Suitable*	
Surgical	5. Local.	
1. May be long and tedious.	*Children*	
2. No relaxation needed.	1. Cyclopropane intratrache- ally.	When respiratory infection is present.
3. Surgeon may use epinephrine in wound.	2. Pentothal basal, nitrous oxide.	When fire hazard is present.
4. Surgeon may use dental drill with elec- tric motor.	3. Halothane-nitrous oxide.	Non-flammable.
5. Room may be darkened.	4. Nitrous oxide-ether intra- tracheally.	
Anesthetic	5. Ether open drop followed by insufflation.	Usual method employed but does not permit control of air- way.
1. Airway not under control unless tube is used.		
2. Head turned to one side and covered by drapes.		

8. Ear—Myringotomy

Problems Encountered	Choices	Remarks
Surgical	1. Cyclopropane.	Use if intratracheal tube is necessary.
1. Brief, requiring a few minutes.		
2. Airway not difficult to control for such a brief period.	2. Pentothal.	If airway may easily be main- tained.
3. Room may be darkened.	3. Vinyl ether-open drop.	Rapid acting-rapid recovery.
Clinical	*Children*	
1. Usually in children.	1. Vinyl ether open drop.	

Fenestration Operation

Problems Encountered	Choices	Remarks
Clinical	1. Cyclopropane intratrache- ally.	
1. Only in adults with few exceptions.		
2. Elective. Subjects in good condition.	2. Thiopental basal nitrous oxide with topical.	
3. Upright position.	3. Ether preceded by nitrous oxide or ethylene.	
Surgical	4. Halothane-nitrous oxide.	Non-flammable.
1. Tedious and meticulous.	*Not Desirable*	
2. Perfect hemostasis required (hypo- tensive anesthesia may be needed).	1. Insufflation ether.	
3. May use dental drill.	2. Hypotensive technique.	Hazard not warranted for such a benign operation.
Anesthetic		
1. Airway difficult to control.		

TABLE II—(continued)

Problems Encountered	Choices	Remarks

9. Mouth—Dental Extractions

Clinical
1. Patients usually in excellent condition.
2. General anesthesia used for children quite frequently.

Surgical
1. Often done in sitting position.
2. May be lengthy, particularly in extracting impacted molars.
3. Jaw must be relaxed.
4. Packs must be used.
5. Surgeon must have access to mouth and head.
6. Oral sepsis often present.

Anesthetic
1. Airway difficult to maintain.
2. Secretions and blood fall backward into pharynx.

1. Nerve blocks.	Best selection for office use.
2. Nitrous oxide with vinethene or Fluromar by nasal mask.	For office use for simple extractions.
3. Nitrous oxide-trichlorethylene with nasal mask.	For office use for simple extractions.
4. Cyclopropane intratracheally.	For extensive and multiple extractions in hospitals.
5. Ether intratracheally preceded by nitrous oxide.	Nausea, vomiting, unpleasant.
6. Nitrous oxide intratracheally and basal pentothal.	Non-flammable.
7. Halothane-nitrous oxide.	Non-flammable.

Less Desirable or Contraindicated

8. Pentothal alone.	Laryngeal spasm and respiratory depression common in postoperative period.
9. Nitrous oxide alone.	Possibility of asphyxia too great.

Children

1. Vinethene by open drop.	Wasteful
2. Nitrous oxide with vinethene or Fluromar.	Permits adequate oxygenation
3. Halothane-nitrous oxide.	Non-flammable.
4. Cyclopropane or ether intratracheally.	For extensive procedures.
5. Ether by insufflation.	

10. Mouth—Operations on Tongue, Salivary Glands, Palate, Gums

Clinical
1. Oral sepsis often present.

Surgical
1. Surgeon must have access to mouth.
2. Blood and secretions pass back into pharynx and larynx.
3. Relaxation of jaw muscles required.
4. May be lengthy.
5. Pharyngeal packs may be used.
6. May use cautery.

Anesthetic
1. Airway difficult to maintain without nasal endotracheal tube.
2. Lesion may offer obstruction.

1. Cyclopropane intratracheally. (nasal)	Allows rapid induction and recovery.
2. Ether intratracheally (nasal) route. Preceded by nitrous oxide or ethylene.	Used when cyclopropane is not desired.
3. Basal pentothal—nitrous oxide intratracheally.	Used when fire hazard exists.
4. Halothane-nitrous oxide.	Non-flammable.
5. Nerve blocks.	Not satisfactory for extensive procedures or patients who are not cooperative.

Less Desirable

6. Insufflation orally.	Not advised—airway difficult to maintain.

11. Lip—Plastic Operations—Resection for Neoplasm, Removal of Scars

Clinical
1. Oral sepsis often present.
2. May be in any age group.

Surgical
1. Surgeon must have access to mouth.
2. Blood and secretions pass into pharynx and larynx.
3. Relaxation of jaw muscles required.
4. May be lengthy.
5. Pharyngeal packs may be used.

Anesthetic
1. Airway difficult to maintain without nasal endotracheal tube.

1. Local or nerve block.	For simple non-extensive procedures.
2. Cyclopropane intratracheally.	Best choice when local cannot be used.
3. Nitrous oxide or ethylene followed by ether.	Used when cyclopropane is not desired.
4. Basal pentothal—nitrous oxide intratracheally.	Used when a fire hazard exists.
5. Halothane-nitrous oxide.	Non-flammable.
6. Insufflation of ether.	Not advised—airway not under control.

Children

1. Cyclopropane or ether intratracheally (oral).	
2. Basal pentothal—nitrous oxide intratracheally.	Used when cautery is required.
3. Halothane-nitrous oxide.	Non-flammable.
4. Local or nerve blocks.	Subjects may not be cooperative.
5. Insufflation of ether.	Airway not under complete control.

TABLE II—(*continued*)

Problems Encountered	Choices	Remarks

12. Jaw—Mandible—Resections, Curettements, Reduction of Fractures, Plastic on Joint, etc.

Problems Encountered	Choices	Remarks
Clinical 1. Fractures common in alcohol addicts. 2. Subjects are most often adults. 3. Oral sepsis often present. *Surgical* 1. Patient may not be able to open mouth due to trauma or disease of joint. 2. Teeth may be wired together. 3. May be prolonged and accompanied by blood loss. *Anesthetic* 1. Airway difficult to maintain without endotracheal tube. 2. Mask may be difficult to apply to face—intubate with local—patient awake.	1. Cyclopropane intratracheally. 2. Ether intratracheally. 3. Basal pentothal—nitrous oxide. 4. Nitrous oxide-halothane. *Less Desirable* 5. Ether by insufflation. *Children* 1. Cyclopropane intratracheally. 2. Ether intratracheally. 3. Basal pentothal—nitrous oxide intratracheally (with topical).	Permits rapid induction and recovery. Used when cyclopropane is not desired. Post anesthetic depression is common and objectionable. Non-flammable. Airway almost impossible to control. Jaws must be fixed after post anesthetic retching and vomiting has ceased. (If jaws are fixed insert oronasal tube before removing naso-endotracheal tube and aspirate secretion through it.)

13. Jaw—Upper—Resection of Maxilla, Reduction of Fractures, Removal of Neoplasms, Curettements

Problems Encountered	Choices	Remarks
Clinical 1. Usually older adults. 2. Fractures associated with other injuries. *Surgical* 1. May be long radical procedures. 2. Considerable blood loss may occur. May require hypotensive anesthesia. 3. Cautery may be used for hemostasis. 4. Surgical site often includes nasal passages. *Anesthetic* 1. Maintenance of airway requires use of intratracheal tube. 2. Presence of lesion does not permit mask to be applied to face. 3. Tracheotomy may be required prior to surgery. 4. Blood and secretions may pass into nasopharynx.	1. Halothane-nitrous oxide. 2. Basal of pentothal, nitrous oxide. 3. Cyclopropane intratracheally. 4. Ether intratracheally. *Less Desirable or Contraindicated.* 4. Nerve blocks or local. 5. Insufflation of ether. 6. Pentothal alone or combined with curare.	Non-flammable. Non-flammable. Flammable. Used if cautery is not. Flammable. Used if cautery is not. Satisfactory relief rarely obtained. Airway not under control. Flammable. Prolonged depression. Airway not under control.

14. Jaw—Upper—Maxilla—Sinuses—Antrotomy—Caldwell-Luc, Removal of Polyps, etc.

Problems Encountered	Choices	Remarks
Clinical 1. Post nasal drainage often present. 2. Nasal passages frequently occluded or distorted. 3. Chronic bronchitis or allergy may be associated with the condition. *Surgical* 1. May be long, and radical. 2. May be traumatic with considerable bleeding. *Anesthetic* 1. Anesthetist must be removed from surgical site. Endotracheal (oral) tube required.	1. Nerve block. 2. Cyclopropane intratracheally. 3. Halothane-nitrous oxide. 4. Pentothal—nitrous oxide intratracheally. 5. Ether intratracheally. 6. Ether by insufflation. *Children* Same as adults.	Best to use but not always feasible. Permits adequate control of airway. Rapid induction and recovery. Non-flammable. Postoperative depression may follow long operations. Slow recovery after long operations. Airway not under control.

TABLE II—(continued)

Problems Encountered	Choices	Remarks

15. Pharynx—Tonsillectomy and Adenoidectomy

Clinical 1. May have chronic respiratory infection. 2. Are usually young subjects. *Surgical* 1. Brief. Time varies with operator. 2. Difficulty in controlling hemorrhage may be encountered. 3. Require postoperative endotracheal suction. 4. Relaxation of jaw required. *Anesthetic* 1. Surgeon must have access to both mouth and nasopharynx. 2. Lymphoid tissue obstructs airway.	1. Local. 2. Cyclopropane oratracheally or nasotracheally if adenoids are not large. 3. Ether as in 2 above. 4. Nitrous oxide, muscle relaxant and basal of pentothal. 5. Insufflation of ether. 6. Halothane-nitrous oxide. *Not Desired* 1. Pentothal alone. *Children* 1. Vinyl ether induction and insufflation of ether with oxygen. 2. Oratracheal intubation with ether or cyclopropane. 3. Basal of pentothal rectally, ether intratracheally. 4. Basal pentothal, ether by insufflation. 5. Halothane-nitrous oxide.	Best choice if patient tolerates it. Surgeons often complain of oozing. Ideal for the purpose, otherwise. Recovery not as rapid as with cyclopropane. Effects of ether on patient. Respiratory depression follows in postoperative period. Difficult to maintain airway and satisfactory depth of anesthesia in adults. Aspiration occurs. Non-flammable. Spasm and obstruction frequent and impossible to obviate. Simple but does not assure adequate airway. Aspiration of blood occurs. Possibility of trauma to trachea and larynx. Aspiration minimized. Respiratory depression objectionable. Airway not maintained adequately. Respiratory depression objectionable. Non-flammable.

16. Pharynx—Drainage of Peritonsillar or Retropharyngeal Abscess

Clinical 1. May not be able to open mouth. 2. Septic with fever. *Surgical* 1. Usually brief. *Anesthetic* 1. Airway difficult to maintain without endotracheal tube. 2. Abscess may rupture during induction or intubation. Aspiration may occur.	1. Local. 2. Cyclopropane nasotracheally. 3. Halothane-nitrous oxide intratracheally. 4. Ether by insufflation.	Best and most frequent choice. Abscess may be ruptured in attempting intubation. Non-flammable. May aspirate. Airway not under control.

17. Larynx—Removal of Polyps, Diagnostic Suspensions, Operations on Cords, etc.

Clinical 1. Dyspnea, orthopnea often present. 2. Common in children. 3. May have tracheotomy. *Surgical* 1. Relaxation required for exposure of larynx. 2. May be long. 3. Surgical procedure may induce bleeding. *Anesthetic* 1. Anesthetist and surgeon both compete for airway. 2. Cough reflex difficult to abolish. 3. Obstruction present prior to inception of anesthesia. 4. Tracheotomy may be advisable prior to anesthesia if airway is inadequate.	1. Local. 2. Topical followed by ultra short-acting barbiturate intravenously with muscle relaxant with chert respirator. 3. Ether by insufflation. 4. Cyclopropane by insufflation. *Children* 1. Ether by insufflation. 2. Cyclopropane by insufflation. 3. Basal of pentothal or avertin followed by 1 or 2.	Useful for simple endoscopic procedures. Not ideal but best available at present time. Spasmogenic. Spasms precipitated by instrumentation, blood and secretions. Distasteful to patient, difficult to maintain at proper depth. Secretions. Not advised. Costly and creates fire hazard. Not best, but safest and simplest to use. For small infants. Spasm may result. Respiratory depression in postoperative period.

TABLE II—(*continued*)

Problems Encountered	Choices	Remarks
18. Larynx—Tracheotomy		
Clinical	1. No anesthesia.	Emergency only.
1. Obstruction and asphyxia are present or eminent.	2. Local.	For elective procedures with obstruction.
Surgical	3. Intratracheal cyclopropane.	Elective without obstruction.
1. May be performed prophylactically.	4. Intratracheal ether.	For elective cases.
2. Urgent in emergencies.	5. Nitrous oxide intratracheally preceded by pentothal.	
	6. Halothane-nitrous oxide.	Non-flammable.
	Children	
	Same.	
19. Larynx—Laryngectomy		
Clinical	1. Cyclopropane intratracheally with topical.	As soon as larynx is removed a tracheal tube is inserted until time of tracheotomy.
1. Are in older age group as rule.		
2. Usually are in fair condition but may be emaciated.	2. Halothane-nitrous oxide.	
3. Dyspnea may be present due to obstruction at larynx.	3. Ether intratracheally.	Used when cyclopropane is not desired.
Surgical	4. Basal of pentothal with nitrous oxide intratracheally and muscle relaxant.	When 1 or 2 are not desired or if fire hazard exists.
1. Are usually long, tedious.		
2. Requires tracheotomy as soon as larynx is removed.	5. Cervical plexus blocks.	
3. Blood loss and shock may occur.	*Not Desired*	
4. Cautery may be used.	4. Pentothal alone.	Spasm, obstruction, prolonged depression follow.
Anesthetic	5. Local.	Difficult to establish complete pain relief.
1. Anesthetist and surgeon compete for operative field.		
2. Possibility of vagal reflexes from manipulation of larynx.	6. Ether by insufflation.	Airway not easily controlled.
20. Bronchi—Bronchograms		
Clinical	1. Topical.	Best choice, but patient may not always be cooperative.
1. Usually performed for diagnosis when suppurative disease of the lung is present.	2. Cyclopropane intratracheally.	Desirable but is flammable. X-ray unit used.
2. May be anemic and emaciated.		
3. Usually have pulmonary disfunction.	3. Ether intratracheally.	Desirable but is flammable. X-ray unit used.
4. Occurs in any age group, but frequently in children.	4. Basal pentothal or avertin, topical with nitrous oxide intratracheally.	Not flammable. Respiratory depression common. Possibility of laryngeal and bronchospasm enhanced by the basal.
Surgical		
1. Requires insertion of cannula and injection of oily opaque substance.	5. Ether by insufflation.	Not advised. Airway not under control.
2. Are not long as a rule.	6. Halothane-nitrous oxide.	Non-flammable.
3. Relaxation and cooperation of patient required.	*Children*	
4. Done in fluoroscopic, room in dark.	1. Ether open drop.	Fire hazard. Excessive secretions.
Anesthetic		
1. Coughing, bronchospasm and diminished ventilation follow injection of contrast media.		
2. Airway must be maintained.		
3. Explosion hazard present.		
4. Must remain anesthetized until x-rays are taken.		
5. Apnea necessary at time of x-ray.		
6. Vagal reflexes may be initiated (administer atropine pre-anesthetically).		

TABLE II—(*continued*)

Problems Encountered	Choices	Remarks
21. Bronchi—Bronchoscopy		
Clinical	1. Topical with sedation.	Best choice but may be unsuitable if patient is uncooperative.
1. May have copious secretions if suppurative disease of lungs is present.		
2. May have hyperactive cough reflex.	2. Basal of pentothal, topical and muscle relaxant used in conjunction with chest respirator.	Simplest to induce, but hazardous from standpoint of bronchospasm and postoperative respiratory depression.
3. Dyspnea and pulmonary dysfunction may be present if done for pulmonary disease.		
4. Pressure symptoms may be present giving rise to obstruction.	3. Ether by insufflation preceded by closed or open drop induction.	Disagreeable, prolonged and difficult induction and difficult maintenance. Safest but not best.
5. Patient not confined to any particular age group.		
Surgical	4. Cyclopropane by insufflation preceded by basal of pentothal.	Expensive and impractical. Explosion hazard greater than with ether.
1. Usually performed for diagnosis, removal of foreign body and therapeutically to remove secretions.	5. Halothane-nitrous oxide.	Non-irritating. Non-flammable.
2. Usually brief in skilled hands.		
3. Massive hemorrhage may be caused by trauma.	*Children*	
4. Relaxation needed for exposure of larynx.	1. Ether open drop followed by insufflation.	Safest, simplest. Ether distorts light and interferes with proper vision.
5. Vagal and cough reflexes are initiated from instrumentation.		
6. Symptoms of anoxia arise if pulmonary dysfunction is present.	2. Cyclopropane by insufflation.	Expensive and impractical Explosion hazard greater than with ether.
7. Performed in a darkened room.	3. Basal and muscle relaxant and topical.	Simplest to induce, but hazardous from standpoint of bronchospasm and postoperative respiratory depression.
	4. Local.	Children are not cooperative for this technique.
22. Esophagoscopy		
Clinical	1. Topical with sedation.	Suitable for cooperative patients.
1. Patient may be emaciated due to poor nutrition.		
2. Patient may be apprehensive (cardiospasm).	2. Cyclopropane intratracheally and muscle relaxant and topical.	Rapid induction and recovery. Ideal for this type of work.
3. Usually in older age group.		
4. Usually performed for diagnosis or removal of foreign bodies.	3. Basal of pentothal, nitrous oxide intratracheally and muscle relaxant and topical.	Suitable but if procedure is prolonged an excess of drug causes respiratory depression.
Surgical		
1. Requires relaxation for exposure.	4. Ether intratracheally and topical.	Ether is disagreeable to patient. Relaxation excellent. Long induction and slow recovery.
2. Cooperation of patient required.		
3. Intratracheal tube distresses most surgeons.	5. Halothane-nitrous oxide.	Non-flammable.
Anesthetic	*Less Desirable*	
1. Surgeon and anesthetist compete for operative field.	5. Ether by insufflation.	Not recommended. Airway not under control.
2. Mucous, vomiting and retching may occur.	6. Pentothal or avertin alone.	Airway not under control. Spasm and respiratory depression result.
3. Vagal reflexes may be initiated by instrumentation.		
	Children	
	1. Vinyl ether—open drop ether, insufflation of ether.	Usual method. Airway not easily maintained.
	2. Cyclopropane intratracheally.	Desirable but surgeon objects to intratracheal catheter.
	3. Basal, with cyclopropane or nitrous oxide with muscle relaxant.	Respiratory depression common from basal.

TABLE II—(*continued*)

Problems Encountered	Choices	Remarks

NECK

23. Anterior—Thyroidectomy (for Toxic and Non-Toxic Goitres)

Clinical
1. May have associated heart disease (in toxic goiter, high pulse pressure, rapid pulse).
2. May have cord paralysis, edema of larynx, tracheitis, deviated trachea.
3. Are apprehensive and highly excitable.
4. Do not withstand epinephrine and sympathomimetic amines.
5. Have a high metabolic rate and are emotionally unstable.
6. Have intrathoracic mass.
7. May have associated myesthenia gravis.

Surgical
1. Relaxation a minor factor.
2. Head must be hyperextended for exposure.
3. Surgeon competes with anesthetist for operative field.
4. Oozing and bleeding commonly occur.
5. May require several hours.

Anesthetic
1. High oxygen consumption and carbon dioxide output.
2. Possibility of heat retention and hyperthermia.
3. Exophthalmos may interfere with application of mask.
4. Airway maintained with difficulty when intubated.
5. Iodides may cause excessive secretions.
6. Circulatory changes such as tachycardia, irregularities, hypertension common.

1. Ethylene, or nitrous oxide followed by ether intratracheally combined with basal narcosis using morphine scopolamine, avertin or intravenous ultra short or short-acting barbiturate.
2. Cyclopropane and basal narcosis described above.
3. Halothane-nitrous oxide.

Less Desirable or contraindicated
4. Local or cervical plexus block.
5. Pentothal-curare; nitrous oxide intratracheally.
6. Open or closed anesthesia without intratracheal tube.

Children
1. Same as adult.
2. Non-toxic—same as above.
3. Intrathoracic—same as above.

Allows maintenance of airway, avoidance of excitement, smooth induction and maintenance.

Increases cardiac irritability in toxic cases.
Non-irritating. Non-flammable.

Apprehension present. Do not tolerate epinephrine and sympathomimetic amines.
Not anesthetic. Depression in the postoperative period.
Airway not under control.

Thyroid crisis and cardiac failure may occur.
Tracheitis and cord paralysis may follow.

24. Anterior—Dissections, Vascular Surgery, Skin Grafts, etc.

Clinical
1. Usually older adults.
2. Usually performed on fair risk.

Surgical
1. Are long procedures and tedious.
2. No relaxation needed.

Anesthetic
1. Airway difficult to maintain unless intubated.
2. Carotid sinuses may be active giving rise to respiratory and circulatory changes.
3. Anesthetist must be away from operative field.
4. Distortion of face from previous surgery may prevent application of mask.

1. Cyclopropane intratracheally.
2. Nitrous oxide or ethylene followed by ether intratracheally.
3. Halothane-nitrous oxide.
4. Pentothal combined with nitrous oxide intratracheally with topical.
5. Infiltration with local anesthesia.
6. Cervical plexus block.

Undesirable
6. Ether open drop and insufflation.
7. Any general anesthetic without intratracheal airway.

Children
1. Cyclopropane intratracheally.
2. Vinethene open drop followed by ether open drop.

Rapid induction and recovery.

Suitable when cyclopropane is contraindicated.

Non flammable.
Suitable for short procedures or when cautery is used.

Minor short procedures in cooperative patients.
Suitable in cooperative non-extensive procedures.

Secretions excessive, airway not maintained safely.
For superficial brief procedures without obstruction.

Advised. As above.

Not advised. Airway not under control.

TABLE II—(continued)

Problems Encountered	Choices	Remarks

25. Anterior—Incisions and Drainages of Phlegmons and Abscesses

Clinical
1. May be "septic" from infection.
2. May be obstructed and orthopneic.
3. May be associated with diabetes, leukemia or other systemic diseases.
4. Inflation may follow dental extractions or mouth lesion.

Surgical
1. Not lengthy.
2. Relaxation not needed.

Anesthetic
1. May have edema of floor of mouth, pharynx, neck, etc. Airway is invariably difficult to maintain.
2. Inability to swallow may be present—saliva accumulates in mouth.

1. Intubation awake with topical anesthesia followed by cyclopropane.
2. Same followed by nitrous oxide or ethylene with ether oxygen sequence.
3. Halothane-nitrous oxide.
4. Same as above but using pentothal—nitrous oxide.

5. Tracheotomy under local followed by cyclopropane, ether or pentothal and nitrous oxide.
6. Local.

Less Desirable or Contraindicated
1. Inhalation anesthesia, basal narcosis without intratracheal airway.
2. Cervical plexus block.

Airway under control at all times—rapid return of reflexes.
Return of reflexes delayed by ether.

Non-flammable.
Respiratory depression prolonged. Possibility of obstruction postoperatively increased.
Mandatory when dyspnea and orthopnea due to obstruction is present.

Suitable for brief superficial operations only.

Asphyxia from obstruction may result.

Not desirable in presence of infections.

26. Posterior—Dissections, Skin Grafts, Incision and Drainages, etc.

Clinical
1. May be septic if surgery is for infection.
2. Patient may be in any age group.

Surgical
1. Relaxation not needed.
2. Usually not long and extensive.

Anesthetic
1. Awkward positions (prone or lateral) is used. Airway difficult to control.
2. Anesthetist must be away from surgical field.
3. Circulatory changes may occur due to positional changes.

1. Cyclopropane intratracheally.
2. Nitrous oxide-halothane.
3. Nitrous oxide or ethylene ether-oxygen sequence intratracheally.
4. Nitrous oxide and a basal of pentothal.
5. Local.

6. Cervical plexus block.

Less Desirable or Contraindicated
6. Inhalation or intravenous anesthesia without an endotracheal airway.

Children
Same as for adults.

Rapid induction and recovery.

Non-flammable.
Delayed return of reflexes in long operations.

Depressed respiration, delayed return of reflexes.
Suitable for brief simple procedures.
Recommended in brief superficial procedures in suitable subjects.

Asphyxia is an ever present danger.

THORAX

27. Chest Wall—Biopsies—Plastic Operations, Excision of Masses, Drainage of Abscesses, etc.

Clinical
1. Physical status usually good.
2. Usually are adults.

Surgical
1. No relaxation required.
2. Vary in duration.
3. May use electrosurgical unit.

Anesthetic
1. Supine position unless operative site is on back for which an endotracheal tube is required.
2. Anesthetist has control of head.

1. Cyclopropane.

2. Halothane-nitrous oxide.
3. Nitrous oxide or ethylene with basal.
4. Nitrous oxide or ethylene followed by ether.
5. Local infiltration.

6. Intercostal or paravertebral block.

Permits rapid induction and recovery.
Non-flammable.
Suitable for short procedures.

Prolonged recovery and undesirable after effects.
Suitable for minor, less extensive procedures.
Can only be used for operations which are in the mid and lower thorax.

TABLE II—(*continued*)

Problems Encountered	Choices	Remarks

28. Chest Wall—Radical Mammectomy

Clinical

1. Usually in middle aged and older women.
2. Disease usually not far advanced in cases selected for radical.
3. Patients often apprehensive and upset by coming ordeal.

Surgical

1. Relaxation not needed.
2. Are long, tedious.
3. May require skin grafting.
4. Blood loss may be considerable.
5. Electrosurgical unit may be used for hemostasis.

Anesthetic

1. Anesthetist has control of airway. No tube needed unless patient is obese or has other factors affecting airway.

Choices	Remarks
1. Cyclopropane.	Rapid acting, rapid recovery.
2. Nitrous oxide or ethylene with basal.	When cyclopropane or ether are not desired.
3. Nitrous oxide or ethylene followed by ether.	When contraindication exists to basal narcosis or cyclopropane.
4. Nitrous oxide-halothane.	Non-flammable.
Not Desirable or Contraindicated	
5. Local infiltration.	Not satisfactory from psychic and surgical standpoint.
6. Intercostal or paravertebral block.	Same as above.

29. Pleura—Drainage of Empyema

Clinical

1. Signs and symptoms of sepsis.
2. Decreased pulmonary reserve usually present.
3. Cough, dyspnea or orthopnea.
4. Possibility of bronchial communications present.
5. Associated pneumonitis is common.
6. Possibility of cerebral abscess.

Surgical

1. No relaxation required.
2. Usually requires rib resection.
3. May be done in sitting position.

Anesthetic

1. Airway may be difficult to maintain due to secretions and position.
2. Respiratory distress may interfere with ventilation.

Choices	Remarks
1. Paravertebral block or intercostal block.	Permits upright position and dependent drainage.
2. Cyclopropane intratracheally.	When block anesthesia is not feasible. Permits rapid induction and high oxygen.
3. Nitrous oxide or ethylene with ether intratracheally.	Possibility of decreased oxygen during induction not desirable.
4. Nitrous oxide intratracheally—basal of pentothal.	Depression of respiration, spasm and prolonged somnolence may occur.
5. Nitrous oxide-halothane.	Non-flammable.
Not Desirable or Contraindicated	
6. Open drop ether.	Insufficient oxygen, excess secretions and lack of adequate airway.
7. Any of above without an endotracheal tube.	Lack of adequate airway.

TABLE II—(*continued*)

Problems Encountered	Choices	Remarks

THORAX

30. Pleura—Thoracoplasty

Clinical
1. Ordinarily performed for tuberculosis or after pneumonectomy to obliterate space in chest.
2. Decreased pulmonary reserve usually present.
3. Anemia, fever, weight loss and other factors incident to disease are present.
4. Tuberculous tracheitis may be present. Intratracheal tube may aggravate it.
5. Tracheobronchial fistulae may be present. Closed system difficult to maintain.

Surgical
1. Shock, due to trauma from removal of ribs and blood loss common.
2. No relaxation needed.
3. May be prolonged.
4. Cautery may be necessary for hemostasis.

Anesthetic
1. Patient is on side—Airway.
2. Circulatory changes due to posture, reflexes, and pleural stimulation.
3. Excessive secretions may be present.
4. Carbon dioxide retention due to inadequate ventilation from posture.
5. Positive pressure or controlled respiration may be required.

1. Cyclopropane intratracheally.

2. Nitrous oxide-halothane.
3. Ether preceded by cyclopropane—ethylene or nitrous oxide.

4. Nitrous oxide or ethylene with basal of pentothal.

5. Paravertebral block.

6. Local.

7. Peridural block.

Not Desirable or Contraindicated.
1. Spinal.

Allows adequate oxygenation, is labile and permits rapid recovery.
Non-flammable.
Used when cyclopropane is not desired.

Accompanied by bronchial spasm. May be followed by respiratory depression.
Not suitable for psychic reasons and from standpoint of duration.
Not always technically feasible.

Complications:
Shock not uncommon at conclusion.
Tension pneumothorax.
Air Emboli.
Respiratory acidosis.

---

31. Lung—Pneumonectomy, Lobectomy, Exploratory Thoracotomy

Clinicial
1. Diminished pulmonary reserve present.
2. Usually sepsis or a neoplasm or both are present.
3. Left vocal cord paralysis (neoplastic) may be present.
4. Atelectasis may be present.

Surgical
1. May be long and tedious.
2. No relaxation needed.
3. Adhesions may give rise to ooze causing considerable blood loss.
4. Shock and hemorrhage likely.

Anesthetic
1. Copious secretions require frequent suctioning.
2. Awkward position interferes with ventilation.
3. Vagal, hilar and tracheobronchial reflexes may cause circulatory disturbances.
4. Mediastinal shift and inadequate ventilation due to open chest may require controlled breathing.
5. Coughing and bronchial spasm make induction difficult.

1. Cyclopropane intratracheally.

2. Cyclopropane followed by ether

3. Nitrous oxide-halothane.
4. Nitrous oxide or ethylene followed by ether intratracheally.
5. Nitrous oxide—pentothal and a muscle relaxant.

Less Desirable or Contraindicated
1. Local or regional blocks.

2. Spinal.

3. Basal narcotics alone or with local.

Children
Same as adults.

Allows quiet breathing. Mediastinum does not move excessively.
Ether causes exaggerated respiratory movements and enhances production of secretions.
Non-flammable.
Induction may be prolonged and difficult and accompanied by sub-oxygenation.
Respiratory pattern disturbed. Respiratory depression follows postoperatively. Bronchial spasm frequent.

Complete block cannot be obtained.
Respiratory paralysis and hypotension cannot be averted or controlled.
Respiratory depression, bronchial spasm and lack of control of airway are objectionable.

Complications
Respiratory acidosis may contribute to shock.
Positional changes may induce shock at conclusion of surgery.
Inadequate ventilation follows due to removal of lung.
Emergence delerium from anoxia not uncommon.
Pulmonary edema from overloading with fluid may occur.
Subcutaneous emphysema.
Pneumothorax or mediastinal emphysema may occur.

TABLE II—(*continued*)

Problems Encountered	Choices	Remarks

32. Lung—Incision and Drainage of Lung Abscesses

Problems Encountered	Choices	Remarks
Same considerations as for pneumonectomy. Secretions may be excessive causing drowning.	1. Cyclopropane intratracheally.	Permits rapid induction and recovery and suctioning through tube.
	2. Ether preceded by rapid induction agent.	Prolonged induction and undesirable after effects objectionable.
	3. Nitrous oxide-halothane.	Non-flammable.
	4. Local.	Does not permit use of intratracheal tube to facilitate suction. Patient cannot cough.

33. Mediastinum—Explorations, Thymectomy, Removal of Aneurysms and Cysts, Excision of Neoplasms, etc.

Problems Encountered	Choices	Remarks
Clinical 1. May be associated with myesthenia gravis (thymus). 2. Symptoms of pressure or obstruction to airway may be present from compression. 3. Not confined to any age group. *Surgical* 1. Requires no relaxation. 2. Ribs must be resected or sternum must be split. 3. May be prolonged depending on procedure. 4. Usually supine position is used. 5. Possibility of massive hemorrhage due to technical error (great vessels). 6. Requires "quiet" mediastinum. *Anesthetic* 1. Open chest requires use of intermittent positive pressure or controlled respiration. 2. Reflexes may arise from periosteum and intrathoracic structures. 3. Bronchial spasm may occur due to manipulation of intrathoracic structures.	1. Cyclopropane intratracheally. 2. Cyclopropane—ether intratracheally. 3. Nitrous oxide or ethylene ether intratracheally. 4. Nitrous oxide or ethylene intratracheally with topical and basal of pentothal with muscle relaxant. 5. Nitrous oxide-halothane. 6. Local. Note: Hypothermia used as adjunct if circulation is interrupted.	Respiration depressed. Provides quiet thorax. Controlled respiration easily induced. Respiratory movements exaggerated. Respiratory depression may occur in postoperative period. For controlled breathings. Non-flammable. Operations are too extensive. Not usually applicable.

34. Heart—Pericardium—Incision and Drainage—Explorations, Resections

Problems Encountered	Choices	Remarks
Clinical 1. Symptoms of cardiac failure may be present. 2. Pulsus paradoxus or cardiac tamponade may be present. 3. Increased venous pressure present. 4. Sepsis is present if due to infection. 5. Increased cardiac irritability may be present. 6. Many patients are children. *Surgical* 1. Requires rib resection or splitting of sternum. 2. No relaxation required. 3. May be prolonged requiring considerable time. 4. Ventricle may dilate and fibrillate. *Anesthetic* 1. Open thorax—intermittent positive pressure may be needed. 2. Reflexes from manipulation of ribs, pleura, great vessels, etc. may be present. 3. Circulatory failure, irregularities of pulse, etc. may occur.	(a) *Incision and drainage* 1. Local. 2. Local with basal. 3. Cyclopropane followed by ether intratracheally. 4. Nitrous oxide or ethylene followed by ether intratracheally. (b) *Resections* 1. Cyclopropane—ether. 2. Nitrous oxide or ethylene followed by ether. 3. Nitrous oxide or ethylene with basal of pentothal. 4. Nitrous oxide-halothane. 5. Local. *Children* Same as under (b).	Suitable for simple incision and drainages. Suitable for apprehensive subjects undergoing simple procedures. For children or apprehensive adults. For children or apprehensive adults. Rapid induction. May be followed by depression postoperatively. Non-flammable. Not adequate.

TABLE II—(*continued*)

Problems Encountered	Choices	Remarks

35. Heart—Myocardium—Correction of Congenital Defects (Tetralogy of Fallot)

Problems Encountered	Choices	Remarks
Clinical 1. May have expanded blood volume. May have high venous pressure. Most subjects are children. 2. Usually have high hematocrit and blood viscosity. 3. Have decreased arterial blood oxygen saturation as a rule. Orthopnea and dyspnea. *Surgical* 1. No relaxation needed. 2. Requires open thorax and rib resection. 3. Meticulous. Are done in supine or lateral position. *Anesthetic* 1. Open chest required—positive pressure or controlled breathing necessary. 2. Attempt to reduce oxygen consumption by (a) relieving apprehension (b) reducing metabolic rate 3. Cardiac irregularities may develop. 4. Cardiac failure may develop. 5. Cerebral thrombosis may develop.	1. Ether intratracheally induced with cyclopropane or nitrous oxide or ethylene with or without basal narcosis. Hypothermia as adjunct. 2. Cyclopropane intratracheally with or without basal. 3. Nitrous oxide-halothane. 4. Pentothal—nitrous oxide. *Not Desired* 5. Local or nerve block.	Most suitable from cardiac standpoint. Increases cardiac irritability. Non-flammable. Depression of respiration common.

36. Heart—Myocardium—Correction of Patent Ductus Arteriosus

Problems Encountered	Choices	Remarks
Clinical 1. Most subjects are children. Decreased diastolic pressure and widened pulse pressure. 2. Cardiac enlargement is present. Symptoms of cardiac insufficiency more common in adults. *Surgical* 1. Open chest. 2. Patient must be on side. 3. Hemorrhage a possibility. 4. Requires quiet mediastinum. *Anesthetic* 1. Lateral position requires use of intratracheal airway.	1. Ether intratracheally. May be induced with cyclopropane, or nitrous oxide or ethylene with or without basal narcosis. 2. Nitrous oxide-halothane. 3. Pentothal basal, nitrous oxide or ethylene intratracheally. *Not Desirable* 4. Cyclopropane alone. 5. Local.	Most suitable from cardiac standpoint. Non-flammable. Depression of respiration common. Increases cardiac irritability.

37. Heart—Myocardium—Valvulotomy and Repairs of Other Intracardiac Defects, Suture of Perforations

Problems Encountered	Choices	Remarks
Same requirements as for correction of congenital defects except that there is increased cardiac irritability due to intracardiac manipulation.	1. Ether intratracheally. Induced with cyclopropane or nitrous oxide or ethylene with or without basal narcosis. 2. Cyclopropane intratracheally. 3. Nitrous oxide halothane.	 Non-flammable.

TABLE II—(*continued*)

Problems Encountered	Choices	Remarks

38. Oesophagus—Resections, Removal of Diverticulae, etc.

Problems Encountered	Choices	Remarks
Clinical 1. Patients are usually adults in older age groups. 2. Cachexia, anemia, etc. due to interference with nutrition may be present. *Surgical* 1. Requires open chest as for thoracic portions. 2. Long, tedious, time consuming. 3. Retention may be present. *Anesthetic* 1. Same as for pneumonectomy and other intrathoracic procedures. In addition presence of stomach tube interferes with application of mask. 2. Possibility of aspiration of contents of diverticuli. 3. Reflex changes due to manipulation of vagi.	1. Cyclopropane intratracheally. 2. Cyclopropane combined with ether intratracheally. 3. Nitrous oxide, or ethylene followed by ether intratracheally. 4. Nitrous oxide-halothane. 5. Pentothal-nitrous oxide. 6. Local or cervical block.	Labile, permits rapid induction and recovery. Suitable when cyclopropane alone cannot be used. Suitable when cyclopropane cannot be used. Non-flammable. Respiratory depression common. Used for surgery upon cervical portion, particularly in diverticulectomy.

39. Diaphragm—Repair of Hernia, Eventrations, etc.

Problems Encountered	Choices	Remarks
Clinical 1. Respiratory distress may be present due to eventration of abdominal contents into thorax. 2. Possible gastric retention due to stasis. *Surgical* 1. May require transabdominal and thoracic approach. *Anesthetic* 1. May require controlled respiration. 2. May encounter troublesome reflexes due to manipulation of phrenics or vagi. 3. Disturbances in ventilation may result from manipulation of diaphragm.	1. Cyclopropane intratracheally. 2. Ethylene or nitrous oxide followed by ether intratracheally. 3. Nitrous oxide-halothane. 4. Nitrous oxide intratracheally. Basal of pentothal. *Not Desired* 5. Local. 6. Spinal.	Labile rapid acting. Causes quiet breathing. Exaggerates breathing. Non-flammable. Suitable if apnea is required for controlled respiration. Depression in postoperative period.

ABDOMEN

40. Upper—Biliary, Gastric, Splenic, Hepatic, Pancreatic Surgery, Repair of Epigastric Hernia, etc.

Problems Encountered	Choices	Remarks
1. Anemia, jaundice, sepsis, weight loss or other factors incident to the disease may be present. 2. Patients may be in any age group. *Surgical* 1. Relaxation required. 2. May be prolonged, tedious 3. "Quiet abdomen" essential. *Anesthetic* 1. Troublesome traction reflexes cause laryngeal and bronchial spasm, and circulatory changes. 2. Possibility of retention in gastric cases. 3. Stomach tube may be required. Interferes with mask. 4. Shock may follow in long cases.	1. Cyclopropane intratracheally with a muscle relaxant. 2. Ether intratracheally induced with ethylene or nitrous oxide with or without a basal. 3. Nitrous oxide-halothane. 4. Nitrous oxide, pentothal and a muscle relaxant. 5. Spinal with basal narcosis or light cyclopropane or ethylene. 6. Field block or intercostal block combined with a splanchnic block. *Children* 1. Ether — non-rebreathing technique. 2. Ether or cyclopropane closed system. 3. Open drop ether.	Provides quiet abdomen. Excellent relaxation obtained. May have prolonged recovery period in long operations. Respiration may be exaggerated. Non-flammable. Depression postoperatively may follow particularly in prolonged operations. Traction causes chest pain, nausea, vomiting. Incidence of atelectasis greater than with other methods. Useful in poor risk subjects but not always satisfactory or of sufficient duration.

TABLE II—*(continued)*

Problems Encountered	Choices	Remarks

41. Lower—Intestinal Operations, Appendectomy, Operations of Pelvic Organs, etc.

Problems Encountered	Choices	Remarks
Clinical 1. Patients may be in any age group. 2. Anemia, weight loss, sepsis and other factors incident to the disease may be present.	1. Spinal. 2. Cyclopropane with a muscle relaxant. 3. Ethylene or nitrous oxide followed by ether. 4. Nitrous oxide-halothane. 5. Nitrous oxide; pentothal and a muscle relaxant. 6. Abdominal field block with basal or gaseous agent.	Yields excellent relaxation. Excellent when spinal is not desired. When 1 and 2 are not desired or contraindicated. Non-flammable. When cautery is used. Depression undesirable. For poorer risk patients.
Surgical 1. Relaxation required. 2. May be long and tedious. 3. Quiet abdomen essential. 4. Performed in supine position.		
Anesthetic 1. Troublesome laryngeal and bronchial reflexes. 2. Possibility of aspiration from obstruction or retention. 3. Stomach tube may be required. Interferes with mask. 4. Shock may occur in long cases.	*Less Desirable or Contraindicated* 7. Open drop ether. 8. Nitrous oxide or ethylene alone. 9. Pentothal alone.	Suitable when nothing else is available. Does not yield relaxation. Insufficient depth and potency with safe limits.
	Children 1. Cyclopropane—ether closed system. 2. Vinethene-ether. 3. Nitrous oxide-halothane.	Non-flammable.

42. Wall—Extra Peritoneal Procedures, Removal of Cysts, Lipomas, Skin Grafts, etc., Plastic Operations

Problems Encountered	Choices	Remarks
Clinical 1. Patients usually in good condition. 2. Patients may be in any age group.	1. Local or field block. 2. Cyclopropane with mask. 3. Nitrous oxide-halothane. 4. Ethylene or nitrous oxide. 5. Basal with nitrous oxide or ethylene. 6. Ethylene or nitrous oxide followed by ether. 7. Spinal.	For brief superficial operation For more extensive procedures. Non-flammable. For procedures not requiring relaxation. For apprehensive subjects. For extensive procedures in which 2 cannot be used. A major anesthetic for a minor procedure.
Surgical 1. Usually superficial or minor. 2. Relaxation not needed. 3. Usually in supine position.		
Anesthetic 1. Anesthetist has ready access to airway.		
	Children 1. Open drop ether. 2. Cyclopropane. 3. Nitrous oxide-halothane.	

43. Wall—Inguinal or Femoral Hernia

Problems Encountered	Choices	Remarks
Clinical 1. Usually in active subjects, but may occur at any age. 2. Are elective except when strangulation is present.	1. Spinal. 2. Cyclopropane. 3. Nitrous oxide-halothane. 4. Nitrous oxide, pentothal basal, with muscle relaxant. 5. Nitrous oxide or ethylene followed by ether. 6. Local.	Suitable for most patients in good health. Suitable for apprehensive subjects who object to spinal. Non-flammable. Desirable, but depression in postoperative period may follow. Traction reflexes may induce spasm. When 1, 2 and 3 are contraindicated. In poor risk subjects. Traction reflexes on cord and peritoneum may cause nausea and vomiting.
Surgical 1. Usually not prolonged. 2. Relaxation of moderate degree required. 3. Peritoneum and abdominal viscera are manipulated.		
Anesthetic 1. Traction reflexes from cord cause laryngeal spasm. 2. Airway easily maintained except in obese subjects.	*Children* 1. Cyclopropane—ether by closed system. 2. Open drop ether. 3. Nitrous oxide-halothane.	When closed system is not available.

TABLE II—(*continued*)

Problems Encountered	Choices	Remarks

44. Intra Abdominal Extra Peritoneal—Bladder Operations, Cystotomy, Cystectomy Resections, Diverticulectomy

Problems Encountered	Choices	Remarks
Clinical 1. May have urinary retention with or without azotemia. 2. More common in older age group. *Surgical* 1. Are usually done suprapubically and extra peritoneally. 2. Require muscle relaxation. 3. May use electrosurgical unit. 4. May require distention of bladder with water—Some may be absorbed or forced intravenously. *Anesthetic* 1. Time variable—resections prolonged; cystotomies brief. 2. Traction reflexes common.	1. Spinal 2. Cyclopropane 3. Nitrous oxide or ethylene followed by ether. 4. Nitrous oxide-halothane. 5. Nitrous oxide and a basal of pentothal, and muscle relaxant. 6. Local. 7. Caudal.	Satisfactory for most subjects because "low" one is required. Rapid recovery and induction. Less desirable. Non-flammable. Depression occurs postoperatively. Not flammable. Suitable for cystotomy or other minor procedures. Satisfactory for transurethral approach only if caudal is high.

45. Bladder—Cystoscopy

Problems Encountered	Choices	Remarks
Clinical 1. Condition of patient variable. *Surgical* 1. Relaxation usually not required. 2. Are performed for diagnosis or for therapy—Removal of stones. 3. Are more painful in males. 4. Patients may be in any age group. 5. Are performed in lithotomy position.	1. Trilene analgesia. 2. Nitrous oxide-halothane. 3. Nitrous oxide and pentothal. 4. Spinal.	For office or outpatient use for diagnosis. For short procedures or for diagnosis. Non-flammable. For longer more extensive procedures in apprehensive subjects. When extensive anesthesia and relaxation is required.

46. Extra Peritoneal—Operations on Kidney and Ureters

Problems Encountered	Choices	Remarks
Clinical 1. Sepsis, tuberculosis or other evidence of infection may be present. 2. Uremia or urinary suppression may be present. 3. Abdominal distention may be present (reflex in colic). 4. Debilitation and other signs of systemic disease. *Surgical* 1. Usually performed in lateral position (prone for lower ureters). 2. Muscle relaxation required. 3. Adrenal gland may be manipulated. 4. Peritoneum may be manipulated. 5. Blood loss may be considerable. *Anesthetic* 1. Intratracheal airway indicated for lateral position. 2. Troublesome reflexes from traction on renal pedicle may cause respiratory and circulatory changes. 3. Hormonal effects from manipulation of adrenal may occur. 4. Nausea and vomiting from traction reflexes (spinal or local). 5. Positive pressure may be needed if pleura is incised.	1. Cyclopropane intratracheally. 2. Cyclopropane combined with ether intratracheally. 3. Spinal—with sedation. 4. Nitrous oxide-halothane. 5. Ether preceded by ethylene or nitrous oxide intratracheally. 6. Basal of pentothal; nitrous oxide intratracheally with a muscle relaxant. *Children* 1. Ether or cyclopropane intratracheally by closed system. 2. Ether open drop. 3. Nitrous oxide-halothane.	Causes little or no metabolic disturbances. Needed for good relaxation. Must be high to abolish reflexes from traction. Non-flammable. Satisfactory when 1, 2 and 3 are not desired. Prolonged depression occurs in postoperative period particularly in chronically ill patients. When closed system is not available. Non-flammable.

TABLE II—(continued)

Problems Encountered	Choices	Remarks

PERINEUM

47. Genitalia (Male)—Orchidectomy, Hydrocelectomy, Vasectomy and Other Operations on Genitalia

Problems Encountered	Choices	Remarks
Clinical 1. Adults most often. 2. Usually good risks. *Surgical* 1. Relaxation not needed. 2. Patient is in supine position. 3. May use cautery. *Anesthetic* 1. Traction reflexes may cause circulatory and respiratory changes.	1. Spinal. 2. Cyclopropane. 3. Nitrous oxide-halothane. 4. Nitrous or ethylene and ether. 5. Pentothal basal; nitrous oxide. 6. Local. *Children* 1. Ether open drop. 2. Ether closed system. 3. Cyclopropane closed system.	Suitable for extensive procedures. Useful for apprehensive non-cardiacs. Non-flammable. When 1 and 2 are contraindicated. When cautery is used and spinal and local cannot be used. For simple procedures or in extremely poor risks. When closed system is not available. If suitable apparatus is available. If suitable apparatus is available.

48. Penis—Circumcision

Problems Encountered	Choices	Remarks
Clinical Elective in young healthy males, as a rule. *Surgical* 1. Brief. 2. No relaxation required. *Anesthetic* 1. Reflex stimulation may occur.	1. Local. 2. Cyclopropane. 3. Spinal. 4. Caudal. 5. Nitrous oxide-halothane. 6. Pentothal alone or pentothal nitrous oxide. *Children* 1. Cyclopropane. 2. Nitrous oxide-halothane. 3. Nitrous oxide or ethylene followed by ether. 4. Ether open drop.	Usual procedure employed. Rapid acting, rapid recovery. A major anesthetic for a minor procedure. Only satisfactory when it is high. Frenulum not blocked. Non-flammable. Priapism and laryngeal spasm may occur. Suitable if satisfactory apparatus is available. Non-flammable. Suitable if satisfactory apparatus is available. Suitable if satisfactory apparatus is not available.

49. Genitalia—Female—Vaginoplasties—Perineal Repairs, Cystocele, Rectocele, Perineorrhaphy and Other Operations on the Vulva, Vagina and Cervix

Problems Encountered	Choices	Remarks
Clinical 1. May be in any age group—usually middle age. 2. Are usually in good physical condition. *Surgical* 1. Patient is placed in lithotomy position frequently (May be in Simms in some cases). 2. Profound relaxation not required. *Anesthetic* 1. Reflexes may cause hypotension accompanied by bradycardia, and respiratory disturbances.	1. Spinal. 2. Cyclopropane. 3. Nitrous oxide-halothane. 4. Ethylene or nitrous and ether. 5. Pentothal, or other basal, and nitrous oxide. 6. Local. 7. Caudal. *Children* 1. Cyclopropane. 2. Ether by closed system. 3. Ether by open drop. 4. Nitrous oxide-halothane.	Abolishes reflexes. Most satisfactory when general anesthesia is indicated. Non-flammable. Suitable when 1 and 2 cannot be used. Laryngeal spasm and respiratory depression occur postoperatively. For simple procedures of a minor nature. Usually not sufficiently extensive unless it is high. Non-flammable.

TABLE II—(*continued*)

Problems Encountered	Choices	Remarks

50. Vaginal Examination

Problems Encountered	Choices	Remarks
Surgical 1. Brief. 2. No relaxation needed. 3. May be ambulatory. *Anesthetic* 1. Manipulation may cause reflex effect on respiration.	1. Nitrous oxide. 2. Ethylene. 3. Cyclopropane. 4. Nitrous oxide-halothane. 5. Pentothal—nitrous oxide.	Pleasant—no nausea. Somewhat nauseating to some patients. Nausea and vomiting which may follow it for such a brief procedure is objectionable. Non-flammable. Laryngeal spasm may occur from stimulation.

51. Cervix—Dilatation and Curettage, Removal of Polyps, Conization, Biopsy, etc.

Problems Encountered	Choices	Remarks
Clinical 1. Patient may be septic, anemic, on verge of shock if post abortal. 2. May be in any age group. *Surgical* 1. Brief. 2. No relaxation required. 3. Performed in lithotomy position. 4. Blood loss may occur. 5. Uterus may be perforated. 6. Cautery may be used. *Anesthetic* Airway easily maintained.	1. Nitrous oxide-halothane. 2. Ethylene. 3. Cyclopropane. 4. Nitrous oxide—pentothal. 5. Local with heavy sedation. 6. Spinal. 7. Caudal	Pleasant, rapid acting, no nausea. Somewhat nauseating to some patients. Rapid acting. Desirable except nausea and vomiting may follow. Satisfactory. Satisfactory in cooperative patient. A major anesthetic for a minor procedure in most cases. Satisfactory procedure if high.

52. Uterus—Vaginal Hysterectomy

Problems Encountered	Choices	Remarks
Clinical 1. Usually performed in middle aged and older females. 2. May be performed in patients not able to stand more extensive surgery. *Surgical* 1. Traction on pelvic vicera. 2. Peritoneal cavity entered. 3. Usually placed in lithotomy position. 4. Technical difficulties may necessitate use of suprapelvic approach in addition to perineal. 5. Moderate relaxation required to avoid bearing down and pushing of abdominal contents outward. *Anesthetic* 1. Traction may cause reflexes, hypotension and bradycardia. 2. Airway maintained easily except in obese patients. 3. Moderately deep anesthesia required.	1. Spinal. 2. Cyclopropane with or without muscle relaxant. 3. Ethylene or nitrous oxide ether. 4. Pentothal, nitrous oxide with muscle relaxant. 5. Nitrous oxide-halothane. 6. Caudal. 7. Pentothal alone.	Ideal but must extend to T 10 Ideal when general anesthesia is desired. Rapid recovery. Suitable if 1 and 2 are contra-indicated. Traction reflexes cause laryngeal spasm. Respiratory depression occurs. Non-flammable. Pelvic peritoneum not anesthetized. Abdominal discomfort follows. Not satisfactory. Large quantities required.

53. Vagina—Incision and Drainage of Pelvic Abscess

Problems Encountered	Choices	Remarks
Clinical 1. Sepsis present. *Surgical* 1. Lithotomy position required. 2. Performed trans-vaginally. 3. Usually brief. 4. Circulatory collapse may follow drainage. *Anesthetic* 1. Anesthetist has access to head. Airway maintained with ease except in obese patients.	1. Cyclopropane. 2. Nitrous oxide or ethylene followed by ether. 3. Halothane-nitrous oxide. 4. Pentothal-nitrous oxide. 5. Open drop vinyl ether. 6. Spinal.	Rapid induction and recovery. Use when cyclopropane is contraindicated. Non-flammable. Suitable, but spasm may occur. Useful in brief and in children. Septic condition may preclude its use.

TABLE II—(*continued*)

Problems Encountered	Choices	Remarks

RECTAL SURGERY

54. Hemorrhoidectomy, Excision of Anal Fissure, Repairs of Prolapse, Removal of Sinus Tracts

Problems Encountered	Choices	Remarks
Clinical 1. Patients are adults most often. 2. Are usually good risk subjects. 3. Anemia may be present in protracted cases of internal hemorrhoids. 4. Fistulous tracts may be associated with tuberculosis infections *Surgical* 1. Relaxation must be extreme. 2. Lithotomy position used by some. Prone jackknife position by others. 3. Cautery may be used. 4. Are usually of short or moderate duration. *Anesthetic* 1. Airway difficult to maintain in prone position. Use intratracheal tube. 2. Hypoventilation accentuated by prone position. 3. Deep anesthesia required to relax sphincters. 4. Laryngeal spasm develops reflexly during general anesthesia.	1. Spinal (saddle) with long-lasting drug. 2. Caudal. 3. Transacral. 4. Intratracheal cyclopropane or nitrous oxide ether. 5. Basal of pentothal, intratracheal nitrous oxide and muscle relaxant. 6. Halothane-nitrous oxide. *Less Desirable* 7. Local. 8. Open drop ether. 9. Basal narcosis alone.	1. Provides desired relaxation and sustained analgesia in immediate postoperative period. 2. Excellent relaxation. Post spinal headache avoided. 3. When caudal canal is inaccessible and spinal is not desired. 4. Flammable: Relaxation not always satisfactory. 5. When cautery is used. Not desirable in prone position because of inadequate ventilation. 6. Non-flammable. 7. Edema, distorts tissues. Satisfactory anesthesia not always obtained. 8. Deep anesthesia required for relaxation. 9. Reflexes not abolished. Relaxation inadequate. Airway not under control in prone position.

EXTREMITIES, BONES, JOINTS

55. Vertebral Column—Cervical Laminectomy, Spinal Fusion, Reduction of Fractures, etc.

Problems Encountered	Choices	Remarks
Clinical 1. Are usually performed for trauma, disks, cord tumors, tuberculosis and other afflictions of cord. 2. May have paralysis or other neurologic lesions. 3. May have paralysis of muscles of respiration. *Surgical* 1. Must be performed in prone position. 2. Shock and blood loss not uncommon. 3. May be long. 4. Usually use electrocoagulation for hemostasis. *Anesthetic* 1. Intratracheal tube necessary to maintain airway. 2. May require artificial respiration throughout procedure. 3. May be unable to flex or extend head—interferes with intubation.	1. Halothane-nitrous oxide. 2. Basal thiopental; nitrous oxide intratracheally with cyclopropane to do intubation. 3. Cyclopropane intratracheally. 4. Nitrous oxide or ethylene followed by ether—oxygen intratracheally. 5. Local or nerve blocks. *Not Recommended* 6. Any type of anesthesia without intratracheal catheter. *Children* 1. Same as for adults.	Non-flammable. Not flammable except in beginning. May be used when coagulation current is not used. When 1 and 2 cannot be used or are not desired. Not satisfactory. Patient experiences discomfort.

TABLE II—(*continued*)

Problems Encountered	Choices	Remarks

56. Vertebral Column—Thoracic Laminectomy—Spinal Fusion, Reduction of Fractures

Problems Encountered	Choices	Remarks
Clinical 1. Are usually performed for trauma, disks, cord tumors, tuberculosis and other afflictions of the cord. 2. May have paralysis of lower part of body including respiratory muscles. *Surgical* 1. Must be performed in prone position. 2. Shock and blood loss common. 3. May be long. 4. Usually use electrocoagulation for hemostasis. *Anesthetic* 1. Intratracheal tube necessary to maintain airway. 2. May require artificial respiration throughout procedure. 3. May be unable to flex or extend head—interferes with intubation.	1. Pentothal basal and nitrous oxide intratracheally. (With cyclopropane to do intubation.) 2. Cyclopropane intratracheally. 3. Nitrous oxide or ethylene followed by ether oxygen intratracheally. 4. Local or regional epidural. 5. Halothane-nitrous oxide. *Children* 1. Same as adults.	Not flammable except in bebinning if cyclopropane is used. When coagulation current is not used. When 1 and 2 cannot be used. Not recommended. Patient experiences discomfort. Flammable.

57. Laminectomy (Lumbar), Spinal Fusions, Operations on Sacrum, Excision of Coccyx, etc.

Problems Encountered	Choices	Remarks
Clinical 1. Are performed for othopedic, neurologic traumatic or for infections. 2. May have paraplegia, sensory changes or other neurologic disturbances. 3. May have decubitus ulcers. *Surgical* 1. Are performed in prone position. 2. May be followed by shock and blood loss. 3. Electrocoagulation may be required. 4. May be long. *Anesthetic* 1. Intratracheal tube is necessary to maintain airway. 2. May require artificial respiration throughout procedure. 3. May be unable to flex or extend head—interferes with intubation. 4. Operation may outlast block if spinal is used.	1. Spinal. 2. Cyclopropane induction followed by nitrous oxide intratracheally and basal of pentothal. 3. Halothane-nitrous oxide. 4. Cyclopropane intratracheally. 5. Nitrous oxide or ethylene with ether intratracheally. 6. Local, nerve blocks and peridural. *Children.* 1. Cyclopropane followed by nitrous oxide intratracheally. 2. Cyclopropane intratracheally. 3. Nitrous oxide or ethylene with ether intratracheally. *Less Desirable or Contraindicated* 4. Open ether.	Ideal when neurologic diseases or psychic state does not preclude its use. When cautery is used. Non-flammable. Flammable. May be used when no fire hazard exists. When 1 and 3 are not suitable. Not easily and adequately maintained. Psychic trauma pronounced. Spinal not suitable. Spinal not suitable. Spinal not suitable. Airway not maintained adequately.

58. Vertebral Column—Sacrum—Excision of Pilonidal Sinus

Problems Encountered	Choices	Remarks
Clinical 1. Subjects usually are young and vigorous. *Surgical* 1. Prone position is required. 2. Infection may be present at site of lesion. *Anesthetic* 1. Airway is difficult to maintain without endotracheal tube. 2. Positional changes cause changes in blood pressure.	1. Spinal. 2. Cyclopropane intratracheally. 3. Ether intratracheally. 4. Nitrous oxide and basal pentothal. 5. Halothane-nitrous oxide.	Ideal unless infection is too near site of lumbar puncture. Rapid induction and recovery assured. Suitable if 1 or 2 are contraindicated. Respiratory depression may occur. Undesirable with patient in prone position. Non-flammable.

TABLE II—(*continued*)

Problems Encountered	Choices	Remarks
59. Upper—Arm—Extremity Upper—Reduction of Fractures, Amputations, Joint Explorations, Osteotomies, Nerve Suture.		
Clinical		
1. May be in any age group.	1. Brachial plexus block.	Suitable for forearm. Upper arm and axilla not anesthetized.
Surgical		
1. Relaxation needed.	1. Cyclopropane.	Most satisfactory. Rapid acting, rapid recovery.
2. Tourniquet may be used, painful with block anesthesia.	2. Nitrous oxide with basal of pentothal.	When cautery or x-rays are used.
3. May be long.	3. Ethylene or nitrous oxide followed by ether.	When 1 and 2 cannot be used.
4. Usually performed in supine but may be done in lateral position.	4. Halothane-nitrous oxide.	Non-flammable.
5. X-ray apparatus may be used.	5. Local.	For minor procedures only.
6. May be shocking and accompanied by blood loss.	*Children*	
Anesthetic	1. Vinethene.	For minor procedures.
1. Anesthetist may be in operators way (shoulder). Endotracheal tube required.	2. Vinethene and ether.	When suitable closed system is not available.
	3. Cyclopropane.	When closed system is available.
	4. Nitrous oxide or ethylene ether.	When closed system is available.
60. Forearm and Hand—Tendon Repairs, Incision and Drainage, Reduction of Fractures, Excision of Nodes, Masses, etc.		
Clinical		
May be in any age group.	1. Cyclopropane.	Suitable if operation outlasts the block.
Surgical		
1. May be long and tedious	2. Brachial plexus block.	Of equal preference to 1 depending upon patient.
2. Relaxation required for larger muscles.	3. Nitrous oxide-halothane.	Non-flammable.
3. Tourniquet may be required.	4. Nitrous oxide and pentothal.	Of equal preference to 1 and 2 depending upon patient.
Anesthetic	5. Nitrous oxide or ethylene with ether.	Only if 1, 2 or 3 are not desired.
1. Airway maintained with ease—patient in supine position.	*Children*	
2. Surgeon and anesthetist do not compete for operative field. Endotracheal tube not necessary.	1. Cyclopropane.	Suitable if closed system is available.
	2. Ethylene or nitrous oxide —ether.	
	3. Vinyl ether followed by ethyl ether.	When closed system is not available.
61. Upper Hand—Digits—Incision and Drainage—Other Minor Procedures		
Clinical		
1. May be in any age group.	1. Cyclopropane.	Rapid induction and recovery.
Surgical	2. Ethylene.	Suitable in well premedicated patients.
1. Little or no relaxation required	3. Halothane-nitrous oxide.	Non-flammable.
2. Are usually short, without shock or blood loss.	4. Nitrous oxide, pentothal.	Suitable in well premedicated patients.
3. Patient may be ambulatory.	5. Brachial plexus block.	Satisfactory in non-apprehensive subjects.
4. Sepsis may be present.	6. Vinyl ether—nitrous oxide or ethylene followed by ether.	For short procedures.
Anesthetic	7. Local infiltration or digital block.	For simple procedures without peripheral vascular disease or infection.
Anesthetist has control of airway.	*Children*	
	1. Vinethene.	For brief simple procedures.
	2. Cyclopropane.	
	3. Vinethene and ether.	When closed system is not available.

TABLE II—(*continued*)

Problems Encountered	Choices	Remarks

62. Thigh and Hip—Osteotomy, Insertion of Pins—Reduction of Fractures, Muscle and Nerve Operations, Bone Grafts

Problems Encountered	Choices	Remarks
Clinical 1. Subjects are often elderly, particularly those with fractured hips. *Surgical* 1. May be long and shocking. 2. Require considerable relaxation. 3. May require tourniquet. 4. Casts may be applied at conclusion of operation. 5. May use electrical saws and X-Ray equipment. *Anesthetic* 1. Patient is in supine position. Airway is accessible.	1. Spinal. 2. Cyclopropane. 3. Nitrous oxide—pentothal. 4. Halothane-nitrous oxide. 5. Nitrous oxide or ethylene followed by ether. 6. Local. *Children* 1. Cyclopropane. 2. Nitrous oxide ether. 3. Vinyl ether followed by open ether.	For healthy subjects without contraindication to spinal anesthesia. Suitable if 1 is not suitable or contraindicated. Not flammable. Use when 1 and 2 cannot. Non-flammable. To be used when 1, 2 and 3 cannot. For brief procedures, of simple nature or extremely poor risk subjects. If closed system is not available.

63. Knee and Leg

Problems Encountered	Choices	Remarks
Clinical 1. May be of varied age group or risk. *Surgical* 1. May be extensive and long. 2. Relaxation required. 3. May be shocking. 4. X-Ray and electric saw used. *Anesthetic* 1. Patient is in the supine position. Airway is accessible.	1. Spinal. 2. Cyclopropane. 3. Nitrous oxide—pentothal. 4. Nitrous oxide-thiopental. 5. Nitrous oxide or ethylene followed by ether. 6. Local.	For healthy subjects without contraindication to spinal. Suitable if 1 is not suitable. Not flammable. Use when 1 and 2 cannot. Non-flammable. To be used when 1, 2 and 3 cannot. For brief procedures, of simple nature or for extremely poor risk subjects.

AUTONOMIC NERVOUS SYSTEM

64. Sympathectomy—Transthoracic and Lumbar

Problems Encountered	Choices	Remarks
Clinical 1. Patients usually have some systemic illness (diabetes, hypertension, arteriosclerosis, etc.). 2. Are usually in upper age group. *Surgical* 1. Require thoracic approach. 2. Patient must be on side. *Anesthetic* 1. May require controlled respiration—intubate. 2. Blood pressure may be very labile.	1. Cyclopropane ether with pentothal induction. 2. Nitrous oxide or ethylene ether with pentothal induction. 3. Nitrous oxide, pentothal. 4. Nitrous oxide-thiopental. *Not Desired* 5. Spinal. 6. Pentothal alone. 7. Local.	Rapid acting easily controlled depth of anesthesia. When use of vasopressors is contemplated. When cautery is to be used. Non-flammable. Anesthesia required is too extensive. Surgical procedure extensive.

65. Lumbar Sympathectomy

Problems Encountered	Choices	Remarks
Clinical 1. Usually have some systemic disease (diabetes, hypertension, etc.) *Surgical* 1. Require lumbar approach. 2. Require relaxation. 3. In semiprone position. *Anesthetic* 1. Blood pressure labile.	1. Cyclopropane ether with pentothal induction. 2. Nitrous oxide or ethylene and ether. 3. Spinal or peridural. 4. Halothane-nitrous oxide. 5. Nitrous oxide—pentothal and muscle relaxant. *Not Desired* 6. Local. 7. Pentothal alone. 8. Lumbar block.	Labile—rapid acting. Rapid recovery. May further eliminate a high blood pressure. When vasopressors are needed. Relaxation excellent. May cause severe fall in blood pressure. Non-flammable. When general anesthesia is required with a cautery.

TABLE II—*(continued)*

Problems Encountered	Choices	Remarks
66. Stellate Ganglionectomy		

Problems Encountered	Choices	Remarks
Clinical 1. Usually performed for vascular disease of head or extremity, causalgia, to relieve angina, excess sweating, status asthmaticus. 2. Patients are usually adults. *Surgical* 1. Operation is in neck area. Anesthetist must be out of operative field. 2. Pleura may be entered—pneumothorax possibility. 3. Many vital structures in area—bleeding may occur. 4. May be long and tedious. *Anesthetic* 1. Airway difficult to control without endotracheal tube. 2. Relaxation not needed. Positive pressure may be needed if pleura is entered. 3. Reflexes due to stimulation of structures in neck (carotid sinus, vagus, trachea) may arise. Atropine needed.	1. Cyclopropane intratracheally. 2. Cyclopropane, ethylene or nitrous oxide followed by ether. 3. Nitrous oxide—pentothal with intratracheal tube. 4. Halothane-nitrous oxide. *Not Desirable* 5. Local. 6. Cervical plexus block. 7. Pentothal alone. 8. Open drop ether, without endotracheal tube.	Rapid acting—rapid recovery. Suitable when #1 cannot be used. Not flammable; suitable when cautery or x-ray unit is to be used. Non-flammable. Not sufficiently extensive or may not last long enough for the purpose. Not extensive for purposes. No control of airway. Large doses needed. Control of airway impossible.

VASCULAR SURGERY

Problems Encountered	Choices	Remarks
67. Cerebral Angiogram		

Problems Encountered	Choices	Remarks
Clinical 1. May have neurological lesion with increased intracranial pressure. 2. May be comatose (see intracranial). *Surgical* 1. Operative site is neck. Anesthetist must be out of operative field. 2. Vessel not easily identified without direct exposure. *Anesthetic* 1. Airway difficult to maintain. Requires intubation. 2. X-ray needed—flammable agents cannot be used. Convulsions and other neurological manifestations occur during or before procedure begins. 3. Disturbances of vascular and respiratory system may occur as dye is injected.	1. Local. 2. Pentothal—nitrous oxide intratracheally with topical. 3. Cyclopropane. 4. Halothane-nitrous oxide. 5. Ether, preceded by nitrous oxide or ethylene. 6. Vinethene.	Not always adaptable to patient. Exploration for artery not always possible. Not flammable. Ideal, but is flammable. Non-flammable. Satisfactory but is flammable. Operation too long. Flammable—secretions copious.

Problems Encountered	Choices	Remarks
68. Renal Angiogram		

Problems Encountered	Choices	Remarks
Clinical 1. Has suspected renal lesion. 2. May be chronically ill. *Surgical* 1. Performed in prone position. 2. Spasm of artery and pain at time dye is introduced. *Anesthetic* 1. Airway difficult to maintain without intratracheal catheter. 2. Analgesia needed at time dye passes into vessel. 3. X-ray unit used—fire hazard. 4. Procedure is a diagnostic one and relatively minor requiring major anesthetic.	1. Pentothal nitrous oxide intratracheally (with relaxant to intubate). 2. Spinal anesthesia. 3. Halothane-nitrous oxide. *Not Desirable* 4. Local anesthesia. 5. Ether. 6. Cyclopropane 7. Pentothal alone with no intratracheal tube.	Not flammable. It is a major anesthetic procedure for minor diagnostic procedure. Suitable but is major anesthetic for minor procedure. Non-flammable. Does not relieve pain at time of injection. Flammable. Flammable. May asphyxiate from obstruction. Airway not under control.

TABLE II—(continued)

Problems Encountered	Choices	Remarks

OBSTETRICS

69. Normal Delivery—Primipara

Clinical
1. Is young and in good health with few exceptions.
2. May have slight decrease in hemoglobin.

Obstetrical
1. Labor may be long and require analgesia.
2. May need episiotomy.
3. May need forceps.
4. May have posterior or other less common presentation.

Anesthetic
1. May have eaten.
2. May have no premedication.
3. Develop stridor when head passes over perineum.

Choices	Remarks
1. Cyclopropane.	Ideal in uncomplicated cases. Baby may be depressed.
2. Ethylene.	Cannot always be given without anoxia.
3. Nitrous oxide or ethylene with ether.	Anoxia obviated, but nausea and vomiting objectionable.
4. Nitrous or ethylene with vinyl ether.	Salivation common unless scopolamine is given.
5. Nitrous oxide with trichlorethylene or halothane.	Tachypnea, cardiac effects and vagal effects common.
6. Saddle block.	Headache and blood pressure drops may follow. May slow up labor increases incidence of instrumental deliveries.
7. Caudal block.	Blood pressure drops, failures common, increased instrumental deliveries. Labor slowed.
8. Pudendal block.	Satisfactory for perineal pain, does not relieve backache and visceral pain.
Less Desirable	
9. Pentothal-nitrous oxide.	Depressed baby common.
10. Nitrous oxide—oxygen.	Rarely can be given without anoxia.
11. Open drop ether.	Nausea, vomiting and depressed baby are common.
12. Trichlorethylene.	Good for analgesia, but not anesthesia.

70. Multipara

Clinical
1. Usually have been in shorter labor than primipara.
2. Are women in child bearing age in good health. Few if any abnormalities encountered.
3. Two individuals to consider, baby and mother.

Obstetrical
1. Usually do not require forceps.
2. Usually do not require epesiotomy.
3. Postpartum hemorrhage may occur.
4. Oxytoxic drugs are used.

Anesthetic
1. May use narcotics, barbiturates and other hypnotics during labor.
2. May have eaten.
3. May have anemia.
4. May have elevated blood pressure.

Choices	Remarks
1. Cyclopropane.	Ideal in uncomplicated cases. Baby may be depressed if delivery is long.
2. Ethylene or nitrous oxide.	Cannot always be given without anoxia.
3. Nitrous oxide or ethylene with ether.	Anoxia obviated, but nausea, vomiting objectionable.
4. Nitrous oxide or ethylene with vinyl ether.	Salivation common unless scopolamine is given. Relaxation poor.
5. Nitrous oxide with trichlorethylene or halothane.	Tachypnea, cardiac and vagal effects encountered.
6. Saddle block.	Post spinal headache and blood pressure drops may be encountered.
7. Caudal block.	Blood pressure drops may occur. Failures common. Incidence of instrumental deliveries increased. Labor slowed.
8. Pudendal block.	Satisfactory for perineal pain, does not relieve uterine and back pains.
9. Vinethene (open drop).	Suitable for short deliveries. Salivation occurs.
10. Pentothal nitrous oxide.	Depressed baby common unless period of use is less than few minutes.
11. Nitrous oxide—oxygen.	Rarely can be given without anoxia.
12. Open drop ether.	Nausea, vomiting and depressed baby are objectionable features.
13. Trichlorethylene.	Good for analgesia, but not anesthesia.

TABLE II—*(continued)*

Problems Encountered	Choices	Remarks
71. Forceps Deliveries		
		Same as for multipara except more profound anesthesia needed.

72. Caesarean Section

Problems Encountered	Choices	Remarks

Clinical
 1. May or may not be in labor.
 2. Have some obstetric complication such as:
   (a) placenta praevia
   (b) disproportion.
   (c) toxemia, nephritis
   (d) prolonged labor due to obstetrical difficulty.
   (e) ruptured uterus.
 3. May be in shock from some obstetric complication or have hypertension.
 	
 Obstetrical
 1. Relaxation of some degree required. The procedure is an abdominal operation.
 2. Usually placed in head down position.
 3. There may be blood loss.
 4. There may be fetal distress.
 	
 Anesthetic
 1. Patient may have eaten—aspiration.
 2. Usually cannot be sedated until baby is born.
 3. Ventilation impaired due to abdominal mass.
	1. Local
	 2. Cyclopropane.
	
	 3. Spinal.
	
	 4. Cyclopropane, ethylene or nitrous oxide followed by ether.
	 5. Pentothal and nitrous oxide.
	 6. Nitrous oxide-halothane.
	
	 Not Suitable
	 7. Caudal block.
	
	 8. Saddle block.
	
	 9. Ethylene alone.
	 10. Nitrous oxide alone.
	 11. Muscle relaxants.
		Not always adequate.
		 Rapid induction and recovery —suitable most of time.
		 Good for the newborn. Blood pressure drop severe and more difficult to control.
		 Has all disagreeable features of ether. Prolonged somnolence for baby in long cases.
		 Depresses newborn.
		
		 Non-flammable.
		
		 Extent of block not sufficient for purpose.
		 Extent of block not sufficient for purpose.
		 Not of sufficient potency.
		 Not of sufficient potency.
		 Not needed. Also pass through placenta to baby.

73. Versions

Problems Encountered	Choices	Remarks
Clinical 1. Usually performed in difficult and complicated situations. 2. Patient may have been in labor long time and be dehydrated or in shock. 3. May be multipara or primipara. *Obstetrical* 1. Relaxation of uterus required. 2. Fetal distress may be present. 3. May use uterine relaxants such as epinephrine. *Anesthetic* 1. Anesthesia must be deep to relax uterus. 2. Relaxation may take some time to accomplish. May have eaten. 3. Shock or hemorrhage may follow.	1. Ether—preceded by cyclopropane, nitrous oxide or ethylene 2. Chloroform. *Not Suitable* 1. Spinal anesthesia. 2. Saddle block. 3. Caudal block. 4. Pudendal block. 5. Muscle relaxants. 6. Cyclopropane (alone). 7. Ethylene or nitrous oxide alone or with pentothal. 8. Vinethene. 9. Halothane.	Only available agent which relaxes smooth muscle which is safe. Relaxes uterus but may depress heart. None of the following relax uterine musculature.

TABLE II—(*continued*)

Problems Encountered	Choices	Remarks
74. Toxemia		
Clinical		
1. May have edema.	1. Local.	Least innocuous but not always suitable.
2. May have liver or renal failure or both.	2. Ethylene—ether.	Ether undesirable because of effect in metabolism and acid base balance.
3. May have elevated blood pressure (diastolic) due to vasospasm.	3. Cyclopropane.	Suitable but may raise blood pressure.
4. May have renal insufficiency.		
5. May have cardiac involvement.	4. Ethylene.	Anoxia—may not be potent enough for operative obstetrics.
6 May have convulsions or other signs of C.N.S. irritability.		
Obstetrical	5. Halothane-nitrous oxide.	Non-flammable.
1. May perform ceasarean section or delivery naturally or aided by forceps.	6. Pentothal—nitrous oxide.	May be used if delivery is rapid.
2. Fetal distress may be present.	7. Caudal.	May cause fall in blood pressure. Technically, not always easily performed.
3. May require heavy sedation to control convulsion.	8. Spinal.	Causes hypotension. Patient awake and apprehensive.
Anesthetic		
1. Avoid obstruction (anoxia and CO_2 excess).	*Avoid*	
2. Avoid pressor substances or drugs which elevate or markedly drop blood pressure.	8. Chloroform	Damages liver.
	9. Trichlorethylene.	Damages liver.
3. Avoid drugs which effect kidney and liver.	10. Vinyl ether.	Not sufficiently potent. May be hepatotoxic.

TABLE III

DRUGS TO USE FOR OR DURING ANESTHESIA FOR THE MORE COMMONLY
ENCOUNTERED CLINICAL CONDITIONS

Diseases	Permissible Drugs	Drugs to Avoid
Acute infections of upper respiratory tract	Cyclopropane, ethylene, nitrous oxide, halothane, spinal, nerve block, local, muscle relaxants.	Ether, ultra short acting barbiturates, chloroform, ethyl chloride, avertin, paraldehyde.
Acute infections of lower respiratory tract	Cyclopropane, ethylene, nitrous oxide, halothane, spinal, nerve block, local.	Ether, vinyl ether, ultra short-barbiturates, chloroform avertin, paraldehyde.
Chronic respiratory tract infections with suppuration or diminished vital capacity	Cyclopropane, ether, ethylene, nitrous oxide, halothane, vinyl ether, spinal, local, muscle relaxants.	Ultra short-acting barbiturates, narcotics, high spinal, chloroform, paraldehyde.
Myocardial disease	Ether, vinyl ether, ethylene, nitrous oxide, pentothal, low spinal, nerve blocks, local, muscle relaxants.	Cyclopropane, chloroform, ethyl chloride, high spinal, pentothal in large amounts, muscle relaxants in large amounts.
Severe valvular disease	Ether, vinyl ether, ethylene, nitrous oxide, pentothal, low spinal, nerve blocks, local, muscle relaxants.	Cyclopropane, chloroform, ethyl chloride, high spinal, pentothal in large amounts, muscle relaxants in large amounts.
Hypotension due to hypovolemia	Cyclopropane, vinyl ether, nitrous oxide, ethylene, local, nerve block.	Ether, pentothal, narcotics, muscle relaxants, chloroform, spinal.
Hypotension (essential)	Ether, cyclopropane, nitrous oxide, ethylene, vinyl ether, local, nerve block.	Spinal, muscle relaxants, nonvolatile basal anesthetics, narcotics.

TABLE III—(*continued*)

Diseases	Permissible Drugs	Drugs to Avoid
Hypertension (essential)	Ether, cyclopropane, nitrous oxide, pentothal, spinal, local, muscle relaxants, halothane.	Vasopressors, high spinal.
Anemia, both primary and secondary and blood dyscrasias causing anemia	Ether, cyclopropane, ethylene, nitrous oxide, halothane, nerve blocks, local, non-volatile agents in small amounts.	Non-volatile drugs in large amounts, spinal, chloroform, muscle relaxants, ethyl chloride.
Acidosis, dehydration	Cyclopropane, vinyl ether, nitrous oxide, halothane, ethylene, spinal, nerve blocks, local.	Ether, chloroform, muscle relaxants, non-volatile drugs, narcotics.
Diabetes, controlled	Cyclopropane, vinethene, ethylene, nitrous oxide, halothane, spinal, local, nerve block, muscle relaxants.	Avertin, pentothal, ether, chloroform, ethyl chloride.
Liver insufficiency, jaundice	Cyclopropane, ethylene, nitrous oxide, halothane, pentothal, spinal, local, nerve block.	Ether, chloroform, ethyl chloride, vinethene, avertin, muscle relaxants.
Renal insufficiency	Cyclopropane, ethylene, nitrous oxide, spinal, local, nerve block.	Ether, vinethene, avertin, chloroform, ethyl chloride, barbiturates, muscle relaxants.
Thyrotoxicosis	Ethylene, nitrous oxide with heavy sedation of avertin, pentothal or morphine, ether.	Cyclopropane, local, nerve block, chloroform, vinethene.
Increased intra-abdominal pressure, due to tumors, acites, distension	Cyclopropane, ether, ethylene, halothane, nerve block, local, muscle relaxants.	Spinal, pentothal, avertin, chloroform, ethyl chloride, vinethene.
Diseases of the heart	Ether, ethylene, nitrous oxide, vinyl ether, non-volatile anesthetics, local, nerve blocks.	Spinal, narcotics.
Increased intra-cranial pressure	Cyclopropane, ether, avertin, pentothal, halothane, local, nerve block, muscle relaxants.	Morphine, nitrous oxide, or ethylene with anoxia.
Mental diseases	Ether, cyclopropane, avertin, ethylene, halothane, pentothal, nitrous oxide, muscle relaxants.	Local, spinal, nerve block.
Alcoholism (acute)	Ether, cyclopropane, ethylene, nitrous oxide, halothane, muscle relaxants.	Spinal, local, nerve block, avertin, pentothal.
Alcoholism (chronic)	Spinal, local, nerve block.	Inhalation, intravenous and rectal anesthesia.

REFERENCES

Adriani, John. The Pharmacologic Basis for the Selection of Anesthesia. New Orleans M. & S. J., 95, 266–273, December, 1942.

Adriani, John. The Pharmacology of Anesthetic Drugs. Charles C Thomas, Springfield, Ill., 4th Ed., 1960.

Adriani, John. Selection of Anesthesia. Charles C Thomas, Springfield, Ill., 1955.

PRELIMINARY EXAMINATION OF THE PATIENT

The patient should be interviewed and his chart examined the day before the operation. The anesthesiologist is not obligated to perform a physical examination if the patient has been studied adequately by an internist. An examination would be desirable for confirmatory purposes.

The following data should be noted on the anesthetic record (see Figs. 1 and 2):

Data	Reasons
1. *Nativity*	Frequently it is an index to emotional status and yields data which influence choice of agent or technique.
2. *Weight of patient*	It may be an index to basal metabolic rate and yield data to be considered in determining type and dose of premedication. Obese patients have poor airway.
3. *History of previous anesthesias. Note* drugs employed, type, duration, complications and operation performed.	Previous difficulties or errors may be avoided.
4. *Risk*, according to classification.	This influences both choice of anesthetic agent and technique of administration.
5. *Body Temperature*	This may be an indication of the metabolic rate and serves as a guide to selection of premedication.
6. *Laboratory Data*	
a. Hemoglobin content hematocrit or erythrocyte count. *Note* anemias.	They are the only reliable indications of the oxygen carrying power of the blood.
b. Leukocyte count and differential.	They indicate presence of infection, sepsis, fever, or toxemia and yield data regarding premedication and choice of agent.
c. Roentgenograms. *Note particularly* views of neck and thorax which show obstruction or distortions of airway.	Advance information regarding abnormalities of airway and other parts of the respiratory tract is desirable.
d. Serological test.	Special precautions to avoid infection may be necessary if patient has syphilis.
e. Urine analysis and renal func-	Abnormal constituents indicate

tion tests.

metabolic disturbances which may be enhanced by anesthesia. Tests reveal renal impairment.

7. Respiratory System

a. Rate, depth, and type of movements. The presence of dyspnoea, hyperpnoea, Cheyne-Stokes respiration, or other abnormalities is significant.

Carbon dioxide excess, anoxia, or respiratory depression should be scrupulously avoided if abnormalities exist.

b. Minute volume exchange. *Note* the extent of any decrease.

If decreased, drugs which cause depression of respiration are contraindicated.

c. Vital capacity. *Note* any decrease.

Anoxemia, carbon dioxide excess, or depression of respiration should be avoided if decreased.

d. Infections of upper or lower respiratory tract (acute or chronic).

Irritating drugs such as ether, chloroform, vinethene, ethyl chloride are not desirable or are contraindicated.

e. Suppurative processes. *Note* history of abscess, bronchiectasis, bronchitis, etc. *Note* character, amount, and frequency of expectorations or the presence of bronchorrhea or purulent material.

Tracheal and bronchial suction or even bronchoscopy may be desirable or necessary before and during and immediately after anesthesia.

f. Airway. *Note* nasopharyngeal abnormalities, bronchial or tracheal obstruction, or the presence of edema or neoplasms anywhere in respiratory tract.

Preparations for intratracheal intubation, tracheotomy, or positive pressure anesthesia and suction (see Part II) may be necessary if abnormalities exist.

8. Circulatory System

a. Myocardial disease. *Note* any change in size of the heart and state of myocardium.

Drugs which increase cardiac irritability (such as chloroform, cyclopropane, and ethyl chloride), or techniques which decrease cardiac output (spinal anesthesia) are contraindicated.

b. Valvular diseases. *Note* type and etiology and state of compensation.

The forementioned objections apply also to valvular disease.

c. Disturbances of rhythm. *Note* type, severity and persistence

Epinephrine, cyclopropane, chloroform and other drugs which in-

of the arrythmia. Record E K G changes.

crease cardiac irritability are objectionable.

d. Disturbances of the vasomotor mechanism. Hypotension or hypertension should be correlated with changes in the heart and kidneys.

Carbon dioxide excess, anoxia, and drugs or procedures which decrease cardiac output (spinal anesthesia, deep anesthesia, avertin, and intravenous barbiturates) may aggravate abnormalities and should therefore be avoided.

e. Peripheral vascular disease and peripheral circulatory failure.

Drugs which cause vasoconstriction, especially in infiltration anesthesia may not be desirable.

f. Abnormalities of cellular elements of blood (dyscrasias) disturbances of clotting mechanism, platelets, etc. Note abnormal pigments. Presence of porphyria.

Special care should be exercised to avoid anoxemia, or carbon dioxide excess. Drugs which cause respiratory depression should be avoided. Bleeding tendencies aggravated by instrumentation.

9. *Metabolism*
   a. Basal metabolic rate.

This may be an index to oxygen requirement and carbon dioxide output during maintenance of anesthesia.

   b. Diabetes, acidosis, or dehydration. *Note* fluid balance.

Drugs which enhance acidosis (such as ether, chloroform, or carbon dioxide excess) are undesirable and should be avoided.

   c. Diseases of the endocrine glands. Correlate with metabolic rate.

They may influence choice of premedication if metabolic rate is altered.

   d. Diseases due to vitamin deficiencies.

They may be accompanied by biochemical disturbances which may influence selection of agent or technique.

10. *Gastro-Intestinal System*
    a. Nausea and emesis. *Note* cause, frequency, and nature of vomitus.

Rapid induction is necessary if present. Precautions to avoid aspiration are to be observed.

    b. Intra-abdominal injuries. *Note* perforation of a hollow viscus, the presence of shock, or abdominal rigidity.

These influence selection of agent. Deep anesthesia may be necessary to overcome abdominal rigidity.

    c. Contour of abdomen. *Note* any distension, gastric dilatation,

Gastric or intestinal decompression and drainage may be neces-

or intestinal obstruction. Investigate fluid balance. Note presence of ascites or large tumor masses.

d. Liver disease or decreased function, jaundice.

Ether, anoxia, chloroform, and certain non-volatile drugs disturb liver function.

e. Colonic inflammations, irritations or neoplasms.

Rectally administered drugs may be undesirable and cause colitis or proctitis. Drug may not be absorbed through diseased mucosa.

f. Time of last meal or fluid.

Postponement of operation if food or fluids were recently ingested is desirable and advisable. Danger of aspiration is great if liquid or solid food is regurgitated.

sary before anesthesia to remove gas and fluid if intestinal obstruction is present.

11. *Genito-urinary System*

a. Renal disease — nephritis, nephrosis, tuberculosis.

Agents such as chloroform, or vinethene should be avoided.

b. Obstruction to urine flow, pyelitis, lithiasis.

Acidosis may be present and be aggravated by certain drugs.

c. N.P.N., blood urea, the presence of anuria, oliguria, or uremia.

Anoxemia, carbon dioxide excess aggravate the acidosis which may be present in renal failure.

12. *Central Nervous System*

a. Intracranial lesions, neoplasms, or cerebral injury. Diseases of the spinal cord. *Note* especially increases in intracranial pressure.

Anoxemia, carbon dioxide excess, and depressant drugs (such as morphine) may cause an increase in intracranial pressure. Depressed respiration or apnoea and circulatory disturbances accompany increased pressure.

b. Infections—syphilis, meningitis, poliomyelitis, myelitis, or encephalitis.

Intrathecal injections of local anesthetic drugs are contraindicated.

c. Mental state. *Note* psychosis, neurosis and whether or not patient is cooperative.

Regional anesthesia may not be advised or large doses of preanesthetic sedation may be required to secure cooperation.

d. Eyes—size, reaction, and abnormalities of pupils.

They are important for future reference in determining depth of narcosis.

e. Convulsions. *Elicit* history and

Anoxia or carbon dioxide excess

note cause and type.

may enhance epilepsy or other cortical irritations.

f. Drug addiction or habituation. *Note* whether due to alcohol or opium alkaloids.

General anesthesia in alcoholic addicts is frequently accompanied by a severe prolonged excitement period. Opiates for "cured" opium addicts are not desirable or large doses may be required for premedication if patient is not "cured."

g. Neuritis, palsies, spasticity of muscles, or other skeletal defects.

Regional anesthesia may be undesirable if pathological changes are present in nerves and muscles.

h. Medication being received.

Drugs may influence choice of anesthesia or decision to operate.

CONTINUANCE AND DISCONTINUANCE OF DRUGS

The procedure should be as follows when drugs in the following categories are being administered preoperatively.

Cortisone and Related Steroids

Continue the administration up to the operative day. On the operative day administer the usual dose intramuscularly if the oral route is not feasible. Resume administration if drug has been discontinued during the 30 days prior to operation. Have parenteral preparation, such as hydrocortisone (100 mgm.) available for intravenous administration during operations.

Reason

Prolonged administration causes hypofunction of the adrenal glands. Adrenal failure may be precipitated by the stress of operation. Characterized by hypotension.

Phenothiazines

Discontinue the day before operation (except promethazine (Phenergan)).

These drugs have an anti-norepinephrine action. Hypotension which does not respond to therapy may develop from stress, blood loss and other factors.

Rauwolfia Alkaloids

Discontinue several weeks prior to operation. Have anticholinergic drug (atropine or hyoscyamine) available to antagonize untoward effects which are characterized largely by varying degrees of hypotension.

These drugs deplete serotonin stores of the body and antagonize the effect of norepinephrine. Not a constant finding. Use norepinephine drug to correct hypotension.

Tranquilizers such as Meprobamate, Hydroxydione (Vistaril), Phenoglycodal (Ultran) and other Non-Phenothiazines

Continue if desired up to time of operation and resume afterward.

These drugs exert no appreciable autonomic effects and may be given without fear of enhancing depressant effects of other drugs to a remarkable extent.

Narcotics and Hypnotics

Use same dose for premedication as patient has been receiving.

Most patients have developed a tolerance if long range use has been practiced and need more than the usual dose.

Antihistaminics

Continue use. Usually cause no adverse effects. Dose of hypnotic and narcotic being used for premedication may have to be reduced.

May cause an additive effect only if they are depressant to the patient; otherwise they cause no effect.

Antibiotics and Sulphonamides

Continue use. If neomycin is used be prepared to combat apnea if used in large doses or if used with ether or muscle relaxants. Kanamycin behaves similarly.

Produces a neuromuscular blockade like curare in large doses when given intravenously or intraperitoneally. Sulphonamides may cause methemoglobinemia which causes cyanosis.

Digitalis and Allied Preparations

Continue administration up to time of operation and resume after operation. Administer intravenously during operation if necessary.

Required in cardiac patients.

Anti-convulsants

Continue administration up to time of operation and resume after operation.

Prevent epileptic attacks preoperatively in patients so predisposed.

Female Sex Hormones

Continue use up to time of operation and afterwards.

These drugs cause no known untoward effects with anesthetics.

Vitamins

Continue administration up to time of operation and resume afterward.

Bear no relationship to anesthesia. Cause no known untoward effects.

Cholinergic Drugs

Discontinue 6 hours prior to operation.

May cause secretion of mucous, bronchospasm, or reflex cardiac effects.

Iodides

Discontinue if possible. If not continue but increase dose of anticholinergic drug used for drying agent.

Usually cause copious secretions of saliva and mucous if infused during operation.

Magnesium Sulphate

Used parenterally for anti-convulsant effects particularly in obstetric cases with toxemia. Proceed with caution using lighter anesthesia.

Magnesium ion has a depressant effect which may act additively with narcotics, hypnotics and anesthetics.

Dextran

Continue but observe patient closely for clotting difficulties or difficulties with typing and matching for transfusions.

Dextran coats platelets and interferes with clotting and testing of blood groups.

Anti-Coagulants

Continue administration if not contraindicated from surgical standpoint.

Hematomas may result from needle punctures or bleeding may commence from trauma by airways, laryngoscopes, etc.

Thiazide Derivatives

Discontinue drugs for four days prior to operation.

Produce hypotensive action. Used as diuretics. Diminish pressor response to epinephrine and cause sodium depletion. May potentiate d tubocurarine.

Guanethedine (Ismelin)

Withdraw drug five days prior to surgery.

Produces hypotensive action by depleting heart of norepinephrine. Used as anti-hypertensive drug.

Bretylium (Darenthin)

Withdraw five days prior to surgery.

Interferes with action of catechol amines at adrenergic nerve endings.

Monamine Oxidase Inhibitors: Ipronazide (Marsalid) Marplan Nardil Monase

Withdraw drug several days prior to surgery.

Depress ganglionic transmission. Produce a hypotensive effect. Potentiate narcotics, hypnotics and anesthetics.

Ilopan, Cozyme: (Alcohol precursor of pantothenic acid, a member of vitamin B complex). For treatment of paralytic ileus.

Withdraw drug for several hours prior to anesthesia. Do not use for 2 hours after anesthesia.

May cause temporary respiratory paralysis with depolarizing drugs.

Polybrene

Used to neutralize heparin effects. Administer slowly during anesthesia.

Produces a hypotensive effect.

PREPARATION OF PATIENT FOR ELECTIVE SURGERY

1. Administer a barbiturate (or opium alkaloid if patient has pain) the evening before to assure a night's rest. Also administer a sedative drug *in the morning* if operation is to be performed late in the forenoon or afternoon.
2. Request enema, and other preparations *the evening prior* to operation for all elective surgery.
3. Omit breakfast and fluids. If operation is to be performed in the afternoon, allow fluids in the morning. Discontinue everything at least four or five hours prior to anesthesia.
4. Order premedication for type of anesthesia selected (see premedication).
5. Examine the patient's chart and be certain all necessary laboratory data such as urine analysis, hematological studies, and examination of heart and lungs, etc., have been performed and are recorded.
6. Examine the patient for recently acquired complications such as "cold," infections, etc., particularly if a time interval has elapsed between previous examinations.

PRE-ANESTHETIC MEDICATION

(A) GENERAL CONSIDERATIONS OF PREMEDICATION

1. *Purpose of Premedication:* There are three chief reasons for administering premedication before anesthesia:
   a. Psychic sedation: This relieves apprehension and to a certain extent decreases length of second stage of inhalation anesthesia.
   b. To secure an additive effect between two depressant drugs of low analgesic or anesthetic potency. Example: Pentothal or morphine combined with nitrous oxide.
   c. Prophylaxis to avoid anticipated undesirable physiological and pharmacological effects produced by certain drugs or procedures:
      (1) Counteracts hypotension in spinal anesthesia (vasopressors).
      (2) Decreases vagal effects accompanying anesthesia with pentothal, cyclopropane, chloroform, and other drugs (atropine).

(3) Minimizes or antagonizes toxic effects of local anesthetic drugs (barbiturates).

(4) Reduces cardiac irritability (procaine amide).

(5) Minimizing or abolishing secretion of saliva and mucous: This prevents respiratory obstruction during anesthesia and respiratory complications after operation.

2. *Drugs Commonly Employed for Premedication:*
   a. For psychic sedation and additive effects.
      a. Alkaloids derived from opium and synthetic narcotics.
      b. Barbiturates and pharmacologically allied hypnotics.
      c. Aliphatic hypnotics and basal narcotics—avertin, trichlorethanol, paraldehyde, etc.
      d. Tranquilizers.
   d. For prophylaxis:
      a. For anticipated hypotension vasopressor drugs such as ephedrine, methoxamine (Vasoxyl) or phenylephrine (Neosynephrine).
      b. For minimizing secretions and vagal effects. Parasympathetic depressants. Notably atropine, levohyoscyamine (Bellafoline) and scopolamine.
      c. For antagonizing local anesthetics. Barbiturates.
      d. Drugs used to decrease cardiac irritability.

3. *Evaluation of Individual Drugs:*
   a. Morphine: Most widely employed because it most satisfactorily performs two of the above functions. Morphine reduces metabolic rate and produces psychic sedation and additive effects.
   b. Dilaudid (Dihydromorphinone): A synthetic drug derived from morphine possessing 8 to 10 times the potency of morphine. Administer 1/8 to 1/10 of a comparable amount of morphine.
   c. Codeine: Infrequently employed for premedication except as a substitute for morphine for children. Possesses approximately 1/4 the potency of morphine.
   d. Pantopon: Aqueous solution of the hydrochlorides of purified opium (10% solution). Contains morphine. Possesses the same action as morphine. 1/3 grain is the equivalent of 1/4 grain of morphine.
   e. Meperidine (Demerol): Synthetic substance derived from pyridine possessing a mild sedative action and analgesic action greater than codeine but less than that of morphine. In addition it possesses an atropine-like action. Employed as a substitute for morphine and related compounds when these are not tolerated or are contraindicated. Average dose gr. $1\frac{1}{2}$ administered simultaneously with atropine or scopolamine in place of morphine in techniques described below.

f. Methadon: Synthetic narcotic possessing same analgesic effects as morphine but less hypnotic and tranquilizing effect. Used when morphine cannot be used. Less effective than morphine.

g. Dromoran: Synthetic narcotic chemically related to morphine, but with a less tranquilizing and hypnotic effect.

h. Barbiturates: Useful for psychic sedation. Depress the cortex and lower centers but have little effect on the metabolic rate. Not satisfactory as substitute for opium derivatives but may be used in conjunction with them. *Barbiturates produce amnesia, but no analgesia.*

i. Paraldehyde: Usually employed as a sedative for chronic alcoholic addicts (see rectal anesthesia).

j. Atropine: Diminishes secretions by paralyzing parasympathetic nerve endings. Stimulates cortex and medullary centers, thereby antagonizing narcotics. Paralyzes vagal nerve endings.

k. Scopolamine (hyoscine): Diminishes secretions by paralyzing parasympathetic nerve endings. Depresses cortex and produces amnesia. Enhances cortical depression of morphine when used with morphine. Possesses a more pronounced effect on secretions than atropine. Does not depress respiration. *Is not an analgesic* and does not accelerate the pulse.

l. l-hyoscyamine (Bellafolline): Diminishes secretions by paralyzing parasympathetic nerve endings. More potent and effective than atropine. Causes less side actions. Accelerates the pulse.

m. Vasopressor drugs: Employed to elevate blood pressure for anticipated "primary shock." Epinephrine, ephedrine, neosynephrine are the most prominent (see spinal anesthesia).

n. Cardiac depressants: Drugs which decrease cordiac irritability such as quinidine, procaine amide and procaine are administered prophylactically to decrease arrhythmias.

(B) Technique of Premedication for Various Types of Anesthesia

1. *Inhalation Anesthesia:* Adults considered to be *average cases:*

a. Administer a therapeutic dose of a barbiturate (secobarbital (Seconal) or pentobarbital or other sedative drug the evening previous to operation.

b. Administer (1) morphine sulphate gr. 1/4, or other narcotic (see Table IV) scopolamine hydrobromide gr. 1/100 (ratio of 25:1) subcutaneously, 1 to 1½ hours prior to induction of anesthesia, or (2) morphine sulphate gr. 1/4, subcutaneously atropine sulphate gr. 1/100 (in a ratio of 25:1) 1 to 1½ hours before induction of anesthesia.

TABLE IV

EQUIVALENT DOSES OF OTHER DERIVATIVES OF OPIUM AND SYNTHETIC
NARCOTICS COMPARED TO DOSE OF MORPHINE

	Grains	Milligrams
Morphine	1/4	15
Codeine	1	60
Dilaudid (Dihydromorphinone)	1/32	2
Demerol (Meperidine)	1 1/2	100
Methadon	1/4	15
Dromoran (Methyl Morphinan)	1/12	5
Nisentil (Alphaprodine)	2/3	40
Oxymorphone (Numorphan)	1/60	1.0
Anileridene (Leritene)	2/3	40
Phenazocine	1/60	1.0
Pimpinadone (Alvodine)	1/60	1.0
Pantopon	1/3	18

2. *Inhalation Anesthesia: Variations from the average:*

   a. Aged subjects: Administer morphine gr. 1/6–1/8 and scopolamine or atropine gr. 1/150–1/200. Metabolic rate decreases with age and less morphine is required (ratio 25:1). Scale dose with age.

   b. Young adults: Administer morphine gr. 1/4 and scopolamine gr. 1/100 if metabolic rate is normal.

   c. Patients in pain: Administer full doses of morphine—gr. 1/4–1/2 and scopolamine gr. 1/100.

   d. Cyclopropane anesthesia: Decrease dose of narcotic.

   e. Fever: Administer full therapeutic dose of morphine and scopolamine. Metabolic rate is increased 7% for each degree (F) of fever.

   f. Diabetes, acidosis, toxemias, etc.: Reduce morphine because it enhances acidosis. Use 2/3 to 1/2 of the usual dose of morphine balanced with scopolamine in proportion of 25 to 1.

   g. Intracranial diseases accompanied by increased intracranial pressure: Omit narcotics because they elevate intracranial pressure. Administer atropine to minimize secretions if inhalation anesthesia is to be employed.

   h. Hyperthyroidism or other conditions accompanied by elevated metabolic rate: Administer morphine gr. 1/4 or other narcotic and scopolamine gr. 1/100 two hours prior to anesthesia. Repeat using half to full dose one hour before anesthesia depending upon the effect first dose has produced.

   i. Hypothyroidism or other conditions characterized by a reduced metabolic rate: Decrease morphine or other narcotic 1/3 to 1/2 the usual adult dose and scopolamine in proportion of 25 to 1.

   j. Emergency surgery: Administer 2/3 to the full dose of morphine with scopolamine in proportion of 25 to 1 intravenously ten minutes prior to anesthesia. Dilute drug well in saline and inject slowly (see intravenous anesthesia page 257).

k. Obstetrics: Administer atropine or scopolamine gr. 1/100–1/150 but omit morphine, other alkaloids of opium or synthetic narcotics.

l. Infants and children: See section on pediatric anesthesia.

m. Highly apprehensive or mentally disturbed patients. Use basal narcosis with an ultra short-acting barbiturate such as pentothal or short-acting barbiturate (seconal or nembutal) intravenously. Avertin may be used rectally. For infants pentothal rectally.

3. *Regional Anesthesia:*

a. Spinal anesthesia

(1) Administer a mixture of morphine and scopolamine in 2/3 quantities and proportion as for inhalation anesthesia. Required for psychic sedation to insure a cooperative patient. Also necessary if anesthesia is unsatisfactory and must be supplemented by general anesthesia. Oversedation results in lack of cooperation in performing the block.

(2) Administer a barbiturate, preferably of short acting type, such as amobarbital, nembutal, secobarbital, or similar drug, in therapeutic doses orally 1 to $1\frac{1}{2}$ hours prior to operation. Barbiturates antagonize toxic effect of local anesthetic drugs. They also act additively in conjunction with morphine as psychic sedatives.

(3) Administer a vasopressor drug (ephedrine gr. 3/4 intramuscularly). Counteracts or prevents the hypotension which accompanies spinal anesthesia. Administer routinely to subjects in whom hypotension is anticipated. In uncomplicated cases, administer I.V. only when indicated after anesthesia has been induced (see spinal anesthesia).

b. Nerve block, infiltration, and topical anesthesia.
   Employ same drugs and technique described for spinal anesthesia but omit ephedrine. Same reasons as for spinal anesthesia.

4. *Intravenous Anesthesia Using thiopental (Pentothal or other short acting barbiturates) with nitrus oxide:*

a. Administer atropine or scopolamine gr. 1/100 1 to $1\frac{1}{2}$ hours prior to anesthesia. Morphine sulfate 1/6 to 1/8 gr. or other narcotic subcutaneously 1 to $1\frac{1}{2}$ hours prior to anesthesia. Belladonna alkaloids diminish vagal effects (laryngeal and bronchial spasm). Narcotics used omitted by many anesthetists because it may enhance the respiratory depression produced by the barbiturate.

5. *Rectal (Avertin):*

    a. Administer atropine or scopolamine gr. 1/100 to 1/150 subcutaneously. Morphine as recommended for inhalation anesthesia may be administered if desired, but is usually omitted. Belladonna alkaloids minimize secretions produced by supplementary inhalation anesthesia necessary to complement narcosis. Morphine enhances respiratory depression produced by Avertin.

6. *Common Errors in Premedication:*

    a. *Premedication administered too soon:* Excess secretions and excitement follow. Both result in a prolongde and difficult induction. Supplement with 1/3 to 1/2 the dose intravenously.

    b. *Insufficient premedication:* Same effects and results as too early administration. Supplement dose intravenously.

    c. *Premedication administered too late:* Drugs do not have time to act. Excess mucus and prolonged excitement follow. Depression of respiration may often occur after anesthesia is established and confuse the anesthetist.

    d. *Over premedication:* Depression of respiration and circulation may occur. Bradycardia, hypotension, and decreased amplitude and rate of respiration are commonly observed. Relaxation is difficult to secure. Antagonize with antinarcotics (nalorphine or levallorphan).

    e. *Premedication omitted:* Induction period prolonged, marked excitement, copious flow of mucus, laryngeal spasm, and poor relaxation may result. Patient may be uncooperative if regional anesthesia is employed.

Comment	*Reason*
1. Do not omit premedication. Administer it intravenously if patient has not had it.	Induction and maintenance of anesthesia become difficult. The patient suffers, the anesthetist is handicapped, and the operation is delayed. Psychic sedation inadequate.
2. Do not order the drug to be administered "on call" or "on the stretcher."	Sufficient time must be allowed for drugs to exert their maximum effects.
3. Do not administer premedication after anesthesia has been started with the exception of anticholinergic to "dry" up secretions.	Its effect is required to facilitate induction of anesthesia. The effects of morphine upon respiration may appear during the course of anesthesia and confuse the anesthetist.
4. When morphine is administered for psychic sedation, scopolamine	Scopolamine augments cortical effects of morphine and antogonizes

is preferred to atropine to minimize secretion of mucus.

5. Administer belladonna alkaloids simultaneously with morphine in a ratio of one part to twenty-five of morphine.

6. Consider body weight as well as age in judging dosage for infants and children.

medullary respiratory depression. Does not elevate pulse.

Clinical experience has demonstrated this to be the optimal ratio for man for surgical anesthesia.

Disproportion between age and body weight is frequently observed in children.

REFERENCES

Adriani, John. Premedication an old idea. New drugs. J.A.M.A, 171, 108–112, 1959.

Cullen, S. C., and Alexander, F. A. D. Preanesthetic Medication, Am. J. Surg., 24, 428–434, 1936.

Guedel, A. E. Inhalation Anesthesia. The Macmillan Company, New York, 1937.

Waters, R. M. A Study of Morphine, Scopolamine, and Atropine And Their Relation To Preoperative Medication And Pain Relief, Texas State J. Med., 34, 294–304, August, 1938.

ANESTHESIA RECORDS

A record should be maintained from time patient arrives in operating room throughout every operation until return to recovery regardless of the type of anesthesia administered. Printed standard anesthesia records (Figs. 1 and 2) are desirable. Regardless of the type of chart employed, a good anesthesia record includes:

1. Significant findings of preoperative examination.
2. Details of conduct of anesthesia drugs used, quantity, mode of administration and a record of unusual events.
3. Post-operative course for a minimum of ten days in major surgery cases. (The anesthetist may use his discretion in the length of the follow-up period in cases of minor surgery.)

Record this data during course of anesthesia:

1. *Preliminary medication:* Time, route of administration, dose and its effect.
2. *Date:* Month, day, and year.
3. *Pulse:* Rate and character. Comment on abnormalities in space for remarks (Fig. 1). Note arrythmias.
4. *Blood pressure:* A record of the blood pressure should be maintained during every operative procedure.
5. *Time:* Induction and start and completion of the operation. Termination of anesthesia. Indicate whether the time is AM or PM.
6. *Anesthetic agents and technique:* Type, time administered, strength, etc. Reason for selection of agent and technique. Supplementary agents or techniques employed in the event that the primary agent is changed and reasons for the change.
7. *Depth:* Depth of inhalation anesthesia in planes of stage III. Extent and

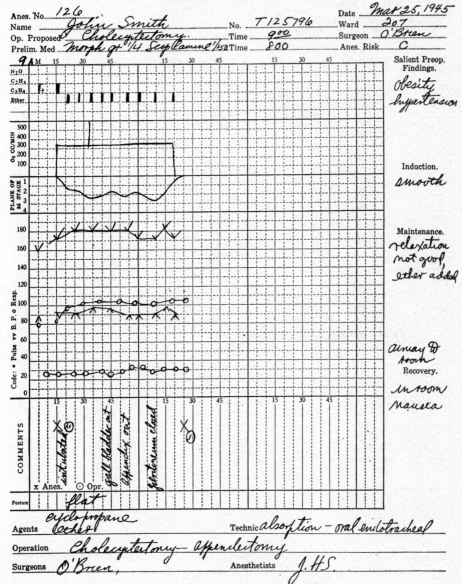

FIG. 1. A suitable chart for anesthesia records.

duration of regional blocks. Level of spinal anesthesia. Mention drug dose, volume, diluent and site of injection.

8. *Oxygen:* Metabolic requirement and any additional amount.

9. *Operation:* Preoperative diagnosis, the proposed operation, the operation performed, and the post-operative diagnosis.

10. *Members of the surgical team:* Surgeon, assistants, anesthetists, and nurses.

Name _John Smith_   (M) F—   Age _47_ Wt. _200_ Nativity _U S_

Address _202 Spring Street_

T.P.R. _98,80_ Hb. _85%_ R.B.C. _5.5_ W.B.C. _10,000_ B.M.R. _+10_ B.P. _160/90_ Special Lab.

Urinalysis _negative_

PREOPERATIVE				POSTOPERATIVE

RESPIRATORY

Tb _____ (None) None _____ Cough

Cough _____ Asthma _____ Emphysema _____ Bronchitis, etc.

Airway _____ Oral sepsis _____ Collapse

Misc. _____ Pneumonia (L B H)

Misc.

CIRCULATORY

C.V. dis. _____ None _____ None _____ Hemorrhage

Tachy _____ Brady _____ Vm. instab. _____ Tachycard _____ Bradycard

(Hypertem) _____ Hypoten. _____ F.C.I.-IIa-IIb-III _____ Circ. Depression _____ Shock

Misc. _____ Misc.

GENITO URINARY

Uremia _____ Incontin. _____ Retent. _____ None _____ None _____ Cystitis

Imp. func. _____ Cyst. _____ Catheterized _3_ days

Misc.

GASTRO INTESTINAL

Obstruct. _____ Distention _____ None _____ None _____ Ileus _____ Peritonitis _____ Dist.

Nau.-Em. Opr. Day _____ Recent _____ Nau.-Em. _1st and 2nd day_

(Began)   Duration   Severity)

Misc. _upper right quadrant pain_ Misc.

CENTRAL NERVOUS SYSTEM

Lues _____ Irrat. _____ Lesion _____ (None) _____ None _____ Emot. Dist.

Headache _____ Headache _____ Paralysis

Misc. _____ Misc.

MISCELLANEOUS

Acidos. _____ Alkal. _____ Diabetic _____ Consciousness returned _in room 1 hr post_

Leuk. _____ Epilep. _____ Anem-s-p. _anes._

Drug addict

Hypomet. _____ Spec. tox.

Malig. _____ Obese _____ Senil.

Other _____ Special medication _non_

Final Comments:

(signed) _J. H. S_

Anesthetist

FORPGGER CO. N.Y.

FIG. 2. The reverse side of the form shown in Fig. 1. Preoperative and postoperative findings are essential for complete records. Data from this record may be transferred to punch cards for statistical studies.

11. *Complications:*

a. *During induction of anesthesia:* Note and record the occurrence, duration, and intensity of any excitement period, spasm, nausea, emesis, cyanosis, anoxia, etc.

b. *During maintenance of anesthesia:* Note and record changes in quality of pulse, degree of muscular relaxation, the occurrence of respira-

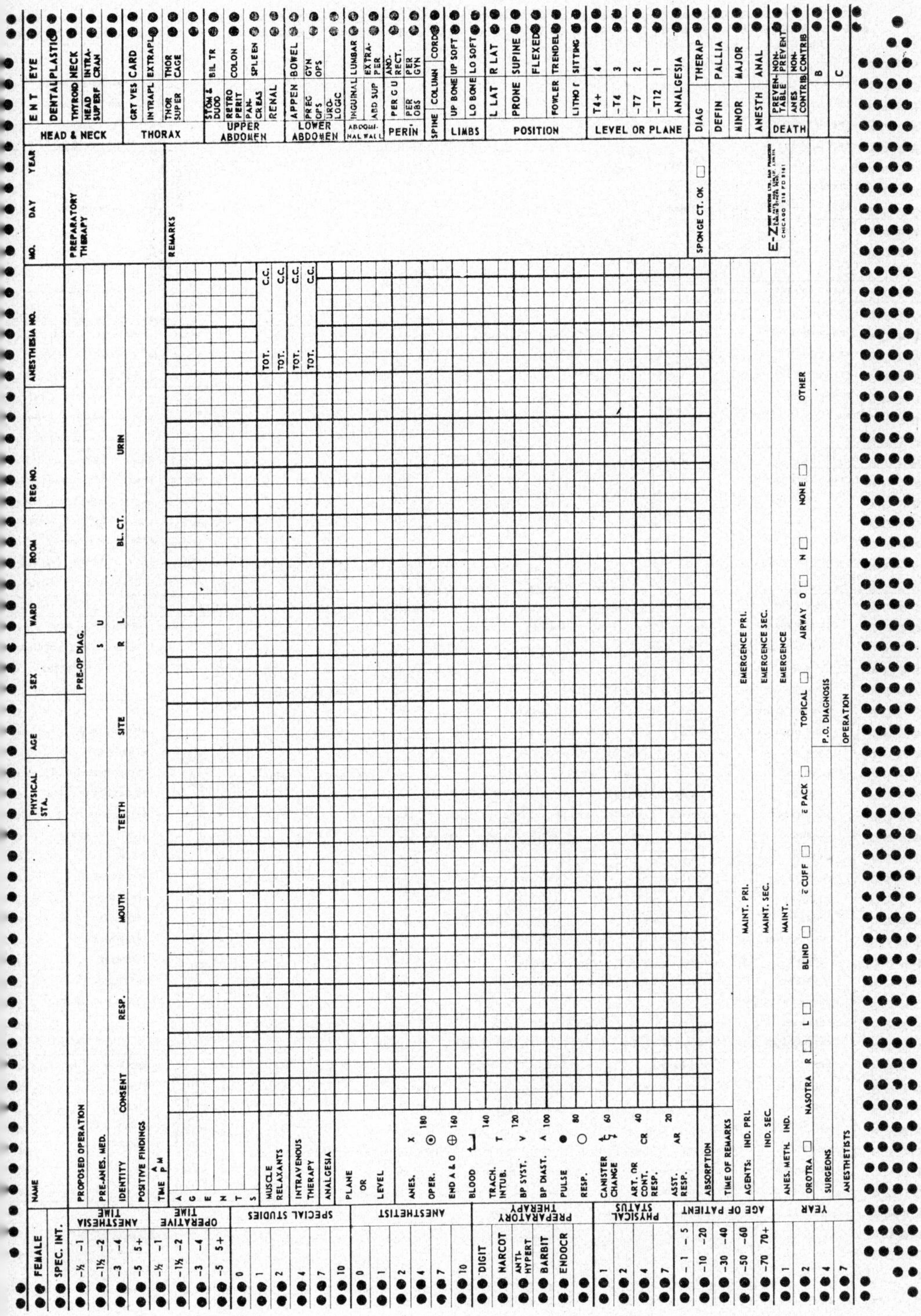

Fig. 2A. Anesthetic record embodying the punch card system using direct coding (Illinois E-Z sort).

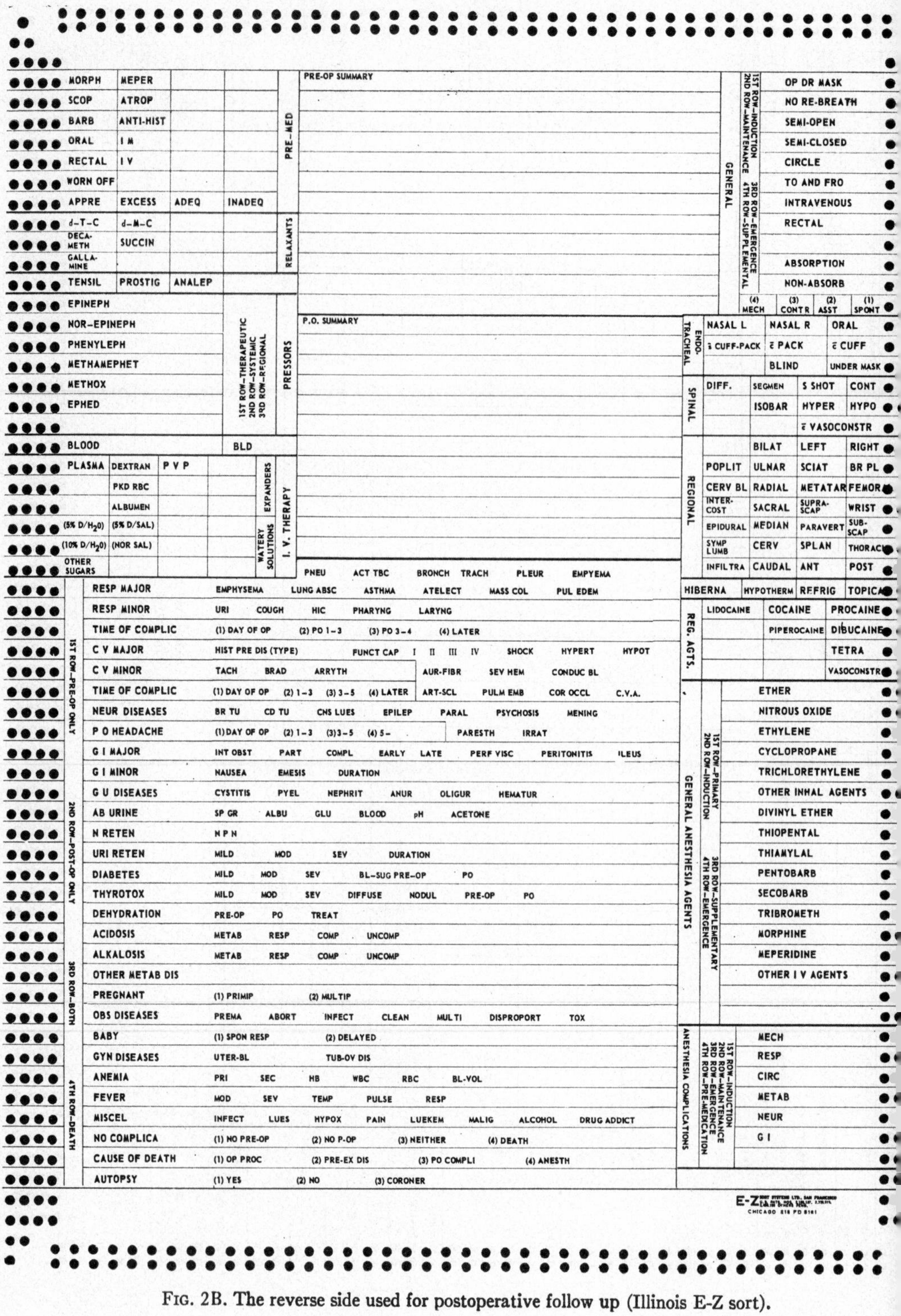

MORPH | MEPER | PRE-MED | PRE-OP SUMMARY
SCOP | ATROP
BARB | ANTI-HIST
ORAL | I M
RECTAL | I V
WORN OFF
APPRE | EXCESS | ADEQ | INADEQ
d-T-C | d-M-C | RELAXANTS
DECA-METH | SUCCIN
GALLA-MINE
TENSIL | PROSTIG | ANALEP
EPINEPH | PRESSORS | 1ST ROW—THERAPEUTIC 2ND ROW—SYSTEMIC 3RD ROW—REGIONAL
NOR-EPINEPH
PHENYLEPH
METHAMEPHET
METHOX
EPHED
BLOOD | BLD
PLASMA | DEXTRAN | P V P | EXPANDERS | I. V. THERAPY
PKD RBC
ALBUMEN
(5% D/H₂0) | (5% D/SAL) | WATERY SOLUTIONS
(10% D/H₂0) | (NOR SAL)
OTHER SUGARS

P.O. SUMMARY

GENERAL — 1ST ROW—INDUCTION 2ND ROW—MAINTENANCE 3RD ROW—EMERGENCE 4TH ROW—SUPPLEMENTAL
OP DR MASK
NO RE-BREATH
SEMI-OPEN
SEMI-CLOSED
CIRCLE
TO AND FRO
INTRAVENOUS
RECTAL
ABSORPTION
NON-ABSORB
(4) MECH | (3) CONTR | (2) ASST | (1) SPONT

ENDO-TRACHEAL: NASAL L | NASAL R | ORAL
c̄ CUFF-PACK | c̄ PACK | c̄ CUFF
BLIND | UNDER MASK
SPINAL: DIFF. | SEGMEN | S SHOT | CONT
ISOBAR | HYPER | HYPO
c̄ VASOCONSTR
REGIONAL: BILAT | LEFT | RIGHT
POPLIT | ULNAR | SCIAT | BR PL
CERV BL | RADIAL | METATAR | FEMOR
INTER-COST | SACRAL | SUPRA-SCAP | WRIST
EPIDURAL | MEDIAN | PARAVERT | SUB-SCAP
SYMP LUMB | CERV | SPLAN | THORAC
INFILTRA | CAUDAL | ANT | POST
HIBERNA | HYPOTHERM | REFRIG | TOPICA
REG. AGTS.: LIDOCAINE | COCAINE | PROCAINE
PIPEROCAINE | DIBUCAINE
TETRA
VASOCONSTR

1ST ROW—PRE-OP ONLY / 2ND ROW—POST-OP ONLY / 3RD ROW—BOTH / 4TH ROW—DEATH
PNEU | ACT TBC | BRONCH | TRACH | PLEUR | EMPYEMA
RESP MAJOR | EMPHYSEMA | LUNG ABSC | ASTHMA | ATELECT | MASS COL | PUL EDEM
RESP MINOR | URI | COUGH | HIC | PHARYNG | LARYNG
TIME OF COMPLIC | (1) DAY OF OP | (2) PO 1–3 | (3) PO 3–4 | (4) LATER
C V MAJOR | HIST PRE DIS (TYPE) | FUNCT CAP I II III IV | SHOCK | HYPERT | HYPOT
C V MINOR | TACH | BRAD | ARRYTH | AUR-FIBR | SEV HEM | CONDUC BL
TIME OF COMPLIC | (1) DAY OF OP | (2) 1–3 | (3) 3–5 | (4) LATER | ART-SCL | PULM EMB | COR OCCL | C.V.A.
NEUR DISEASES | BR TU | CD TU | CNS LUES | EPILEP | PARAL | PSYCHOSIS | MENING
P O HEADACHE | (1) DAY OF OP | (2) 1–3 | (3) 3–5 | (4) 5– | PARESTH | IRRAT
G I MAJOR | INT OBST | PART | COMPL | EARLY | LATE | PERF VISC | PERITONITIS | ILEUS
G I MINOR | NAUSEA | EMESIS | DURATION
G U DISEASES | CYSTITIS | PYEL | NEPHRIT | ANUR | OLIGUR | HEMATUR
AB URINE | SP GR | ALBU | GLU | BLOOD | pH | ACETONE
N RETEN | N P N
URI RETEN | MILD | MOD | SEV | DURATION
DIABETES | MILD | MOD | SEV | BL-SUG PRE-OP | PO
THYROTOX | MILD | MOD | SEV | DIFFUSE | NODUL | PRE-OP | PO
DEHYDRATION | PRE-OP | PO | TREAT
ACIDOSIS | METAB | RESP | COMP | UNCOMP
ALKALOSIS | METAB | RESP | COMP | UNCOMP
OTHER METAB DIS
PREGNANT | (1) PRIMIP | (2) MULTIP
OBS DISEASES | PREMA | ABORT | INFECT | CLEAN | MULTI | DISPROPORT | TOX
BABY | (1) SPON RESP | (2) DELAYED
GYN DISEASES | UTER-BL | TUB-OV DIS
ANEMIA | PRI | SEC | HB | WBC | RBC | BL-VOL
FEVER | MOD | SEV | TEMP | PULSE | RESP
MISCEL | INFECT | LUES | HYPOX | PAIN | LUEKEM | MALIG | ALCOHOL | DRUG ADDICT
NO COMPLICA | (1) NO PRE-OP | (2) NO P-OP | (3) NEITHER | (4) DEATH
CAUSE OF DEATH | (1) OP PROC | (2) PRE-EX DIS | (3) PO COMPLI | (4) ANESTH
AUTOPSY | (1) YES | (2) NO | (3) CORONER

GENERAL ANESTHESIA AGENTS — 1ST ROW—PRIMARY 2ND ROW—INDUCTION 3RD ROW—SUPPLEMENTARY 4TH ROW—EMERGENCE
ETHER
NITROUS OXIDE
ETHYLENE
CYCLOPROPANE
TRICHLORETHYLENE
OTHER INHAL AGENTS
DIVINYL ETHER
THIOPENTAL
THIAMYLAL
PENTOBARB
SECOBARB
TRIBROMETH
MORPHINE
MEPERIDINE
OTHER I V AGENTS

ANESTHESIA COMPLICATIONS — 1ST ROW—INDUCTION 2ND ROW—MAINTENANCE 3RD ROW—EMERGENCE 4TH ROW—PRE-MEDICATION
MECH
RESP
CIRC
METAB
NEUR
G I

E-Z SORT SYSTEMS LTD. SAN FRANCISCO CHICAGO 818 PD 8161

FIG. 2B. The reverse side used for postoperative follow up (Illinois E-Z sort).

tory obstruction, laryngeal spasm, or cyanosis. Record significant manipulations or points of interest in progress of operation.

c. *During immediate recovery period:* Note the occurrence of retching, vomiting, respiratory depression, spasm, excitement, delirium, circulatory collapse, etc.

12. *Medication:* Fluids and other treatment administered during operation: Note time of administration, route, quantity, and therapeutic effect (if any).

13. *Position of patient:* Indicate the time and nature of changes in posture, i.e., prone, supine, lateral, Trendelenburg, lithotomy, sitting, etc. (Table V, p. 108).

CLASSIFYING THE PATIENT AS AN OPERATIVE RISK

Risks are classified as A, B, C, or D, or as 1, 2, 3, or 4 according to the following criteria. Note the class on the anesthesia record:

1 or A Risk: A patient having no systemic defects who is undergoing a "minor" or "major" surgical procedure. *Example:* Young healthy adult undergoing hemorrhoidectomy or appendectomy.

2 or B Risk: A patient having a minor or not significant systemic defect who is undergoing a "major" surgical procedure. *Example:* An adult undergoing appendectomy who has uncomplicated essential hypertension.

3 or C Risk: A patient who is undergoing a "major" surgical procedure but who has in addition to the surgical condition another disease which would not in itself prove immediately fatal. *Example:* Appendectomy in a subject who has a hypertension with moderate cardiac hypertrophy.

4 or D Risk: A patient who is undergoing a "major" surgical procedure but who has in addition to his surgical condition a disease which itself might be immediately fatal. *Example:* Cardiac decompensation in a patient undergoing cholecystectomy for acute cholecystitis.

Comment: The demarcation between "minor" and "major" surgical procedures is difficult to define. Therefore the distinction is purely arbitrary. The classification of risk is a matter of opinion and can only be an approximation of an arbitrary nature.

The American Society of Anesthesiologists in 1962 adopted the following classification:

1. A patient having no systemic disease who is undergoing a surgical procedure. Example: A young, healthy adult undergoing hemorrhoidectomy or appendectomy.

2. A patient having a minor and not significant systemic defect who is undergoing a surgical procedure. Example: An adult undergoing appendectomy who has uncomplicated essential hypertension.

3. A patient undergoing a surgical procedure who has in addition to the surgical condition a systemic disease which is serious but is not one which might be immediately fatal. Appendectomy in a subject who

has hypertension and coronary sclerosis with definite evidence to myocardial disease.

4. A patient who is undergoing a major surgical procedure who has in
   addition to his surgical disease, a disease which in itself might be immediately fatal. Example: Cardiac decompensation in the patient
   undergoing cholecystectomy for acute cholecystitis.
5. A patient who is moribund who needs urgent surgery.

In the event of an emergency the number is preceded by an "E."

CODING (PUNCH CARD) SYSTEMS

1. *Manual Classifying and Sorting* (Keysort Punch Card—McBee Company)

Features: The anesthetic record is printed on a card bearing a double line of
holes on its borders. A hand punch is used to extend the hole corresponding to the factor which is to be recorded to the edge to form a V shaped
slot. Each hole corresponds to an agent technique or complication. Data
is recorded directly or indirectly.

(a) Direct recording—The various factors and details of anesthesia are
    assigned a particular hole on the perimeter. When a factor is present
    the hole is punched out into a V shaped slot. The cards are sorted by
    placing a spindle through the hole corresponding to the factor being
    studied. The positive cards drop out of the stack since the hole has
    been punched out and are thereby separated from those in which the
    factor is negative.
(b) Indirect recording—Numbers are assigned to various factors and to
    the holes in the card. This system permits the recording of many
    more factors than the direct coding method. The cards are punched
    and sorted in the same manner as in direct coding.

2. *Mechanical Punching and Sorting* (Hollerith)

The various factors to be recorded are assigned a number in a code
book (prepared by the American Society of Anesthesiologists). Data are
transferred from the anesthetic record in code to a card $3\frac{1}{4} \times 7\frac{3}{8}$ and holes
punched by a machine corresponding to the numbers written on the
card. This system permits mechanical sorting and recording of many
more factors than the manual system. The anesthetic record is separate
from the statistical record.

3. Illinois E-Z-sort devised by Max Sadove (pages 51 and 52).

Uses: To record data for statistical analysis.

Comment: The data is as reliable as the least conscientious member of the
staff and is as correct as the opinion of the least experienced member of
the staff.

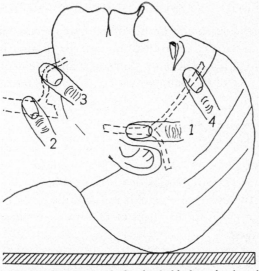

Fig. 3. Sites about the head suitable for palpation of
the pulse listed in the order of their importance:
(1) External temporal artery.
(2) Carotid artery.
(3) External maxillary artery.
(4) Frontal branch of external temporal artery.

PULSE RATE

The quality of the pulse when correlated with blood pressure offers the
best index of the status of the circulation during surgery. Sites for palpation
of the pulse during anesthesia are as follows (Fig. 3):

1. External temporal artery anterior to meatus of the ear (most accessible,
   desirable, and commonly employed site).
2. Carotid artery at level of thyroid cartilage. Palpation not always satisfactory in anesthetized subjects.
3. External maxillary artery as it crosses mandible. Simultaneous palpation of pulse and traction on jaw may be achieved while holding
   mask, if this vessel is prominent.
4. Frontal branch of external temporal artery.
5. Radial artery if either arm is accessible (on an arm board).

Comment:

1. Always use a watch to count the pulse rate.
2. Palpate pulse frequently and if necessary continuously (especially
   when administering cyclopropane, chloroform, ethyl chloride, or during
   shock, or other circulatory disturbances).
3. Record pulse rate on graph every five minutes in uncomplicated anesthesia. *Note* quality and volume of the pulse as well as the rate and
   rhythm.
4. Pulse rate unless correlated with blood pressure is not always a satisfactory guide to state of circulatory system.

BLOOD PRESSURE DURING ANESTHESIA

The arterial tension should be determined at regular intervals on all patients undergoing surgery regardless of the type of anesthesia employed or nature of the operation performed. Repeated measurements correlated with the rate and quality of the pulse are *the best criteria of the status of the circulatory system.*

Reasons for determining blood pressure:

1. Forewarns of circulatory failure—shock, hemorrhage, deep anesthesia, vasomotor instability, or reflex circulatory changes.
2. Warns of excess carbon dioxide in the inhaler.
3. Indicates the presence of anoxia or asphyxia.
4. Serves as a guide to the effect of therapy or medication administered during surgery.

Materials required for determining blood pressure:

1. Mercury or aneroid sphygmomanometer. These are mounted on a stand with a broad base or fastened directly to the anesthesia machine.
2. Stethoscope of diaphragm type provided with a long extension tube.
3. Towel and safety pin (for obese subjects).
4. Arm board (for obese subjects).

Procedure	*Reasons*
1. Abduct and extend the patient's right arm so that the palm rests in either of the anesthetist's axillae (Fig. 4).	The anesthetist may thus hold the patient's arm to his side. Both his hands remain free for application of cuff and stethoscope.
2. Palpate brachial artery in the cubital fossa with forefinger.	The artery is on side closest to body (medial).
3. Arrange the bell of the stethoscope over the artery so that the tube leads towards the head of patient. Secure tightly with the tape provided for the purpose.	Sounds are often indistinct if bell is not placed and securely fastened *directly over the artery.*
4. Wind cuff securely about the arm above the cubital fossa. Arrange tubings so that they point towards the head of the table.	Tubing becomes kinked if it is not properly arranged.
5. Test apparatus once or twice before anesthesia is started to ascertain if it is applied correctly and functioning properly.	Readjustment is simpler before patient is draped and surgery started.

Frequency of Readings:

1. A pre-anesthetic reading should be recorded and compared with the blood pressure recorded during the physical examination.

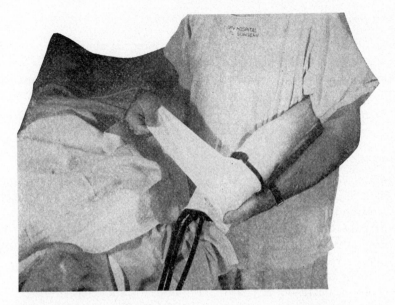

FIG. 4a. Applying cuff of sphygmomanometer. The patient's palm is held in the anesthetist's axilla to allow use of both hands for winding the cuff.

2. A reading should be recorded as soon as the patient passes into third stage. (*Do not inflate cuff during second stage. Stimulation may cause excitement.*)

3. A reading should be recorded at 3 or 4 minute intervals if all is well; and more frequently if all is not well.

4. A reading should be noted at 1 or 2 minute intervals or oftener if there has been any notable fall or pronounced elevation of blood pressure or if pre-operative blood pressure was not with normal limits.

5. A reading should be noted at two or three minute intervals during the first fifteen minutes of spinal anesthesia.

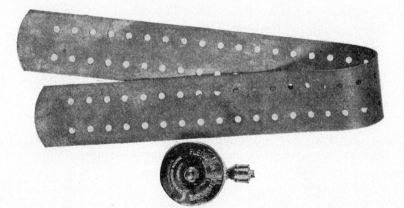

FIG. 4b. Stethoscope bell with nipple on back and perforated rubber strap for securing to the arm.

Care of Apparatus:

1. Fold stethoscope neatly and place in cabinet of anesthesia machine or other designated place.
2. Fold rubber tubing neatly and wrap cuff and arm band around it to form a neat compact bundle.
3. Remove covering from the cuff and sterilize by boiling if soiled by secretions or blood.

Comment	*Reasons*
1. Apply cuff to left arm before patient is turned when the prone position is contemplated.	The attachments to the manometer will lead to the right side of the table during the operation.
2. Arrange cuff on uppermost arm when the patient is to lie on his side.	Compression of artery of undermost arm frequently occurs. Sounds are inaudible or indistinct.
3. Extend and abduct the arm of obese subjects on a board and fasten loosely.	Auscultation is more satisfactory if arm is abducted.
4. Deflate the cuff completely between readings.	*Ischemia of the extremity may be disastrous.*
5. Do not apply the cuff to the arm being used for intravenous therapy.	Stasis, even though intermittent, causes a clot to form which results in plugging of the needle.
6. When a pulse of good volume is palpated but sounds are inaudible, check apparatus before notifying the surgeon that a hypotension exists.	The bell of the stethoscope may have shifted so that it is no longer over the artery.
7. *Do not hang stethoscope about the neck between readings.* Tuck it beneath the pad of the operating table when not in use.	The instrument usually becomes tangled at the most inopportune moments and restricts the anesthetist's movements.
8. Place manometers mounted on stands well behind the head of the table.	The stand interferes with the movements of surgical team when placed along side the table
9. Do not allow the bulb which inflates the cuff to fall to the floor.	The valve and air release screw are sensitive structures and easily damaged.
10. For pediatric patients less than one year old use 1″ arm band.	The larger cuff is ineffective.
11. For pediatric cases and in adults with upper extremities missing the bell of stethoscope may be placed in popliteal space and cuff above knee.	The tibial arterial is larger and sounds are louder.

CARDIAC AND PULMONARY AUSCULTATION

Principle

Auscultation of cardiac and respiratory sounds during anesthesia by means of a stethoscope. The device ordinarily used consists of a monaural earpiece, a receiver of the diaphragm type applied to the precordium (Fig. 4c) or to an oesophageal stethoscope (Fig. 4d).

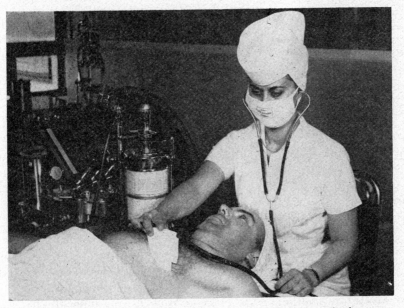

FIG. 4c. Attaching diaphragm type stethoscope for cardiac auscultation

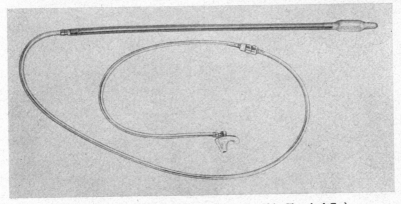

FIG. 4d. Oesophageal stethoscope. (Courtesy Ohio Chemical Co.)

Purpose

To monitor heart and breath sounds in addition to pulse and blood pressure during anesthesia. (See Monitoring)

Materials

1. Monaural earpiece of type used for hearing aids. These may be obtained custom made of plastic at surgical supply houses supplying hearing aids (about $8 to $10).
2. Flat diaphragm type receiver (Becton-Dickinson or other type). Catheter the tip of which is covered with Penrose drain approximately $\frac{1}{4}$" in diameter to be used for oesophageal auscultation when thoracic procedures are performed.
3. Three-way stopcock to permit shifting from stethoscope to syngmomanometer to read blood pressure.
4. Rubber or plastic tube $3\frac{1}{2}$–4 ft. long to connect receiver, a stopcock and earpiece.

Procedure

1. Fix receiver snuggly over precordium at point of maximum intensity of heart sounds.
2. Strap snuggly with adhesive so that diaphragm is close to chest to prevent shifting and to obtain maximum intensity of sounds.

Comment	*Reason*
1. Sounds may be distant and hard to follow in adults.	Thorax is often barrel chested and lung emphysematous.
2. Procedure of greater effectiveness in infants and children.	Both breath and heart sounds more easily heard due to relative smallness of thoracic cage.
3. Auscultate continuously.	Moment to moment changes in heart sounds. Sounds faint and more high pitched as anesthesia deepens. Important changes are missed if the procedure is not continuous.
4. Use oesophageal receiver, for thoracic or chest wall operation.	Extraneous sounds make auscultation impossible in operations above diaphragm.

MONITORING

The term *monitoring* as applied to anesthesia refers to the overall surveillance of the patient by methods employing the senses (touch, sight, hearing or smell) or by means of devices which operate chemically, physically or electrically to measure the adequacy of various physiological functions. The primary objective during anesthesia is to determine the adequacy of perfusion of the tissues by the blood. Adequacy depends upon proper blood flow and composition. Adequacy can only be determined by indirect means since no direct method is available. The gaseous content of the blood, the blood pressure and the pulse pressure offer indirect evidence of the adequacy of blood flow, carbon dioxide removal, oxygenation. Depth of anesthesia is proportional to the concentration of the drug in the cell. Drug concentration is estimated by determination of nervous and autonomic reflex activity or by variations in biophysical activity (electrical activity of the heart and brain).

The following are the conventional methods of monitoring based upon the senses and the instrumental methods employing mechanical, chemical or electronic principles.

Simple Methods Employing the Senses

The information readily gathered by the senses is confined largely to the following three organ systems:

Central Nervous System

1. Reflex activity (eye signs—pupils, lid reflex, corneal reflex).
2. Muscle tone (degree of relaxation—eyeball movements).

Respiratory System

1. Rate, depth and character of ventilatory movements.
2. Degree of oxygenation (color of blood, skin).
3. The presence of hypercarbia (blood pressure).

Cardiovascular System

1. Pulse (digital palpation).
2. Blood pressure (sphygmomanometric—direct and indirect).
3. Heart sounds (aural, auscultation and by use of the phonocardiogram).

Instrumental Methods of Monitoring

Functions amenable to monitoring by instrumentation during anesthesia are:

Central Nervous System

1. Cortical activity of cerebrum (electroencephalography).
2. Muscle tone (myography).

Respiratory System

1. Minute volume exchange (spirometry, ventilation meters).
2. Blood gases
   a. pCO_2 (end expired CO_2 analysis, CO_2 electrodes, pH meters).
   b. pO_2 (oxyhemograph, oximeters, polarographs).
3. Inhaled and blood anesthetic concentrations (analyzers—measuring moment to moment end expired anesthetics).

Circulatory System

1. Pulse (R- Wave monitors, plethysmographic methods).
2. Blood pressure measurements
   a. Direct (transducers).
   b. Indirect (plethysmography).
3. Heart sounds (phonocardiography).
4. Electrical activity of the heart (electrocardiography).

TACTILE PULSE

Palpation manually of radial, carotid, external maxillary, and pre-auricular arteries since these are readily accessible.

Reveals

1. Cardiac rate and rhythm.
2. Pulse pressure.

Does Not Reveal

1. Blood pressure.
2. Blood flow.
3. Sounds made by extraneous beats of insufficient force to create a wave or feeble efforts of failing heart.

Limitations

1. Ties up one hand so that other duties are neglected.
2. Difficult to palpate when pressure is low, in the obese, in infants or when peripheral vessels are constricted or in spasm.

Comment: Provides basic observations and essential data familiar to both the expert and the novice.

STETHOSCOPE

Principle: Auscultation of heart and breath sounds directly or electronically using a precordial or esophageal receiver connected to monoaural leads.

Reveals

1. Cardiac rate and rhythm.
2. Intensity and quality of heart sounds. These may be index of cardiac force and quite revealing if employed continuously.
3. Murmurs and adventitious sounds.
4. Ventilatory activity.

Does Not Reveal

1. Changes in arterial and pulse pressure.
2. Adequacy of perfusion.

Limitations

1. Not a substitute for "finger on pulse," but is a most useful adjunct.
2. Variations in size and contour of thorax modify intensity and quality of sounds.
3. Extraneous sounds interfere with audibility.
4. More useful in adults than children.

Comment: Useful as adjunct to tactile pulse and sphygmomanometry. Only of benefit when used continuously to follow changes occurring in sounds from moment to moment.

SPHYGMOMANOMETRY

Principle: Indirect manometry of intra-arterial pressure.

Method: Utilizes the conventional cuff and stethoscope.

Reveals

1. Constricting force necessary to overcome pulsation of artery (systolic pressure).
2. Force artery exerts overcoming externally applied pressure (diastolic).
3. Pulse pressure.

Does Not Reveal

1. Precise pressure within the artery.
2. Pulse wave contour.
3. Blood flow.

Limitations

1. Pressure not detectable when severe vasoconstriction is present (hypothermia) or when pulse pressure is low.
2. Readings vary with positioning and size of cuff or bell of stethoscope, diameter of arm or leg.
3. Unreliable or non-functional for infants and small children.

Comment: Provides essential comparative information in simple, effective manner for routine use when peripheral pulse pressure is of sufficient magnitude to create audible sounds in a partly filled artery.

CARDIAC MONITORS (PLETHYSMOGRAPHIC TYPE)

Principle: Converts energy of arterial pulsation in an extremity into a visible or an audible signal. Plethysmograph encloses a digit or a hand. Volume changes occurring with pulsation cause current to flow into amplifier in proportion to volume of the pulsation. Amplifier operates a light or sound reproducing device such as lamp, buzzer or loud speaker.

Reveals

1. Cardiac rate and rhythm.
2. Gross irregularities in rhythm.

Does Not Reveal

1. Cardiac output.
2. Pulse pressure.

Limitations

1. Signal absent when peripheral pulse is feeble or not palpable due to intense vasoconstriction or peripheral circulatory failure.
2. Subject to artefacts from extraneous movements.

Comment: Data provided is merely confirmatory and not as revealing as tactile pulse. Signals absent when pulsation is adequate.

CARDIAC MONITORS (R-WAVE TYPE)

Principle: The conversion of the R-Wave of the QRS complex of the heart into a current of a magnitude to create an audible or visible signal by amplification.

Reveals

1. Cardiac rate and rhythm.
2. Gross irregularities of the heart.
3. Gross changes in contractile force of the heart.

Does Not Reveal

1. Changes in cardiac output.
2. Changes in blood pressure.
3. Effectiveness of perfusion of the tissues.

Limitations

1. Signals may persist even though cardiac output is zero and effective cardiac action has ceased.
2. Mechanical failure—signals disappear but the cardiac action is still normal.
3. Electrical interference introduces artefacts.
4. Annoying and alarming to members of the surgical team.

Comment: Data obtained is merely confirmatory and not as revealing as the tactile pulse. Useful when pulse cannot be palpated or anesthetist must use hands for other duties.

DIRECT BLOOD PRESSURE MANOMETRY

Principle: Direct manometry of arterial pressure by means of catheters communicating with strain gauges (transducers) operating continuously recording visual devices (oscilloscope) as well as devices scribing a permanent record.

Reveals

1. Actual blood pressure in vessel or cardiac chamber.
2. Moment to moment variations in pressure.
3. Contour of pulse wave.
4. Gross variations in rhythm.

Does Not Reveal

1. Cardiac output.
2. Blood flow and degree of perfusion of cells.

Limitations

1. Clotting in cannula modifies result or renders instrument inoperable.
2. Cannulation of artery often difficult and not desired.
3. Strain gauges fragile and easily deranged.
4. Requires technician in constant attendance.

Comment: Applicable when peripheral vasoconstriction precludes indirect manometry (hypothermia causing vasospasm). Precise determination possible at extremes of pressure scale. Permits determination of pressure in great vessels and cardiac chambers. More accurate than indirect methods.

ELECTROCARDIOGRAPHY

Principle: Galvanometric detection of electrical activity by heart.

Reveals

1. Status of conducting mechanism of the heart.
2. Cardiac rate and rhythm.
3. Site and extent of myocardial or pericardial injury.

Does Not Reveal

1. Cardiac output and pulse volume.
2. Cause of derangement in conduction.

Limitations

1. Extraneous electrical interference and somatic tremors may obliterate signal.
2. Signals persist even though cardiac action is ineffective and not of sufficient force to create significant pulse wave.
3. Abnormality of electrical pattern does not necessarily correlate with functional activity of the heart.

4. Abnormality of electrical pattern may be due to remote cause and not within the heart itself.

Comment: Data may be superfluous or merely confirmatory in routine situations. Misleading if sole reliance is placed upon the device for monitoring the circulation.

PALPATION OF BREATHING BAG

Reveals

1. Alterations in minute volume exchange.
2. Character of respiratory pattern and moment to moment changes involving ventilatory movements.
3 Resistance to inflation and deflation (changes in compliance).
4. Patency of airway.

Does Not Reveal

1. Adequacy of gaseous exchange.
2. Adequacy of distribution of gases through lungs.

Limitations

1. Observations are intermittent.
2. Ties up one hand, usually the right, which is required to perform other necessary functions.

Comment: Simplest, expeditious and most effective means of evaluating ventilatory efforts. May increase pressure in system and prevent venous return which may be detrimental in borderline cases.

VENTILATION METERS

Principle: The volume of respired gases is measured by bellows, turbine or Venturi flow meters.

Reveals

1. Volume of gas moved in and out of lungs.
2. Moment to moment changes in tidal volume.

Does Not Reveal

1. Effectiveness of gas transfer across alveolar membranes.
2. Composition of respired mixture.
3. Distribution of gases in the lung.

Limitations

1. May add resistance and increase respiratory effort.
2. The device is subject to mechanical difficulties and may thus introduce artefacts.

Comment: Information gained is superfluous per se and of little value under ordinary circumstances unless correlated with other data

MECHANICAL VENTILATORS

Principle: Two basic types. (1) Pressure fixed, volume variable or (2) pressure variable, volume fixed devices which insufflate lungs and maintain respiration artificially during anesthesia.

Reveals

1. Volume of inspired gas delivered at lips.
2. Pressure developed at lips.

Does Not Reveal

1. Adequacy of gaseous distribution and transport of gases across alveoli in lungs.
2. Adequacy of gaseous exchange at alveoli.
3. Pressure in alveoli.
4. Degree of mixing of gases in alveoli.

Limitations

1. Reduce cardiac output by increasing intrathoracic pressure, particularly if insufflation time occupies more than one-half of total respiratory cycle.
2. Over-ventilation may cause alkalosis.
3. Excessive pressure may rupture alveoli.
4. Does not overcome changes in compliance.
5. May cause bronchi to collapse.

Comment: Not a monitoring device in the strict sense. It is merely an aid which relieves the burden of continuous manipulation of breathing bag manually.

ANALYSIS OF EXPIRED CARBON DIOXIDE

Principle: Determination of end expired carbon dioxide by analyzing last portion of expired air using a physical or chemical analyzer. This reading is a reflection of arterial CO_2 tension.

Method: The air is collected in a sampler, such as the Rahn sampler, and analyzed by infra-red absorption (Liston-Spinco).

Reveals

1. Moment to moment approximation of alveolar carbon dioxide tension.

Does Not Reveal

1. Actual *blood* carbon dioxide tension since diffusion may be inhibited at membrane.
2. Actual state of carbon dioxide combining power or the state of acid base balance.
3. Adequacy of volume distribution of pulmonary gases.
4. Adequacy of ventilation.

Limitations

1. Most carbon dioxide analyzers are cumbersome, are not easily managed and are easily deranged. This applies to infra-red devices.

Comment: Provides valuable confirmatory information on adequacy of carbon dioxide elimination.

OXYHEMOGRAPH

Principle: Measurement of differential absorption of red light transmitted through the pinna of the ear by oxy and reduced hemoglobin.

Reveals

1. Changes in blood oxygen content.
2. Moment to moment gross variations in per cent oxygen saturation.

Does Not Reveal

1. Absolute quantity of oxygen in blood.
2. Cause of sub-oxygenation.

Limitations

1. Cumbersome and tedious to calibrate.
2. Pigments in skin introduce error.
3. Low degree of accuracy.
4. Ear piece may cause burns.

Comment: Data obtained is comparative, relative and merely confirmatory. Same data may be available by simpler means. Color of blood, mucous membrane, and nail beds equally as informative.

REFLEX ACTIVITY

Principle: Observation and testing by clinical means (non-instrumental) the superficial and deep reflexes.

Reveals

1. Degree of depression (concentrations of anesthetic in the neurons).

Does Not Reveal

1. Adequacy of perfusion in organ systems other than the brain.
2. Status of circulatory and respiratory systems.

Limitations

1. Changes may lag behind inhaled or injected fractions of anesthetic.
2. Changes are modified by age, non-volatile drugs, anoxia, hypercarbia and duration of anesthesia. Sluggish in the aged.

Comment: Provide essential information in a simple and expeditious manner when properly interpreted and correlated with other data.

ELECTROENCEPHALOGRAPH

Principle: The detection, amplification and recording of cortial electrical activity. Intensity (voltage) and frequency (times per second voltage rises and falls) is an index of activity of the brain.

Method: Two electrodes, one in occiput and one on midline of the scalp collect the current and deliver it into an amplifier which activates a current of external source in proportion to the current produced by the neurons. The wave contour is visualized on the screen of an oscilloscope or recorded in a tracing by inkwriting levers.

Reveals

1. Electrical activity in brain. This is an index of adequacy of perfusion and composition of perfusate. Correlates well with concentration of drug in the cell or absence of oxygen or metabolites.
2. Moment to moment variations in level of activity. Little or no lag.

Does Not Reveal

1. State of perfusion in organs, other than the brain.
2. Distinction between inactivity due to drugs and other factors (anoxia, carbon dioxide excess hypotension, etc.).
3. Degree of muscle relaxation.

Limitations

1. Require skill for operation and interpretation.
2. Complex, highly sensitive and often rendered useless by A.C. interference.

Comment: Provides confirmatory data. In routine cases effort required to obtain data does not justify means. Useful when other methods of monitoring are not available (extracorporeal).

BODY THERMOMETRY

Principle: Continuous recording of rectal or esophageal temperatures by the use of electronic devices.

Method: Two types available: (1) The changes in temperature at a bimetal junction (thermocouple) cause a current to flow proportional to the disturbance. This is amplified and recorded in a galvanometer and translated in terms of temperature. (2) A current flowing through a wire varies in intensity with the resistance. Resistance is decreased by decreases in temperature and increased by an increase. Wire is placed in contact with tissues and warmed to temperature of the tissues.

Reveals

1. Moment to moment changes in temperature at region of application of thermometer.

Does Not Reveal

1. Temperature in other areas of body. Water conducts heat slowly and body, being mostly water, does not conduct heat uniformly.
2. Amount of "drift" which may be anticipated after coolant is removed.

Limitations

1. Erroneous temperatures recorded due to malfunctioning of instrument.

PART II

INHALATION ANESTHESIA

A. TYPE AND METHODS

Available Drugs

Gases: Nitrous oxide, ethylene, cyclopropane.

Volatile liquids: Ether, vinethene, chloroform, ethyl chloride, halothane, methoxyflurane and trichlorethylene.

Methods of Administration: Inhalation anesthesia is administered by the open or closed methods as follows:

1. Open
   a. Insufflation: The drug in gas or vapor form is mixed with air or oxygen and is conducted into the nostrils, mouth, nasopharynx, or trachea.
   b. Open Drop: The drug in liquid form is vaporized on a gauze or other type of mask, mixed with air or oxygen and inhaled.
2. Semi-open
   a. Insufflation: Same as open insufflation, except that a towel or other protecting device is wrapped about mouth and nose to prevent escape of gases or vapors.
   b. Drop: Same as open drop method, except that a towel or other enclosing device is wrapped about mask to minimize the escape of gases or vapors.
3. Semi-closed: Mixtures of gases or vapors are enclosed in an inhaler equipped with an expiratory valve to allow the escape of excess gases and carbon dioxide.
4. Closed: Mixtures of gases or vapors are enclosed in an inhaler and completely rebreathed. The patient's metabolic requirement of oxygen is added from an external supply and carbon dioxide is removed by chemical absorption.

Apparatus and Equipment for Inhalation Anesthesia

Inhalation anesthesia is administered by means of open masks, insufflators, or inhalers. Inhalers are usually parts *of machines*. All appliances for administering inhalation anesthesia (from the simplest mask to the most complex inhaler) have these essential features:

1. A source of oxygen.
2. A device or means for the disposal of carbon dioxide.
3. A device to vaporize liquid anesthetic drugs.

Open Masks

Definition: Open masks are devices, usually fashioned from wire or screen, to fit over the face and nose of the patient. Layers of gauze, flannel or similar substances, upon which the drug may be vaporized, are draped and fastened over the metal framework. Many types have been devised

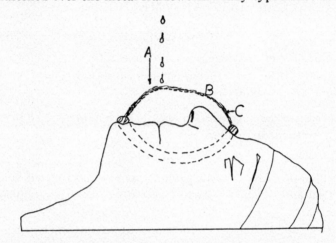

Fig. 5. The open drop technique, simple as it is, embodies the three cardinal features of all inhalation anesthesia appliances: (A) a source of oxygen which in this case is air; (B) a means for the unimpeded disposal of carbon dioxide which is the meshes of the gauze screen; and (C) a device for vaporizing the liquid agent which in this case is the gauze covering.

but all serve the same purpose (Fig. 5). The air supplies the oxygen, and carbon dioxide escapes through the mesh of the cloth.

Insufflators

Definition: An insufflator is a device so arranged that air, oxygen, or other gases may be bubbled through certain volatile liquids. The resultant vapor becomes mixed with the gas and is conducted to the upper portion of the respiratory tract through a catheter or other conduit and inhaled (Fig. 6).

Anesthesia "Machines"

Definition: An anesthesia machine is an apparatus for the administration of anesthetic gases and vapors by inhalation.

Constant features which appear on anesthesia machines:

1. An inhaler composed of a mask and rebreathing bag and necessary connecting pieces, carbon dioxide filter, escape valves etc.
2. A flowmeter for metering gases, pin valves and connecting tubes for leading gases to the inhaler (see flowmeters).
3. A vaporizer for volatile liquid anesthetic drugs (see vaporizers page 86).

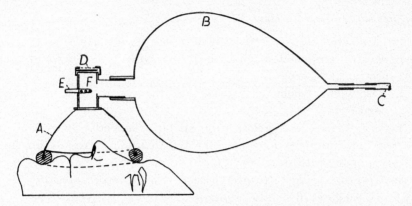

FIG. 6. Cross section of a semiclosed inhaler composed of (A) a closed mask and (B) a breathing bag. A continuous flow of gases is admitted from a flowmeter through the (C) inlet tube. Exhalations, excess gases and vapors escape through (D) the adjustable valve. A variable amount of rebreathing occurs, depending upon the flow of gas, size of the mask, and the bag, tidal volume of the patient, and patency of the valve. The bag may be closed from the mask by (E) the obturator, which allows the patient to breathe room air through (F) the vents.

4. An expiratory valve or other outlet for the elimination of exhaled gases, particularly carbon dioxide (Fig. 6).

5. A yoke and reducing valve for attachment of one or more cylinders of oxygen (Fig. 11).

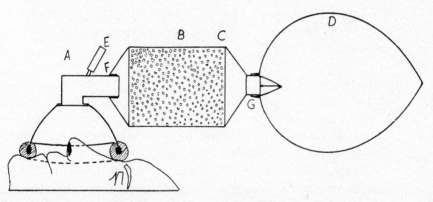

FIG. 7. Simplified form of to and fro inhaler composed of (A) a mask, (B) a canister charged with (C) soda lime, and (D) a five liter rebreathing bag. Gases and vapors are admitted into the inhaler through the (E) inlet. During expiration, gases pass over the soda lime to the breathing bag; during inspiration, the direction is reversed. The contents of the inhaler are exposed to the absorbent twice. The slip joints (F) and (G) allow the inhaler to be dismantled or the canister to be removed.

6. A yoke and reducing valve for attachment of one or more cylinders of nitrous oxide (or ethylene).

7. A yoke and reducing valve for attachment of one cylinder of carbon dioxide.

8. A yoke and reducing valve for a cylinder of cyclopropane.

Features not constantly present, but desirable:

1. Flowmeters for coarse and fine flows for a given gas.
2. A valve for quickly flooding the inhaler with oxygen in event of emergency.
3. A sphygmomanometer attached to the apparatus at a convenient point.
4. An automatic mixing flowmeter capable of delivering gases on demand in certain fixed percentages (the McKesson-Nargraff machine is equipped with such a meter).
5. A pressure gauge attached to each yoke to record pressures of compressed gases in supply cylinders.
6. A cabinet, drawers, writing table, etc.
7. A water, mercury, or diaphragm type of manometer for measuring and controlling the pressure in the inhaler.

Inhalers

Description: Inhalers are devices from which a subject breathes gases or vapors. Two types are employed for anesthesia: (a) the semi-closed, and (b) the closed.

   a. *The semi-closed inhaler* is composed of a mask, a breathing bag, an exhalation valve, and necessary slip joints and sleeves. A continuous flow of gases and vapors must be delivered into the bag which acts as a reservoir. The excess and the exhaled gases escape through the exhalation valve (Fig. 6).

   Two types are defined:

   1. The *non-return* or non-rebreathing type in which valves are interposed between the supply of gas and the external atmosphere.
   2. The *rebreathing* type in which the valve between the breathing bag and the mask is omitted and gas is returned to the system.

   b. *The closed inhaler* is composed of a snugly fitting mask, an absorption system for carbon dioxide, a rebreathing bag, and necessary slip joints and sleeves. The exhaled gases are rebreathed after carbon dioxide is removed (Fig. 7). A flow of oxygen for the metabolic requirements of the patient is provided from a storage cylinder.

Face Pieces

Description: A face piece, often referred to as a mask, is composed of a metal, celluloid, or hard rubber body (Fig. 8) and a soft rubber, usually inflatable, face cushion (Fig. 9). The body communicates with the rebreathing bag by means of a slip joint.

Uses: The face piece acts as a closed mask for semi-closed and closed inhalers.

Features:

1. Face pieces should be as small as possible to minimize "dead space."
2. Face pieces should have wide apertures leading to the other portions of the inhaler (at least 2.5 cms.).
3. Face pieces should be shaped so that they may be held comfortably in one hand by the anesthetist.

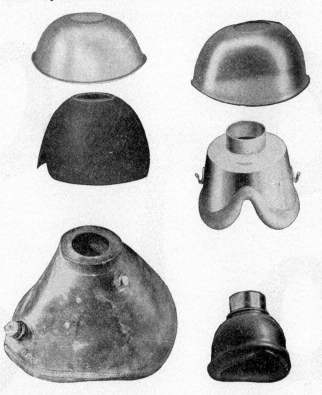

Fig. 8. Face pieces used to form the mask for inhalation anesthesia. Some are made of plastic substances, others of rubber, still others of metal. (Courtesy of Richard Foregger, Ph.D.)

4. The cushion should be soft and fit snugly and comfortably over the face.
5. The cushion should be well inflated and leakproof if of the inflatable type.

Care of Face Pieces:

1. Immediately after use, disconnect the face piece from remainder of inhaler. Scrub with soap and water (soak in Wescodyne solution), 70% alcohol, wipe dry, and wrap in a clean dry towel.

Comment

1. Always select a face piece which fits the patient's face snugly to assure an airtight fit.

2. Never use creosol or other disinfectants of the phenol type to disinfect rubber. *Rubber becomes impregnated with the phenol and may cause burns.*

Head Bands

Definition: Head bands are straps composed of sheet rubber, plastic, or other elastic substances. They are shaped to fit about the occiput, and pass along side the face to the face piece (Fig. 10).

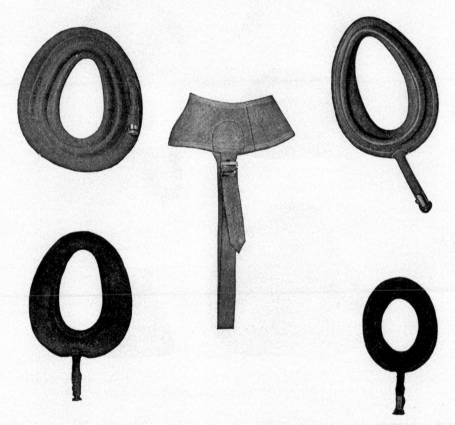

FIG. 9. Face cushions used to complete the mask for inhalation anesthesia. These cushions slip over the edges of the face pieces shown in Fig. 8. (Courtesy of Richard Foregger, Ph.D.)

Synonym: Mask retainer, mask harness.

Uses: They hold the face piece securely and comfortably to the face.

Features:

1. Head bands should possess sufficient resilience to allow as loose or snug an application of the face piece as desired.
2. They should be composed entirely of conductive rubber or covered with a substance which is easily cleaned in event of soiling.
3. They should be free from sharp hooks or prongs or other metal pieces which may injure the patient or anesthetist.

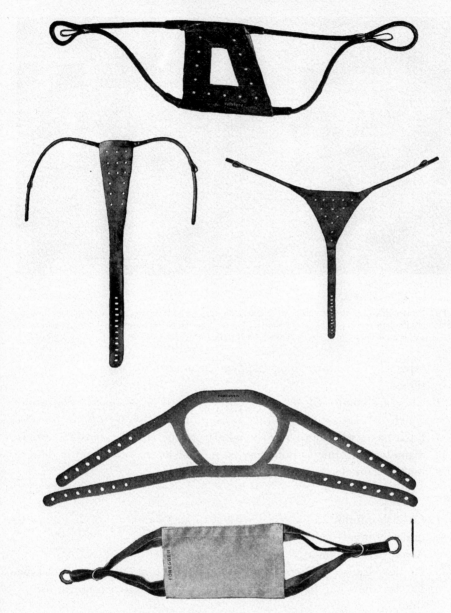

Fig. 10. Various types of head bands used to secure masks to the patient's face. (Courtesy of Richard Foregger, Ph.D.)

Breathing Bags

Description: Breathing bags for inhalation anesthesia are composed of conductive rubber. They are placed at some convenient point in the inhaler and act as reservoirs for mixtures of vapors and gases.

Features:

1. They are usually ovoid in shape and vary between one and five liter

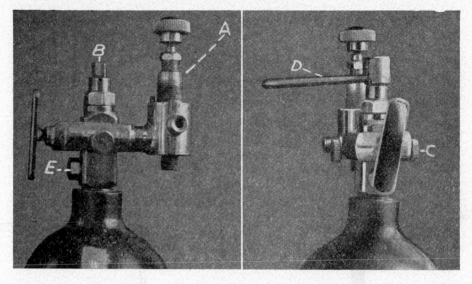

a   b

FIG. 11(a) and (b). (A) Reducing valve and yoke. (B) Cylinder valve. (E) Bolt containing core of soft metal which melts and acts as a safety plug in the event of exposure to high temperatures. (C) Screws for securing cylinder to the yoke. (D) Handle for cylinder valve.

capacity, depending upon the type of inhaler for which they are designed.

2. They are composed of light gum or other type of conductive rubber which will not offer resistance to respiration.
3. Each has a wide outlet to the inhaler at one end (2.5 cms or more in diameter). An inlet nipple may be present at the other end in designs for the semi-closed inhaler.

Care of Bags:

1. Cleanse interior and exterior with soap and water Rinse and allow to drain by inverting the wide outlet downward.
2. Always store rubber pieces in a cool place when not in use.
3. Do not cleanse with creosol or other disinfectants of the phenol type.
4. Do not allow bag to remain distended with gases, when not in use.

Comment:

1. Anesthetic gases diffuse through rubber and hasten its deterioration.
2. Perforations or tears should be patched immediately with rubber cement and strips of gum rubber. *Do not use adhesive plaster.*

Cylinders for Storage of Gases

Anesthetic and other gases employed for anesthesia are compressed into steel cylinders for storage and transportation.

Features of Cylinders:

1. The walls, constructed of 3/8″ steel, are capable of withstanding pressures which vary between 3000 to 4000 pounds per square inch. They must resist 1⅔ of the currently used or *service* pressure.

2. All possess a valve which is a permanent part of the cylinder. This controls the flow from the cylinder to the reducing valve on the machine (Fig. 11).

3. All are provided with a safety plug containing a metal which melts and releases the contained gases in the event the cylinder is exposed to excessively high temperatures (Fig. 11).

4. All have the following identifying marks engraved upon the shoulder: Type, serial number, date cylinder was commissioned, date tested, insignia of testing laboratory, service pressure, and name and address of the manufacturer of gases owning it (Fig. 12).

5. Refilled cylinders are sealed at the valve port, tagged with weight of gas, equipped with a new washer, and labeled.

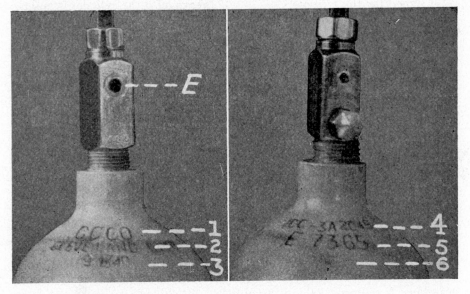

a   b

Fig. 12(a) and (b). Markings on the shoulder of storage cylinders for compressed gases:
(1) Name or initials of manufacturer.
(2) Location of the manufacturer.
(3) Symbol of the laboratory which tested the cylinder after five years, use and date of test. (E) Port for exit of gases.
(4) Interstate Commerce Commission cylinder type (3A) used for anesthetic gases. Service pressure 2025 lbs. per square inch.
(5) Size of cylinder, and manufacturer's number
(6) Symbol of original testing laboratory.

Care of Cylinders	*Reason*
1. Always close valves after using a machine or before removing cylinder from a yoke.	The cylinder may not be empty and gases will escape if they are jarred loose in the yoke or if one attempts its removal.
2. Replace worn washer with the new one provided with each newly filled cylinder.	Gases leak if a durable washer is not interposed between port of the valve and nipple of the yoke.
3. Store all cylinders in a cool place away from combustible materials.	Gases expand when warmed, and the pressure in the cylinder becomes excessive.
4. Label exhausted cylinder "empty" with chalk or other erasable marking substance.	Storing empty with full cylinders may cause confusion and lead to accidents.
5. Close valves on all empty cylinders.	Dirt, moisture, and other deleterious agents must be excluded from the interior of the cylinder.
6. Fasten cylinders in an upright position or place in a rack designed for the purpose.	The valve is the most vulnerable part of the cylinder. It easily breaks off if the cylinder is upset.

Identification: Cylinders are identified by the color of their exteriors as well as by their labels. The following colors have been adopted by the U. S. Bureau of Standards.

	Color	State of Drug in Cylinder
Cyclopropane (C_3H_6)	orange	liquid
Ethylene (C_2H_4)	red (violet W.H.O.)	gas
Nitrous oxide (N_2O)	blue	liquid
Helium (He)	brown	gas
Oxygen (O_2)	green (white W.H.O.)	gas
Carbon dioxide (CO_2)	grey	liquid
Carbon dioxide-oxygen	grey-green	gas
Helium-oxygen	brown-green	gas

Reducing Valves

Definition: A reducing valve is a valve usually of the diaphragm type interposed between main cylinder valve and pin valve on flowmeter.

Purpose: Permits the expansion of a gas from a relatively high (2000 lbs. per sq. in.) but variable pressure to an area of lower and more constant pressure (40–60 lbs.).

Types:

    a. *Fixed pressure.* Variations due to changes in cylinder pressures cannot be corrected.

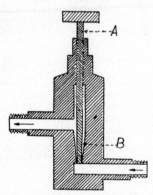

Fig. 13A. Cross section of a reducing valve of the "pin type." (A) The pin fits into (B) the seat. If the pin is screwed too tightly, the seat is damaged and the fine adjustment is lost.

b. *Variable pressure*. Changes due to changes in cylinder pressure are corrected by varying tension on diaphragm by varying the tension on a spring.

Pin Valves

A device which permits variation in size of an orifice for altering flow of gases discharged from a point of higher pressure to a lower one. Usually consists of a pin which screws into a tapered slot. Flow varies as the tapered needle is screwed in and out of the seat (Fig. 13A).

Comment

In the Foregger apparatus the pin valve serves dual purpose of regulating gas flow and reducing pressure. It is the only valve between main cylinder valve and flowmeter.

Care of Pin Valves:

1. Turn pin valves until flow of gas ceases.
2. Never tighten (screw in) valves of the pin type. The seat or the pin (whichever is softer) becomes worn and the valve develops a leak or loses its fine adjustment.
3. Do not oil or grease any reducing valve on any high pressure gas system.
4. Always close pin valves before turning on the cylinder valve. The high pressure from the cylinder may suddenly be transmitted to the flowmeter or inhalers.
5. Always turn off pin valves (after turning off the main valves) when the anesthesia apparatus is not in use.
6. Wipe pin valves and seats with ether or acetone to remove dirt. Dry with clean gauze.

Yokes

Definition: Yokes are metal clamps with adjustable screws which secure the cylinders to the apparatus or reducing valves. They are equipped with nipples which fit snugly into the inlet socket or port of the cylinder valve (Fig. 11).

Pin Index System

The pin index system consists of a combination of two pins projecting from the yoke assembly and arranged to fit into matching holes on the cylinder valve. Each gas has a certain combination of positioning of holes and pins so that no interchange is possible on yoke designed to accommodate a specific (Fig. 13B).

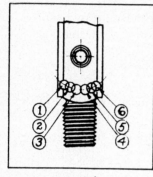

Master Index

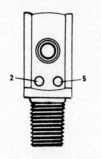

Oxygen

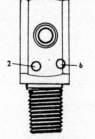

Carbon dioxide—
Oxygen mixtures
(CO2 not over 7%)

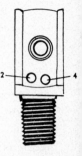

Helium-Oxygen
mixtures
(He not over 80%)

Ethylene

Nitrous oxide

Cyclopropane

Helium and
Helium-Oxygen
mixtures
(O2 less than 20%)

Carbon dioxide
and Carbon dioxid
—Oxygen mixtures
(CO2 over 7%)

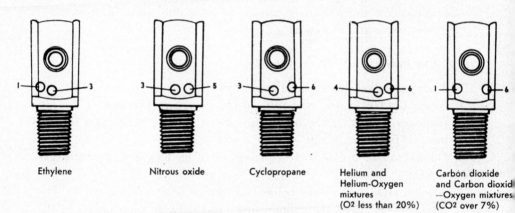

FIG. 13B. The pin index system designed to prevent accidental interchanging of cylinders and the administration of the incorrect gases. The pins on the yoke match the holes on the valve of the cylinder. (Courtesy Ohio Chemical Company.)

Flowmeters

Definition: A flowmeter is a device for measuring volumes of gases or vapors under pressure as they effuse from storage cylinders or other containers.

Two basic types are recognized:

a. *The variable orifice—fixed pressure type.* A float in a tapered tube is suspended by a fixed pressure. Increases in flow increase the pressure in the tube and elevate the float thereby increasing the cross-sectional area of the orifice until the pressure falls to that necessary to suspend the float.

b. *Fixed orifice.* As the flow of gas is increased the pressure proximal to the orifice is increased in proportion to the flow rate. Pressure changes measured by manometers or gauge and translated into terms of volume.

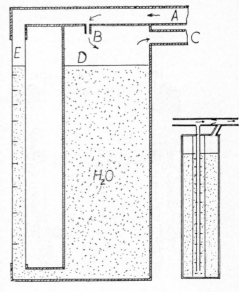

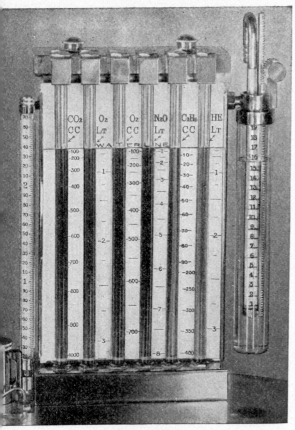

a

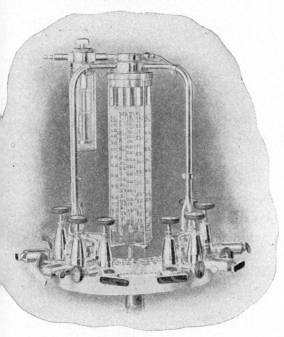

b

Fig. 14a, b, c. (a) A typical flowmeter head of the hydraulic ("Outside") type. (Courtesy of Richard Foregger, Ph.D.)

(b) A typical flowmeter head of the hydraulic ("Inside") type.

(c) Schematic diagram illustrating the operation of the hydraulic flowmeter. The gas passes from the cylinder and reducing valve into (A) the inlet tube, through (B) a narrowed orifice to (C) the delivery tube leading to the inhaler. The passage of gas through the narrow orifice causes the pressure in (A) to exceed that over the water in (D). This difference in pressure causes a depression of the column of water in (E). The greater the amount of gas flowing through orifice (B), the greater the pressure developed in (A), and the greater the depression of the meniscus in (E). (E) is calibrated in such a manner that the amount of depression indicates the flow in liters or fractions of a liter per minute. Calibrations apply to the gas indicated or to a gas of identical molecular weight. Inset shows principle of the inside type of flowmeter. The principle of operation is identical in both types. The tubes on the inside type are enclosed in the jar, on the outside type they are individually mounted on a scale placed in front of the water reservoir.

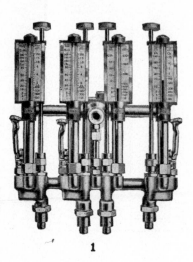

1

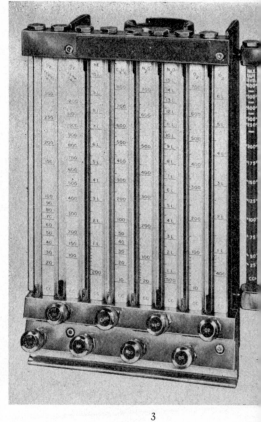

3

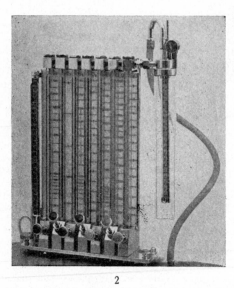

2

Fig. 15a. 1. Flowmeter used on Heidbrink. 2. Rotameter (Foregger). 3. Flowmeter constructed on rotameter principle on Heidbrink anesthesia apparatus.

Types: Three types are commonly employed for anesthesia:

1. *Hydraulic type.* Also known as the "wet" flowmeter. A constriction in the inlet tube causes an increase in pressure of the flowing gas. This increase in pressure is transmitted to a column of water which is depressed in a calibrated tube in proportion to the flow of gas (Fig. 14).
2. *Dry or floating gauge type.* The flow of gases suspends a spherical or cylindrical float in a transparent tube, the sides of which are calibrated in liters or gallons per minute (Fig. 15). The rotameter is of this type.

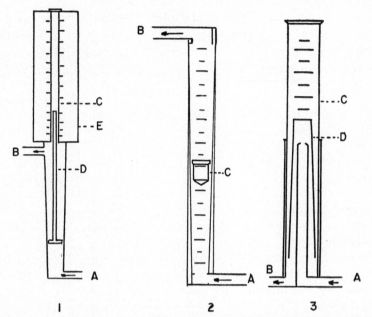

FIG. 15b. Dry types of flowmeters constructed on the "variable orifice" principle. (1) Type used on Heidbrink. The gases enter at A into tapered tube. As flow increases plunger is elevated higher into tube to permit gas to flow around edge and the stem D is pushed further into transparent tube C along scale E. (2) Rotameter type of flow meter. Plastic rotating bobbin C is suspended in transparent tapered tube by the stream of gases which enter at A and leave at B. The bobbin is spherical in certain types of units. (3) Type used on the McKesson apparatus operated on the same principle. The gases pass through the nozzle type orifice B into tapered tube which is elevated into calibrated transparent tube C in proportion to flow of gases. The gases enter the apparatus at A and leave at B.

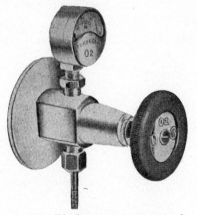

FIG. 16a. Diaphragm or gauge type of flowmeter.

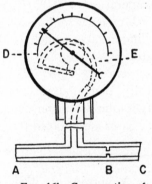

FIG. 16b. Cross section of gauge type of flowmeter. The gases enter (A) the tube through (B) the orifice to (C) the delivery tube. The narrow orifice causes a difference in pressure between (A) and (C) which is transmitted to (D) the diaphragm. The diaphragm operates a clockwork mechanism (E). The dial is calibrated in liters or fractions of a liter per minute.

3. *Gauge type.* A constriction in the inlet tube increases the pressure of flowing gases. The increased pressure is transmitted to a diaphragm which works a clocklike mechanism and records flow of gases in liters or gallons per minute (Fig. 16).

Care of Flowmeters	Reason
1. Never lubricate valves or other parts of a flowmeter with grease or oil.	Explosive mixtures may form.
2. Always close the reducing valve before the cylinder valve is turned on.	The high pressure from the cylinder is transmitted to the flowmeter.
3. Always maintain the water in a hydraulic flowmeter at its prescribed level.	Incorrect volumes of gases are metered if water level is low.
4. Cleanse flowmeter jars with diluted hydrochloric acid *once a month.* Rinse and refill with distilled water.	Water becomes discolored and jar coated with film in due time.

Comment

1. *Each flowmeter is calibrated only for that gas which it is to measure.* Substitution of one gas for another may result in inaccurate measurement of volumes unless corrections are allowed.
2. The flow is gauged at atmospheric pressure (76 cm. Hg.) and room temperature (25°C).
3. Each meter must have a reducing valve interposed between it and the cylinder valve to deliver the gases at a safe pressure and a constant rate.
4. Gases are measured in terms of the metric system in *liters* or fractions of liter per minute.
5. Hydraulic flowmeters do not humidify the gases they measure unless the gases are bubbled through the water.

Vaporizers

Definition: Vaporizers are devices used to volatilize low boiling liquid anesthetic drugs.

They may be placed (1) at some point in the inhaler so that vapor-

Fig. 18. Schematic diagram of a typical "bubble type" vaporizer. The (A) motor driven pump delivers a stream of compressed air whose volume may be controlled by (B) the valve through the (C) container for the volatile liquid. The air is divided into fine bubbles which facilitates vaporization. The air and the vapor are conducted through (D) the trap which prevents the accidental passage of liquid to the patient. The (C) container is surrounded by the (E) water bath which is warmed in (F) the container by (G) electric heater.

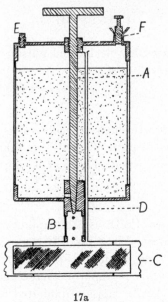

17a

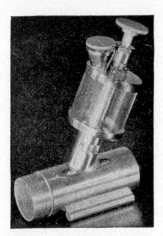

17b

FIG. 17a. Ether vaporizer of dropper type. (A) The pin valve adjustment controls the size, rate and drop formation which may be observed through (B) the window. The drug drops upon the (C) copper screen and is vaporized by the gases in the inhaler. (D) The tube allows the pressure over the surface of the liquid to be equalized with that in the inhaler. (E) The vent is opened when the cup is filled through (F) the funnel to allow displacement of air by the liquid.

(b) Type used for to and fro filter. (Courtesy Richard Foregger Ph.D.)

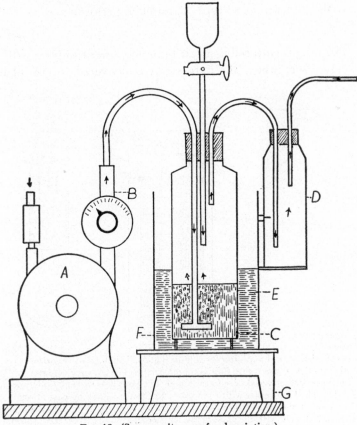

FIG. 18. (See opposite page for description.)

ization occurs in the inhaler or (2) they may be located outside the inhaler so that the vapors must be delivered to it.

Types:

1. *Dropper Type* (Fig. 17):
    a. The liquid contained in a cup passes through a needle valve and drops on a copper screen placed in the path of inhaled or exhaled gases. The vapors are caught in the current. The heat is supplied from the environment.

2. *Bubble Type* (Fig. 18):
    a. Gases, usually air, oxygen, or mixtures of nitrous oxide and oxygen, are bubbled through the liquid contained in a jar. The vapor and gases are conducted to the inhaler (see insufflators page 87). The source of heat is variable and percentage of vapor delivered fluctuates and is inconstant. The copper kettle supplies unlimited heat, however.

3. *Gauze or Wick Type* (Fig. 19A):
    a. Exhaled or inhaled gases are conducted over a gauze or wick which is continually soaked by partial immersion in the liquid. Also known as the "drawn over" type. Variable in performance.

4. *Heater Type:*
    a. The drug is enclosed in an air tight container equipped with a needle valve from which the pure vapor is delivered to the inhaler. The

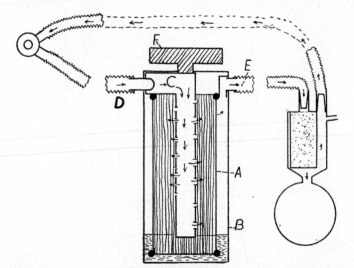

FIG. 19A. The wick type of vaporizer for volatile liquids. This type of vaporizer is usually introduced into either the delivery or return tube of the circle filter. The (A) wick dips into the (B) partially filled jar and is thus constantly soaked with the liquid. The gases pass through from tube (D) over the wick and out through (E) together with the vapor. (F) Control allows by-pass of some of the gases to regulate the amount of drug added to the inhaler. If the vaporizer is on the exhalation side of the inhaler, the vapor is diluted with the gases in the canister and the bag. If on the inspiratory side, the "strong" vapor passes into the mask and mixes with the gases in the lungs first.

drug is vaporized by warm water or a chemical heater (Oxford) which surrounds the container.

Comment	*Reason*
1. Discard unused liquid at the end of each day.	Most liquid drugs are decomposed after exposure to light, air, or heat.
2. Close the vent (bubble type) except when filling the vaporizer.	The vent is a source of a leak. The back flow of gases prevents proper dropping of the liquid.
3. Remove wicks from the jar and allow to dry when machine is not in use.	Condensed water vapor from patient's exhalations often wets wick and reduces efficiency
4. Tighten ether jars securely in their sockets.	The rim of the jar is frequently a source of leaks.

Fluotec Vaporizer

Definition

A calibrated vaporizer for halothane which is temperature compensated and delivers a uniform and unvarying concentration of vapor ranging from

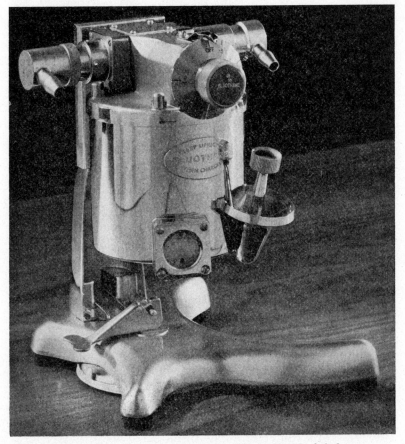

FIG. 19B. The fluotec is a precision controlled vaporizer for halothane.
(Courtesy Fraser Sweatman.)

0.1% to 4%. A flow of nitrous oxide or oxygen passes into the vaporizer at flow rates varying from 4 to 15 liters (Fig. 19B).

Features

1. Vernier control which permits variation in concentrations to be made in increments of 0.1%.
2. The per cent composition is self-adjusting and, therefore, the per cent composition remains constant as the flow rate to the ambient gas is varied.
3. A bimetalic valve expands and contracts as the temperature of the liquid varies due to evaporation and environmental changes. This permits a proportionate increase or decrease of vapor to pass from the device.

Uses

1. Designed specifically for use of halothane by semi-closed technique.
2. May be used to vaporize Fluoromar.

Copper Kettle

Definition:

A bubble type vaporizer composed of a copper container which absorbs heat from the environment and conducts it in amounts to provide a constant percentage of vapor (Fig. 19C).

COMPUTING PROPORTIONS OF GASES AND VAPORS WHEN USING THE COPPER KETTLE

1. Determine the vapor pressure of the liquid at temperature of room from a prepared table or from the vapor pressure curve for the agent.
   Example: Ether—400 m. Hg. at 20° C.
2. Determine the per cent of vapor issuing from the copper kettle by dividing the normal atmospheric pressure into the vapor pressure and multiplying by 100.
   Example: $760 \overline{)\ 440} = 58\%$
3. Determine the volume of vapor delivered by each 100 cc. of oxygen bubbling through the vaporizer.
   Example: 100% (ether and oxygen)—58% (ether) = 42% (oxygen)

   $$\frac{42\%\ O_2}{100\ cc\ O_2} = \frac{58\%\ ether}{x\ cc.\ ether} \quad X = 139 \text{ cc. of ether vapor delivered by each 100 cc. } O_2$$

4. Determine the value of agent necessary to make up the desired volume of mixture at the desired percentage.
   Example: 5 liters of 4% ether-oxygen mixture is desired. This means 40 cc. of ether are required per liter or 200 cc. total for the 5 liters.

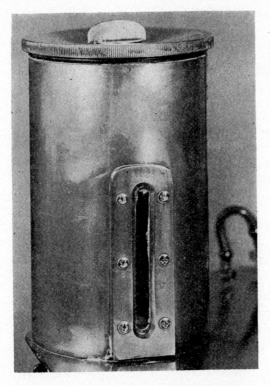

Fig. 19C. New bubble type of vaporizer commonly referred to as the "copper kettle." The high thermal conductivity of copper permits transfer of heat from the environment to the liquid. The efficiency of this vaporizer is increased if it is mounted on a brass table top from which it readily absorbs the necessary heat.

5. Determine volume of O_2 required to vaporize the desired amount of ether. This is done by dividing the vapor delivered by 100 cc. of oxygen into the required amount of vapor to make the desired mixture.

Example: 100 cc. delivers 139 cc. of ether

$$139 \overline{)\ 200.0} \quad 1.35 = 1.35 \text{ increments of } 100 \text{ cc. or } 135 \text{ cc. of } O_2$$

6. Determine volume of diluent necessary by subtracting the volume of oxygen delivered from the total volume of anticipated mixture.

Example: 5000 cc. of O_2 − (135 cc O_2 + 200 cc. ether)
= 4665 cc. O_2 from flow meter

Thus: 4665 cc. of oxygen flow into the apparatus directly bypassing the vaporizer.

135 cc. of oxygen pass into the copper kettle to vaporize the ether.

200 cc. of ether issues from the kettle.

335 cc. of combined ether and oxygen issue from the kettle.

5 liters of a 4% mixture pass into the apparatus.

The Chemical Absorption of Carbon Dioxide

Principle: The carbon dioxide is absorbed by the passage of the patient's exhalations over strong alkalis in a canister. The gases, freed of carbon dioxide, are then returned to the mask and are rebreathed.

Apparatus: The devices employed to accomplish absorption are called filters. Filters are of two types:

1. The *to-and-fro filter* which consists of a mask, canister, and rebreathing bag (page 77).
2. The *circle filter* which consists of two tubes, two valves, a mask, a canister, and a rebreathing bag (page 75).

Absorbent: Hydroxides of alkali and alkaline earth metals are the only available absorbents. Two types are employed:

1. *Soda lime.* A mixture of sodium and calcium hydroxides. This is the most popular and widely employed absorbent (see page 92).
2. *Barium-lime* (Baralyme). A mixture of barium and calcium hydroxides. This mixture has recently been introduced into anesthesia but is not as widely employed as soda lime.

Advantages of Carbon Dioxide Absorption:

1. It allows complete rebreathing of exhaled gases *which results in considerable reduction in the cost of anesthesia.*
2. It allows complete enclosure of inflammable mixtures and, therefore, minimizes the hazard of explosion.
3. It allows inhalation of a mixture of nearly constant composition. Thus an even level of anesthesia is maintained.
4. It allows the inhalation of warmed gases and vapors.
5. It allows the carbon dioxide tension in the alveoli to be maintained at a constant value.

Disadvantages:

1. The "dead space"* in the mask and connecting pieces is difficult to eliminate and so some carbon dioxide is rebreathed.
2. Resistance to inspiration or expiration, or both, may be introduced by valves, tubing, and other parts of the machine or inhaler.

Soda Lime

Definition: Soda lime is a mixture of sodium and calcium hydroxides moulded into the form of granules. It is commonly employed to absorb acidic gases, such as, carbon dioxide.

Composition: Two varieties of soda lime are available for anesthesia: (a) the high moisture type; (b) the low moisture type. The high moisture type should be used. The low moisture type is unsatisfactory.

The composition of soda lime for anesthesia is as follows:

(a) *Low moisture*

Sodium hydroxide	5%
Water	2% or less
Calcium hydroxide	To make 100%

* Dead space is that space containing gases which are rebreathed without coming into contact with the absorbent and are, therefore, not freed of carbon dioxide.

(b) *High moisture*

Sodium hydroxide	5%
Potassium hydroxide	1%
Water	14–19%
Calcium hydroxide	To make 100%

Necessary Qualities of Soda Lime for Anesthesia:

1. It should be non-hygroscopic: A low sodium hydroxide content insures this feature.
2. It should not "cake": Non-hygroscopic properties insure this feature.
3. It should be of proper size for the filter employed. A mixture of granules not larger than will pass through a four-mesh standard screen nor smaller than will pass through an eight-mesh is the most satisfactory size for clinical anesthesia.
4. It should be free from alkaline dust and sufficiently hard to prevent fragmentation of the granules. Hardness is obtained by adding small amounts of silica.

Process of absorption: The reaction of absorption is a *neutralization.* During the reaction the following phenomena occur:

1. Forty-four grams (22.2 liters) of carbon dioxide unite with the alkali yielding sodium carbonate, calcium carbonate, and eighteen grams of water.
2. Heat (known as the heat of neutralization) is generated. This amounts to 13,700 calories for every forty-four grams of carbon dioxide absorbed. The temperature of the reacting mass in an 8×13 cm. canister during clinical anesthesia in an adult with a normal metabolic rate averages approximately 50–60° C. in the to and fro filter and 45-55° C. in the circle filter.

Absorption Efficiency of Soda Lime:

1. Maximum efficiency is secured when the tidal volume is equal to the air space in the charged canister. (An 8×13 cms. canister averages 425 cc. of air space.)
2. A charge of 500 grams (one pound) totals an absorption period with intermittent use of 6–7 hours.
3. Absorption is more efficient if a charge is used intermittently due to interaction between the sodium and calcium compounds in the granule.

Signs of Exhaustion of Absorbent	*Reason*
1. *Absence of heat production.* The canister is cold when palpated.	The heat evolved during absorption warms the walls of the canister. May not be a reliable sign in the circle filter if the canister is inside the inhaler.

2. *Elevation of the blood pressure.* The pulse rate is not altered to any appreciable extent. Pressure returns to normal when absorbent or canister is changed.

Excess carbon dioxide stimulates the vasomotor center even under anesthesia.

3. *Hyperpnea.* If unnoticed or is not pronounced, depression of respiration may be only respiratory sign.

Excess carbon dioxide stimulates the respiratory center. Depression follows stimulation, the hyperpnea disappears and respiration assumes a gasping quality.

The Circle Filter

Description: Circle filters consist of a face piece connected to a canister and a rebreathing bag by two tubes of corrugated, non-kinking rubber. Flutter valves at the inlet and outlet of the canister insure a unidirectional flow of gases over the absorbent (Fig. 20, 21).

Features:

1. They possess a bypass valve allowing for partial rebreathing and partial or complete absorption of carbon dioxide.
2. They possess two canisters with a valve for changing from one to the other or a bypass for rebreathing without absorption. Canisters vary in size; but average 500 grams capacity.
3. They possess an exhalation valve. This may be either at the face piece or at the canister and allows conversion to a semiclosed inhaler.
4. They possess an inlet tube which conducts gases from the flowmeter. This is usually located at the canister.
5. They possess an obturator which is usually placed at the face piece slip joint. Obturators prevent loss of mixture from the inhaler.
6. They possess a vaporizer for ether or other drugs which may be either of the dropper or wick type. It may be placed at the inlet or outlet of the canister.

Technique:

1. Inflate rebreathing bag with the desired gases.
2. Fasten the mask in the routine manner, allowing tubes to the canister to lead off from right side of mask.
3. Turn head slightly to right side.
4. Turn filter to "on" to initiate absorption of carbon dioxide.

Advantages of Circle Filters:

1. Alkaline dust is not inhaled because it accumulates in the rubber tubes.
2. The inspired air is warmed, but not excessively (31–33° C.).

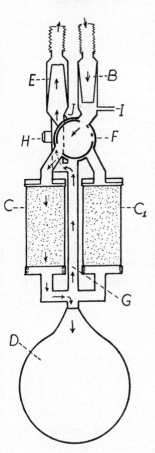

Fig. 20. Diagram of a "two canister" circle filter. During expiration the gases pass from the (A) mask through the (B) valve through (C) the absorbent in the canister into (D) the bag. During inspiration they pass from the bag to (E) the valve, to the mask. The unidirectional flow causes them to pass over the absorbent only once. (F) The valve allows a shift from canister (C) to (C_1) during course of anesthesia. Rebreathing without filtering carbon dioxide is accomplished by adjusting valve (F) allowing gases to pass through (G) the tube into the bag without passing over the absorbent. The exhalation valve (H) allows filter to be converted to a semi-closed inhaler. Gases are admitted through (I) the inlet. The ether vaporizer of dropper type may be fastened at (J).

Fig. 21. A double canister circle filter. (Courtesy of Richard Foregger, Ph.D.)

3. A snug application of the face piece is easily secured and maintained, particularly by inexperienced individuals.

4. Carbon dioxide is removed gradually after rebreathing, during induction, or at other times over a period of several minutes.

5. The air space between the mask and the absorbent in the canister does not act as a "dead space" if the valves function properly.

6. The efficiency of the apparatus is not decreased when the tidal volume is less than air space of the canister (this is not so in the to and fro).

Disadvantages:

1. They are composed of numerous parts, some of which may become deranged.

2. The surface of the tubes, the large canister and the valves create added resistance to respiration.
3. The possibility of cross infection, if tubing, valves and other parts are not carefully cleansed, is greater than in the to and fro.
4. Absorption efficiency is not as satisfactory as in the to and fro over long periods of time. Apparently exhaustion of the absorbent occurs. This must be followed by periods of rest to regenerate activity.

Comment

Reason

1. All tubes should be as wide and as short as possible. All apertures should be wider than the trachea.

Long or narrow tubes create resistance to respiration.

2. Inspect valves frequently for efficiency.

Old rubber valves become rigid and useless. Metal valves may adhere to parts.

3. Cleanse tubes with soap and water between cases.

Tubes may be responsible for cross infection.

4. Double canisters are desirable.

One charge may "rest" without being removed from the inhaler while the other is being used.

5. Clamp or screw top of canister tightly after filling.

The top is the source of many large leaks.

Circle Filter—Canisters in Series

Principle

1. The gases pass from the exhalation tube to the canister and into the breathing bag. They then pass from the breathing bag upward through the second canister and into the inhalation tube (Fig. 21A), (Fig. 21B).
2. The bulk of the carbon dioxide is absorbed by the first canister. No carbon dioxide filters through into the bag when the charge is fresh.
3. As the absorbent becomes exhausted increasing amounts of carbon dioxide gradually pass into breathing bag, but these are filtered by the second canister.

Procedure

1. Use the inlet canister (#1) until all the charge in the indicator has changed color from top to bottom (Fig. 21A).
2. Discard this charge and refill canister with fresh soda lime.
3. Shift partly exhausted canister (#2) to position which has been occupied by exhausted canister on outlet side.
4. Place freshly charged canister on the inhalation side which has just been occupied by the partly exhausted canister.
5. Repeat. Use canister on exhale side until exhausted and shift once again.

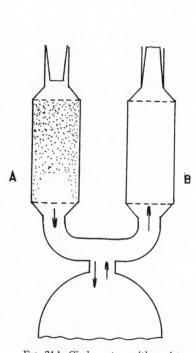

FIG. 21A. Circle system with canisters in series. The charge in canister 1 (left) in position A is used until indicator dye changes color throughout the charge. At this point charge in canister 2 (right) is only partly exhausted. Canister 2 is placed in position A and canister 1 is replenished and placed in position B and used until indicator changes color. Partly used 1 is returned to position A and refilled 2 to position B. Gases are filtered on inspiration and expiration.

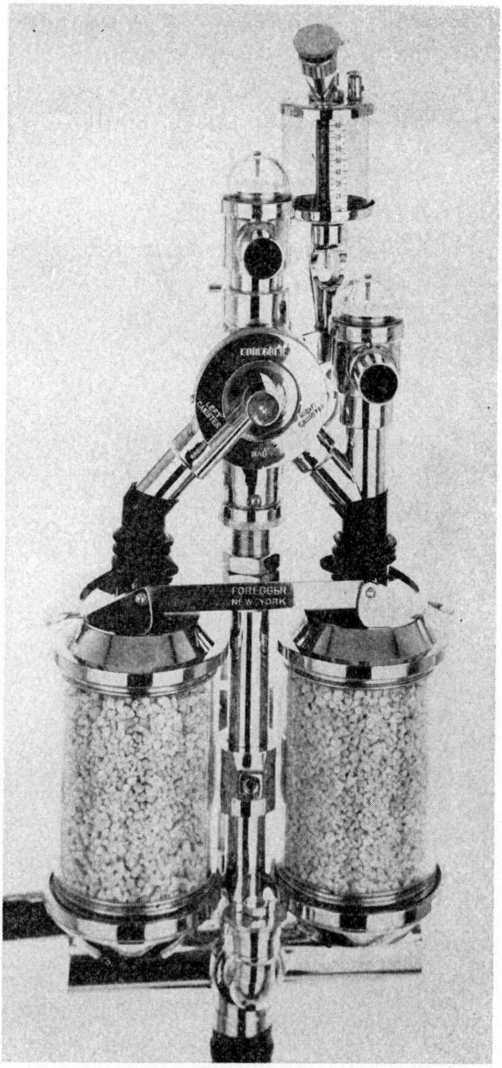

FIG. 21B. Adriani filter using canisters in series. Traces of unabsorbed CO_2 passing into breathing bag on expiration are absorbed during inspiration by second canister. See legend 21C.

Comment	*Reason*
1. Process goes on ad infinitum without any carbon dioxide filtering through to the patient.	The second canister absorbs all unfiltered carbon dioxide coming from the first canister.
2. Permits using the indicator which heretofore was of no service.	Physiological end point and chemical end point do not coincide when single canister is used.
3. Set selector valve (on Adriani	Gases pass from patient through

filter) in left hand (exhale) position and leave there permanently.   left hand side canister and back up right hand side from breathing bag.

4. Fill canisters and pack tightly.   Tight packing prevents channeling.

Advantages

1. Permits use of smaller canisters which in turn reduce resistance.
2. All of alkalai completely utilized.
3. Canisters can be quickly interchanged during the operation if necessary.

Circle Filter—Divided Canisters

Principle

1. The absorbent at the inlet portion of a canister is totally exhausted before that in the outlet portion is neutralized. This lower portion of the charge would be wasted if rejected (Fig. 21C, 21D, 21E).
2. Carbon dioxide in traces begins to filter through before the charge is absorbed giving rise to varying degrees of hypercarbia.
3. By increasing the size of the canister to 1800 or 2000 grams of soda lime capacity and dividing the canister into two sections, the inlet half can be discarded and refilled with fresh absorbent when it becomes exhausted.
4. The partially exhausted lower half of the charge is moved up to the inlet and the recharged half is placed below at the outlet.

Procedure

1. Use charge until indicator in upper half has completely changed color and there is no change or slight change in lower half.
2. Remove upper half of the canister. Discard soda lime and refill.
3. Move partly exhausted half to upper space (position 1).
4. Replace replenished half in lower space (position 2).

Advantages of Divided Canisters

1. Permits complete utilization of absorbent.
2. Permits complete removal of carbon dioxide at all times.
3. Permits long use of canister without frequent changes at inopportune times.
4. Permits utilization of indicators.

Disadvantages

1. Construction of canisters with gaskets at dividing points favors development of leaks.
2. Some increase in resistance occurs from large bulk of alkali.
3. Not sanitary. Many more patients exhale into a given charge.
4. Settling in each canister creates space between absorbent in canister 1 and 2.

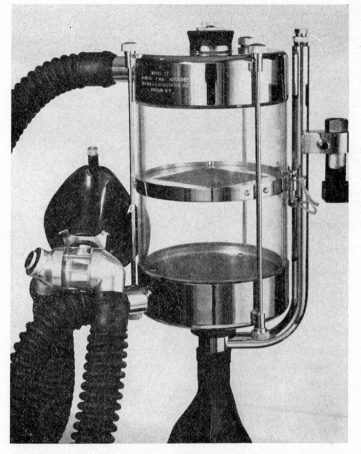

Fig. 21C. The Roswell Park circle filter employs divided canisters.

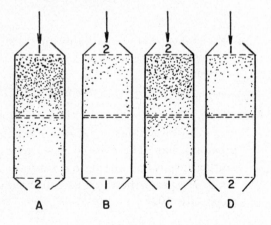

Fig. 21D. The alkali in the absorbent may be utilized to its fullest extent in the circle filter by dividing the canister into two sections. Absorbent in upper section (1) is terminally exhausted as evidenced by change in color of indicator while that in lower half (2) is partly exhausted. (A) Absorbent is utilized to its fullest extent by shifting lower section 2 to upper position and recharging section 1 and placing in lower position (B). Absorbent in section 2 changes color when terminally exhausted, but that in 1 is only partly used (C). Section 2 is replaced by 1 and 2 is recharged (D). The process is carried on ad infinitum.

5. Canister unwieldy and large.
6. Large quantity of absorbent may become impregnated with vapors, such as those of ether.

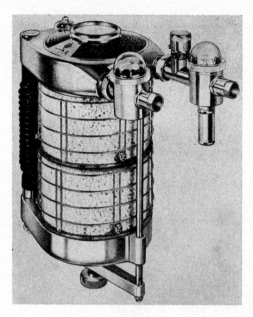

FIG. 21E. Divided canister for circle filter. Design of Ohio Chemical Company.

7. The charge is difficult to replenish during operation.
8. Water condenses at lower portion of absorbent at bottom of canister which may lead to caking.

Comment

1. Process goes on ad infinitum without any carbon dioxide filtering through.	Fresh absorbent in lower canister filters traces which come through.
2. Takes advantage of indicator.	Indicator of no benefit in small single canister because physiological and chemical end points do not coincide.
3. Pack canisters tightly.	Channeling may occur and gases will seep through without being absorbed.
4. Resistance not remarkably increased by large volume of absorbent.	Most of the resistance due to valves.

To and Fro Filter

Description: The to and fro filter consists of a mask which slips into the inlet of a cylindrical canister. The canister in turn slips into the inlet of the breathing bag. The exhaled gases pass over the soda lime to the bag. During inspiration the flow is reversed and the gases pass from bag to mask. The gases, therefore, pass over the absorbent twice (Figs. 22 and 23, pages 101, 102).

Features:

1. All have a face piece, interchangeable canister, and interchangeable bag with an inlet nipple for gases and vapors (simplest).

2. Some possess an exhalation valve at the slip joint on the face piece or the bag or canister which allows their conversion to a semi-closed inhaler if desired (Fig. 22).

3. Some may possess an obturator at the face piece which prevents loss of gases during intubations, insertion of airways, etc (Fig. 22).

4. Some may have an ether vaporizer, usually of the dropper type, interposed between the face piece and the canister, or the bag and canister (Fig. 22).

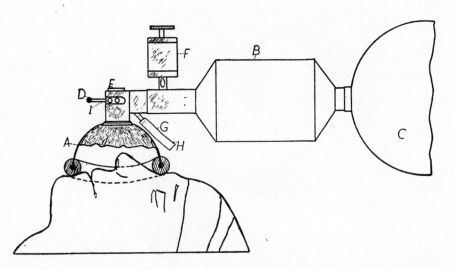

FIG. 22. To and fro inhaler composed of (A) a face piece (B) a canister and (C) a breathing bag. The unit is complete with (D) the obturator which allows the mask to be closed from the remainder of the inhaler. (E) an adjustable exhalation valve and (F) a vaporizer of the dropper type are also provided. Gases are admitted into the inhaler through the (G) inlet attached to (H) the delivery tube. The patient breathes room air through the (I) vents when obturator is turned on and the inhaler is closed from the mask.

Canister Sizes: Canisters are usually cylindrical, brass containers with wide inlets averaging 2.5 cms. (Fig. 23). They vary in size as follows:

1. 8×13 cms. (capacity 500–550 gm.). For adult subjects whose tidal volume averages 500 cc. The inter- and intra-granular air space in the canister, when charged by 4-8 mesh soda lime, averages 425 cc.

2. 7×12 cms. (capacity (350–400 gm.). For young adults and subjects whose tidal volume approximates 350 cc.

3. 6×8 cms. (capacity 250–275 gm.). For children and subjects whose tidal volume ranges between 100–200 cc.

Technique:

1. Choose the canister of proper size for patient to be anesthetized. The size depends upon the tidal volume of the patient.

2. Place a pillow approximately 3″ thick under the occiput. No other form of support works satisfactorily.
3. Blow the dust from the absorbent as follows: Hold the palm of the hand tightly over the outlet and blow into inlet of canister. Suddenly release palm. Repeat several times.
4. Apply the mask of the inhaler in the usual manner and hold with left hand. Support the canister in the right.
5. Induce anesthesia in desired manner. As soon as canister is inserted

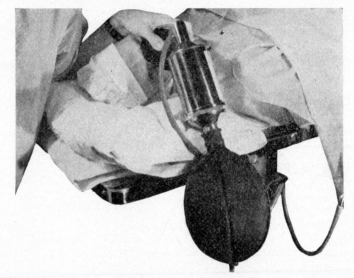

Fig. 23. The satisfactory management of the to and fro inhaler requires that the head be supported upon a pillow and inclined to the right. The end of the canister rests upon the edge of the pillow and the bag remains alongside the operating table.

tilt head towards right side so that the canister end rests on pillow and bag hangs over the right side of operating table (Fig. 23).

Advantages of the To and Fro Filter:

1. Gases pass over the absorbent twice—during inspiration and during expiration. The efficiency of absorption is thereby increased.
2. Resistance to respiration is low (2.5–3 mm. H_2O).
3. The apparatus is relatively simple because it consists of so few parts. It is difficult to derange.
4. Cross infection is minimized because the parts are easily cleansed.
5. Carbon dioxide is quickly removed (45 to 60 seconds) when the filter is introduced into the inhaler after the patient has been rebreathing without it.

Disadvantages:

1. Inspired gases may be warmed above body temperature (37°–41° C. as a rule).

2. Alkaline dust from the absorbent may be inhaled because the filter is next to the face piece. The dust causes severe irritation to the respiratory tract.
3. A snug fit of face piece is frequently difficult to secure and maintain.
4. The apparatus is in the operative field in operations about head or neck.
5. As the charge becomes exhausted, the space at the mask end of the canister acts as a "dead space." This "dead space" is quite pronounced if a large canister is employed when the tidal volume is low.

Comment	*Reasons*
1. Do not drop canisters.	The canister develops leaks at the joints and seams.
2. Do not prop canisters with pads, towels, etc.	Improperly balanced canisters cause leaks about the face piece.
3. Replace the canister with a fresh one approximately every hour even though absorption is proceeding satisfactorily.	This prevents overheating of gases. Temperature in mask rises to 39–41°C., at the end of an hour.
4. Do not wet or moisten soda lime.	The porosity of the granules is disturbed and resistance to respiration is increased by wetting.
5. Always have a freshly charged canister in reserve.	The "used" canister may suddenly become exhausted.
6. Always pack canisters tightly.	Fragmentation of the granules and dust formation is thereby minimized. "Channeling" is also prevented.
7. When filling canisters, screen the absorbent if it appears dusty or fragmented.	The dust is difficult to remove completely by blowing out the canister if the amount is excessive

Clinical Use of Carbon Dioxide Absorption

The filter should be in use during induction and maintenance of all types of anesthesia and particularly in the following circumstances:

Circumstance	*Reasons*
1. Diabetes, nephritis, or acidosis from any cause.	Carbon dioxide enhances acidosis and should not be allowed to accumulate in the inhaler.
2. Cardiac disease.	Carbon dioxide causes circulatory disturbances, enhances arrythmias, and increases the respiratory effort.
3. Hypertension.	Carbon dioxide excess causes an elevation of blood pressure due to stimulation of the vasomotor center.

4. Thoracic surgery, respiratory obstruction, dyspnoea, and cyanosis.

Carbon dioxide excess may disturb the central control of respiration. It stimulates the respiratory center and increases the amplitude of respiration.

5. Fever or high metabolic rate.

The output of carbon dioxide is above normal in these subjects and an excess may rapidly accumulate in the inhaler if rebreathing is tolerated.

6. Cyclopropane anesthesia.

Hyperpnea is not necessary to facilitate induction. It may contribute to the elevation of blood pressure often observed with this drug.

7. Anesthesia for children.

Children appear to be more susceptible to effects of excess carbon dioxide than adults.

8. Administration of oxygen during spinal anesthesia and other similar circumstances.

The respiratory effort is increased and movements of the diaphragm interfere with the work of the surgeon.

Comment

1. The filter should be turned on slowly and gradually if carbon dioxide is allowed to accumulate during induction of anesthesia.

2. Always record the time a charge of soda lime is used at the end of each case (Fig. 24).

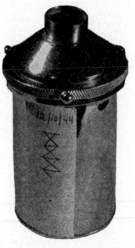

Fig. 24. Marking the time sode lime has been used to filter carbon dioxide. Each X indicates one hour's use. Each portion of the X indicates one quarter hour or fraction thereof.

Reasons

Carbon dioxide possesses anesthetic properties. Patient may "lighten" and often cough if it is removed too rapidly if patient is not deep.

The record provides an index of the state of the absorbent so that long operations will not be started with almost completely exhausted canister.

REFERENCE

Adriani, J. The Chemistry and Physics of Anesthesia, Chapter V. Charles C Thomas, Publisher, Springfield, Ill., 1962.

Cleansing Equipment

Contaminated parts of anesthetic apparatus include: face masks, connectors, airways, endotracheal tubes, laryngoscope blades, suction catheters, delivery tubes, breathing bags, breathing valves, cannisters, slip-joints, vaporization bottles and mask retainers. They should be removed and cleansed and sterilized.

Procedure

1. In routine cases remove parts to be cleansed and wash with soap and hot water. Sterilize as follows:
   (a) Metal objects—by autoclaving.
   (b) Endotracheal catheters and other rubber objects—immerse in 70% alcohol or 1-1000 Zephrian or 1-1000 mercuric chloride for 12 hours.
2. In heavily contaminated or contagious cases immerse all parts in Wescodyne solution (a detergent-iodine complex) composed of $\frac{1}{2}$ oz. to one gallon of water. Allow to remain immersed in this solution at least 5 minutes. Scrub and rinse with tap water.

Comment

1. Wescodyne is both bactericidal and virucidal being lethal to all resistent organisms including the tubercle bacilli.
2. Moisten all parts by immersing in cleaning solution or water to prevent drying of secretions and formation of crusts.
3. Use Wescodyne if pathogenic bacteria are present for the scrubbing process in order to protect personnel.
4. Clean and scrub lumena of endotracheal, pharyngeal and nasal airways with malleable (test tube type) brushes.
5. Wash metal suction tips by forcing water under pressure through them. Wash with soap and water and rinse.
6. Remove adhesive and oily lubicants from parts with ether or other solvent.
7. Hang breathing tubes and rubber bags in dependent position to drain and dry after rinsing with water.
8. Cleanse exposed parts of the anesthesia machine with 70% alcohol, Wescodyne or other solution known to be lethal to bacteria.
9. Store catheters, masks, airways, etc., in sterile towels or sterile plastic bags or tubes.
10. Perishable items not sterilizable by heat are effectively handled in chemical (ethylene oxide) sterilizer. Entire machine or filter and tubes may be sterilized by this method.

B. TECHNIQUES OF INHALATION ANESTHESIA

PREOPERATIVE INTERVIEW OF PATIENT

1. Note psychic make-up of patient. Explain in non-technical terms, details of anesthetic procedure which appear to be pertinent to make patient at ease. Explain plans of anesthesia such as medication, type of drug to be used, reaction afterward.
2. Acquaint patient with immediate preoperative and postoperative events which he will encounter which will be a new experience.
3. Explain purpose of recovery room and that a delay in returning to the room will ensue because of variable stay in this unit.
4. Determine any particular anxiety patient may have, the reason behind it and reassure him to allay fears.
5. Relay to the surgeon or other proper person any data patient relates which is not necessarily related to anesthesia which other physicians have not obtained in their examination.

PREPARATION FOR INHALATION ANESTHESIA

The anesthetist should complete all preparations for anesthesia well in advance of the operating time to avoid delaying the surgical team.
His duty is to:

1. Assemble all necessary equipment and to be positive that the following details are in order:
   a. Each cylinder on the machine should contain an adequate supply of gas.
   b. The reserve oxygen cylinder should be full.
   c. The inhaler should be complete in all its parts and there should be no leaks.
   d. An adequate supply of each anesthetic agent or gas should be on the machine or within immediate reach.
   e. The soda lime should be fresh or, if only partially exhausted, a freshly charged reserve canister should be available.
   f. The desired type of artificial airway should be within reach.
   g. The suction apparatus should be in working order and available for instant use.
2. Examine the chart, check the identity of patient, contemplated operation, signature for permission for operation, report of the examination of the heart and lungs, urine report, and whether or not premedication has been given.
3. Arrange the patient, machine, and other equipment as shown in Fig. 25.
4. Remove loose dentures, bridges, and other objects which may cause obstruction to respiration or which might be aspirated.
5. Loosen gown and all bandages or tight dressings on thorax or neck. Remove gown for thoracic operations.

6. Apply blood pressure apparatus and intercoupler to patient.
7. Apply leg strap and wrist cuffs loosely. Fasten them at time of induction, but not so tightly as to embarrass circulation in the extremities.
8. Dim glaring lights and turn off those which are directed toward the patient. Talking and loud noises should be avoided until patient is anesthetized.
9. Request an attendant, nurse, or a member of the surgical team to remain in the anesthetic room during the induction period.

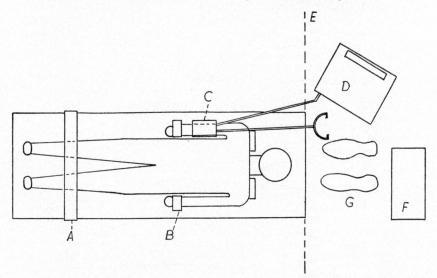

FIG. 25. General arrangement of the patient and anesthesia apparatus. The patient is placed upon the table in the center of its long axis. The (A) strap is adjusted above the knees. The arms are secured by means of (B) wrist cuffs. The (C) blood pressure apparatus is adjusted to the right arm. The (D) anesthesia apparatus is placed on the right side beyond the line of the (E) end of the table. (F) Suction apparatus is within ready reach of the (G) anesthetist.

Comment

1. Do not anesthetize patients on stretchers, rollers, in bed, or in situations in which one cannot cope with emergencies instantly.

2. Do not anesthetize patients in the operating room if special anesthesia rooms are available.

3. Do not anesthetize any patient who does not have properly applied restraints.

4. Do not anesthetize any patient unless an attendant is present as an assistant.

Reasons

The "head down" position so necessary in the event of emesis is difficult to secure on rollers or in bed. Fire hazards are usually greater in such circumstances.

Quiet surroundings contribute to the tranquility of both the anesthetist and patient.

Many patients exhibit remarkable strength during excitement stage and may suffer injury.

The attendant may help restrain the patient. A second person should be present for protection of the anesthetist from a medicolegal standpoint.

TABLE V

TERMINOLOGY FOR POSITIONS OF PATIENTS ON OPERATING TABLE*

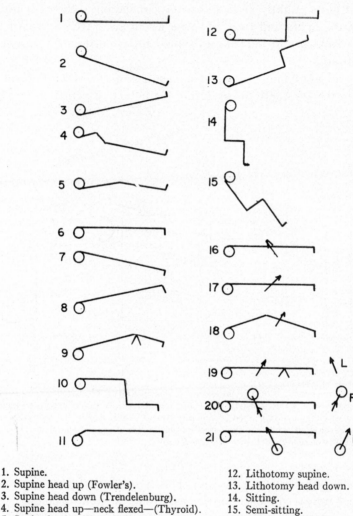

1. Supine.
2. Supine head up (Fowler's).
3. Supine head down (Trendelenburg).
4. Supine head up—neck flexed—(Thyroid).
5. Supine lumbar lift (gall bladder.)
6. Prone.
7. Prone head up.
8. Prone head down.
9. Prone—pelvis lift.
10. Prone—thighs flexed.
11. Prone—head flexed (Cerebellar).

12. Lithotomy supine.
13. Lithotomy head down.
14. Sitting.
15. Semi-sitting.
16. Lateral—left supine.
17. Lateral—right supine.
18. Lateral flexed.
19. Lateral lumbar lifted (Kidney).
20. Lateral left head elevated.
21. Lateral right head down.

* Symbols in diagram above may be used to designate position if desired.

Positioning the Patient

1. The position that least possibly interferes with respiration is the supine.
2. Arms should be along side of the patient. If out on an arm board they should not be abducted beyond 90°.
3. The arms should not hang over the edge of the table otherwise injury to the radial and other nerves may result.

4. When Trendelenburg position is used place knees slightly below break in the table. Lower foot of table and support body by calves.
5. Shoulder braces should be well padded. Do not allow shoulder braces to bend medially, where brachial plexus may be injured.
6. When prone position is used place pads at symphysis, anterior superior spines and shoulders to minimize pressure.
7. Steep Trendelenburg, prone and extreme lithotomy position may cause severe circulatory depression or interference with respiration.
8. Lateral flexion of patient may interfere with adequate ventilation.
9. Elevation of gall bladder bars in the prone or lateral position may cause precipitous drops in blood pressure.
10. Changing from prone to supine position may cause drops in pressure.
11. Blood pressure may fall when legs are lowered from lithotomy position.

Application of Masks and Inhalers

Masks should be snugly applied and firmly held to the face for successful inhalation anesthesia by the closed method. Masks for anesthesia by the drop method are held in the same manner as for the closed system. Consequently, the majority of the remarks below apply to all types of masks.

Procedure	*Reasons*
1. Select a mask which fits the patient's face snugly.	A snug fit is necessary for successful inhalation anesthesia. The mask is the source of 90% of the leaks in the closed system.
2. Center the headband under the occiput. The retaining hooks should be in line with the prongs on the mask.	Leaks result if the mask is not properly applied.
3. Cover the eyes with a thin flat piece of moistened cotton.	This protects the conjunctiva from mask and secretions from the mouth.
4. Ventilate apparatus by filling and emptying the breathing bag several times with oxygen until all odors of previously employed gases or vapors are dispelled.	Extraneous gases or vapors, particularly ether, may cause excitement or coughing.
5. Warn patient as mask is being applied to the face. Allow him to breath through it with obturator closed. Request that patient breathe in a normal manner.	The patient cannot see movements of the anesthetist because he stands behind the patient. Sudden movements and unexpected maneuvers may cause excitement in apprehensive subjects.
6. Grasp the mask in the left hand so that the thumb rests along	This grasp permits distribution of pressure to proper points on face to

margin at its back, the second digit on the front (Fig. 26).

7. Wrap the third, fourth, and fifth digits around the chin, below the mandible, and extend chin so that it points directly upward (Fig. 26).

maintain a snug fit.

This grasp allows traction to be made on the chin to maintain a free airway.

8. Distribute the forearm along the left side of the head and rest elbow on the table (Fig. 23).

The forearm does not become tired in this position.

9. Add 600 or 700 cc. of oxygen or gas mixture to the inhaler and start the flow of mixture.

The patient should never be permitted to breath from an empty inhaler.

10. Explain to the patient that he may feel the mask pressing tightly on his face for a few minutes.

Reassuring the patient establishes confidence in the anesthetist and avoids excitement.

11. Adjust the right strap of the headband to the mask and then the left. *Adjust the right side first.*

Breathing tubes and canister are connected on the right side of the mask. Therefore this side is more difficult to fasten if the left side is fastened first.

12. Turn the head slightly to the right as soon as the patient is in stage III.

a. The "head on the side" position allows mucous and other secretions to gravitate to the side of the mask and not backward.

b. This position is necessary to correctly balance the canister in the to and fro system.

Comment

1. Always select the mask of smallest capacity particularly for children.

Reasons

Minimize "dead space" as much as possible. The tidal volume of children is relatively small. These subjects therefore may rebreathe the contents of a large mask over and over again.

2. The pointed end (narrow) of the mask should be placed over the bridge of the nose.

The wide portion of the mask is intended to fit over the mouth.

3. Hold all masks with the left hand. Never use both hands.

The right hand should remain free for other manipulations.

4. Always wipe the mask dry and be certain it is free from odors before applying it to the patient's face.

Wet masks are uncomfortable and annoy the patient. They may contribute to the formation of pressure marks.

5. If a patient is extremely apprehensive, hold mask lightly and touch him as little as possible until he passes into stage III.

Tight feeling of the mask about the face may further stimulate the patient and cause excitement in stage II.

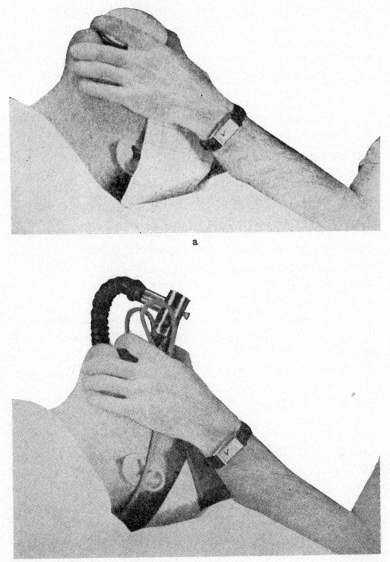

a

b

FIG. 26a and b. Techniques for holding masks. The thumb and index finger of the left hand hold the mask firmly to the face; the remaining three fingers maintain the airway by supporting the chin and jaw. The same technique applies to holding both open and closed masks. Closed masks must be held regardless of the fact that they are secured by head bands. Note that the Yankauer mask in Fig. 26a is entirely open and the gauze trimmed to fit the edges. Towels and superfluous gauze contribute to the obstruction to respiration.

6. In edentulate persons, insert the pharyngeal airway, then pad cheeks with a gauze pack in each side of the mouth.

The mask may be applied more satisfactorily if the cheeks and angles of mouth bulge outward.

7. During long operations, loosen the mask at least once every hour.

Tight headbands frequently interfere with the circulation to the forehead and scalp.

8. At termination of anesthesia, re-

It may become soiled if post anes-

move the headband from beneath the occiput as soon as the mask is disconnected.

thetic emesis occurs.

9. Do not clean masks (or other rubber appliances) with lysol, creosol, or other necrotizing disinfectants.

The chemical soaks into the rubber and may burn the face.

Judging Depth of Inhalation General Anesthesia

Anesthesia affects all the physiological systems of the body to some degree. However, the anesthetist relies chiefly upon certain physical signs and symptoms in the following three systems as guides to the status of the patient and depth of narcosis:

1. The central nervous system: The behavior of superficial and deep reflexes and muscle tone are observed. The eyes, because they are accessible and have reflexes which undergo graded changes, are used as a guide.
   Lid reflex: The presence of voluntary control of the eye lid is noted.
   Ocular motion: Position and movements of the eye balls in response to stimulation by light are noted.
   Pupillary change: Size and response to light are observed.
2. The respiratory system: Respiratory rate, tidal volume, character of inspiration and expiration, and intercostal and diaphragmatic activity are observed continuously.
3. The circulatory system: Rate and volume of pulse and variations in blood pressure are noted at intervals (see page 51).

Inhalation General Anesthesia Is Divided into Four Stages

Stage I. Analgesia: From the beginning of the administration of anesthesia to the beginning of loss of consciousness. Use of this stage is limited to obstetrics, dental extractions, and other superficial operations.

Stage II. Delirium: From the loss of consciousness to the loss of the lid reflex. This stage is of brief duration and is often unnoticed in well premedicated subjects. It may be of long duration and accompanied by marked excitement in apprehensive, unpremedicated subjects, and alcohol addicts. No well demarcated line of transition exists between stages I and II.

Stage III. Surgical: From the loss of lid reflex to cessation of respiratory efforts. This lack of respiratory effort must be due to the effect of the drug. Surgery is performed in this stage. The zone is wide and for the sake of convenience is divided into four strata called planes.*

Stage IV. Overdosage: From cessation of respiratory efforts to circulatory failure. Death supervenes unless artificial respiration is instituted immediately to supply oxygen and remove the excess drug from the alveoli and blood.

* Indicate stages by Roman numerals and planes by Arabic numerals: Thus the fourth plane of third stage is stage III, plane 4.

Signs in the Three Systems

	Nervous System	Respiratory System	Circulatory System
First Stage	1. Reflexes remain active, but sensation to pain is diminished or lost. 2. No changes occur in eye reflexes, ocular movements, or pupillary size. 3. Muscle tone is unchanged. 4. The subject remains conscious and aware of his surroundings.	1. Normal—No change occurs in rate or amplitude of respiratory movements.	1. No change occurs in the rate or character of the pulse. 2. Blood pressure is not changed if subject is not apprehensive.
Second Stage	1. The cerebral cortex is depressed and consciousness is gradually lost. 2. Muscle tone increases and rigidity usually appears. 3. Superficial reflexes are active, and may be exaggerated or hyperactive (react to stimulation of skin). 4. Excitement, as characterized by semi-voluntary struggling, singing, crying, loud talking. It may appear or be precipitated by stimuli on touching the patient. 5. Pupils may dilate, react to light and possess a regular outline. 6. Eyeball movements remain active, but voluntary control gradually disappears. Occasionally, pupils are eccentrically placed. 7. Voluntary control of lid is retained (when lid is touched, patient closes eye voluntarily). 8. Ability to vomit, cough, and swallow persists.	1. Respiratory rate and rhythm are irregular. Apprehensive subjects may breathe deeply or hold their breath. Acapnia from deep breathing may produce brief periods of apnea. 2. Intercostal muscles and diaphragm remain active.	1. Blood pressure may rise from excitement. 2. Pulse rate increases due to excitement and probable sympathetic stimulation.
Third Stage Plane 1	1. "Lid reflex" is inactive (tone as well as voluntary control of the lid disappears). 2. Superficial reflexes are obtunded (active stimulation of the skin). 3. Eyeballs are active. When the lids are lifted, both move synchronously in a horizontal plane (occasionally motion may be vertical). The motion is preceded by a latent period of inactivity of several seconds. The reflex soon becomes obtunded and the motion ceases, but reappears if the lids are closed to exclude light momentarily and then reopened.	1. Respiratory rhythm becomes regular and automatic. 2. Amplitude remains unchanged with some drugs (ether). 3. Intercostal muscles are active. 4. Full diaphragmatic activity is present. 5. Inspiration and expiration are of approximately equal duration. The thorax expands as diaphragm expands.	1. Blood pressure and pulse rate gradually return to preanesthetic levels from relief of excitement, unless altered by other factors such as anoxia, carbon dioxide excess, premedication, trauma, etc.

Signs in the Three Systems—(Cont.)

	Nervous System	Respiratory System	Circulatory System
	4. Pupils revert to preanesthetic size. 5. The reflex in the pharynx disappears, and the patient usually tolerates a pharyngeal or nasal airway without retching, coughing, or swallowing. 6. Muscle tone decreases but relaxation is not sufficient for abdominal surgery.		
Plane 2	1. Eyeballs become progressively less active and finally are centrally fixed as the lower border of this plane is attained. 2. There is a slight increase in size of pupils as compared to plane 1. 3. Corneal reflex is gradually obtunded. 4. Laryngeal (glottic) reflex disappears or is obtunded. 5. Muscle tone decreases and relaxation is improved.	1. Intercostal muscles are still active. 2. Inspiration is quickened, expiration slightly prolonged. 3. Interrespiratory pause is lengthened. 4. Thorax still expands as diaphragm contracts.	1. No noteworthy change occurs in blood pressure or pulse rate, unless modified by other factors such as trauma, shock, hypercapnia, etc.
Plane 3	1. Eyeballs remain fixed as in plane 2. Dilatation of pupils is more pronounced. Light reflex becomes progressively obtunded. 2. Muscle tone is decreased markedly. Relaxation of abdominal muscles is usually sufficient for surgery.	1. Intercostal muscles are paralyzed progressively from above downward. 2. Rocking motion of the thorax gradually becomes apparent. 3. Inspiration is quickened, expiration prolonged more than in plane 2. 4. Interrespiratory pause is prolonged further. 5. Thorax and intercostal muscles may retract as diaphragm contracts.	1. No alteration in either blood pressure or pulse rate occurs unless modified by other factors such as trauma, shock, anoxia etc.
Plane 4	1. Eyeballs remain centrally fixed. 2. Pupils dilate widely, become irregular, and do not react to light. Conjunctiva may have a glassy appearance. 3. Flaccidity of muscles and other tissues occurs. 4. Bronchial reflexes obtunded.	1. Respiration is maintained almost entirely by the diaphragm. It may be characterized by a gasping type inspiration, prolonged period of expiration and a long pause at end of expiration. 2. Decreased ventilation may cause cyanosis.	1. Blood pressure decreases. 2. Pulse pressure decreases. 3. Pulse rate increases, volume decreases.
Fourth Stage	1. There is absence of all reflex activity. 2. There is complete flaccidity of tissues. 3. Pupils are widely dilated. 4. Sphincters are relaxed.	1. Failure of respiratory movements is due to medullary depression. 2. Cyanosis is frequently but not always observed.	1. Circulatory failure follows respiratory failure unless artificial respiration is instituted.

The above table merely serves as a general guide to the depth of anesthesia by currently employed inhalation anesthetics drugs. Variations occur with each agent or in using the same agent and another technique of administration. These are described under the discussion of individual techniques. Variations frequently occur in different individuals. However a certain group of signs persist for a particular individual throughout anesthesia. The following factors may cause considerable modification of many of these signs.

Anoxia: Dilatation of pupils, vomiting, rigidity of muscles, and an elevation of blood pressure are common sequelae.

Respiratory Obstruction: The character of respiratory movements, intercostal and diaphragmatic activity are altered.

Hypercapnia: Character of respiration is modified by the accompanying hyperpnoea or respiratory depression. Elevation of blood pressure invariably occurs.

Increased Intracranial Pressure: Pupillary signs are modified. Eye reflexes, pharyngeal and laryngeal reflexes are frequently obtunded.

Reflex Stimulation: Traction reflexes may contribute to laryngeal spasm, coughing, retching.

Age of the Patient: Pupillary activity decreases with age and is often not a reliable guide after the fifth decade. Pupillary size is subject to greater variation in children. Reflex activity decreases with age.

Status of Patient: Reflexes persist for a longer period in robust subjects than in the weak and infirm. Frequently, they are obtunded in debilitated, comatose, or cachectic subjects.

Non-Volatile Drugs: Superficial and deep reflexes are obtunded as a rule by non-volatile drugs. Ocular reflexes and movements are unreliable when drugs such as avertin, pentothal and barbiturates of a similar type are employed for narcosis or as the sole agent.

Comment

1. Size of pupils is not always a reliable guide to depth of anesthesia, and is of little significance in stage III unless they are dilated.

2. Signs often reappear in different sequence in the ascent from stage IV to I during recovery, than in the descent from stage I to IV.

3. The patient should not be prepared, moved, or disturbed in any manner before the lid reflex disappears (patient is in stage III).

Reasons

Pupillary size is modified by the opium and belladonna alkaloids employed for premedication. The effects of the combination are unpredictable.

Certain signs, therefore, may not be reliable guides to changes in depth during maintenance of anesthesia.

Avoid excitement as struggling may ensue under such circumstances if stage II has not been traversed.

4. Tilt the mask forward and away from the eyes when observing pupillary and other eye reflexes.

The pressure on the eyes, which may obscure the signs, is thus released without loss of mixture from the inhalator.

5. Examine both eyes simultaneously in studying ocular movements and reflexes.

Although eyes oscillate synchronously in stage III they may not always do so in other stages.

6. When doubt exists regarding activity of ocular signs allow the eyes to close momentarily to exclude light and then reexamine them.

The oscillation reflex "wears off" after lengthy exposure to light, but reappears after a few seconds rest in the absence of light.

7. Never judge depth of anesthesia by determining the activity of the corneal reflex.

Ulceration often results from even the gentlest stimulation of the cornea.

8. Cyanosis or "color" should never be an index of depth of anesthesia.

Cyanosis merely indicates anoxemia. It may appear during light or deep anesthesia.

9. When several signs are characteristic of a certain plane they do not necessarily appear simultaneously or with equal rapidity.

Signs vary in onset according to the mechanism which produces them and the degree of saturation of tissues by the agent employed.

Depths of Anesthesia Desired for Various Types of Surgery

1st plane: Incision and drainages of superficial abscesses, superficial operations on skin, plastic surgery, suture of tendons of small muscles, mastectomy, mastoidectomy, thyroidectomy, craniotomy, reduction of fractures of small bones, and normal obstetrics.

2nd plane: Surgery of the large bones, gynecological, urological, and perineal operations, tonsillectomy and other pharyngeal surgery, thoracic surgery, hernioplasties, amputations, laminectomies, operative obstetrics, lower abdominal and eye surgery.

3rd plane: Upper abdominal surgery, ventral hernioplasties, rectal surgery, intratracheal and intra-laryngeal surgery, obstetrical surgery requiring relaxation of the uterus.

4th plane: Not employed under any circumstances.

USE OF THE ELECTROENCEPHALOGRAM TO DETERMINE DEPTH OF ANESTHESIA

Basic Principles

The brain produces electrical activity quantitatively measurable in terms of potential (volts). The Electroencephalogram (E.E.G.) is a graphic record of the sum of the voltages developed by individual neurons in a particular area of the cerebral cortex. Usually the activity of an area of the cortex is measured. The current is of such small magnitude that it is measured in microvolts (millionths of a volt). The minute electrical impulses pass through the intact skull, through the scalp, and are gathered by a pair of electrodes. They then are conducted through amplifiers which magnify the current millions of times. The amplified current operates a system of levers which records variations in intensity of current graphically on a moving roll of paper with ink-writers. The current rises from zero to a maximum and then reverts back to zero many times per second. The resulting tracing consists of waves called *cycles*. The height (amplitude) of wave is governed by the voltage developed. The number of waves (frequency, also cycles) varies with different stages of activity of the neurons.

Normal Patterns

Normally in unanesthetized patients three wave patterns are noted.
(1) Alpha (awake with eyes closed)—about 10 cycles per second, 50 millivolts—obtained from occipital areas.
(2) Beta—20 to 50 cycles per second, 5–10 millivolts.
(3) Delta—1 to 5 cycles per second, voltage increased 20 to 200 microvolts—occurs in sleep and in pathologic states in awake persons.

Characteristic Modifications Caused by Anesthesia

The cortical potentials are altered (suppressed) by central nervous system depressants. The suppression becomes more marked as depression increases. The suppression is proportional to the quantity of drug in the brain.

The changes produced have the following characteristics:
(1) Are reproductible for a given drug in a given patient.
(2) Vary little from person to person for a given drug.
(3) The discharge is serial—it disappears and reappears in same manner as the concentration is varied.
(4) The response is rapid and occurs on a moment to moment basis.
(5) Clinical signs of reflex activity (Guedel) lag behind cortical activity.
(6) The brain discharges as a unit. Local differences from one area of the cortex to the next disappear and synchronization of activity of the cortex appears.
(7) The rhythm simplified. It is the same in all areas.
(8) The stages of depression are correlated with blood concentration (volatile drugs).
(9) Applicable to techniques using volatile, non-volatile or combinations of volatile and non-volatile drugs.

Basic Charges in Pattern During Anesthesia

Certain basic changes in pattern are common to the majority of drugs. These are: (Fig. 26A)

(1) An increase in frequency up to 20–30 cycles per second. No change in voltage (as consciousness is lost).

(2) The small, rapid waves are replaced by larger (5–300 microvolts) waves at slower rhythm (1–5 cycles per second) as consciousness is lost.

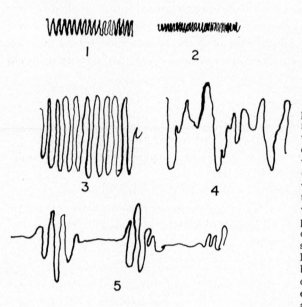

FIG. 26A (1) (See text.) Awake pattern 18-13 cps.—50 or less microvolts. (2) Fast frequency-low voltage. Activity of 20–30 cps. (loss of consciousness) and 20 microvolts or less. (3) Slower frequency (4-8 cps.), rhythmical, increased voltage (100–200 u.v.) (light anesthesia). (4) Mixed pattern, low voltage, fast frequency, superimposed on high voltage, low frequency. (5) Periods of inactivity separated by periods of activity of less than 3 seconds. Referred to as burst suppression (moderate depth). (6) Periods of inactivity exceeding three seconds (deep anesthesia).

(3) Fast low voltage waves appear and become superimposed on a background of high voltage, low frequency waves. This pattern is known as a *mixed pattern*.

(4) The voltage decreases and the frequency decreases. Periods of inactivity are interposed between periods of activity. The periods of activity separated by inactivity are called *burst suppression*. The interval of inactivity becomes longer and number of waves in the active phases decreases as anesthesia deepens.

(5) A complete loss of activity appears. A flat tracing of low voltage and very slow rhythm appears. This occurs in overdosage.

Uses of the Electroencephalogram for Anesthesia

(1) During whole body perfusion to detect adequacy of cerebral perfusion.

(2) To assess cerebral damage after anesthetic accidents (cardiac arrest).

(3) To detect changes in cortical activity during hypothermia.

(4) To detect changes in depth of anesthesia when other methods are not feasible.

(5) For use in clinical and laboratory study of new agents.

Technical Difficulties

The electroencephalogram is not wholly practical because of technical difficulties. Satisfactory results not obtained because the current is amplified a million or more times and interference from power lines produce strong potentials and cause artefacts or obliterate the cortical pattern. Some of the difficulties encountered are:

(1) Movements of electrodes.

(2) Improper placement of the electrodes (one is usually placed in midline and one over occipital region).

(3) Mechanical defects of apparatus.

(4) Sixty cycle interference caused by "house" current.

(5) Electrical activity due to muscular movements of patient are picked up by the electrodes and obliterate the basic pattern.

(6) Movement of the patient causes extraneous electrical activity.

(7) Movement of the cables causes variations in potential.

(8) Cardiac current is superimposed and amplified to produce artefacts.

Variations in Pattern Noted with Individual Agents

I. VOLATILE ANESTHETICS

A. Gases

Nitrous Oxide—70% N_2O—30% O_2 produces wave forms of 5–70 cycles per second and increased amplitude. Waking frequencies are replaced by slow waves 2–4 cycles per second and an increase in amplitude up to 40 to 70 microvolts. Burst suppression does not occur.

Ethylene—Suppression similar to nitrous oxide.

Cyclopropane—Six levels of activity. The first five are similar to those of ether (see below). Amplitude is less. In Level VI a flat line results instead of waves.

B. Liquids

Ether—Seven levels are described.

Level I—The alpha waves are converted to a low amplitude wave form of approximately 30 microvolts with an increased frequency of 20–30 cycles per second (lasts 7 minutes).

Level II—An abrupt appearance of slow waves 2–8 cycles per second of high amplitude (200–300 microvolts). (This lasts about 60 seconds).

Level III—The rhythmicity is lost and a mixed pattern appears.

The slow waves of high voltage are superimposed by faster waves of decreased amplitude. No evidence of suppression.

Level IV—Burst suppression appears. Periods of inactivity are of maximum duration of 3 seconds. The wave frequency is 2–4 cycles per second. Average amplitude is 150 microvolts.

Level V—The suppression time is increased to 3–10 seconds. The intervening waves are single and of smaller amplitude.

Level VI—The activity is reduced to less than 1 per 10 seconds. An irregular amplitude of about 70 microvolts appears.

Level VII—Complete suppression occurs. The activity is less than 20 microvolts. Waves are absent.

Divinyl Ether (*Vinethene*)—Classification of levels not available in humans.

Trifluoroethyl Vinyl Ether (*Fluoromar*)—Six levels are described.

Level I—The alpha rhythm is replaced by a wave form whose activity is 15–25 cycles per second. The voltage is decreased below 25 microvolts.

Level II—The frequency becomes 4–6 cycles per second. Low voltage up to 50 microvolts appears. Spindles of 6–8 per second appear are superimposed on the fast activity of previous level.

Level III—The fast background activity ceases. The dominant waves increase in voltage and frequency. Regular waves of 3–5 cycles predominate. The amplitude ranges between 75–125 microvolts.

Level IV—Irregular, large slow waves (100–300 microvolts) of 2–4 cycles per second appear.

Level V—The dominant forms are fairly regular. They are of high voltage and of long duration, every 1–2 seconds. Spread of 1 second. Voltage from 100–150 microvolts. Superimposed on faster waves of 3–5 cycles per second in amplitude of 25–75 microvolts.

Level VI—Dominant slow wave frequency disappears to one every 2 seconds. Superimposed waves of 3–5 cycles per second are present. Voltage decreased from 25 to 15 microvolts.

Chloroform—Six levels are described.

Level I—A slow frequency wave pattern of higher amplitude than normal superimposed against fast-low amplitude of background activity.

Level II—A low voltage wave of rapid activity appears.

Level III—A low voltage wave of an activity 20–30 cycles per second is present.

Level IV—Delta type waves appear. Rhythm is slow with a high voltage.

Level V—The 20–30 cycles rhythm ends and the dominant wave is a slow one.

Level VI—A decrease in the amplitude and decrease in frequency appears.

Trichloroethylene with Nitrous Oxide—Three levels are described.

Level I—The amplitude diminishes from that seen in the awake tracing. The frequency is increased as analgesia and unconsciousness ensue.

Level II—Pattern is rhythmic. Large, slow waves of an amplitude of 100–300 microvolts and a frequency 3–5 cycles per second appear.

Level III—The frequency is low and the amplitude is high. The rhythmicity disappears.

Ethyl chloride—Decreased frequency and increased amplitude. No levels have been described.

Halothane (Fluothane)—Seven levels are described.

Level I—The waking wave pattern changes to a fast, low voltage rhythm of 15–20 cycles per second of 10–25 microvolts.

Level II—Slow waves 3–6 cycles per second appear with an amplitude 50 microvolts. Waves of fast, low voltage activity are superimposed on these.

Level III—Slow waves averaging 4 cycles per second appear with an amplitude of 5–100 microvolts. The fast activity disappears.

Level IV—Fast activity has disappeared completely. Slow waves of an amplitude 100–300 microvolts and a frequency 2–3 cycles per second appear. They may be notched and irregular.

Level V—Slow waves 1 cycle per second and an amplitude of 100–200 microvolts appear. Intervening smaller and faster waves of an amplitude of 25–50 microvolts and a frequency 6–8 cycles per second are seen.

Level VI—Slow waves of a frequency of 1 cycle per 2–3 seconds. Upon these are interposed and superimposed waves of 6–8 cycles per second with an amplitude of 25 microvolts. Burst suppression appears.

Level VII—Complete suppression and absence of wave forms are observed.

II. NON-VOLATILE DRUGS

A. Hypnotics

Barbiturates—Sedative doses cause no change.

Thiopental (Pentothal)—Five levels are noted.

Level I—A wave form of high amplitude (75–80 microvolts) and fast frequency 10–30 cycles per second appear. The wave forms are spiked.

Level II—Complex. Composed of slow waves with an irregular contour and random occurrence of frequency ranging from 2 cycles per second and upward and an amplitude of about 150 microvolts. "Spiky" waves with irregular amplitude and frequencies of 10 cycles are superimposed on slow waves.

Level III—Suppression of less than 3 seconds duration appears. Biphasic bursts also appear. The first phase lasts 1 second. The frequency of these is 10 cycles per second. The second phase is of 2 cycles per second merging into the next suppression.

Level IV—A marked suppression lasting 3–10 seconds appears. The activity is similar to that in Level III but less in amplitude.

Level V—The activity occurs every 10 seconds of an amplitude of less than 25 microvolts.

Hydroxydione (Viadril)—Four levels are observed.

Level I—Alpha activity is suppressed. Slow waves 4–5 cycles per second appear. These are of an increased amplitude.

Level II—A compound pattern of 8–12 cycles per second appears. The amplitude is 6–100 microvolts. Superimposed upon these is a pattern of low voltage, fast activity waves with "spiky" contour.

Level III—Burst suppression of several seconds duration appears.

Level IV—Widely spaced bursts of activity of less than 20 microvolts merging into a flat tracing as anesthesia deepens.

B. Narcotics and Premedicants

Morphine—Causes no significant effect in analgesic doses.

Methadon—Causes no significant effect in analgesic doses.

Meperidine—No effects in analgesic doses.

Chlorpromazine—(25 mgm) Fast activity induced by intravenous injection. Oral administration causes no effect. Decreased amount of ether necessary for level IV when this drug is used for premedication.

Atropine—1/100–1/150 grain intravenously causes a decrease in voltage of all waves, followed by burst waves of high voltage at 10 cycles per second. Bursts appear at 10 second intervals and last 1–3 seconds.

C. Analeptics

Bemegride—Causes a revertion of pattern produced by sleep doses of barbiturates to patterns of light narcosis. Used alone causes similar effects as other convulsants.

Levallorphan—Further slowing of frequencies when used with nitrous oxide and meperidine. No reversal of cortical pattern.

Caffeine—Causes no effects.

D. Muscle Relaxants
   Curare—Causes no remarkable effects.
   Erythroidine—Causes no remarkable effects.
   Gallamine (Flaxedil)—Causes no remarkable effects.
   Decamethonium—Causes no remarkable effects.
   Succinyl Choline—Causes no remarkable effects.

E. Anoxic Anoxia—Causes an increase in rate and of amplitude of waves
   followed by pronounced slowing. Then a great increase in amplitude occurs. Finally a decline to a flat tracing appears.
   Stagnant Anoxia—Causes same changes as anoxic anoxia. Inhalation
   of 6–11% oxygen causes small, fast activity within 60 seconds replaced by slow, large waves. Recovery occurs in reverse order.

F. Hypotension—Inadequate cerebral perfusion results in changes
   characteristic of anoxia. A depression of high voltage with fast
   activity occurs as pressure declines. Cortical activity ceases at levels
   of 50 mm. Hg systolic. Vasopressors restore rhythm toward normal.

G. Hypothermia—Usually causes negligible change at 25–28°C. A tendency towards slowing of frequency occurs but not greater than
   25%. Occlusion of circulation results in waves of low voltage and
   fast frequency superimposed on the usual pattern and persisting
   after cessation of lower frequencies. The pattern becomes isoelectric
   for the duration of the occlusion. After release of clamps activity reappears and gradually returns to pre-occlusion level. Low voltage,
   fast frequency activity (file pattern) occurs during recovery from
   occlusion.

H. Hypoglycemia—Cause a decrease in alpha activity which is reversible
   with ingestion of sugar. Insulin coma causes abrupt appearance of
   large, slow waves as consciousness is lost. Severe hypoglycemia
   abolishes cortical activity.

I. Hyperglycemia—Causes no change.

J. Hypercapnia—Suppression of activity. In conjunction with anesthetics the blood concentration necessary to obtain a given level is less
   than if the drug were used alone.

PROCEDURE FOR USE OF THE ELECTROENCEPHALOGRAPH

Description

The electroencephalograph is an apparatus consisting of one or more units
(channels) each of which is composed of:
   1. Two electrodes for attachment to the skin of the scalp (occipital area
   and midline) to collect the current developed by the cerebral cortex.

2. An amplifying circuit relying on an external power source (usually house current or batteries) to amplify the cortical potential a million or more times.
3. A transducer which converts this amplified electrical energy to light which is visible on a screen (Oscilloscope) or to mechanical energy which operates an ink writing lever.
4. A moving paper recorder for scribing a continuous record. Paper is ruled in seconds on horizontal line and microvolts on vertical line.

Comments

1. No specific instructions can be outlined since each apparatus varies with the design of the manufacturer. Instructions of the manufacturer must be followed.
2. One skilled in the basic principles of electroencephalography must interpret tracings, otherwise artefacts may be confused with actual findings and lead to error.
3. The apparatus is not "explosion proof" and must be elevated five feet from the floor and be away from the operating table or in an adjacent room which permits observation through a window.
4. The apparatus is expensive and requires expert attention for maintenance and repairs.

REFERENCES

1. Faulconer, A., Bickford, R. The Electroencephalogram in Anesthesiology. Thomas, Springfield, 1959.
2. Brechner, V., Dillon, J. Clinical Use of the Electroencephalogram in Anesthesiology. Thomas, Springfield. 1962.
3. Adriani, J. Chemistry and Physics of Anesthesia. Pp. 585–590, Thomas, Springfield, 1962.
4. Adriani, J. Pharmacology of Anesthetic Drugs. Pp. 167–169, Thomas, Springfield, 1960.
5. Guedel, A. E. Inhalation Anesthesia. Pp. 15–39. The Macmillan Co., New York, 2nd Ed., 1951.
6. Gillespie, N. A. Signs of Anesthesia—Anesth. & Analg. 22, 275–282, September, 1943.

ETHER ANESTHESIA

Description: Ether is a volatile inflammable liquid whose vapor possesses marked narcotic potency, a pungent odor, and is highly irritating to the mucous membranes.

Uses:

1. For surgery of all types particularly that requiring relaxation of muscles.
2. For fortifying mildly potent anesthetic drugs.
3. As a complemental agent to basal narcosis obtained from drugs such as avertin, various barbiturates, or morphine.

Cost: Relatively inexpensive (approximately 90¢ per lb.).

Concentration:
  (a) For surgical anesthesia: approximately 4% by volume in the alveoli.
  (b) For respiratory failure: approximately 8% by volume in the alveoli.

Premedication: Morphine and scopolamine or morphine and atropine in standard doses.

Methods of Administration:
  1. *By open masks.* With air as a vehicle.
  2. *By semi-open mask.* With air or oxygen as a vehicle.
  3. *By insufflation.* With air or other gases as a vehicle.
  4. *By semi-closed or closed inhaler.* With oxygen or other gases.

Induction of Ether Anesthesia: Induction is prolonged because of the irritating effects of ether (Fig. 27). In order to simplify and shorten the induction period the patient is anesthetized with a non-irritating rapid acting drug. Under this narcosis the anesthetic concentration of ether is attained as rapidly as possible. The first and second stages of ether anesthesia are thereby shortened (Fig. 39).

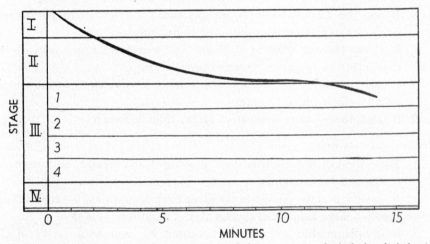

Fig. 27. Curve showing the rate of transition through the stages of anesthesia during the induction period, using ether by the "open drop technique." The high air blood ratio, the irritating qualities and its comparatively high solubility in water are responsible for the prolonged period of induction which ether requires.

The following are some common methods of induction:
  1. Nitrous oxide-oxygen induction, ether vapor and nitrous oxide-oxygen sequence by the semi-closed method.
  2. Nitrous oxide-oxygen induction by semi-closed method, ether-oxygen sequence by the closed method.

3. Ethylene-oxygen induction, ether vapor and ethylene-oxygen sequence by the semi-closed method.

4. Ethylene-oxygen induction, by semi-closed method and ether vapor-oxygen sequence by the closed method.

5. Cyclopropane induction by the closed method; ether-oxygen sequence by the open or closed method.

6. Vinethene induction by the open method, ether vapor sequence by the open method.

7. Ethyl chloride induction, by the open drop method, ether vapor sequence by the open method.

8. Avertin or other types of basal narcosis, followed by any of the above methods of induction and ether sequence.

9. Chloroform induction, ether sequence by either the open or closed methods.

Advantages of Ether:

1. It is a potent agent useful for all types of surgery.
2. It possesses a wide margin of safety.
3. It is relatively inexpensive.
4. It is chemically stable and easily preserved.
5. It may be administered with very simple apparatus if necessary.
6. It may be administered by inexperienced individuals under surveillance of an experienced anesthetist in emergencies.
7. It allows the use of air as a diluent and source of oxygen because the concentration required for anesthesia is low.
8. It does not affect circulation appreciably at the levels of anesthesia usually employed for surgery.
9. It tends to stimulate respiration rather than depress it.

Disadvantages of Ether:

1. The period of induction is slow, prolonged, unpleasant, and often accompanied by excitement.
2. Recovery is slow, particularily after long operations, because tissues absorb a large amount of the agent and desaturation is slow.
3. It is inflammable and therefore cannot be used with safety in the presence of cautery, x-ray units, or nonspark-proof electrical equipment.
4. It is irritating to respiratory passages and causes coughing, secretion of mucus, and salivation.
5. It disturbs important metabolic functions. Liver function, acid-base balance, and carbohydrate metabolism are affected particularly.
6. Nausea common.

Contra-Indications to Ether   *Reasons*

1. Acute or chronic infections of the   Secretions may assist the spread of
   upper or lower portions of the   infection from one portion of the

respiratory tract (pulmonary tuberculosis, active or latent).

respiratory tract to another.

2. Diabetes, or acidosis from any cause.

Elevation of blood sugar and lowering of carbon dioxide combining power accompany anesthesia even though the duration is short.

3. Nephritis; renal insufficiency.

Transient decrease in renal function accompanies and follows anesthesia.

4. Decreased liver function, diseases of the liver, jaundice.

A transient decrease in liver function accompanies and follows anesthesia.

5. Diseases or injuries to the brain accompanied by increased intracranial pressure.

Increased intracranial pressure accompanies anesthesia, particularly in the presence of anoxemia or carbon dioxide excess.

Ether by the Open Drop Method

Principle: Ether is dropped on a gauze held away from nose and mouth of the subject so that it may be readily vaporized, mixed with air, and inhaled.

Uses:

1. For surgery on children and young adults.
2. For anesthesia which must be administered by inexperienced individuals or in the absence of adequate apparatus.
3. As a preliminary to ether by insufflation methods.
4. As a necessity in the event other agents or equipment for their administration are not available or impractical.

Concentration:

1. Surgical anesthesia: approximately 4% by volume in the alveoli.
2. Respiratory failure: approximately 8% by volume in the alveoli.

Premedication:

1. Morphine and scopolamine, or morphine and atropine, in standard doses (see premedication).

Apparatus:

1. Wire mask: Yankauer, Ferguson, or other type (Fig. 28).
2. 6–12 layers of gauze or stockinet to cover mask.
3. Pharyngeal airway of size required for the subject.
4. One eye protector consisting of a piece of rubber-dam to cover both eyes.
5. Mineral or castor oil for eyes (The castor oil must not be rancid).
6. Two surgical towels.

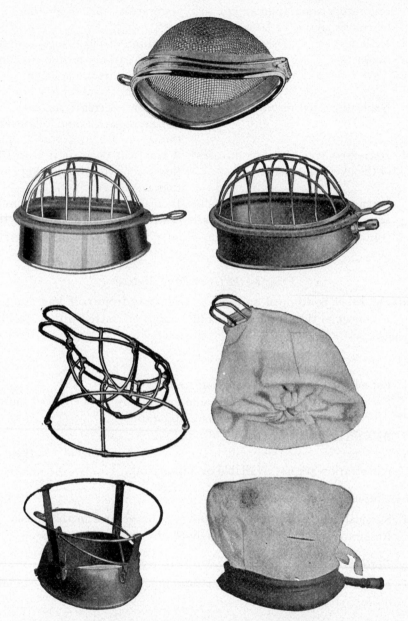

FIG. 28. Various types of open masks for the open drop administration of volatile drugs. (Courtesy of Richard Foregger, Ph.D.)

7. Suction apparatus, tubing, and metal pharyngeal tip (Fig. 85).
8. Container of ether ($\frac{1}{4}$ or $\frac{1}{2}$ lb.) arranged to act as a dropper (Figs. 29, 30).
9. Vaseline to lubricate eye protector and skin.

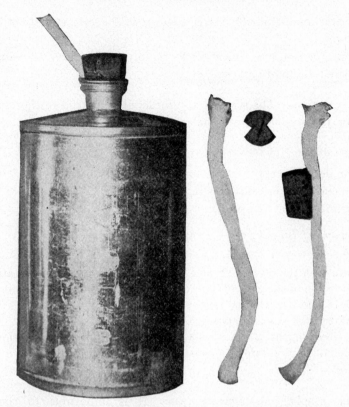

FIG. 29. The original container may be improvised as a dropper by cutting two longitudinal wedges in a cork and placing it in the opening of the can. A wick of rolled gauze passes through one wedge, the other acts as a vent.

Technique:

1. Prepare mask, ether dropper and lubricate one side of the eye protector (with Vaseline Petroleum Jelly) in the desired manner.
2. Arrange patient in usual manner described for inhalation anesthesia. Apply blood pressure cuff, leg strap, and wrist cuff in routine manner.
3. Cover eyes with protector and drape the forehead and eyes with a folded towel.

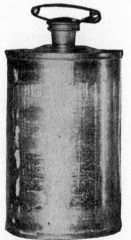

FIG. 30. The original container may quickly be converted into a dropper by piercing the soft metal top with a large safety pin and enlarging the holes to adjust the rate of flow.

4. Apply mask to face. Hold in same manner as other masks (see holding masks and Fig. 26).
5. Allow ether to flow at the rate of one drop every three or four seconds

at first and gradually increase to as fast a rate as patient tolerates vapor.

6. Continue dropping the ether as rapidly as necessary to maintain the desired depth of narcosis.

Signs of Anesthesia: The signs of anesthesia are identical to those described under Judging Depth of Inhalation Anesthesia (page 112).

Advantages of Ether by the Open Drop Method:

1. The dead space in mask is small (important in children)
2. No elaborate apparatus is required.
3. Air may act as the source of oxygen.

Disadvantages of Ether by Open Drop Method	*Reasons*
1. Induction period is long and disagreeable to the patient, averages 10–15 minutes whether or not the anesthestist is experienced.	The drug possesses irritating properties and high air-blood distribution co-efficient.
2. Desired depths of anesthesia are difficult to maintain at a constant level.	The rate of vaporization fluctuates with changes in respiratory volume and the temperature of the mask.
3. The escaping vapors create a fire hazard.	It is impossible to confine the vapors.
4. Disturbances in carbon dioxide tension in the lungs are frequent.	Hyperventilation from respiratory stimulation may cause a decrease of carbon dioxide in the alveoli.
5. It is wasteful and expensive.	The major portion of the ether escapes into the air. Closed methods are more economical.
6. Vaporization is not adequate to maintain anesthesia in most adults, particularly in warm climates.	The semi-open method must be employed in these circumstances.
7. Cold ether vapor is inhaled.	This may enhance secretion of mucus and may lower body temperature.
8. Mild anoxemia is not uncommon.	Oxygen in the air is diluted by the ether. The tension in the alveoli is thereby reduced.

Complications:

1. Excess mucus secretion: Commonly occurs in poorly premedicated subjects. Some mucus forms during induction regardless of premedi-

cation. Administer atropine or scopolamine before anesthesia to minimize secretions.

2. Laryngeal spasm: Usually appears early during anesthesia from strong concentrations of ether or is initiated by mucus in the larynx or pharynx.

3. Overdosage: Occurs after anesthesia is well established. Rare during the induction period unless the patient is non-resistant from debilitation, shock, coma, etc.

4. Conjunctivitis: Ether, blood, or secretions may pass into the eye as result of careless technique.

5. Blistering of the skin. Caused by a combination of ether, moisture, and pressure applied over an area of skin.

Comment	*Reasons*
1. Drop ether slowly at first and increase rate gradually, steadily, and as fast as patient tolerates the vapor.	If concentration of the vapor is increased too rapidly, spasm, mucus, and coughing invariably result.
2. Turn the head to one side after patient has passed into stage III.	Mucus and saliva collect at the side of the mouth and do not flow over face into the eyes.
3. If coughing occurs during the induction period, or concentration of ether is increased too rapidly, lift mask momentarily and replace it after the patient takes several breaths of air.	The concentration in the pharynx is diluted by this maneuver and spasm is avoided.
4. Replace wet mask covers with dry gauze.	Water vapor from the lungs condenses on the cold mask. Vaporization is retarded and obstruction to respiration is increased by wet gauze.
5. Do not apply traction to chin or lower jaw while patient is conscious during induction (stage II and stage I).	Such stimulation precipitates excitement which ordinarily can be obviated.
6. Do not cease dropping ether if patient becomes excited. Continue the administration as rapidly as it is tolerated.	The excitement stage will be prolonged or the patient may pass back into first stage if administration is halted. The object is to increase the concentration and pass into stage III as soon as possible.
7. Do not wrap towels about the mask when anesthetizing children	Excess carbon dioxide may accumulate and symptoms of carbon

unless absolutely necessary and then only loosely.

8. Use the suction freely and remove all secretions as often as necessary.

9. Increase and decrease dropping of ether gradually and administer it continuously during maintenance.

10. If signs of suboxygenation appear, insert a nasal catheter into one nostril—administer oxygen at the rate of 500 cc. or more per minute.

dioxide excess develop.

A patent airway must be maintained. Incidence of postanesthetic complications is increased when secretions are excessive.

A constant concentration of ether vapor is necessary under the mask to maintain a proper alveolar tension for the desired plane of anesthesia.

When air alone is a vehicle for the vapor, the oxygen tension may be reduced.

Ether by the Semi-Open Method

Principle:

1. The technique and principle are similar to the open drop method except that ether vapor is confined by wrapping a towel about the mask. Some degree of rebreathing thereby is instituted (Fig. 31).

Uses:

1. When vaporization by the open method is inadequate.
2. In warm climates when vaporization proceeds rapidly.

Technique:

1. Same as for ether by open drop with the exception that a towel is wrapped about the mask in a chimney-like fashion.

Advantages:

1. It allows a greater concentration of ether to be inhaled than by the open method.
2. It is the only satisfactory method of obtaining anesthesia in an adult by the drop method.

Disadvantages:

1. Rebreathing may increase carbon dioxide tension to undesired and perhaps dangerous levels.
2. Oxygen tension is decreased by interference of ventilation by the towel.
3. The possibility of overdosage is increased.
4. Hyperpnea from carbon dioxide excess often exaggerates abdominal movements and handicaps the surgeon.

Comment

1. Always begin administration by the open method and gradually wrap towel about mask as anesthesia progresses.
2. The towel should be applied in a chimney-like fashion about the mask.
3. The top should be opened widely

Reasons

Rebreathing from outset may cause patient to struggle and cough because the concentration of ether is too strong.

Ether vapor is heavier than air and will thus be confined over the mask.

This allows free passage of carbon

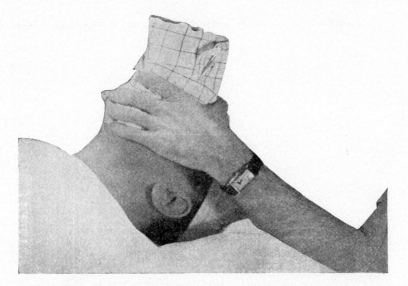

Fig. 31. Semi-open technique of anesthesia by the drop method. Note that the towel is arranged in a chimney like fashion about a Fergusen mask.

and the entire mask should form the floor of the enclosure (Fig. 31).

4. Do not cover any portion of the mask with the towel.
5. Always administer oxygen with nasal catheter under mask (1–1½ liters per min.).

dioxide and oxygen through the mask.

Obstruction to respiration results. Prevents anoxia.

Minimizes excitement.

Ether by Insufflation

Principle:

1. A current of air, of oxygen, or a mixture of nitrous oxide or ethylene and oxygen is propelled over the surface of liquid ether or through it in the form of fine bubbles, and the mixture of gases and vapor is conducted into the nose or mouth and trachea through a tube or cannula.

Types:

1. *Intranasal insufflation:*

> The mixture is conducted into the oropharynx by a single or double nasal catheter (Fig. 32a).

2. *Intraoral insufflation:*

> The mixture is conducted into the oropharynx by a cannula or "ether hook" placed in the mouth (Fig. 32b).

3. *Intratracheal insufflation:*

> The mixture is conducted into the trachea by inserting a lubricated

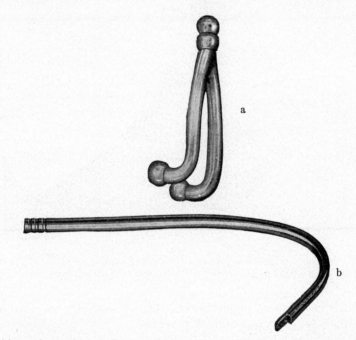

FIG. 32. (a) Nasal piece for nasopharyngeal insufflation of anesthetic gases and vapors. (b) "Ether hook" for oral insufflation of anesthetic gases and vapors. (Courtesy of Richard Foregger, Ph.D.)

> catheter into the lumen of an intratracheal tube (see artificial airways, page 247).

Uses:

> 1. For operations about the head or face, pharynx, larynx, trachea, or esophagus.

Premedication:

> 1. Morphine and scopolamine, or morphine and atropine, in standard doses (same as for open ether).

Materials:

1. Ether vaporizer and connecting tubes.
2. Mechanical air compressor or other source of compressed gas.
3. Reducing valve if cylinders are used as a source of gas.
4. Nasal catheters 14–18 F. The size varies with the subject (if intranasal insufflation is to be employed).
5. "Ether hook" (if oral route is contemplated) (Fig. 33).
6. Vaseline to lubricate the catheter (nasal route).

Technique (Oral):

1. Test the vaporizer and place it in a convenient position which in no way interferes with the surgical team.
2. Anesthetize the patient with ether by open drop technique and attain the level of anesthesia desired to complete the operation.
3. Commence vaporization of ether. Be positive the mixture is flowing through the cannula or catheter. Test the flow of gas by holding the cannula against palm of the hand or by cautiously smelling for ether.
4. Remove mask and immediately insert hook or cannula into the mouth.
5. Suction pharynx if secretions are present.
6. Proceed as described under "open drop" technique for signs of anesthesia, maintenance of airway, and precautions.

Technique (Nasal):

1. Anesthetize patient as described under *Oral Insufflation.*
2. Mark off a distance equivalent to the distance between the ala of nose and tragus of the ear on the catheter.
3. Commence the vaporization of ether and insert the well lubricated catheter the measured distance into the nostril.

Advantages of Insufflation:

1. "Dead space" is minimal or negligible.
2. It may be employed when intratracheal anesthesia is not feasible, practical, or desirable for oropharyngeal surgery and operations about head, face, or neck.

Disadvantages:

1. Airway is frequently maintained with difficulty particularly if the head is not accessible to the anesthetist.
2. The quantity of ether vapor delivered by the vaporizer is frequently insufficient to maintain anesthesia for adults.
3. The air-ether mixture is an explosive and a fire hazard.
4. The method is wasteful and expensive.

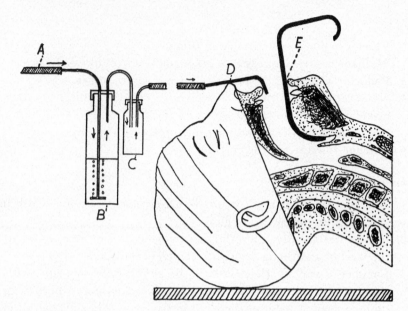

Fig. 33. Diagram illustrating oral insufflation of volatile liquids. (A) Source of compressed gas, usually air or oxygen. (B) Jar containing volatile liquid. (C) Trap to prevent liquid from accidentally passing over into the mouth. (D) Hooked cannula. (E) Blade to support the tongue and provide a patent airway.

5. Liquid ether may be propelled into the pharynx if the vaporizer is not equipped with a trap.
6. Objectionable quantities of ether are inhaled by members of the surgical team.

Comment	*Reasons*
1. Always start and test vaporizor before placing the hook or catheter in the mouth or in the nose of the patient.	Leaks or other mechanical defects may decrease the output of vapor even though the apparatus appears to function well. High concentrations of ether, liquid ether, or gases under pressure may be blown into the upper respiratory tract if apparatus is defective.
2. Judge depth of anesthesia by the responses of the patient to the ether and not by the size of the stream or the rate of vaporization of the liquid.	Vaporization varies as the temperature of the ether changes.
3. Lower head below the level of the shoulders in performing intraoral, intranasal, or intrapharyngeal operations or if secretions are excessive.	Prevent aspiration of secretions or blood into trachea or bronchial tree

4. Remove hook from mouth or catheter from nose when ether is discontinued.

If apparatus is equipped with a warming device, pure ether vapor may be distilled into pharynx and cause spasm or overdosage.

5. If vaporization is inadequate surround the ether container with warm water to assist in vaporization.

Ether becomes progressively cooler and does not vaporize so well as the operation proceeds.

6. Add sufficient oxygen to whatever gas is employed to propel the vapor.

The oxygen tension may be reduced to dangerously low levels unless extreme care is exercised.

Variations of Insufflation Technique

1. *Insufflation into pharyngeal airway:*
   a. The delivery tube from the vaporizer is attached to an oropharyngeal airway equipped with a nipple designed for the purpose, or a catheter may be threaded through its lumen into the pharynx. Anesthesia then proceeds as in the foregoing techniques.

2. *Insufflation into tracheotomy cannula:*
   a. A loose fitting lubricated catheter attached to the insufflation tube may be inserted for a distance of one to two inches into the cannula. The patient is first anesthetized by the open drop method by placing the mask on the neck over the cannula and then gentle insufflation is practiced at a positive pressure not to exceed 25 mm. Hg.

Ether Analgesia

Description: Use of Stage I anesthesia obtained by inducing stage III anesthesia and permitting patient to pass back into lower strata of stage I.

Uses:

1. For surgery in which the patient's constitution forbids use of deep anesthesia (poor risk patients for cardiac surgery).

Preparation:

1. Explain contemplated procedure to patient and assure that no pain or discomfort will ensue.
2. Administer scopolamine, atropine or other anticholinergic agent one hour before induction time.
3. Administer pentothal in divided doses to induce light basal narcosis. Technique is best carried out in anesthesia room.

Procedure:

1. Anesthetize patient deeply with ether, using open drop, nitrous oxide or ethylene ether oxygen sequence.
2. Intubate using succinyl choline and topical anesthesia.
3. Discard ether mixture and allow patient to pass back into first stage.
4. Add sufficient amount of ether to maintain patient in this Stage I.

Comment

1. Maintain level at point at which patient barely responds to questioning.
2. Remember nausea and vomiting may occur if analgesic state is too light.
3. "Bucking" and gagging are prevented by use of topical anesthesia.
4. Not suitable for states requiring muscle relaxation.
5. Be sure to induce surgical anesthesia (Stage III) then permit reversal into stage I.
6. Some patients not suitable for the technique—become unruly and uncooperative.

REFERENCES

Gwathmey, J. T. Anesthesia. 2nd Ed. The Macmillan Co., New York, 1929.

Adriani, J. The Pharmacology of Anesthetic Drugs. 4th Ed. Pp. 33–36. Charles C Thomas, Springfield, 1960.

Goodman, L., and Gilman, A. The Pharmacological Basis of Therapeutics. 2nd Ed. Pp. 56-64 The Macmillan Co., New York, 1955.

Artusio, J. F. Ether Analgesia During Major Surgery. J.A.M.A., *57:* 30, 1955.

NITROUS OXIDE ANESTHESIA

Description: A non-irritating, sweet-smelling, non-flammable, inorganic gas which possesses a mild narcotic potency. The anesthesia it produces is characterized by a rapid induction and rapid recovery but is rarely deeper than first plane (Fig. 34).

Uses:

1. For operations not requiring profound anesthesia or muscle relaxation.
2. As an induction agent for ether.
3. As a supplemental agent to basal narcosis or intravenous anesthesia.
4. For operations requiring use of cautery, endotherm, endoscopes, or other electrical equipment which may be a source of fire hazard.
5. For analgesia for obstetrical or dental surgery.
6. For thoracic surgery.

Cost: Relatively inexpensive, 1¢ to 1½¢ per gallon.

Concentration:

1. Analgesia, 35–50% by volume in the alveoli.
2. Anesthesia, 80–90% by volume in the alveoli.

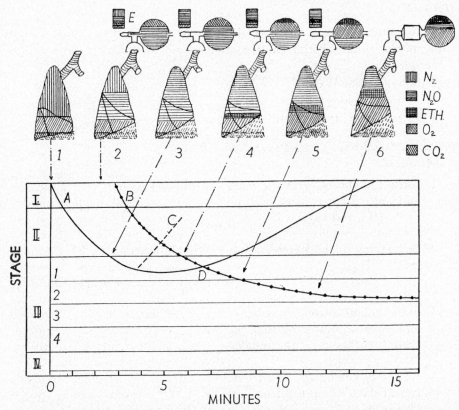

FIG. 34. Changes in gas tensions in the lungs, inhaler, and expired gases during the induction and maintenance of nitrous oxide-ether sequence anesthesia by the semi-closed technique. The subject breathes from an inhaler into which is admitted a mixture of oxygen and nitrous oxide. (1) The air in the lungs is mixed with the gas. (2) The nitrogen normally present in the lungs is eliminated through the exhalation valve. The patient passes into surgical anesthesia (Curve A), as soon as the nitrogen is replaced by nitrous oxide (85%) (3) When first plane anesthesia is attained, addition of ether is started (Curve B). The ether concentration required for surgical anesthesia can be more rapidly attained during the easily induced anesthesia of the non-irritating nitrous oxide. The flow of nitrous oxide must be maintained while ether is being added, otherwise recovery occurs (Curve C) before sufficient drug is present in the alveoli to maintain third stage ether anesthesia. (4) The concentration of ether is sufficient for surgical anesthesia. (5) The flow of nitrous oxide may be gradually diminished since enough ether is added to maintain first plane anesthesia (Point D). (6) Rebreathing with a closed inhaler is then instituted. During induction some nitrous oxide and ether are also lost through the exhalation valve along with carbon dioxide and nitrogen (E). Some nitrous oxide remains in the inhaler and lungs during maintenance. Although the lungs are depleted of nitrogen in the beginning of maintenance, some is gradually eliminated from the tissues and accumulates in the inhaler. (6) Ether must be added from time to time, or even continuously in large subjects, to replace the drug absorbed by the tissues. Oxygen is added to satisfy metabolic needs; carbon dioxide is absorbed by soda lime.

3. Respiratory failure, 90–100% by volume in the alveoli (due to the combined effects of anoxia and the drug).

Premedication:

1. Morphine and scopolamine or morphine and atropine in full therapeutic doses (see premedication). The doses employed should be large enough to decrease reflex irritability and metabolic rate.

Materials:

1. Machine having a flowmeter for nitrous oxide and oxygen, a closed inhaler equipped with an exhalation valve (circle filter), and a vaporizer.
2. Sphygmomanometer.
3. Artificial airway.
4. Intercoupler (if the addition of ether is contemplated).

Procedure for Nitrous Oxide-Oxygen Anesthesia

Reasons

1. Close the obturator at the mask and fill inhaler with nitrous oxide 85% and oxygen 15%.

A full bag is employed at the outset to more quickly dilute and displace the air in the apparatus and lungs with anesthetic gas.

2. Adjust, but do not fasten mask to face.

Stimulation created by the pressure may cause patient to become excited as he passes through stage II.

3. Turn on carbon dioxide absorber and open obturator so that patient breathes from the inhaler.

Carbon dioxide should be removed to prevent the feeling of suffocation which patients frequently experience during induction.

4. Adjust flowmeter to deliver oxygen at 1200 cc. and nitrous oxide at 4 liters per minute (or 80% N_2O 20% O_2 if automatic, demand type mixing meter is employed).

A mixture of 80% nitrous oxide and 20% oxygen is thus assured in the inhaler (Table VI).

5. Open exhalation valve sufficiently to allow excess gases to escape from inhaler but not so wide that the bag becomes deflated.

Nitrogen, some nitrous oxide, and carbon dioxide are eliminated during each exhalation. Ultimately most of the nitrogen in the alveoli is replaced by nitrous oxide and oxygen and the patient passes into stage III.

6. Increase or decrease the flow of nitrous oxide to the amount required to obtain and maintain anesthesia.

The alveolar tension of the gas necessary for anesthesia varies according to the individual, the state of the patient, and effectiveness of premedication. No fixed percentages can be recommended.

7. As soon as the patient is in stage III fasten mask securely to face.

A snug fit prevents inhalation of air about the face cushion and subsequent dilution of the mixture.

8. Allow mixture to flow until patient is in stage III then decrease

The mixture in the inhaler and lungs tends to become diluted from

the flow of nitrous oxide to approximately 1000 cc. per minute or less according to the needs of the patient. Add O_2 according to Table VI.

9. Close exhalation valve almost entirely but allow for escape of excess gases which would accumulate in the apparatus.

leaks, nitrogen, oxygen, etc., and patient will recover from anesthesia at an inopportune moment if nitrous oxide is not added in small amounts.

Overdistension of the breathing bag causes a positive pressure in inhaler which disturbs respiration.

TABLE VI

PROPORTIONS OF NITROUS OXIDE AND OXYGEN WHICH MUST BE FLOWN INTO A SEMI-CLOSED INHALER TO ASSURE 20% OXYGEN IN THE MASK ON INSPIRATION

N_2O	O_2
400 cc.	600 cc.
500	625
750	675
1000	750
1500	800
2000	850
2500	925
3000	1000
3500	1100
4000	1200
4500	1400
5000	1550
5500	1700
6000	2000

Comment:

1. An 80–20%-O_2 mixture does not assure adequate oxygenation unless supplied at the minute volume exchange of the patient. Enrich the mixture when using flows at less than this rate (Table VI).
2. Always turn soda lime absorber on. Carbon dioxide accumulates unless mixture is supplied at minute volume exchange. A volume of gas equivalent to the expired tidal volume must be ejected to the outside if no soda lime absorber is used.

Signs of Anesthesia:

1. Without anoxia the signs of nitrous oxide anesthesia conform to those enumerated in the table Judging the Depths of Inhalation Anesthesia (p. 112).

If anesthesia cannot be maintained in stage III without decreasing the oxygen to less than 20%, ether or other desired drug should be added to the mixture and oxygen tension increased as described below.

Nitrous Oxide-Ether Oxygen Sequence
(Fig. 34)

Reasons

1. Begin as for nitrous oxide-oxygen anesthesia.

   Induction is same as for nitrous oxide-oxygen.

2. As soon as patient passes into stage III turn off carbon dioxide filter.

   Carbon dioxide is desirable to stimulate respiration and increase tidal exchange to facilitate absorption of ether.

3. Start vaporizing ether gradually and increase concentration as rapidly as patient tolerates the vapor.

   Additions of ether must be gradual and in amounts which patient can tolerate. Excess ether causes cough, mucus secretion, or spasm of the larynx.

4. Continue flow of nitrous oxide and oxygen allowing exhalation valve to remain open during the introduction of ether.

   Anesthesia with nitrous oxide must be maintained while ether is being raised to the concentration necessary for surgical anesthesia (Fig. 34).

5. When the necessary concentration of ether is attained, gradually decrease flow of nitrous oxide. Decrease at rate of 1000 cc. every two minutes. Ultimately the entire flow will be off (within 5 minutes as a rule).

   All concentrations of gases and vapors should be raised or lowered gradually.

6. Close exhalation valve when the flow of nitrous oxide is stopped and adjust oxygen to 400–500 cc. per minute.

   This institutes rebreathing of ether and carbon dioxide because the filter is still off.

7. Allow a hyperpnea to develop. Continue to add ether as rapidly as tolerated during the hyperpnea.

   The absorption of ether in the alveoli is facilitated during the increased ventilation.

8. As soon as the hyperpnea becomes maximal and respiratory excursions begin to decline from the depression caused by carbon dioxide, gradually turn on the filter. Doing it in steps taking 3 or 4 minutes to go from off to on.

   Remove carbon dioxide to prevent deleterious effects on circulation and respiration. Carbon dioxide in high concentrations causes depression of the central nervous system.

9. If, after carbon dioxide is removed, the patient does not tolerate the ether concentration present in the inhaler, dilute mixture with a few hundred cc. of nitrous

   Carbon dioxide possesses some anesthetic properties and its rapid removal causes lightening of anesthesia. If the concentration of ether in the inhaler is too high, the

oxide. Discontinue carbon dioxide absorption, reestablish a hyperpnea, and gradually increase the ether once more.

patient may hold his breath or cough as soon as the carbon dioxide is removed.

10. Gradually turn on the filter. This time the ether concentration is usually tolerated. If not, repeat the process once again or as often as necessary for the concentration to be tolerated.

Carbon dioxide reestablishes the hyperpnea necessary to facilitate absorption of ether.

11. Continue addition of ether and adjust oxygen to the patient's metabolic requirement (250–300 cc. per minute)

Ether must be added throughout the operation to replace the portion absorbed by tissues from the blood.

Signs of Anesthesia:

1. The signs of anesthesia are identical with those described for ether.

Advantages of Nitrous Oxide:

1. It is non-inflammable.
2. It is non-irritating to the respiratory tract.
3. It is inexpensive if carbon dioxide absorption technique is employed.
4. Induction and recovery are rapid (2–3 minutes).
5. It does not depress the respiratory or circulatory system.
6. It disturbs physiological functions only slightly if oxygenation is adequate.
7. Post anesthetic nausea and emesis are not common.
8. It is useful for analgesia, either continued or intermittent.

Disadvantages of Nitrous Oxide:

1. It does not ordinarily yield anesthesia below first plane unless accompanied by some anoxia.
2. Relaxation of muscles is inadequate for major surgery.
3. Danger of asphyxia is always present, particularly when administered by inexperienced individuals.

Complications

1. Failure to obtain third stage anesthesia.

2. Apnea—usually lasts 10 or 15 seconds.

Cause

Usually due to unsatisfactory premedication or dilution of the gas by oxygen, air, or nitrogen.

Follows the addition of oxygen during anoxia. Due to the loss of carotid body stimulation by the anoxemia.

| 3. Retching and vomiting during anesthesia. | Usually follows dilution of the mixture with air or oxygen with subsequent lightening of the anesthesia. Most common when anoxia has been present. |
| 4. Anoxia. | Due to reduction of oxygen tension by excess nitrous oxide. |

Signs of Anoxia with Nitrous Oxide:

1. Increased rate and depth of respiration, frequently irregular and jerky, often accompanied by phonation, "crowing," or groaning on inspiration or expiration.
2. Slow, bounding pulse (approximately 60).
3. Elevated blood pressure.
4. Increased pulse pressure.
5. Cyanosis of skin, mucous membranes, nail beds, and conjunctival vessels. *Blood in the operative wound appears dark.*
6. Rigidity of the muscles of the body, followed by twitchings of small muscles, gradually merging into convulsive movements of large muscles as the anoxia increases.
7. Sweating and coldness of the skin.
8. Dilated pupils, which do not react to light.
9. Secretion of small amounts of thick glairy mucus.

Overdosage:

1. *Signs:*

   a. *Without anoxia:* Overdosage is a remote possibility unless the subject is debilitated or moribund, or basal narcosis or large doses of nonvolatile drugs are employed in conjunction with the agent.
   b. *With anoxia:*
      1. Respiratory failure. Usually preceded by irregular, stertorous, spasmodic, or very rapid breathing.
      2. Marked cyanosis of mucous membranes and skin.
      3. Bradycardia.
      4. Hypertension—a rapid fall in blood pressure soon supervenes if not relieved.
      5. Widely dilated pupils.
      6. Spasticity of muscles (in early stages) followed by twitchings and convulsive movements. Complete flaccidity soon appears.
      7. Loss of all reflexes.

Treatment of asphyxia:

   a. *Artificial respiration:*
      1. Insert an artificial airway (oropharyngeal).

2. Hold mask firmly on face and secure a snug fit.
3. Fill rebreathing bag of the inhaler with pure oxygen.
4. Inflate thorax by alternately compressing and relaxing breathing bag. If spasm is present, force oxygen into lungs. Even a small amount may assist in relieving the anoxia and overcoming the spasm.

Contra-Indications   *Reasons*

1. Nitrous oxide without any reduction in the normal alveolar oxygen tension:
   None, if depth of anesthesia obtained by this technique is satisfactory.
2. Nitrous oxide with a slight or moderate decrease in alveolar oxygen tension:
   a. Hypertension and associated cardiovascular diseases. — Anoxia causes an elevation of blood pressure and increases cardiac irritability.

   b. All types of diseases of the respiratory tract, but particularly if vital capacity is lowered. — The decrease in oxygen tension, even though slight, may cause severe anoxemia in pulmonary disease.

   c. Diabetes, renal insufficiency, or acidosis from any cause. — Anoxia enhances acidosis regardless of its etiology.
   d. Impaired liver function. — Anoxia markedly disturbs liver function.

   e. Fever, toxemia, or diseases accompanied by an increase in metabolic rate. — The basal oxygen requirement is increased in these conditions. A decrease in efficiency of the agent is observed.

   f. Shock, hemorrhage, or anemias. — Anoxia increases capillary permeability and enhances peripheral circulatory failure.

3. Nitrous oxide with ether:
   The contra-indications are identical with those described for ether (see ether). — The addition of ether to nitrous oxide immediately converts the anesthesia to an ether anesthesia.

Comment   *Reasons*

1. Do not expect the impossible of nitrous oxide. — The gas is satisfactory for induction of ether anesthesia or first plane anesthesia but not for deeper anesthesia.

2. Do not expect satisfactory anesthesia without proper premedication.

Premedication facilitates non-asphyxial anesthesia with this drug.

3. Do not tolerate leaks about the face piece or in other parts of the inhaler.

Air aspirated into the apparatus reduces potency of the mixture by decreasing the partial pressure of nitrous oxide in the alveoli.

4. Avoid introducing an artificial airway during nitrous oxide anesthesia unless it is absolutely necessary to do so.

Anesthesia is so light that often the patient inhales room air during the insertion and recovers before the airway is properly placed.

5. Observe nail beds, mucous membranes, and conjunctival vessels for cyanosis in Negroes or other heavily pigmented subjects.

These structures lack the usual skin pigment and best reveal the presence of excess reduced hemoglobin.

6. Record blood pressure and palpate pulse frequently during nitrous oxide anesthesia.

Circulatory changes offer excellent criteria for detecting the presence of anoxia.

7. Do not rely upon cyanosis as a symptom of anoxemia.

Cyanosis may not be apparent in severe anemias. The appearance of cyanosis depends upon (1) the hemoglobin content of blood, (2) amount of pigment in the skin, (3) caliber of the peripheral vessels, and (4) thickness of the skin.

8. Rely upon physiological responses as guides to depth of anesthesia and degree of oxygenation rather than the proportions of gases registered by flowmeters.

Discrepancies frequently exist between the flow of gases registered and concentrations delivered because these flowmeters are subject to mechanical derangements.

9. Always employ the semi-closed method for induction of anesthesia (Fig. 34).

The nitrogen in the alveoli must be replaced by nitrous oxide to obtain anesthesia and can be eliminated only by ejecting it through the exhalation valve.

10. Revert to the closed system for the maintenance of anesthesia.

The closed system affords a saving of gas and better control of carbon dioxide tension.

11. Add oxygen cautiously during induction and maintenance.

Sudden or excessive dilution of the mixture may cause the patient to pass from stage III to stage II.

REFERENCES

Adriani, J. The Pharmacology of Anesthetic Drugs. 4th Ed. Pp. 21–23. Charles C Thomas, Springfield, Ill., 1960.

Clement, F. W. Nitrous Oxide Oxygen Anesthesia. Lea and Febiger, Philadelphia, 1939.

Goodman, L., and Gilman, A. The Pharmacological Basis of Therapeutics. Chap. VI The Macmillan Co., New York, 1955.

ETHYLENE ANESTHESIA

Description: A non-irritating, inflammable, gaseous hydrocarbon which possesses an ethereal odor and a mild narcotic potency. The anesthesia it produces is characterized by a rapid induction and recovery but is rarely deeper than first plane (Fig. 34).*

Uses:

1. For operations requiring approximately first plane anesthesia.
2. As an induction agent for ether.
3. For thoracic surgery, because of its non-irritating qualities.
4. As a supplemental agent for intravenous anesthesia or basal narcosis.
5. For analgesia for obstetrical or dental surgery.

Cost:

1. Relatively inexpensive: $1\frac{1}{2}$¢ to 2¢ per gallon.

Concentration:

1. Analgesia: 35% to 50% by volume in the alveoli.
2. Anesthesia: 80% to 85% by volume in the alveoli. In well premedicated subjects, less than 80% may be effective.
3. Respiratory failure 90% to 100% by volume in the alveoli (due to the combined effects of anoxia and the drug).

Premedication:

1. Morphine and scopolamine or morphine and atropine in full therapeutic doses (see premedication). The doses employed should be large enough to decrease reflex irritability and metabolic rate.

Materials:

1. Machine having a closed inhaler equipped with an exhalation valve.
2. Sphygmomanometer.
3. Artificial airway.
4. Intercoupler (at all times).

Procedure for Ethylene-Oxygen Anesthesia	*Reasons*
1. Fill breathing bag (5 liter) with an 80%-20% mixture. Close obturator at mask.	A bag filled with the gas is employed at the outset to more quickly dilute and displace the air in the appartus and lungs with anesthetic gas.
2. Adjust, but do not fasten mask to face.	If the mask is fastened, the stimulation may cause excitement in passing through stage II.

* Ethylene has potency, pharmacological properties, and uses similar to nitrous oxide.

3. Turn on carbon dioxide filter and open obturator so that patient breathes from the inhaler.

Carbon dioxide should be removed to prevent the feeling of suffocation which patients frequently experience during induction.

4. Adjust flowmeter to deliver 1200 cc. of oxygen and 4 liters of ethylene per minute.

A mixture of approximately 80% anesthetic gas and 20% oxygen is thus assured in the inhaler.

5. Open exhalation valve to allow excess gas to escape but not so wide that bag becomes deflated.

Nitrogen and some ethylene are thus eliminated with each expiration. Ultimately the nitrogen in the alveoli is replaced by ethylene and oxygen and the patient passes into stage III.

6. Increase or decrease the flow of ethylene to the amount required to obtain and maintain anesthesia.

The alveolar tension of the gas necessary for anesthesia varies according to the individual patient and effectiveness of premedication. No fixed percentages can be recommended.

7. As soon as patient is in stage III, fasten mask securely to the face.

A snug fit prevents inhalation of air around face cushion and subsequent dilution of the mixture.

8. Reduce flow of ethylene to 1000 cc. or less per minute according to needs of patient. Add oxygen according to Table VII.

Small amounts of ethylene must be added continuously because mixture in inhaler tends to become diluted by nitrogen and oxygen from leaks and other causes.

9. Close exhalation valve almost completely but allow for escape of excess gases.

Overdistension of the breathing bag causes positive pressure in the inhaler which disturbs respiration.

TABLE VII

PROPORTIONS OF ETHYLENE AND OXYGEN WHICH MUST BE FLOWN INTO A SEMI-CLOSED INHALER TO ASSURE 20% OXYGEN IN THE MASK ON INSPIRATION

Ethylene	Oxygen
400 cc.	600 cc.
500	625
750	675
1000	750
1500	800
2000	850
2500	925
3000	1000
3500	1100
4000	1200
4500	1400
5000	1550
5500	1700
6000	2000

Signs of Anesthesia: If anoxia is not present, signs of anesthesia with ethylene conform to those enumerated in the table under Judging Depths of Anesthesia (page 112). If anoxia complicates the anesthesia, the signs are altered and not at all reliable.

Comment

1. If anesthesia cannot be maintained in stage III without reducing the oxygen tension to less than 20% ether should be added to the mixture and the oxygen tension increased as described below.
2. An 80-20%-O_2 mixture does not assure adequate oxygenation unless supplied at the minute volume exchange of the patient. Enrich the mixture when using flows at less than this rate (Table VII).
3. Always turn soda lime absorber on. Carbon dioxide accumulates unless the mixture is supplied at the minute volume exchange.

Procedure for Ethylene-Ether Oxygen Sequence (Fig. 34)

Reasons

1. Begin as for ethylene anesthesia.

   Induction is same as for ethylene-oxygen.

2. As soon as stage III has been attained with the ethylene-oxygen mixture, turn off carbon dioxide filter.

   Carbon dioxide produces a hyperpnea and also a certain amount of depression, both of which hasten induction.

3. Start vaporizing ether slowly at first and increase the concentration as fast as patient tolerates it.

   If ether concentration is raised too quickly, cough, and laryngeal spasm may result.

4. Continue to flow ethylene-oxygen. Allow the exhalation valve to remain open during introduction of ether.

   Anesthesia from ethylene must be maintained while the concentration of ether is being raised to the level necessary for surgical anesthesia.

5. Gradually decrease flow of ethylene in steps of 1000 cc. per 1–2 minute intervals. as the ether tension necessary to maintain third stage anesthesia is attained. Ultimately shut off entire flow (usually within five minutes).

   All concentrations of gases and vapors should be raised or lowered gradually.

6. Close exhalation valve as soon as flow of ethylene is stopped and allow hyperpnea to develop. Add ether as rapidly as tolerated during the hyperpnea.

   The hyperpnea increases tidal exchange and hastens absorption of ether.

7. As soon as hyperpnea is maximal and respiratory excursions begin to decline from the depressant action of carbon dioxide, gradu-

   Carbon dioxide exerts deleterious effects on circulation and respiration if not removed when signs of depression appear.

ually turn on soda lime filter taking 2–3 minutes to go from "off" to "on."

8. If, after carbon dioxide is removed, patient does not tolerate ether concentration present in inhaler, dilute mixture with several hundred cc. of ethylene. Discontinue ether and carbon dioxide absorption and reestablish a hyperpnea. Resume ether, and gradually turn on filter as in the previous step.

Removal of carbon dioxide causes lightening of anesthesia because carbon dioxide possesses anesthetic properties. Carbon dioxide should be removed gradually during induction.

9. Continue the addition of ether and adjust the flow of oxygen to the patient's metabolic requirement.

Tissues constantly absorb ether from the blood which must be replaced.

Signs of Anesthesia:

1. The signs of anesthesia are identical to those described under Judging Depths of Anesthesia.

Advantages of Ethylene:

1. Induction and recovery periods are rapid (2–3 minutes).
2. It is nonirritating to the respiratory tract.
3. It disturbs physiological functions only slightly if adequate oxygenation is maintained.
4. It is more potent than nitrous oxide when employed in similar circumstances.
5. It does not notably disturb respiratory or circulatory systems.
6. It is inexpensive if the carbon dioxide absorption technique is employed.

Disadvantages:

1. It does not ordinarily yield anesthesia below first plane unless anesthesia is accompanied by some anoxia.
2. Its odor is unpleasant to some patients.
3. Post anesthetic nausea and emesis are not uncommon.
4. Relaxation of muscles is not adequate unless followed by ether or employed in conjunction with some other agent.
5. Its range of inflammability varies from 1.5% to 80% with oxygen at the usual room temperatures and atmospheric pressures.
6. Danger of asphyxia is always present if the concentration is increased.

Complications:

1. Failure to obtain third stage. Supplement with ether and oxygen. Ineffective premedication or the mixture contains too much oxygen.
2. Vomiting during maintenance of anesthesia. Due to lightening of anesthesia from dilution of mixture with air or oxygen.
3. Coughing. Due to reducing the flow of ethylene too soon during ether induction.
4. Anoxia. Symptoms, similar to those observed when it occurs with nitrous oxide. Due to reduction of oxygen tension by ethylene.

Signs of Anoxia with Ethylene:

1. The signs of anoxia are identical in most respects to those described under nitrous oxide (page 144).

Overdosage:

1. Signs of overdosage are identical to those described under nitrous oxide (page 144).

Contra-Indications	*Reasons*
1. *Without anoxia:* None, save operations requiring cautery and high frequency units.	The gas is highly inflammable when mixed with either air or oxygen.
2. *With a mild degree of anoxia* (the usual method):	
(a) Hypertension and associated cardiovascular diseases.	Effects of anoxia on circulatory system are deleterious.
(b) Acute or chronic pulmonary diseases, particularly if vital capacity is lowered.	Decreased oxygenation even of slight degree may be deleterious.
(c) Diabetes, renal insufficiency, or acidosis from any cause.	Anoxia enhances acidosis regardless of its etiology.
(d) Diseases accompanied by decreased liver function.	Anoxia disturbs liver function.
(e) Fever, toxemia, or diseases accompanied by increased metabolic rate.	The basal oxygen requirement is increased.
(f) Shock, hemorrhage, or anemias.	Anoxia increases capillary permeability and enhances peripheral circulatory failure.
3. *Ethylene-Ether:* The contraindications are identical to those described for ether.	The addition of ether immediately converts an ethylene anesthesia to an ether one.

Comment	*Reasons*
1. Do not expect the impossible from this agent.	The drug is a satisfactory induction agent for ether and first plane

2. Do not tolerate leaks about the face piece.

The patient aspirates air which dilutes the ethylene and reduces its potency.

3. Refrain from employing an artificial airway if possible.

If it is necessary, insert it as quickly as possible to avoid ascent into stage II and return of pharyngeal reflex.

4. Add oxygen cautiously during induction or maintenance of anesthesia.

Sudden or excessive dilution of ethylene by oxygen may cause patient to revert into stage II from stage III.

5. Always employ the semi-closed method for induction.

Nitrogen in the alveoli must be replaced by ethylene to obtain anesthesia. This is best accomplished by eliminating it through the exhalation valve

6. Revert to the closed system during maintenance of anesthesia (the semi-closed system if desired, may be employed throughout).

The closed system affords a saving of gas and a decrease in fire hazard.

Nitrous Oxide Using Demand Type Apparatus (McKesson)

The McKesson apparatus (Nargraff head) is a semi-closed inhaler. Several models are available with the following features.

1. Automatic mixing device (Nargraff Head) which supplies preformed mixtures of nitrous oxide and oxygen.
2. An automatic feeding device activated by reduced pressure in the inhaler caused by escape of gas or inspiratory negative pressure. Replaces gas lost from inhaler.
3. Device for adjusting pressure in the inhaler. Pressure ranges from atmospheric to 40 mm. Hg. in the system.
4. A bellows type breathing bag adjustable to permit partial to complete rebreathing. Notches on side limit excursions of bellows. Each notch = 100 cc. (This is present on dental models.)
5. Key for adjusting pressure in bellows. Each figure on side indicates one mm. Hg. 10 = 10 mm. Hg. (on dental models).
6. Indicator dial on top for:
   (a) rebreathing volume (red pointer)
   (b) tidal volume (black pointer)
       (also on dental models.)
7. Variable reducing valves at each yoke which permits pressure in mixing device to be constant as cylinder becomes exhausted. (All models.)

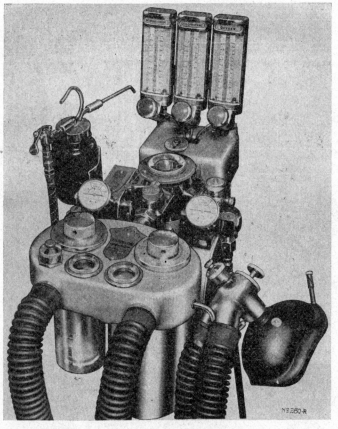

A

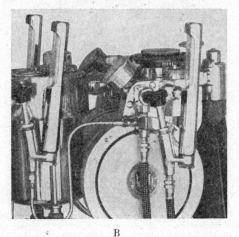

B

FIG. 35. The McKesson anesthetic apparatus. A. Recent model with Nargraff (automatic mixing demand supply) unit and flow meters for nitrous oxide, cyclopropane and oxygen. B. Older model embodying same features with old style flow meter and without flow meter for nitrous oxide.

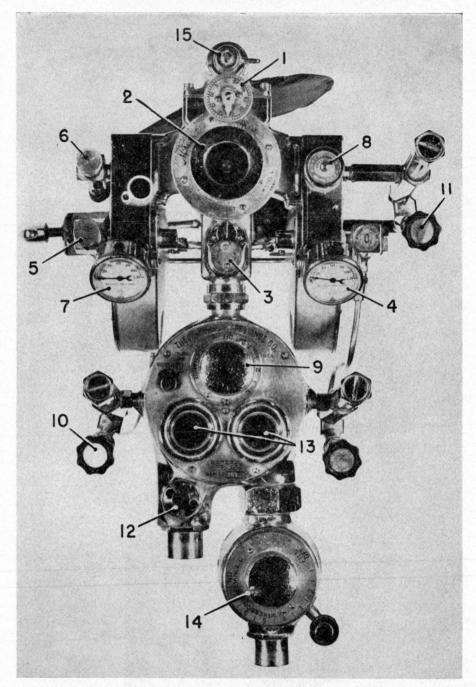

Fig. 36. Top view of McKesson anesthetic apparatus showing the various parts described in the text. (1) Vernier oxygen control valve on automatic mixer. (2) Coarse adjustment oxygen control valve on automatic mixer. (3) Positive pressure control gauge. (4) Oxygen pressure gauge to automatic mixer. (5) Nitrous oxide valve to automatic mixer. (6) Ethylene valve to automatic mixer. (7) Nitrous oxide pressure gauge to automatic mixer. (8) Energizing oxygen flush valve. (9) Carbon dioxide absorber control. (10) Cyclopropane flow meter. (11) Oxygen flow meter. (12) Exhalation valve. (13) Flutter valves on soda lime canister. (14) Ether vaporizer.

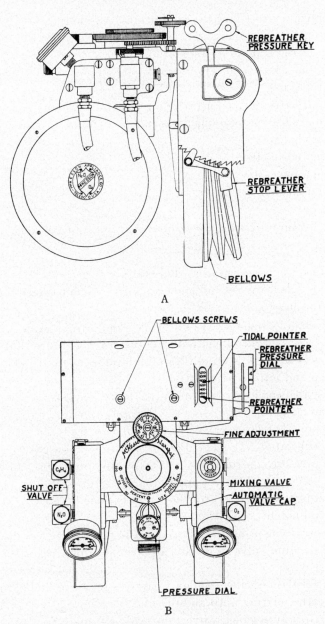

FIG. 37. A. Side view of the McKesson anesthetic apparatus of semi-closed type with automatic mixing device with demand flow, rebreathing bellows. B. Top view. (Courtesy E. I. McKesson, Toledo, Ohio.)

8. Gauges for indicating pressure of oxygen and nitrous oxide supplied to mixing meter. (All models.)

9. Exhalation valve (adjustable). (All models.)

10. Valve to shut off ethylene and admit nitrous oxide and vice-versa.

11. Vaporizer for volatile liquids—type varies with agent used.

12. Emergency direct flow oxygen button. (All models.)

The combined semi-closed and closed apparatus (Fig. 35) has the following features minus the bellows for rebreathing:

13. Soda lime canister for absorption of carbon dioxide.
14. Breathing bag.
15. Shut off valve device for excluding bag from system.
16. Auxilliary bag for retaining gases and maintaining anesthesia when soda lime is changed.
17. Oxygen flowmeter.
18. Cyclopropane flowmeter.
19. Carbon dioxide flowmeter.

Technique Using Semi-Closed Apparatus and Bellows

Technique:

1. Set pressure gauge on off (3, Fig. 36).
2. Close ethylene (5, Fig. 36) and open nitrous admit valve (6, Fig. 36) on Nargraff head.
3. Open main cylinder valves for oxygen and nitrous oxide entirely.
4. Turn screws controlling reducing valves downward until pressure gauges (4 and 7, Fig. 36) on Nargraff head registers 40–60 lbs. for both oxygen and nitrous oxide.
5. Adjust the small circular (fine adjustment) oxygen valves (1, Fig. 36) to read 20%.
6. Ascertain that large valve (2, Fig. 36) also reads 20% (not 80%).
7. Open exhalation valve (12, Fig. 36) partly to allow gas to escape.
8. Turn pressure control valve (3, Fig. 36) to 5 mm. Hg. and allow some gas to escape to flush out apparatus.
9. Adjust bellows (Fig. 37) to 200 cc. rebreathing by putting bellows stop into 2nd notch.
10. Set rebreathing pressure key to equal pressure at pressure dial (Fig. 37).
11. Open pressure valve to register between 0–5 mm. Hg. until gas flows.
12. Adjust mask to face.
13. Open exhalation valve to allow excess gas to escape and permit patient to breathe mixture until anesthetized.
14. Adjust pressure gauge valve to provide adequate flow and excursions of the bellows.

Comment

1. Rebreathing is not desirable because it is not physiological.
2. Vinyl ether, ethyl ether, halothane, Vinamar, Fluromar, trichlorethylene or chloroform may be added to fortify mixture. Increase oxygen to 25%.

Technique Using Nargraff, Bag and Soda Lime Absorber

1. Set pressure gauge on off (1, Fig. 36).
2. Close ethylene (5, Fig. 36) and open nitrous admit valve (6, Fig 36) on Nargraff head.
3. Open main cylinder valves for oxygen and nitrous oxide entirely.
4. Turn screws controlling reducing valves downward until pressure gauges on Nargraff head registers 40–60 lbs. for both oxygen and nitrous oxide.
5. Close obturator of Y mask holder.
6. Turn pressure gauge (3, Fig. 36) to read five or more mm. Hg. to allow bag to fill with mixture.
7. Close to zero as soon as bag is full.
8. Turn soda lime absorber to "on position."
9. Adjust mask to face and open obturator.
10. Open exhalation valve sufficiently to allow excess gas to escape.
11. Turn pressure valve between 1 and 5 until gas flows and permit patient to breathe mixture until anesthetized.

Nitrous Oxide Ether-Oxygen Sequence Using Bag and Filter

12. Allow patient to pass into Stage III using above procedure.
13. Turn on ether (14, Fig. 36) without disturbing nitrous oxide mixer setting or the pressure setting.
14. Advance ether gradually but as rapidly as patient tolerates.
15. After 3–5 minutes gradually decrease pressure setting by turning valve slightly and close exhalation valve partially with each decrease so that automatic gas flow is reduced but is sufficient to keep bag full. Take 3 or 4 minutes to reduce flow until nitrous oxide oxygen is off completely.
16. Set oxygen (metabolic) at 300 cc. per minute.
17. Turn absorber to off position and allow hyperpnea to develop.
18. Increase ether gradually as hyperpnea develops.
19. Allow hyperpnea to develop until maximal and depression of respiration appears.
20. Turn ether control back half way.
21. Gradually, over a period of several minutes, turn on soda lime absorber until it is in "on" position.
22. Advance ether gradually to point which maintains desired depth of anesthesia.

Comment

1. Manipulations and reasons are basically same as those described for nitrous oxide-ether sequence for standard flow meter technique.
2. Positive pressure of 15 mm. Hg. theoretically increases efficiency of nitrous oxide but in actual practice is of little value.

Nitrous Oxide Oxygen-Demand Principle for (McKesson) Dental Surgery

Materials: McKesson semi-closed apparatus with rebreather and oronasal mask to be followed by nasal attachment.

Preparation:

1. Patient should be fasting and be premedicated.

Procedure:

1. Sit in dental chair.
2. Restrain legs and wrists.
3. Loosen collar.
4. Apply mask and commence flow of nitrous oxide as described above for semi-closed apparatus with rebreather until 3rd stage is attained.
5. Set exhale valve at 5 mm. Hg.
6. Set pressure valve at 5 mm. Hg.
7. Quickly remove mask and substitute nasal piece and fit over nose.
8. Increase nitrous oxide to 90% and decrease oxygen to 10%.
9. Adjust pressure in apparatus to permit adequate flow.
10. Set rebreather at pressure of 12 and rebreath at 300.
11. Pack mouth.

Comment

Without premedication using this technique third stage cannot be obtained without anoxia. Reinforce with:

(a) Vinyl ether.
(b) Trichlorethylene.
(c) Basal narcotic such as pentothal.

Ethylene Oxygen Using Demand (McKesson) Principle

1. Follow procedure outlined for nitrous oxide oxygen by same method (page 107) with following exceptions:
   (a) Close nitrous oxide inlet valve (3, Fig. 36) and open ethylene valve (2, Fig. 36).
   (b) Maintain pressure for mixing at 60 lbs. for ethylene and 60 lbs. for oxygen.
   (c) Follow same precautions outlined for ethylene by standard technique.
2. Follow procedure outlined for nitrous oxide oxygen ether by same method (see nitrous oxide page 110).

REFERENCES

Adriani, J. Pharmacology of Anesthetic Drugs. 4th Ed. Pp. 24–26. Charles C Thomas, Springfield, Ill., 1960.

Goodman, L., and Gilman, A. The Pharmacological Basis of Therapeutics. Pp. 75–93. The Macmillan Co., New York, 1955.
Luckhardt, A. B., and Carter, J. B. Ethylene As an Anesthetic. J.A.M.A., p. 807, 1923.

Nitrous Oxide or Ethylene Using the To and Fro Unit

The above mentioned procedures apply to the use of nitrous oxide or ethylene if the circle filter is employed. When the to and fro inhaler is employed, the principles are the same, but manipulations vary in some respects. Manipulations also vary with the type of to and fro inhaler employed. The to and fro inhaler may be composed in one of the following ways:

1. A mask, bag, and canister with no obturator or exhalation valve. The ether vaporizer possesses no by-pass so that all the gases from the flow-meter pass through or over the ether (Fig. 7). The technique is as follows:

    a. Adjust the nitrous oxide or ethylene flow to 6 liters and the oxygen to 1500 cc. per minute.

    b. Adjust the mask to the face and fasten securely. If necessary, increase the flow of gases or add oxygen from the emergency valve so that the patient does not breathe from a collapsed bag at the outset.

    c. Allow the bag to fill with the mixture.

    d. After the bag is filled, allow the patient to rebreath from the inhaler for thirty to sixty seconds. Then quickly tilt mask backward and manually express all the mixture from the breathing bag. This eliminates the nitrogen which has diffused from the lungs together with the ethylene and oxygen.

    e. Fill the bag with fresh nitrous oxide-oxygen mixture and repeat the maneuver once or twice more or until the patient is in stage III.

    f. Retard the flow of nitrous oxide and adjust oxygen at metabolic flow (see Table VI).

    g. Insert the canister into the inhaler. To accomplish this as quickly as possible without loss of the mixture, the following routine should be followed:

        (a) Place the canister along the side of the patient's head so that mask end rests squarely against the right shoulder.

        (b) Grasp the breathing bag tightly about the neck in such a manner that there is no loss of mixture and slide it in to the sleeve of the bag end of the canister.

        (c) Pick up both the bag and canister and connect it to the mask, still maintaining the grasp about the neck.

        (d) Balance the canister as described on page 79. The operation should be completed in several seconds.

    h. Replenish the mixture which may have been lost from the inhaler with nitrous oxide or ethylene.

    i. From time to time at intervals of several minutes, add several hundred cc. of nitrous oxide or ethylene and allow excess gases to escape by slightly tilting the mask.

For nitrous oxide-oxygen-ether (or ethylene-oxygen-ether sequence), proceed as follows:

(a) Begin addition of ether when stage III has been attained with the gas and gradually increase rate of vaporization by increasing oxygen flow.

(b) As soon as the patient is in stage III, turn off nitrous oxide or ethylene completely and adjust oxygen to the metabolic flow (250–300 cc. per minute).

(c) Allow the patient to rebreathe the mixture without the canister until the hyperpnoea reaches its maximum.

(d) Introduce the canister in place. Immediately afterward, dilute the mixture in the inhaler with several hundred cc. of nitrous oxide or ethylene to avoid the lightening of anesthesia which results from removal of carbon dioxide.

(e) Continue to add ether and carry anesthesia to the desired depth.

2. A mask, bag, and canister with no obturator or exhalation valve, but a dropper type vaporizer on the inhaler (Fig. 17). The gases do not pass through the liquid.

The same technique as above is followed except that ether is added by controlling the dropper.

3. A mask, bag, and canister with an obturator and exhalation valve. The vaporizer is of the bubble type and possesses no by-pass so that all the gases from flow meter pass through the liquid (Fig. 18).

The technique is same as in 1 except that nitrogen is eliminated through the exhalation valve which is allowed to remain partially open rather than by tilting the mask.

4. A mask, bag, and canister, with an obturator, exhalation valve, and dropper vaporizer (Fig. 22).

The technique is similar to that described for the circle filter except that the canister is not introduced into the inhaler until the hyperpnoea is maximal.

Analgesia with Nitrous Oxide or Ethylene for Obstetrical Use:

1. Close obturator, set the soda lime filter for absorption.
2. Fill inhaler with 80% nitrous oxide or ethylene and 20% oxygen and have it in readiness.
3. Ask patient to raise her hand at the first suggestion of a uterine contraction.
4. Apply the mask to the face, open obturator, and ask the patient to breathe deeply during the contraction.

5. Turn on the flow of gas mixture to keep inhaler filled.
6. At the height of the contraction, ask her to hold her breath and "bear down."
7. Remove the mask when contraction is over, fill the inhaler, and have it in readiness for the next contraction.

Comment	*Reasons*
1. Begin inhalation as soon as first sign of pain appears.	A latent phase of 10 or 15 seconds elapses before the onset of analgesia. Analgesia will be of no avail if inhalation begins at the height of the contraction.
2. Use a high concentration of gas at the outset.	The possibility of oxygen want is remote because the gas is diluted with the air in the alveoli.
3. If administration is sustained over a period of several minutes, add oxygen to satisfy the metabolic rate.	The possibility of anoxemia increases if the period of inhalation of mixtures of low oxygen tension is prolonged.

Analgesia for Other Purposes:

1. Follow the procedure for nitrous oxide anesthesia, but employ a concentration of 50% oxygen and 50% nitrous oxide at the outset.
2. Increase or decrease the flow of nitrous oxide according to the requirement of the patient and maintain the stage of analgesia between the zone of pain relief and the zone of loss of consciousness.

Nitrous Oxide or Ethylene with Other Volatile Agents: Both gases may be employed with volatile drugs such as chloroform, trichlorethylene or vinyl ether. Proceed in the same manner as for nitrous oxide-ether or ethylene-ether.

1. Place the liquid in the vaporizer.
2. Fill the inhaler with a mixture of 3 liters of the gas to one of oxygen.
3. Open the exhalation valve and allow the gas to pass into the inhaler in the same manner as for the gas-ether sequence technique.
4. Begin the vaporization and continue the administration by the semi-closed technique. Add O_2 according to Table VI.

Nitrous Oxide or Ethylene with Non-volatile Agents:

1. Nitrous Oxide-Pentothal. The gas provides analgesia; the pentothal unconsciousness and moderate relaxation. Less pentothal and a lower concentration of gas are required than if each were used alone.
    (a) Induce narcosis as described under pentothal (Part IV).
    (b) Follow procedure above using nitrous oxide or ethylene in proportions outlined in table VI or VII.

    (c) Increase flow of gas according to requirement of patient, but in no case exceeding 80%–20% O₂.

    (d) Add pentothal as needed.

2. Nitrous Oxide or Ethylene-Avertin.

    (a) Establish basal narcosis with avertin (Part V).

    (b) Proceed with nitrous oxide or ethylene using a 75%–25% O₂ mixture at outset.

    (c) Decrease or increase gas concentration according to the needs of the patient, but in no case exceeding an 80–20% O₂ mixture.

3. Nitrous Oxide or Ethylene-Curare. The gases provide the analgesia and anesthesia; the curare the muscle relaxation.

    (a) Administer adequate premedication.

    (b) Induce anesthesia with the gas in the routine manner.

    (c) Administer curare in 20 unit fractions intravenously, pausing 3 or 4 minutes between fractions until desired degree of muscle relaxation is secured.

    (d) Intubate (if necessary) to maintain a free airway.

4. Nitrous oxide-pentothal-muscle relaxant.

    (a) Premedicate patient in usual manner with a narcotic and scopolamine or atropine.

    (b) Induce pentothal basal narcosis as described in Part IV.

    (e) Commence flow of nitrous oxide or ethylene-oxygen using semi-closed technique with flows according to table V or VI.

    (d) Add muscle relaxant as described in Part IV. Curare 60 units or equivalent of other muscle relaxant is administered intravenously.

5. Nitrous Oxide or Ethylene-Regional. The relaxation and analgesia are secured by the regional block; the gases are merely used for securing unconsciousness in uncooperative patients.

    (a) Proceed in the routine manner described above.

CYCLOPROPANE

Description: A stable, inflammable, and pleasant smelling gaseous hydrocarbon which is easily inhaled and quickly produces unconsciousness and surgical anesthesia.

Uses:

1. For anesthesia for all types of surgery. Depth may be varied from 1st to 4th plane of stage III with adequate oxygenation.

2. For rapid induction of anesthesia or a preliminary agent to ether. Shortens stages I and II.

3. As a supplemental agent to regional, rectal, intravenous, or other forms of anesthesia.

4. For thoracic surgery (because of its potency and non-irritating properties).

Cost: Expensive, 35–40 cents per gallon.

Method of Administration: Cyclopropane can be satisfactorily administered only in a closed inhaler. The cost and flammable nature of the drug prohibit the use of any but the rebreathing techniques.

Concentration:

1. Analgesia: approximately 8% by volume in the alveoli.
2. Anesthesia: 20–25% by volume in the alveoli.
3. Respiratory failure: 35–39% by volume in the alveoli.

Premedication:

1. Morphine and scopolamine or morphine and atropine $\frac{1}{2}$ to $\frac{2}{3}$ of the usual therapeutic doses employed for ether.
2. Basal narcosis using pentothal, seconal or nembutal intravenously (Part IV).

Materials:

1. Machine with closed inhaler and flowmeter calibrated for cyclopropane. Either the circle filter or the to and fro may be employed. The technique is similar in both instances.
2. Artificial airway.
3. Intercoupler (if floor is not conductive).
4. Sphygmomanometer.

Procedure (see Fig. 38)

Reasons

1. Arrange the patient and equipment in the routine manner described for ether or other gases.

Preparations differ in no way from those required for other gas anesthetics.

2. Turn on carbon dioxide absorber if the circle filter is employed or insert the canister into the system if the to and fro is used.

The hyperpnea of carbon dioxide is not necessary to accelerate induction. Carbon dioxide may cause an elevation of blood pressure.

3. Close the exhalation valve.

Nitrogen need not be eliminated because the concentration required for anesthesia is low.

4. Adjust and hold mask lightly to face.

Avoid loss of gas into the room without causing discomfort by pressure.

5. Partially fill system with 400 or 500 cc. of oxygen, fasten mask and turn on obturator.

Patient should not breathe from an empty bag or inhaler.

6. Adjust flow of oxygen to 1000 cc. and cyclopropane to 600 cc. per minute.

A concentration of 37% by volume is delivered to the inhaler. However, this becomes diluted by the air in the inhaler and lungs to approximately the anesthetic concentration.

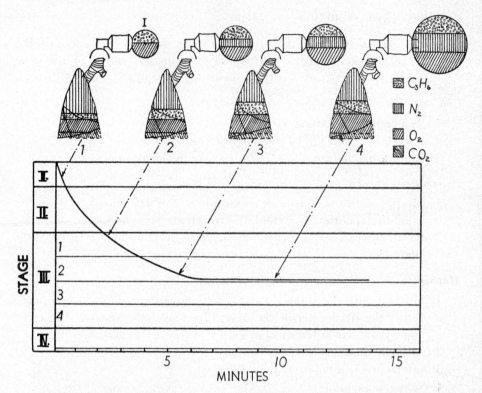

Fig. 38. Induction and maintenance of anesthesia by the closed technique using cyclopropane. This can only be accomplished when potent anesthetic agents, which produce surgical anesthesia at low partial pressures, are employed. Nitrogen need not be eliminated. During the induction, (1) a high concentration (40% ±) of cyclopropane and oxygen is admitted into an almost empty inhaler. As the inhaler fills, the gases mix with the air of the lungs and dilution occurs. The inhaler then contains nitrogen, oxygen and cyclopropane (2) and (3). When surgical anesthesia is fully established, the inhaler is full and an equilibrium exists between the gases in the alveoli and those in the inhaler (4). The concentration of cyclopropane, if an inhaler of approximately 5 liters capacity is employed, averages 25% by volume.

7. As soon as patient is in stage III or if bag fills before he is in stage III, discontinue flow of cyclopropane. Then reduce the oxygen to metabolic rate (300 cc. per minute). Observe signs of anesthesia closely.

The anesthesia becomes deeper for a number of seconds following the termination of flow of gas due to a delay in establishing equilibrium between the alveolar and blood gases.

8. If the bag fills before patient is in stage III, resume flow of cyclopropane after 30 seconds to 400 cc. Maintain oxygen at the metabolic flow. Observe patient closely.

Cyclopropane concentration is being very rapidly increased when it flows into the inhaler at this rate.

9. Add cyclopropane as necessary at the rate of 400–600 cc. per

Tissues absorb drug from blood and thus cause the anesthesia to

minute for ½ to 1 minute at a time as required to maintain the desired depth. Be guided by the signs and symptoms of narcosis shown by the patient.

lighten. The drug absorbed by the tissues must be replaced.

10. Deepen the anesthesia prior to making the incision and before peritoneum is sutured or cut or other painful stimulation occurs.

Painful stimuli tend to lighten the anesthesia.

Cyclopropane—Alternate Method

Procedure:

1. Empty breathing bag completely and close obturator.
2. Turn on oxygen to 1000 cc. and cyclopropane to 600 cc.
3. Allow bag to fill completely with this mixture.
4. Turn on soda-lime absorber.
5. Adjust metabolic flow of oxygen to 300 cc. per minute and cyclopropane to 400 cc. per minute.
6. Apply mask to patient's face and allow him to begin to breathe the mixture.
7. As soon as patient is in third stage turn off cyclopropane and wait several minutes before adding more.
8. Continue to add cyclopropane at 400 cc. per minute at required intervals.

Comment

1. Beware of the concentration.

Reason

This concentration may be excessive for a non-resistant patient.

Cyclopropane—Oxygen Using McKesson

Procedure:

1. Shut off all valves on automatic mixer and turn on cyclopropane and oxygen.
2. Turn soda lime absorber to "on."
3. Close obturator.
4. Flush in oxygen, approximately 700 cc.
5. Turn cyclo flowmeter to 600 and oxygen to 1000 cc. per minute.
6. Apply mask and adjust.
7. Open obturator.

Comment

All other preparations and details same as for cyclopropane administered by other apparatus.

Signs of Anesthesia: Signs of anesthesia differ in certain respects from those characteristic of ether described in the table under Judging Depths of Anesthesia. The following deviations are common:

1. *Nervous System:* Oculomotor activity is present until the third plane of stage III. Pupils remain constricted and do not react to light. Dilation is uncommon unless anoxia is present. Lachrymation is common. No sharp line of demarcation exists between planes 1 and 2.
2. *Respiratory System:* Amplitude and rate of thoracic movements are slightly decreased in first and second planes. As third plane is attained, the amplitude and rate markedly and progressively decrease. Diaphragmatic activity disappears in fourth plane.
3. *Circulatory System:* Bradycardia and arrhythmia may appear in third and fourth planes, but are not necessarily an index of depth of anesthesia. Arterial tension is unchanged but may be elevated in any plane.

Complications	*Reasons*
1. *Overdosage:* respiratory failure precedes circulatory failure.	Eye signs may not be fully established at outset but pupils may be dilated. Thorax is easily inflated. Pulse is slow. Tissues relaxed. Reflexes are absent.
2. *Apnea:* Caused when high oxygen is employed in conjunction with morphine. Also caused by inherent properties of the drug on the respiratory center.	Patient may be light, but respiratory depression prevents adequate absorption of drug and attainment of satisfactory anesthesia. Change to ether or use controlled respiration.
3. *Cardiac arrhythmias:* Many types may be observed: extra systoles, coupled beats, auricular fibrillation, ventricular tachycardia, etc. Due to increase in irritability of automatic tissue of the heart.	Lighten anesthesia by adding oxygen. If persistent, change to ether or other agent.
4. *Unsatisfactory relaxation* (especially of abdominal muscles).	Change to ether or other anesthetic agent. May be due to respiratory depression which prevents absorption of agent, to inherent property of drug, or to a resistant subject.
5. *Laryngospasm.*	Possibly due to parasympathetic stimulation or reflex stimulation of other types. Apply pressure to bag to inflate chest. Spasm may disappear with deepening of anesthesia. Intubate, if spasm persists.

Continuous Flow Cyclopropane

Induce anesthesia as described in previous paragraphs. Turn cyclopropane flow to 50 cc. Observe response of patient increasing or decreasing flow to meet needs of patient and adjusting metabolic requirements of oxygen at 200 cc. adjusting flow to meet needs of patient also.

Contra-Indications to Cyclopropane:

1. Cardiac disease characterized by severe arrythmias cardiac irritability.
2. Operations requiring use of cautery, high frequency units, or other equipment which may cause sparks or produce flames.
3. When epinephrine or norepinephrine are necessary.
4. When bronchospasm is anticipated as a possibility

Advantages:

1. It is rapid acting (3–5 minutes), pleasant, and non-irritating in anesthetic concentrations.
2. The anesthesia may be quickly lightened or deepened during the maintenance phase.
3. Recovery is rapid; most of the drug is eliminated in ten minutes.
4. The concentration required for anesthesia allows use of high partial pressures of oxygen (up to 60%–70% by volume).
5. Elimination of nitrogen is unnecessary so that the closed system may be used from the outset.
6. It possesses a wide margin of safety.
7. It is non-irritating to the respiratory tract.
8. It tends to maintain blood pressure at normal levels in shock, hemorrhage by offsetting vasodilatation.
9. It does not enhance acidosis, elevate blood sugar, or decrease renal or hepatic function.
10. It decreases tidal volume and produces quiet respiration.

Disadvantages:

1. It is expensive, particularly if a completely closed system is not employed.
2. It increases cardiac irritability and causes arrythmias.
3. The patient may pass to stage IV if one does not observe him closely.
4. Muscle relaxation is secured with difficulty in some cases.
5. It is inflammable; anesthetic concentrations are explosive when mixed with air or oxygen.
6. It occasionally produces an elevation of blood pressure.
7. Postanesthetic nausea and vomiting not unusual.

Comment

Reasons

1. Decrease morphine approximately 1/3 to 1/2 of usual dose when administering premedication for cyclopropane anesthesia.

Overpremedication enhances respiratory depression frequently observed with the drug.

2. Do not allow the patient to recover until the skin is sutured and the dressing is in place.

Patient reacts very rapidly, and may emerge from anesthesia before the operation is completed.

3. Be prepared to restrain the patient on the stretcher or in the room.

Excitement or emergence delirium may occur during the recovery period. Administer morphine intravenously to relieve it.

4. The gas may be used in uncomplicated hypertension without fear of increase of pressure or other deleterious effects.

The hypertension appears to be more pronounced in subjects with normal blood pressure. It may be due to a retention of carbon dioxide in the tissues.

5. Employ the gas for short minor surgical procedures.

Induction and recovery are rapid and anesthesia is easily induced and controlled by this agent.

6. Treat any apnea whose cause is not determined as an *overdose* of the drug and institute artificial respiration immediately.

Overdosage is dangerous because the drug is a cardiac depressant and cardiac failure may quickly follow respiratory failure.

7. Do not administer epinephrine for any purpose during cyclopropane anesthesia.

Irritability of cardiac automatic tissue is increased by both drugs. Ventricular fibrillation or serious arrhythmias may occur if they are used together.

8. Beware of an extremely rapid or very slow pulse (below 60). Add ether if cardiac effects persist.

Each is a sign of cardiac irritability. Ether exerts a protective action on the heart.

9. Insert an intratracheal airway if abdominal surgery is to be performed.

The laryngeal spasm frequently prevents adequate ventilation and absorption of sufficient amount of agent for satisfactory relaxation.

Changing to Ether:

1. Light anesthesia: If the anesthesia is light, empty the bag and fill with nitrous oxide 80% and oxygen 20% and start ether (ethylene and oxygen may be employed instead of nitrous oxide).
2. Deep anesthesia: Begin to drop the ether as fast as the patient tolerates it. Change to nitrous oxide or ethylene is not necessary.

Comment

Reason

1. Do not add ether if the anes-

Ether tends to lighten the anes-

thesia is light without adding thesia further and causes a spasm
ethylene and oxygen. of the larynx.

Cyclopropane-Muscle relaxants: Cyclopropane provides analgesia and unconsciousness, the relaxant relaxes the muscles. Light cyclopropane anesthesia may thus be employed in major surgical procedures.

1. Anesthetize patient as described above.
2. Administer curare (tubocurarine) intravenously at the time the skin
   incision is made in 20 unit doses waiting 3 minutes between doses until
   desired muscle relaxation is obtained.
3. Intubate (if necessary) to maintain a free airway.

Comment

Other muscle relaxants may be used as described (see Part IV).

Cyclopropane-ether Combination

Ether added to the cyclopropane "stimulates" breathing, provides relaxation without relaxants and precludes against development of arrhythmias.

1. Anesthetize with cyclopropane to deep level.
2. Gradually introduce ether, but maintain cyclopropane flow so that
   level does not change. Ether tends to "rouse" patient.
3. Alternate additions of fraction between ether and cyclopropane. Add
   ether when respiratory depression characteristic of cyclopropane appears. Add cyclopropane when quantity of ether being used is excessive.

Uses:

1. In long operations when relaxation is required.
2. When respiratory depression is severe due to the cyclopropane.
3. When arrhythmias appear and persist.

Advantages:

1. Permits minimal quantities of ether to be used so that its advantages
   are utilized.
2. Prevents respiratory acidosis—stimulates respiration.
3. Avoids arrhythmias.
4. Avoids prolonged somnolence.
5. Averts objectionable oozing.
6. Dispenses with controlled respiration.
7. Minimal metabolic disturbances.
8. Averts post-anesthesia hypotension.

REFERENCES

Adriani, J. The Pharmacology of Anesthetic Drugs. 4th Ed. Pp. 27–29. Charles C Thomas,
Springfield, Ill., 1960.

Goodman, L., and Gilman, A. The Pharmacological Basis of Therapeutics. Pp. 90–93. The Macmillan Co., New York, 1956.

Robbins, B. H. Cyclopropane Anesthesia. Williams & Wilkins Co., Baltimore, 2nd Ed. 1959.

Waters, R. M., and Schmidt, E. R. Cyclopropane Anesthesia. Jour A.M.A., *103*, 975–983, 1934.

VINYL ETHER

Description: A highly volatile, inflammable liquid whose vapor is easily inhaled, quickly produces unconsciousness and surgical anesthesia. The drug is an unsaturated ether.

Synonyms: "Vinethene,"*—*divinyl ether*, or vinyl oxide.

Uses:

1. As preliminary agent to shorten the first and second stage of ether anesthesia.
2. For anesthesia or analgesia for brief minor surgical procedures such as dental extractions, incision and drainage, reduction of fractures, obstetrics, etc.
3. As a complemental agent to nitrous oxide, ethylene, or other inhalation anesthesia.

Cost: Relatively expensive—25 cc. cost approximately 90 cents. Usually available in 10, 25, or 50 cc. bottles provided with plastic dropper caps to facilitate use.

Methods of Administration:

1. *Open drop.* This is the safest and simplest method of administration by inexperienced individuals and is the method recommended.
2. *Semi-closed.* This method allows use of the drug with other gases, particularly oxygen. It is less expensive than the open method.
3. *Closed.* This method affords considerable saving and insures adequate oxygenation, but an even level of anesthesia is often maintained with difficulty by inexperienced individuals.

Concentration:

1. Analgesia: 2% by volume or less in the alveoli.
2. Anesthesia: approximately 4% by volume in the alveoli.
3. Respiratory failure: 8–10% by volume in the alveoli.

Premedication: May be administered without premedication, but morphine and atropine or morphine and scopolamine in doses similar to those employed for ether are preferred (see premedication).

Materials: The same equipment required for ethyl ether by the open drop technique may be employed.

1. Artificial airway.

---

* A patented name for vinyl ether containing 4% absolute ethyl alcohol and .01% alpha phenyl naphthylamine. The latter substance acts as a stabilizer.

2. Mask and 6–10 layers of gauze.
3. Towels.
4. Vaseline or cold cream.
5. Eye protector.
6. Bottle of vinethene with dropper cap.
7. Suction equipment.

Technique of Open Drop Method (see Fig. 39):

1. Arrange patient in manner described for ether by the open drop technique.

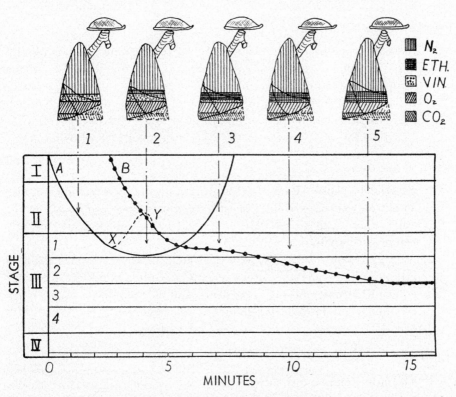

FIG. 39. Changes in gas and vapor tensions in the lungs during induction of anesthesia with a rapid acting potent liquid agent and maintenance with ethyl ether by the open mask technique. Curve A represents anesthesia obtained by vinyl ether. The partial pressure in the alveoli required for surgical anesthesia with this agent is comparatively small but does cause a slight decrease in both nitrogen and oxygen tensions if the vapor inhaled is mixed with air (1). As soon as first plane anesthesia is attained (point X) ethyl ether vapor is added (Curve B) together with vinyl ether. The presence of both vapors causes a still further decrease of oxygen and nitrogen tensions in the alveoli (2). If administration of vinyl ether is halted when the ethyl ether vapor is started, its elimination begins. Recovery from vinyl ether anesthesia occurs (upswing of Curve XY) before sufficient ethyl ether is present in the alveoli to maintain surgical anesthesia. Consequently administration of vinyl ether should continue until enough ethyl ether is present in the alveoli to maintain surgical anesthesia. (Y) The vinyl ether is quickly eliminated during the maintenance of ethyl ether anesthesia (3, 4, 5). Upswing of Curve A.

The same principles apply to the use of other volatile rapid acting drugs (chloroform, ethyl chloride) when used as a preliminary to ethyl ether.

2. Lubricate the skin with vaseline and apply the protector over the face and eyes in the manner described for ether.
3. Apply mask arranged with stockinet or 6–10 layers of gauze (as for ethyl ether anesthesia).
4. Commence to drop drug slowly on the mask, increasing the rate to 40 or 50 drops per minute. Hold the tip of the dropper approximately one inch from the mask and drop the drug continuously at an even rate.
5. As soon as patient passes into stage III, adjust rate of dropping according to the physiological requirements of the patient and the depth of anesthesia desired.

Vinethene-Ether Sequence:

1. As soon as the patient is in stage III, begin dropping ether as rapidly as patient allows without soaking the mask. Continue to add vinethene while concentration of ether necessary for anesthesia is being attained. If patient becomes "light" or coughs, add vinethene until cough disappears and then resume ether.
2. Continue the anesthesia after the ether is begun as described for ether.

Signs of Anesthesia:

1. *Respiratory system:* Rate of respiratory movements may increase, and amplitude decreases in light anesthesia, otherwise it is the same as for ethyl ether in all stages. Watch respiration closely. Respiration fails before circulation.
2. *Nervous system:* Ocular movements remain active until third plane is attained. Eye signs are not as reliable a guide as they are for ethyl ether. Rhythmic rolling movements and horizontal nystagmus are commonly observed during induction and recovery.
3. *Circulatory system:* Changes are similar to ether.

Advantages:

1. The induction and recovery are rapid and pleasant. The period usually occupies 2–3 minutes.
2. It may be administered by means of simple apparatus or even the use of a piece of gauze as a vaporizer.
3. The low partial pressure necessary for surgical anesthesia allows use of air as a vehicle for the vapor.
4. It does not affect the circulatory system.
5. It does not depress respiration.
6. Postanesthetic nausea and vomiting are not common.
7. The vapors may be inhaled directly without causing discomfort.
8. Reflexes quickly return. Postanesthetic depressions are slight or absent.

Disadvantages:

1. It is not chemically stable and requires a preservative and protection from light, heat, and air to maintain its stability.
2. It is highly volatile (B.P. 28°C.). Evaporation occurs readily at room temperature. (Keep tightly stoppered).
3. It may cause convulsions (during reduction).
4. It frequently causes copious salivation and secretion of mucus.
5. The depth of anesthesia is difficult to maintain at a constant level.
6. The vapor forms explosive mixtures with air or oxygen.
7. Muscle relaxation is inadequate for major surgery.
8. It is expensive, in comparison to other volatile liquids.
9. It may cause burns or blisters to skin.
10. It causes physiological disturbances, such as elevation of blood sugar and decrease in CO_2 combining power, but not so profoundly as ethyl ether.
11. It may cause hepatic or renal damage, particularly if administered over a long period of time or if administration is accompanied by anoxia.

Nitrous Oxide Oxygen Fortified with Vinethene

Materials:

1. Either the apparatus which permits the use of pre-mixed oxygen nitrous oxide mixtures to be delivered on demand (McKesson) or standard type (Heidbrink, Foregger) may be used.
2. Special vaporizer designed for vinethene. Usually a squat, wide mouth jar with wick.

Procedure:

1. Adjust the flow of nitrous oxide to deliver a 75%–25% oxygen mixture at the rate of 6 liter flow. On demand (McKesson) apparatus set positive pressure gauge for 3–4 mm. Hg. and mixing device for 75% N_2O and 25% O_2.
2. Adjust mask to the patient's face and commence flow of gas.
3. Open the exhalation valve partially to allow excess gas to escape. Permit the patient to breathe this mixture for 3 to 4 minutes, then gradually add vinethene until the superficial reflexes disappear and patient is in stage 3.
4. Turn on carbon dioxide absorber and continue anesthesia with this mixture.

Comment

For lengthly procedures decrease opening in exhalation valve reduce flow of nitrous oxide to 2 liters and increase oxygen to 850 cc. and vinethene in proportion to maintain surgical anesthesia.

Contra-Indications:

1. For long operations or operations of undetermined duration.
2. For procedures requiring muscle relaxation.
3. The presence of hepatic or renal insufficiency or diseases.
4. The presence of acute infections of the respiratory tract.
5. Procedures requiring use of cautery or other types of apparatus which may be a source of ignition.

Complications	*Cause*
1. Respiratory obstruction.	It is usually the result of salivation and secretion of mucus. Prevent by adequate premedication of atropine or scopolamine.
2. Overdosage.	The drug is administered too rapidly. Respiratory movements cease before circulation fails. Treat with artificial respiration.
3. Postanesthetic nausea and vomiting.	The cause is probably the same as with other anesthetic drugs and procedures.
4. Headache.	The cause is not determined. Not common or serious if it occurs.
5. Convulsions.	These are probably due to the effect of the drug upon the central nervous system. They occur less frequently if premedication of morphine and scopolamine is employed. Control them with ultra-short-acting barbiturates intravenously administered.

Comment	*Reasons*
1. Do not induce anesthesia until all preparations for surgery have been made.	The period of anesthesia should be as short as possible. The use of the drug for periods exceeding thirty minutes is not recommended.
2. Regulate the number and size of the drops by adjusting the cap on the dropper.	No vent is required on the bottle because the drug is so volatile that the vapor forces it out of the bottle.
3. Use the semi-open method for anesthesia in adults.	Vaporization occurs so rapidly it may not be adequate in robust subjects.
4. Store the drug in a cool place away from acids and fumes.	Heat and acids hasten its deterioration.
5. Do not use the drug beyond its expiration date.	The drug is stable in the container for two years.

6. Select vinyl ether in preference to ethyl chloride as an inhalation anesthetic agent.	The scope and utility of the two agents are similar, but the cardiac effects of ethyl chloride are absent with vinyl ether.
7. When this drug is employed do not tolerate anoxia or obstruction under any circumstances.	The possibility of hepatic damage is markedly enhanced by lack of oxygen.
8. Do not administer the drug too rapidly or in too high a concentration.	Salivation and secretion of mucus are more pronounced. The possibility of overdosage is increased.
9. Drop the drug continuously on the mask during induction and maintenance of anesthesia.	The drug is so volatile that intermittent dropping causes uneven anesthesia.
10. Do not allow the liquid to drop on or come into contact with the skin.	Burns and blisters may result, particularly if pressure is applied to the area involved.

Variations in Technique

1. *For Analgesia:* Proceed with the induction until patient feels a sensation of dizziness; then decrease the rate of administration as stage II is approached. Instruct the patient to raise his hand when he feels pain during the surgery and increase the rate of administration.
2. *For Anesthesia by Closed Methods:* Place the vinyl ether in the ether vaporizer and allow oxygen or mixtures of oxygen and nitrous oxide or ethylene to flow over the liquid or bubble gently through it. Proceed as described for ether by closed system.

REFERENCES

Adriani, J. The Pharmacology of Anesthetic Drugs. 4th Ed. Pp. 37–40. Charles C Thomas, Springfield, Ill., 1960.

Lyons, S. S., and Frank, H. P. Vinethene Analgesia. Jour. A. Dental A., *26*, 580–584, April, 1939.

Martin, S. J., and Rovenstine, E. A. Vinethene, Recent Laboratory and Clinical Evaluation. Anesthesiology, *2*, 285–299, May, 1941.

Ravdin and others. Divinyl Ether. Jour. A. M. A., *108*, 1163, April, 1937.

FLUOROMAR (TRIFLUOROETHYL VINYL ETHER) ANESTHESIA

Synonyms—"Fluroxene" (generic name)

Description

Fluoromar is a clear, colorless, flammable liquid having an unobjectionable, ethereal odor. The odor resembles that of vinyl ether. The drug is a halogenated ether chemically allied to vinyl ether but differing from it in having one ethyl group with three fluorine atoms on the terminal carbon and a vinyl group. The boiling point is 42.7°C. and the air blood ratio is 5.0. The absorption distribution and elimination are intermediate between gases such as cyclopropane and the vapors of ether and chloroform.

Uses

1. To fortify nitrous oxide for procedures not requiring relaxation.
2. As a sole agent for minor procedures not requiring profound muscle relaxation.
3. For major procedures in conjunction with a muscle relaxant.
4. As an analgesic for obstetrics, dentistry, etc.
5. As an induction agent for ethyl ether.

Cost

Relatively expensive. A 100 cc. bottle costs approximately $10.00.

Methods of Administration

1. Open drop technique (not recommended due to the high vapor pressure required at room temperature and expense).
2. Semi-open technique using Fluotec copper kettle, or other bubble type vaporizer and a gas machine utilizing a reservoir bag and a nonrebreathing valve of the Stephen-Slater or Fink type or demand principle (McKesson).
3. Semi-closed technique using circle filter with exhalation valve with vaporizers listed above.
4. Closed technique using draw-over, Verni-trol, or copper kettle vaporizers.

Concentration

	Volume % Inspired	Mgms. % Arterial Blood
Analgesia	2.0	9.3
Plane 1	3.2	15.0
Plane 2	5.0	20.0
Plane 3	8.2	29.0
Plane 4	12.0	39.0
Apnea	—	49.0

Vapor pressure: At 28°C. 395 m. Hg.

Premedication

Morphine and atropine or morphine and scopolamine in the usual therapetutic doses for adults. Seconal-hydroxyzine (Vistaril) combination and levohyoscyamine (Bellafoline) or Demerol and Bellafoline for children in standard doses. (See premedication.)

Materials

1. Anesthesia gas machine with either a to and fro or a circle absorber convertible to semi-closed, flow meters calibrated for oxygen, cyclopropane, and nitrous oxide, plus a suitable vaporizer. (The draw-over type, verni-trol, Fluotec or copper kettle may be employed.)
2. Artificial airways.
3. Sphygmomanometer.

4. Precordial stethoscope.
5. Suction machine.
6. Intercoupler if conductive floor is not available.

CYCLOPROPANE-FLUOROMAR OXYGEN SEQUENCE

Cyclopropane is used to expedite induction. Maintenance is with Fluoromar-Oxygen.

Technique

Reasons

1. Arrange the patient and apparatus in the routine manner described for ether or other gases.

Preparations differ in no way from those required for other inhalation anesthetics.

2. Turn on carbon dioxide absorber if the circle filter is employed or insert the cannister into the system if the to and fro is used.

The hyperpnea of carbon dioxide is not necessary to accelerate induction. Carbon dioxide may cause an elevation of blood pressure.

3. Empty breathing bag completely and close obturator.

Patient must breathe anesthetic mixture from outset to facilitate induction.

4. Turn on oxygen to 1000 cc. per minute and cyclopropane to 600 cc. per minute and allow bag to fill completely with this mixture.

A concentration of 37% by volume is delivered to inhaler. However, this becomes diluted by the air in inhaler and lungs to approximately the anesthetic concentration.

5. Adjust metabolic flow of oxygen to 300 cc. per minute and cyclopropane to 300 cc. per minute.

Any mixture of cyclopropane stronger than 50% may produce irritation with resultant laryngospasm.

6. Apply mask lightly to face and allow patient to breathe the cyclopropane mixture.

Avoid loss of gas into the room without causing discomfort by pressure.

7. As soon as patient is in third stage fasten mask securely to patient's face, turn off cyclopropane and wait several minutes before adding more.

Undue depression is thus avoided.

8. Commence to add Fluoromar. If employing the Ohio number 8 drawover vaporizer the valve is opened about two positions every three or four breaths. (If the vernitrol or copper kettle is used, delivered concentrations of agent may be computed using the Ohio flow calculator).

Because of the mild odor of Fluoromar this rate of increase of concentration of vapor does not irritate patient or cause breath holding or laryngospasm.

9. Allow the patient to breathe the mixture with the valve set at the

Higher than maintenance concentrations are required during induc-

ninth or tenth (wide open) position until the desired depth of anesthesia is obtained as evidenced by respirations becoming slower and deeper (cyclopropane is added as needed until this depth is attained).

10. For maintenance set the valve on the third or second position, depending upon the particular patient's requirements.

tion. If depth is increased further until tachypnea develops, undesirable effects may ensue, such as hypotension, bradycardia, decreased tidal volume and respiraatory acidosis.

For maintenance of anesthesia a "cut back" must be made from concentration required for induction. The required concentration is markedly reduced.

NITROUS OXIDE-FLUOROMAR OXYGEN SEQUENCE (CLOSED SYSTEM)

Technique

1. Close the obturator at the mask and fill inhaler with nitrous oxide 80% and oxygen 20%.

2. Adjust but do not fasten mask to the patient's face.

3. Turn carbon dioxide absorber to "on" position and open obturator so that patient breathes from the inhaler.

4. Adjust flow meter to deliver oxygen at 1200 cc. and nitrous oxide at 4 liters per minute.

5. Open exhalation valve sufficiently to allow excess gases to escape from inhaler but not so wide that the bag becomes deflated.

6. As soon as patient passes into stage III, gradually commence vaporizing Fluoromar and increase as rapdily as the patient tolerates it. (Vaporization may commence sooner if stage II is prolonged.)

7. Continue flow of nitrous oxide and

Reasons

A full bag is employed at the outset to more quickly dilute and displace the air in the apparatus and lungs with anesthetic gas.

Stimulation created by the pressure may cause patient to become excited as he passes through stage II.

Carbon dioxide should be removed to prevent the feeling of suffocation which patients frequently experience during induction if rebreathing occurs.

A mixture of 80% nitrous oxide and 20% oxygen is thus assured in the inhaler.

Nitrogen, some nitrous oxide, and carbon dioxide are eliminated during each exhalation. Ultimately most of the nitrogen in the alveoli is replaced by nitrous oxide and oxygen and the patient passes into stage III.

The non-irritating qualities of Fluoromar may be used to advantage to shorten induction.

Anesthesia with nitrous oxide (as

oxygen allowing exhalation valve to remain open during the introduction and "build-up" of Fluoromar to concentration necessary for maintenance.

is the case with ether) must be maintained while Fluoromar is being raised to desired concentration.

8. When the desired concentration of Fluoromar is attained, gradually decrease the flow of nitrous oxide. Decrease at rate of 1000 cc. every two minutes. Ultimately the entire flow will be off. (Within 5 minutes as a rule.)

All concentrations of gases and vapors should be raised or lowered gradually to insure a stabilized depth of anesthesia.

9. Close exhalation valve when the flow of nitrous oxide is stopped and adjust oxygen to 300–400 cc. per minute and Fluoromar to maintenance concentration.

With system closed and metabolic requirements of oxygen being furnished, rebreathing of Fluoromar is instituted.

10. System need not be closed off if Fluoromar is used only to fortify the nitrous oxide.

This technique is useful for short procedures, such as teeth extractions in children.

Comments

1. Closed system administration is the most advantageous in using this agent.

Reasons

Economy-wise far less Fluoromar is used and desired level of anesthesia can be maintained and controlled with greater ease.

2. When using the draw-over type vaporizer, wick need consist only of 5–8 strands of absorbent material.

This is sufficient for adequate vaporization and the salvage rate of Fluoromar is greatly increased.

3. Close observation of the blood pressure is essential due to liability of the agent and the ease with which anesthesia may be deepened.

Hypotension is directly related to the concentration of Fluoromar. Lightening the level of anesthesia produces a prompt return of the blood pressure to normal or near normal levels.

4. Respirations should be observed closely and assisted when necessary.

Tachypnea and decreased tidal volume may occur during deep anesthesia.

5. The classical signs for ether are not usually apparent. "Eye signs" are not a reliable guide to depth of anesthesia.

Fluoromar is comparable to vinyl ether in this respect.

6. Fluoromar may be used as an induction agent for ethyl ether.

Not recommended due to the high boiling point of Fluoromar which may be reflected in prolonged inductions.

Advantages of Fluoromar

1. Rapid, pleasant induction.
2. Rapid recovery.
3. Excitement uncommon.
4. Non-irritating to respiratory tract.
5. Nausea and vomiting uncommon.
6. Does not depress respiration in lighter planes.
7. Does not depress circulation.
8. Does not sensitize heart to epinephrine.
9. Respiration ceases before circulation in overdosage.
10. May be combined with ether or nitrous oxide.
11. Does not notably interfere with important physiological functions.
12. Control of respiration is achieved easily.

Disadvantages of Fluoromar

1. Relatively expensive (compared to ether).
2. Inflammable—fire hazard.
3. Muscle relaxation unsatisfactory.
4. "Eye signs" not reliable guide to anesthesia.
5. Not satisfactory with open technique.

Contraindications

1. Operations requiring muscle relaxation.
2. The presence of cautery or other source of ignition.
3. Shock from trauma or hemorrhage.
4. Acidosis from any cause.

REFERENCES

Adriani John. Chemistry and Physics of anesthesia, 2nd Ed. Chap 15, Springfield, Thomas, 1962.
Adriani John. The Pharmacology of Anesthetic Drugs, 2nd Ed. Pp. 42–45. Springfield, Thomas, 1960.

METHOXYFLURANE (PENTHRANE)

Description

Methoxyflurane is a clear, colorless, non-flammable liquid with a characteristic fruity odor. The drug is a halogenated ether having a methyl group on one oxygen atom and an ethyl group on the other. The two hydrogen atoms on the carbon atom next to the oxygen on the ethyl group are replaced by two fluorine atoms. The hydrogen atoms on the terminal carbon atom of the ethyl group are replaced by two chlorine atoms.

The boiling point is 104.6°C. at normal atmospheric pressure. The vapor is non-flammable at room temperature. The absorption distribution and elimination are similar to those of ether except that absorption and elimination requires longer time. Air-blood ratio is 13.0.

Uses

1. As an analgesia for obstetrics, dentistry or minor procedures.
2. To fortify nitrous oxide when non-flammable anesthetics are required.
3. As a sole agent for major surgical procedures when relaxation is required and relaxants are not desired.

Cost

Relatively expensive. 100 cc. bottles costs approximately $10.00.

Concentration

Approximately 3% for induction; 0.5–1% for maintenance. Maximum possible concentration at 23°C. is approximately 4%.

Methods of Administration

1. Semi-closed technique with oxygen in the copper kettle (or Vernitrol on the Heidbrink).
2. Closed technique using draw-over or bubble type of vaporizer (Heidbrink No. 8 on inspiratory side).

Premedication

Morphine and scopolamine or morphine and atropine in the usual therapeutic doses recommended for adults for ether.

Secobarbital, hydroxyzine (Vistaril) combination or levohyoscyamine (Bellafoline) or meperidine and levohyoscyamine (Bellafoline) for children in standard doses (see premedication).

Materials

1. Anesthesia gas machine equipped with circle filter, copper kettle (or other suitable desired type of vaporizer) flow meters calibrated for oxygen and nitrous oxide.
2. Artificial airways.
3. Sphygmomanometer.
4. Precordial stethoscope.
5. Suction machine.

Procedure Using Semi-Closed Technique

1. Arrange the patient and apparatus in the routine manner described for ether and other types of anesthesia. Add drug to vaporizer.
2. Commence oxygen at 6 liter flow. Partly fill breathing bag and apply mask.
3. Open exhale valve to allow excess gas to escape.
4. Turn vaporizer (Heidbrink No. 8) to No. 1 position. Then gradually open by small increments as rapidly as vapor is tolerated. Open to the wide open position (No. 10) if necessary.

5. Allow vaporizer to remain in open position until surgical anesthesia is established (15–20 min.).
6. Gradually cut back vaporizer to 3 or 4 position for maintenance concentration.
7. Induce anesthesia with thiopental in the usual manner to shorten induction if desired.

Procedure Using the Copper Kettle and Semi-Closed Technique

1. Commence with a mixture obtained by flowing 1000 ml. of oxygen through the copper kettle.
2. Gradually increase oxygen flow through liquid in kettle in increments tolerable to the patient to 3000 cc. per minute.
3. As soon as induction is complete decrease flow for maintenance to 1000–2000 cc. (15 minutes).
4. Induce anesthesia with thiopental to shorten induction time if desired.

Procedure Using Closed Method

1. Use apparatus with draw-over type of vaporizer.
2. Induce anesthesia with
   (a) thiopental intravenously followed by nitrous (semi-closed) oxide 3 liters to 1 oxygen
   or (b) cyclopropane closed technique.
3. Gradually introduce methoxyflurane by opening vaporizer in small increments to patient until necessary concentration to maintain anesthesia has been attained.
4. Withdraw nitrous oxide gradually as in the case of ether.
5. Close the system and cut back methoxyflurane to 3 or 4 position or whatever concentration is necessary for anesthesia.

Comment	Reason
1. Use induction agent such as thiopental or cyclopropane.	Averts excitement and shortens induction time. Absorption and elimination of the drug is similar to ether; induction slow, recovery slow.
2. Vapor concentration of drug maximal at 23° at 4%.	Vapor pressure at room temperature is low.
3. Do not store methoxyflurane in contact with copper, brass, bronze or aluminum.	Becomes discolored and forms a precipitate with metals.
4. Use high carrier gas flow during induction and a cut back during maintenance.	High concentration of drug needed to saturate tissues at outset.
5. Use vital signs (blood pressure, pulse rate and respiration) as guide to depth of anesthesia.	The signs of Guedel are not applicable to methoxyflurane.

6. Assist respiration.	Respiratory depression accompanies anesthesia.
7. Monitor blood pressure frequently.	Methoxyflurane causes drop in blood pressure due to myocardial depression, vasodilatation and other factors.
8. Do not use epinephrine in conjunction with methoxyflurane.	Produces arrhythmias, as does cyclopropane, chloroform and halothane.
9. Discontinue anesthesia 10 to 15 minutes prior to end of operation.	Allow time for recovery since it is slow due to slow elimination.

Contraindications

1. Liver disease or insufficiency.
2. Situations in which rapid recovery is mandatory.
3. Hypotensive states.

Advantages of Penthrane

1. Non-flammable at room temperature.
2. Produces excellent relaxation as sole agent without aid of relaxants. Useful when relaxation without relaxants is desired.
3. Not unpleasant to inhale.
4. Analgesia extends into the period of emergence and lasts several hours postoperatively.
5. Compatible with other inhalation anesthetics and non-volatile central nervous system depressants.
6. Chemically stable with soda lime.
7. Salivation not excessive.
8. Not laryngospasmogenic or bronchospasmogenic.
9. Augments the action of non-depolarizing muscle relaxants (tubocurarine).

Disadvantages

1. Characterized by a prolonged induction and excitement period.
2. Prolonged somnolence during emergence and recovery period.
3. Headaches during the postoperative period (some patients).
4. Depresses the heart muscle, produces hypotension and arrhythmias.
5. Not compatible with epinephrine.
6. Signs of Guedel not suitable as a guide to depth of anesthesia.
7. Traces persist in plasma (released from fat depots) for several days after administration.
8. Depresses respiration during maintenance.
9. Invariably produces hypotension in deeper phases of anesthesia.

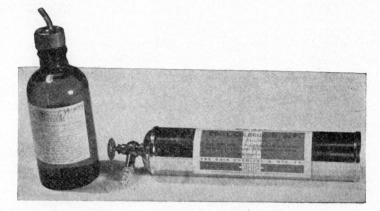

Fig. 40. Dropper bottle for vinyl ether with an adjustable tip to control the rate and size of drops, and ampule for storage of ethyl chloride.

REFERENCES

Artusio, J. F. Clinical Evaluation of Methoxyflurane in Man. Fed. Proc. *19:* 273 (Mar. **1**), 1960.

Van Poznak, A., Artusio, J. F. Methoxyflurane as an Anesthetic for Neurological Surgery, J. Neurosurg. *17:* 477 (Mar.), 1960.

ETHYL CHLORIDE

Description: A highly volatile, inflammable liquid whose vapor is pleasant smelling, easily inhaled and quickly produces unconsciousness and surgical anesthesia and analgesia. The drug is a halogenated hydrocarbon.

Synonym: "Kelene."

Uses:

1. As an induction agent to shorten the first and second stage of ether administered by the open mask techniques.
2. To secure anesthesia and analgesia for operations or minor surgical procedures of not more than several minutes duration.

Cost: Relatively inexpensive (100 cc. cost approximately 50 cents).

Methods of Administration:

1. *Open drop:* Safest and simplest and the recommended technique for the novice.
2. *Closed:* This method allows the use of oxygen and affords considerable saving of drug, but the depth of anesthesia is difficult to maintain at a constant level. Not recommended for inexperienced individuals.

Concentration:

1. Analgesia: 2 or 3% by volume in the alveoli.
2. Anesthesia: 5–6% by volume in the alveoli.
3. Respiratory failure: not determined.

Premedication: Morphine and scopolamine or morphine and atropine in doses similar to those employed for ether anesthesia.

Materials: The same equipment employed for ethyl ether by the open drop technique:

1. Artificial airway.
2. Wire mask with 6–10 layers of gauze or a stockinet.
3. Towels.
4. Eye shield.
5. Ethyl chloride. The drug is usually packed in metal or glass ampules equipped with a capped nozzle (Fig. 40). The liquid may be sprayed or dropped from the nozzle by manipulation of the cap.

Technique of Open Drop Method (see Fig. 41):

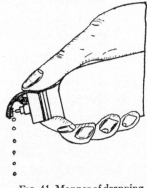

1. Arrange patient in a manner similar to that described for ether anesthesia by the open drop method.
2. Protect the face and eyes. Apply and hold the mask as described for ether anesthesia.
3. Hold the ampule in the right hand several inches above the mask and tilt it so that the liquid gravitates to the outlet. Lift the cap from the nozzle sufficiently to allow the stream of liquid to strike and glance off it to the mask in form of drops (do not spray). Hold nozzle of ampule several inches from the mask (Fig. 41).

FIG. 41. Manner of dropping drug for inhalation anesthesia by the open mask technique is shown.

4. Allow a few drops of the drug to fall upon the mask to accustom patient to odor.
5. Ask patient to begin counting out loud (if he is cooperative).
6. Commence to drop the drug at the rate of one drop every three or four seconds and gradually increase the rate to one every two or three seconds.
7. As soon as consciousness is lost (between one to two minutes) change the rate but continue to drop the drug until a hyperpnea develops.
8. Quickly begin to drop ether as rapidly as the patient tolerates the drug.

Signs of Anesthesia: These are similar to those described for vinyl ether.

Advantages:

1. The period of induction and recovery are rapid. Usually occupy several minutes.
2. It shortens the length of stages I and II of ether anesthesia when used as a preliminary to it.
3. It may be administered with a simple apparatus.
4. The low partial pressure required for surgical anesthesia allows the use of air as a vehicle and source of oxygen.

5. It does not cause respiratory depression.
6. It is pleasant to inhale and is not irritating to membranes of the respiratory tract.
7. It is chemically stable.
8. It causes little postanesthetic nausea and vomiting.

Disadvantages:

1. It possesses a narrow margin of safety.
2. It depresses the circulatory system and frequently causes cardiac failure. Circulation may fail before respiration.
3. It forms explosive mixtures when mixed with air or oxygen.
4. It frequently causes stridor or muscle rigidity.
5. The depth of anesthesia is difficult to maintain at a constant level.
6. It may cause renal or hepatic damage if administered over a prolonged period of time.
7. A cold vapor is inhaled when it is employed; this may be irritating.

Contraindications:

1. The presence of any circulatory disturbances or disease.
2. Procedures requiring more than several minutes for completion.
3. The presence of acute respiratory infections.
4. Procedures requiring use of cautery or other apparatus which may be a source of ignition.

Complications	*Reasons*
1. Stridor or laryngeal spasm.	These are usually of reflex origin. Discontinue the drug and administer oxygen under slight positive pressure to relieve it.
2. Syncope.	It is caused by cardiac failure from overdosage or the depressant action of the drug upon the heart.
3. Respiratory failure.	It is due to overdosage. Institute artificial respiration immediately.
4. Spasm of muscles: Usually manifested by opisthotonus, rigidity, or twitchings.	Discontinue the drug immediately, remove mask from face, and allow the patient to recover from anesthesia.

Comment	*Reasons*
1. Avoid use of this drug for inhalation anesthesia unless absolutely necessary.	The deleterious cardiac effects render this a dangerous drug even when administered by expert individuals.
2. Remember that a latent phase of 30 or 40 seconds follows cessation	The drug in the lungs continues to be absorbed into the blood even

of administration of ethyl chloride. During this interval the patient becomes more deeply anesthetized.

3. Do not spray the drug on mask.

The spray is so fine that it passes through the gauze and causes excitement if it falls on the patient's face. High concentrations collect under the mask if the spray passes through it.

4. Do not wrap towels about the mask.

The drug is not sufficiently diluted with air and a dangerously high concentration collects around the mask.

5. Begin dropping ether as soon as the patient is narcotized by the ethyl chloride.

Recovery begins almost immediately after cessation of administration of ethyl chloride. The drug is eliminated even though ether is being inhaled.

6. Remove the frost which collects on mask.

Water vapor of exhaled air freezes because a low temperature is produced by the vaporization of ethyl chloride. The frost may cause obstruction.

7. Do not return to the administration of ethyl chloride once the administration of ether has been instituted.

The possibility of overdosage is increased if this is done.

8. Do not tolerate anoxia or respiratory obstruction under any circumstances.

Cardiac irritability caused by this drug is enhanced by anoxia. Ventricular fibrillation may follow.

9. Drop the drug continuously onto the mask during induction period and maintenance.

The drug is so volatile that intermittent dropping results in an uneven plane of anesthesia.

10. Do not administer epinephrine in conjunction with ethyl chloride.

Both drugs increase irritability of cardiac tissues.

REFERENCE

Adriani, J. The Pharmacology of Anesthetic Drugs 4th Ed. Pp. 49-51. Charles C Thomas Springfield, Ill., 1960.

CHLOROFORM

Description: Chloroform is a colorless, volatile liquid whose vapor is sweet smelling, easily inhaled, and non-inflammable. Chloroform is one of the most potent inhalation anesthetic agents available.

Uses:

1. For all types of surgery in which a potent anesthetic agent is required.

2. As preliminary induction agent for shortening the first and second stages of ether anesthesia.
3. As an analgesic agent for obstetrical and other uses.
4. For operations in which a non-inflammable inhalation anesthetic is necessary.

Cost: Relatively inexpensive.

Methods of Administration:

1. *Open drop:* This is the most commonly employed, simplest, and safest technique and the one which is recommended.
2. *Semi-closed:* This technique allows the drug to be administered with oxygen or other gases.
3. *Closed:* This technique allows rebreathing with high oxygen concentration but is only recommended for experienced individuals.

Concentration:

1. Analgesia: less than 1% by volume in the alveoli.
2. Anesthesia: approximately 1.5% by volume in the alveoli.
3. Respiratory failure: 2% by volume in the alveoli.

Premedication: Morphine and atropine or morphine and scopolamine in the usual therapeutic doses employed for ether (see premedication).

Materials (open method):

1. A large mask provided with four to six layers of gauze or a stockinet. The edge should be cut to the shape of the mask.
2. An artificial airway.
3. A protecter for the eyes.
4. Chloroform in a bottle equipped with dropper.
5. Petrolatum or cold cream for the skin.
6. Castor oil for the eye and a dropper.
7. Inhaler to supply oxygen and artificial respiration if necessary.
8. Nasal catheter for the oxygen.

Technique of Open Method:

1. Arrange and prepare the patient in the same manner described for ether by the open method.
2. Place the eye protector over eyes and lubricate the face well with petrolatum or cold cream.
3. Apply the mask to the face and hold it in the same manner as described for ether by the open method.
4. Begin to drop chloroform on the mask as rapidly as patient tolerates it. Start with three drops the first minute and double the rate each succeeding minute for the first four or five minutes.

5. As soon as patient is in stage III, instill two drops of castor oil into each eye.
6. Insert a nasal catheter into one nostril and replace the mask. Supply oxygen at approximately 1000 cc. per minute from inhaler.
7. Continue to drop the drug at rate necessary for desired plane of anesthesia.

Signs of Anesthesia: The signs of anesthesia are in general similar to those outlined under Judging Depth of Anesthesia.

Advantages of Chloroform:

1. It is the most potent inhalation anesthetic agent available. The relaxation it yields is excellent.
2. The period of induction is rapid and does not necessitate the use of a preliminary agent such as nitrous oxide or ethylene.
3. It forms non-inflammable mixtures with air or oxygen.
4. It possesses a degree of volatility (B.P. 61°C.) which allows its use in the tropics or warm climates.
5. It may be administered by means of very simple equipment.
6. It does not unduly stimulate respiration. A "quiet abdomen" follows.
7. Its extreme potency and the low partial pressure necessary for anesthesia allow the use of air as a vehicle.
8. It is chemically stable if preserved by alcohol away from heat, air, or light.

Disadvantages:

1. It possesses a narrow margin of safety. The transition through the upper to lower stages of anesthesia is rapid.
2. It may cause hepatitis to appear postoperatively.
3. It may cause severe derangement of liver function, without hepatitis.
4. It causes cardiac depression which is manifested by syncope, ventricular fibrillation, arrhythmias or other disturbances.
5. It causes serious biochemical disturbances, such as elevation of blood sugar, decrease in acid-base balance or dehydration.
6. It may decompose if exposed to flames or cautery in the presence of air to form phosgene.
7. Its elimination is slow.
8. It is frequently accompanied by postanesthetic nausea and vomiting.

Contra-Indications	*Reasons*
1. Diseases of the heart.	Chloroform increases irritability of cardiac automatic tissue.

2. Hypertension or hypotension or "shock."

The vasomotor center is depressed, and cardiac output is decreased by the drug.

3. Diabetes mellitus or acidosis from any cause.

Carbon dioxide combining power is decreased and blood sugar is elevated during anesthesia.

4. Diseases of the liver.

It decreases liver function and predisposes to or causes hepatitis.

5. Diseases of the kidney.

It causes oliguria or anuria.

6. Acute or chronic diseases of the respiratory tract.

It increases production of mucus and other secretions which disseminate infection from one part of the respiratory tract to another.

Comment

1. Never allow liquid chloroform to come into contact with the skin.

Reasons

If chloroform remains in contact with the skin it causes burns or blisters, particularly if pressure is applied to the area.

2. Do not tolerate anoxia during the administration of chloroform. Supply oxygen if possible.

The possibility of liver damage is increased. Anoxia augments cardiac irritability and hastens cardiac failure and shock.

3. Do not expose chloroform vapor to naked flames or sparks.

Phosgene, which is irritating to pulmonary epithelium, may form. Pulmonary edema occurs.

4. Drop the drug slowly and at a constant rate rather than intermittently.

This insures a constant level of anesthesia. Overdosage can only be avoided by extreme care.

5. Do not administer chloroform to starved, debilitated, or emaciated individuals.

The possibility of hepatitis is greater in these subjects. Preoperative administration of glucose is desirable if possible.

6. Do not use epinephrine for any purpose during chloroform anesthesia.

Both drugs increase cardiac irritability. Ventricular fibrillation may result.

7. Do not omit premedication. Administer both an opium and a belladonna derivative.

Avoid any and all excitement. Epinephrine may be liberated into the blood during the period of excitement and the patient may die of ventricular fibrillation during the induction.

8. Palpate the pulse continuously and record blood pressure readings frequently.

Circulatory failure may precede respiratory failure at any time.

9. Remember that as the operation continues smaller amounts of

As time goes on an equilibrium becomes established between the

drug will be necessary to maintain the desired depth of anesthesia.

10. Do not delay instituting artificial respiration in the event respiratory failure occurs.

The margin between respiratory failure and circulatory failure is narrow. Delays may be fatal.

11. Decrease the rate of administration should the patient suddenly breathe deeply. Raise the mask from the face if the patient holds his breath

The amount of drug necessary for anesthesia is so small that a sudden concentrated breathful may lead to overdosage and cardiac arrest.

12. Do not stimulate the patient in any way during the induction and recovery periods.

May cause excitement.

13. Discontinue the drug if the pulse becomes slow (50 or less) or irregular.

Such changes indicate cardiac depression, irritability, or shift of the pace maker.

14. Never pour chloroform onto the mask.

The danger of overdosage is ever present and is increased by such a technique.

REFERENCES

Adriani, J. The Pharmacology of Anesthetic Drugs. 4th Ed. Pp. 45–48. Charles C Thomas, Springfield, Ill., 1960.

Goodman, L., and Gilman, A. The Pharmacological Basis of Therapeutics. Pp. 75–93. The Macmillan Co., New York, 1955.

TRICHLORETHYLENE

Description: Trichlorethylene is a colorless, slowly volatilizing liquid whose vapor is sweet smelling, easily inhaled and not inflammable. The odor resembles that of chloroform.

Synonyms: Trilene, trimar.

Uses:

1. As an analgesic agent for obstetrics, skin grafting and other minor forms of surgery.
2. To fortify nitrous oxide.
3. For operations in which a non-inflammable inhalation anesthetic may be necessary. The use of the drug for general anesthesia has been abandoned.

Cost: Relatively inexpensive, approximately 1 cent per cc.

Methods of Administration:

1. Open drop. This is the most commonly employed, simplest technique

and the one which is recommended for surgical anesthesia.

2. Semi-closed. This technique allows the drug to be administered with oxygen or nitrous oxide.
3. Closed. This technique cannot be used because the drug is unstable in the presence of soda-lime.

Concentration:

1. Analgesia—less than 1% by volume in the alveoli.
2. Anesthesia—approximately 4% by volume in the alveoli.
3. Respiratory failure—exact concentration not established.

Premedication:

Morphine combined with atropine, bellafoline or scopolamine in the therapeutic doses recommended for ether anesthesia (see premedication).

Materials:

1. A large open drop mask provided with 4 to 6 layers of gauze or stockinet. The edge should be cut to fit the shape of the mask.
2. An artificial airway.
3. A protector for the eyes.
4. Trichlorethylene in a bottle equipped with a dropper.
5. Petrolatum or cold cream for the skin.
6. Castor oil for the eyes and a dropper.
7. Inhaler to supply oxygen and artificial respiration if necessary.
8. Nasal catheter for oxygen and oxygen supply.

Technique of
the Open Method:

1. Arrange and prepare the patient in the same manner described for ether by the open method.
2. Place the eye protector over the eyes and lubricate the face well with petrolatum or cold cream.
3. Apply the mask to the face and hold it in the same manner as described for ether by the open method.
4. Begin to drop the trichlorethylene on the mask as rapidly as the patient tolerates it. Start with two or three drops the first half minute and double the rate each succeeding minute for the first four or five minutes.
5. As soon as patient is in stage III, instill two drops of castor oil into each eye.
6. Insert a nasal catheter into one nostril and replace the mask. Supply oxygen at approximately 1000 cc. per minute from the inhaler.
7. Continue to drop the drug at a rate necessary for the desired depth of anesthesia.

Signs of
Anesthesia:

The signs of anesthesia are in general similar to those outlined under Judging depths of anesthesia.

Complications:

1. Tachypnea. This is due to stimulation of the alveolar nerve endings and indicate a dangerous intense vagal stimulation.
2. Salivation: This occurs frequently when premedication is not used.
3. Cardiac irregularities: The drug is like chloroform in its behavior on the heart.
4. Poor relaxation. Absorption is slow.

Advantages of
Trichlorethylene:

1. It may be administered by means of simple equipment.
2. It is a potent analgesic agent which can be administered by simple means.
3. The low partial pressure necessary for anesthesia allows the use of air as a vehicle.
4. It is accompanied by little post-anesthetic nausea and vomiting.
5. In concentrations less than 10% it forms nonflammable mixtures with air or oxygen.
6. It is inexpensive.

Disadvantages:

1. It causes cardiac depression manifested by arrhythmias.
2. It is decomposed in the presence of soda-lime and cannot be used in the closed system.
3. Induction is slow.
4. It may cause derangement of liver function.
5. It may be confused with chloroform because it possesses a chloroform-like odor.
6. It volatilizes slowly. This contributes to the slow induction.
7. It causes a very rapid rate of respiration, sometimes up to 50 or 60 per minute.
8. Its margin of safety is somewhat like that of chloroform when used for surgical anesthesia.
9. It cannot be used in the closed system. Toxic products form.
10. Muscle relaxation is poor.
11. It may cause burns on the skin.

Comment

Reason

1. The drug is not recommended for surgical anesthesia.

1. The drug induces deleterious cardiac effects, the effects on respiration are undesirable and relaxation is poor.

2. Do not use the drug in the closed system.

2. It is not stable in the presence of soda-lime.

3. Do not expose the vapor to flames or sparks.

3. Phosgene which is irritating to the pulmonary epithelium may form and pulmonary edema may form.

4. Drop the drug slowly at a constant rate rather than intermittently.

4. This insures a constant level of anesthesia. Overdosage can thus be avoided.

5. Do not administer to starved, debiliated or emaciated individuals.

5. The possibility of hepatitis is greater in these subjects. Preoperative administration of glucose is desirable.

6. Do not use epinephrine during the anesthetic.

6. Epinephrine increases cardiac irritability and causes serious arrhythmias.

7. Discontinue the drug if the pulse becomes slow or irregular.

7. Such changes indicate cardiac depression, irritability or shift of the pace-maker.

8. Never pour trichlorethylene on the mask.

8. The danger of over-dosage is ever present, and increased by such a technique.

9. Discontinue administration if tachypnea occurs.

9. This indicates possible intense vagal stimulation.

Contra-Indications

1. Diseases of the heart.

1. Trichlorethylene increases irritability of the cardiac automatic tissue.

2. Hypotensive states.

2. The drug may depress the vasomotor center and affects the heart.

3. Acidosis from any cause.

3. Carbon dioxide combining power may be elevated.

4. Diseases of the liver.

4. The drug is a halogenated hydrocarbon and these compounds predispose to hepatitis.

5. Diseases of the kidney.

5. Causes decrease in urinary output.

6. Acute or chronic disease of the respiratory tract.

6. The drug tends to produce mucus and other secretions

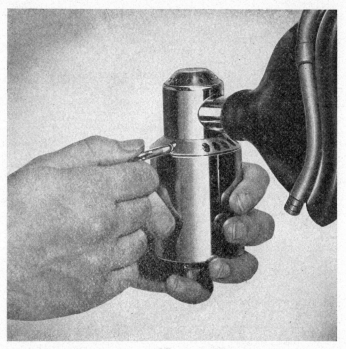

FIG. 42. A. Cyprane inhaler for self-administration of vapors of vapors of volatile liquids.

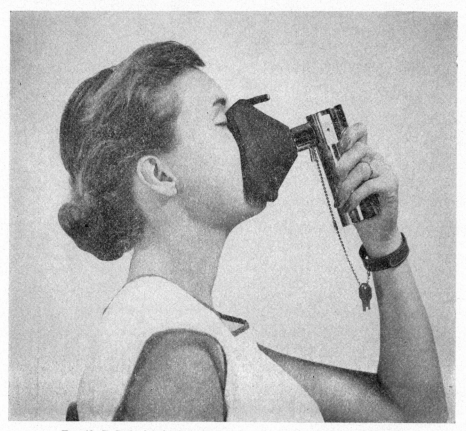

FIG. 42. B. Duke inhaler for self-administration of vapors of volatile liquids.

which may disseminate infection from one part of the respiratory tract to the other.

*Variations in
Technique:*

1. For analgesia. Proceed with the induction until the patient feels a sensation of dizziness, then decrease the rate of administration as stage II is approached.
2. Instruct the patient to raise his hand when he feels pain during the surgery and increase the rate of administration.

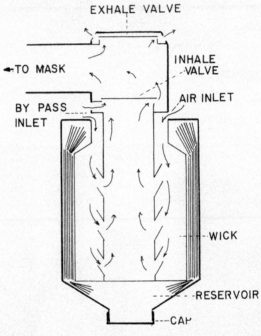

Fig. 43A. Cross section of semi-closed inhaler (Duke, Cyprane type) used for administering mixtures of air and volatile liquids. On inspiration air is drawn through the ports over the surface of the wick which lines the cylindrical container, mixes with vapor which volatilizes from the wick and passes through the inhale valve to the mask. On expiration the exhaled gases pass from the mask through the exhalation valve. Thus, with the exception of the gases in the mask, there is no rebreathing. The adjustable ports permit the by-passing of the anesthetic so that the percentage of vapor and air can be varied. The liquid is stored in the bottom of the container.

ANALGESIA USING THE CYPRANE OR DUKE INHALER

Description: The Cyprane and the Duke inhalers (Figs. 42 and 43) are devices which can be held by the patient for the self-administration of vapors mixed with air. Each consists of a cylindrical container attached to a mask. A device for evaporation of the volatile liquid is in the cylindrical portion of the container. Air drawn by the patient over the vaporizer is mixed with the vapor, passes through a valve into the mask. The gas is then exhaled through another valve on top the mask. Only the vapor and air in the mask is rebreathed.

Technique:

1. Load the chamber with the trichlorethylene to saturate wick (15 cc.)
2. Empty excess liquid.
3. Attach mask to face.
4. Set vaporizer at minimum.
5. Commence administration and gradually rotate vapor control from minimum mark towards maximum until optimum concentration is reached.
6. Lock device at this point.

Comment

The wick holds about 15 cc.

NITROUS OXIDE—TRICHLORETHYLENE OXYGEN

Material: Same as for nitrous oxide-vinethene.

Premedication: Morphine—scopolamine, hyoscyamine or atropine.

Procedure: Same as outlined for nitrous-oxide oxygen-vinethene, except that special vaporizing jar without a wick must be used for trichlorethylene. No rebreathing must be permitted.

1. Adjust mask to the patient's face.
2. Commence a flow of 6 to 8 liters of nitrous oxide 75%–25% oxygen.
3. Allow patient to breathe this mixture for several minutes until maximum depth the mixture can give is attained. It is uncommon to go beyond second stage.
4. Increase vaporizer control gradually trichlorethylene and permit vapor to mix with nitrous oxide until patient passes into 3rd stage. Turn in trichlorethylene slowly.
5. Maintain concentration at this point.

Comment	*Reason*
1. Do not use carbon dioxide absorber.	Soda-lime decomposes trichlorethylene and forms dangerous biproducts.
2. Use a high flow of gas mixture with adequate oxygen.	Carbon dioxide must be washed out of the inhaler. It will not be removed unless the tidal exchange of the patient is flown into apparatus.
3. Do not maintain anesthesia below first plane.	Cardiac irregularities and tachypnea may develop.

4. If demand type apparatus is used merely set mixing device for 75% nitrous oxide 25% oxygen and add trichlorethylene as described above.

The tidal exchange of the patient will be supplied by the apparatus.

5. Do not use vaporizer with wicks of type used for ether.

The concentration of vapor delivered will be excessive.

REFERENCES

Adriani, J. Selection of Anesthesia. Charles C Thomas, Springfield, Ill., 1955.

Goodman, L., and Gilman, A. The Pharmacological Basis of Therapeutics. Macmillan, New York, pp. 55–75, 1955.

HALOTHANE (FLUOTHANE) ANESTHESIA

Description

Fluothane is a volatile, non-flammable liquid whose vapor possesses marked narcotic potency, an ethereal odor and is not pungent nor irritating to the mucous membranes.

Uses

1. When a non-flammable anesthetic in combination with a relaxant is desired for major surgery.
2. As a fortifying agent for nitrous oxide.
3. As a rapid induction agent for ethyl ether.

Cost

Relatively expensive (approximately $3.66 per ounce).

Concentration

1. For induction 0.2–2.5% by volume in the alveoli.
2. For maintenance 0.4–1.5% by volume in the alveoli.
3. Vapor pressure at 20°C.= 241.5.

Premedication

1. Morphine or meperidine (Demerol) and atropine for adults.
2. Secobarbital (Seconal)—hydroxyzine (Vistaril) combination and Bellafoline or Demerol and Bellafoline for children in standard doses (see Table under premedication).

Methods of Administration

1. By semi-closed, non-rebreathing techniques using a precision calibrated heat compensated vaporizer (Fluotec) and the non-heat compensated vaporizer (Ohio type, F.N.S. and Copper Kettle).

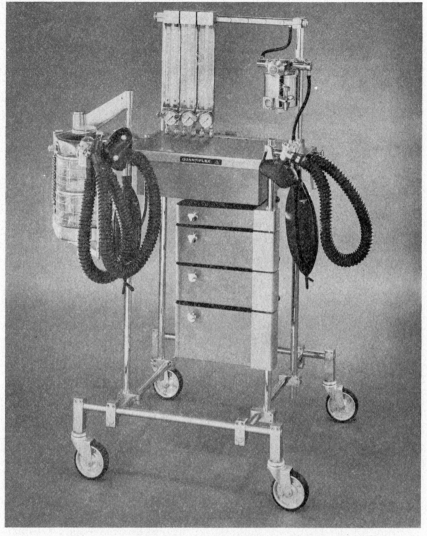

FIG. 43B. Fluotec assembly for administration of halothane by
the non-return semi-enclosed technique.

2. By closed, rebreathing techniques using the atomizer or injector type
of vaporizer.
3. By insufflation with oxygen or oxygen-nitrous oxide mixture as vehicle.

Materials

1. Machine with a semi-closed inhaler, circle or to and fro filter and flow
meters calibrated for oxygen and nitrous oxide.
2. A vaporizer such as Fluotec, F.N.S. or Copper kettle interposed between the gas source and the filter. Device must permit the quantita-
tive shunting of a vehicular gas through a vaporizer containing liquid

Fluothane. (Any of the precision calibrated heat compensated and non-heat compensated vaporizers will suffice). (Fig. 43B).

3. Artificial airways.
4. Sphygmomanometer.
5. Precordial stethoscope.
6. E.K.G. if desired.

Technique

1. Arrange the patient and equipment in the routine manner described for ether or other inhalation anesthesia.

Preparations differ in no way from those required for ether gas anesthetics, except inclusion of vaporizer.

2. Close the obturator at the mask and fill inhaler with 100% oxygen, 50% oxygen and 50% nitrous oxide, or 37.5% oxygen and 62.5% nitrous oxide mixture.

These concentrations should be derived from a 4 liter per minute flow rate of gases to insure accurate percentage concentration delivery from vaporizer. The additive effect of nitrous oxide may be utilized if desired. (If copper kettle is used, follow directions supplied with machine concerning flow rates.)

3. Adjust, but do not fasten mask to face.

Stimulation created by the pressure may cause patient to become excited as he passes through stage II.

4. Turn on carbon dioxide absorber and open obturator so that patient breathes from the inhaler.

Carbon dioxide should be removed to prevent the feeling of suffocation which patients frequently experience during induction and to avoid hypercarbia.

5. Open exhalation valve sufficiently to allow excess gases to escape from inhaler but not so wide that the bag becomes deflated.

Nitrogen, some nitrous oxide, and carbon dioxide are eliminated during each exhalation. Ultimately most of the nitrogen in the alveoli is replaced by nitrous oxide and oxygen.

6. Turn on halothane (Fluothane) vaporizer to deliver 0.1% concentration, and gradually increase concentration by 0.1–0.2% increments until patient is in stage III. (Blood pressure should be checked frequently during this period.)

Due to potency of agent and relatively high concentration required for induction patient must not be rushed into stage III.

7. As soon as consciousness is lost fasten mask securely to face.

A snug fit prevents inhalation of air about the face-cushion and

8. Allow mixture to flow until patient is in stage III, then decrease concentration gradually to that required for maintenance.

subsequent dilution of the mixture. Usually nearly twice the concentration is required for induction compared to that needed for maintenance. Some degree of hypotension may be encountered at the end of induction, but is usually corrected by the lower maintenance concentrations required.

9. If hypotension occurs decrease concentration until blood pressure is restored to desired level. If blood pressure fails to respond, agent should be discontinued.

The drug is a myocardial depressant. Degree of hypotension bears direct ratio to concentration.

Comments

1. Atropine or Bellafoline should be administered as a premedicant.

2. Do not allow the patient to recover until the skin is sutured and the dressing is in place.

3. Be prepared to restrain the patient on the stretcher or in the operating room.

4. Treat any hypotension whose cause is not determined as an overdose of the drug. Decrease concentration or discontinue its use until hypotension is reversed.

5. Regard as ominous signs any extremely rapid or very slow pulse.

6. Continual monitoring of pulse and frequent blood pressure determinations are mandatory. (At least every five minutes during maintenance and more frequently during induction and hypotensive episodes.)

7. Do not use epinephrine in conjunction with halothane.

8. Do not rely upon the drug to yield muscle relaxation. Use

Reasons

Obviates the bradycardia and decreases in cardiac output which is due to vagal effects.

Drug is rapidly eliminated and the patient reacts quickly and emerges from anesthesia before the operation is completed.

Excitement or emergence delirium may occur during the recovery period particularly if effects of narcotic used for premedication have subsided and patient feels pain.

Overdosage is dangerous because the drug is a cardiac depressant and cardiac arrest may quickly ensue.

Each is a sign of marked cardiac irritability.

Due to potency of drug its rapid action and its cardiovascular effects, arrhythmias, hypotension or both may be disastrous unless promptly detected and corrected.

The combination may cause ventricular tachycardia or fibrillation.

Deep anesthesia is necessary which may result in overdosage.

succinyl choline or other relaxant.

9. Decrease concentration after period of induction (cutback).

Higher concentration required for body saturation during induction than in maintenance because of variable degree of water solubility (air-blood ratio 2.3).

Children are easily overdosed by the drug.

10. In pediatric patients use the concentration which will just prevent movements of patients.

11. Do not use ordinary vaporizers intended for ether, vinyl ether, etc. Precision micro-vaporizers required.

The drug is potent and overconcentration easily results.

Contraindications to Fluothane

Reasons

1. Presence of cardiac disease or irregularities of rhythm.

In healthy hearts arrhythmias appear in deep anesthesia with all techniques.

2. The simultaneous use of epinephrine and related drugs.

Heart sensitized to pressor amines, particularly epinephrine and norepinephrine, resultant use of which may be ventricular fibrillation.

3. Hypotension (shock).

Vasomotor center and myocardium depressed by the drug. Unless hypotensive technique is desired, agent is to be avoided in patients susceptible to shock or who are in shock.

4. In emaciated, cachectic, "toxic," anemic or acutely ill patients.

Percentage of agent required to produce anesthesia may cause severe hypotension. The drug has a narrow margin of safety in these patients.

5. In hands of the inexpert.

Due to potency and cardiotoxicity of agent, administration by the unskilled may quickly result in overdosage and cardiac arrest.

6. Surgical procedures requiring relaxation.

Adequate muscle relaxation is not obtained consistently unless a muscle relaxant concomitantly used.

Advantages of Fluothane

1. Non-flammable.
2. Non-irritating to the upper respiratory tract.
3. Non-spasmogenic to larynx and bronchi.
4. Characterized by rapid induction and recovery.
5. Potent—more potent than chloroform in regards to rapidity of induction.

6. Suitable for fortifying nitrous oxide.
7. Chemically stable if protected from light and not in prolonged contact with metals.

Disadvantages of Fluothane

1. Over-concentration leads to circulatory collapse.
2. Expensive.
3. Difficult to use in closed systems with draw-over type of vaporizers, or by open-drop method.
4. Depresses respiration and circulation. May be hepatotoxie.
5. Enhances ganglionic blockade.
6. Adequate muscle relaxation not obtained consistently without relaxants.
7. Increases irritability of cardiac automatic tissue predisposing to arrhythmias.
8. Decomposed and forms toxic product on prolonged contact with copper and oxygen.

HALOTHANE (FLUOTHANE) BY THE CLOSED METHOD

Principle

Small amounts of vaporized Fluothane are added to a closed rebreathing system according to patient's requirements. Only the metabolic requirement of oxygen is used. The vaporizer is outside the circuit.

Materials

1. Same as for semi-closed technique, except that a micro-atomizer replaces the previously mentioned vaporizers.
2. The micro-vaporizer has the following features:
   (a) Slender calibrated jar of 20 cc. capacity so that the number of cubic centimeters or fraction thereof of fluid vaporizer can be visualized.
   (b) A bulb which draws gas from the circle system and forces it through the fluid in fine bubbles.
   (c) An outlet from the vaporizer back into the circle system.

Procedure

1. Place atomizer filled to the full mark between delivery tube and EXHALATION valve of Foregger machine.
2. Prepare machine in same manner as for semi-closed induction.
3. Adjust flow meters to deliver a mixture of 80% nitrous oxide and 20% oxygen.
4. Apply mask to patient's face and add halothane in small increments to oxygen-nitrous oxide mixture by compressing the bulb of atomizer.
5. Upon entrance of patient into stage III, gradually reduce flow of the nitrous oxide and oxygen until nitrous oxide is no longer required to maintain anesthesia. Reduce the oxygen flow to metabolic requirements and close off system.

6. Continue adding halothane in increments as needed for maintenance of desired level of anesthesia.

Advantages

1. Far less halothane consumed in the closed system compared to the semiclosed system.
2. Substantially less oxygen is used than with the closed system.
3. Nitrous oxide is required for induction, but not for maintenance.
4. Closed system permits freer use of controlled and assisted respiration.
5. May be used as an induction agent for ether.

Disadvantages

1. Maintenance of an even level of anesthesia requires close observation and expert technique.
2. Unsuitable for infants because of ease of occurrence of overdosage.
3. Exact concentration of agent delivered is unknown.

Comments	*Reasons*
1. Blood pressure must be determined frequently.	Blood pressure reponse (hypotension) provides clue to overdosage.
2. Always place atomizer on the exhalation side of circuit.	The inhaled gas will vary widely in concentration of Halothane with resultant untoward cardiovascular effects.

Alternate Method for Closed System Fluothane

Omit the nitrous oxide as an induction agent and simply induce anesthesia as described above by adding small quantities of halothane to the system filled with oxygen and flowing the metabolic oxygen requirement.

HALOTHANE (FLUOTHANE) BY INSUFFLATION

Principle

A current of oxygen, or a mixture of nitrous oxide and oxygen is propelled over the surface of liquid Fluothane or through it in the form of fine bubbles. The mixture of gases and vapor is then conducted into the nose, mouth or trachea through a tube or cannula.

Types

1. Intra-oral insufflation. The mixture is conducted into the oropharynx by a cannula or "ether hook" placed in the mouth.
2. Intra-nasal insufflation. The mixture is conducted into the nasopharynx through a catheter.
3. Intratracheal insufflation. The mixture is conducted into the trachea by inserting a small intratracheal tube directly into the trachea using the Ayre's T piece or into tracheotomy cannula.

Uses

1. For operations about the pharynx, larynx, trachea, or esophagus.

Materials

1. Fluothane vaporizer (Fluotec, F.N.S., etc.) and connecting tubes for conducting mixture into appropriate device.
2. Anesthetic machine.
3. "Ether hook" if oral route is contemplated, nasal catheter, if oronasal route is contemplated or appropriate sized intratracheal tubes if intratracheal route is contemplated.
4. Basic equipment for any anesthetic induction (artificial airways, masks lubricants, etc.).

Technique (Oral):

1. Test the vaporizer and place it in a convenient position on the anesthetic table or machine.
2. Anesthetize the patient with halothane using the semi-closed technique and attain the level of anesthesia necessary to complete the operation.
3. Remove mask and immediately insert hook or cannula into the mouth.
4. Proceed as described under semi-closed technique to maintain anesthesia.

Comments

1. Be positive the mixture is flowing through the cannula or catheter. Test the flow of gas by holding the cannula against palm of the hand or by cautiously smelling for halothane.
2. Attach hook or cannula to tube leading from outlet of vaporizer.
3. Maintain flow at sufficient rate to provide necessary volume of ambient mixture to hold anesthesia at the desired level.

Technique (Intratracheal)

1. Assemble equipment necessary to perform intratracheal intubation.
2. Anesthetize the patient in the same manner as described under oral insufflation.
3. Remove the mask, expose the larynx, and insert intratracheal catheter into the trachea.
4. Attach delivery tube from vaporizer to T piece and intratracheal tube.

Comment

1. Insert a "bite" block in patient's mouth after intubation to avoid having the patient bite down on the intratracheal tube.

Advantages

1. "Dead space" is minimal and insignificant.

2. It may be employed when intratracheal anesthesia is not feasible, practical or desirable for oropharyngeal and laryngeal surgery.

Disadvantages

1. Airway is frequently maintained with difficulty particularly during intra-oral and head and neck surgery.
2. The method is wasteful and expensive.
3. Halothane (Fluothane) may be inhaled by members of the surgical team.

Variations

1. Insufflation into pharyngeal airway. The delivery tube from the vaporizer is attached to an oropharyngeal airway equipped with a nipple designed for attachment of a tube, or a catheter may be threaded through its lumen into the pharynx. Anesthesia is then conducted as in the foregoing techniques.
2. Insufflation into bronchoscope. The delivery tube from the vaporizer is attached to a bronchoscope equipped with a side arm and a nipple designed for the purpose. Anesthesia then proceeds as previously described.

REFERENCES

Adriani, J. Pharmacology of Anesthetic Drugs. Pp. 51–53. Springfield, Thomas, 1960.
Adriani, J. Chemistry and Physics of Anesthesia, Chap. 15. Springfield, Thomas, 1962.

ARTIFICIAL AIRWAYS

Definition: Artificial airways are rigid or semi-rigid tubes composed of rubber or metal. They are designed to fit into the upper portions of the respiratory tract.

Purpose:
1. They provide an unimpeded pathway for respired gases.
2. They facilitate removal of secretions from the respiratory tract.
3. They conduct anesthetic mixtures to the respiratory tract.

Types:
1. *Oropharyngeal:* These are metal, plastic or rubber tubes which are inserted through the mouth into the pharynx.
2. *Nasopharyngeal:* These are soft rubber catheters which are inserted into the pharynx through the nostrils.
3. *Orotracheal:* These are rubber, metal, plastic or silk woven catheters which are inserted into the trachea through the mouth, usually by the aid of a laryngoscope.
4. *Nastracheal:* These are soft rubber or plastic catheters which are inserted through the nostrils into the trachea.

Oropharyngeal Airways

Description: Oropharyngeal airways are tubes shaped in such a manner that they conform to the curvature of the palate. They extend from the lips to the pharynx and serve either as pathways for respired gases or support the tongue and pharyngeal structures so that the natural airway remains patent (Fig. 44).

Types:

1. *All metal:* These are curved flat tubes with a flange or disk at the oral end to fit over the lips. Many designs are available, all of which accomplish the same purpose (Fig. 45).
2. *Wire cage type:* These are similar in design to the metal type except that they are woven from ewire (Fig. 45).
3. *All rubber:* These are curved tubes of semi-hard rubber similar in design to the metal type. They serve the same purpose and are introduced in the same manner (Fig. 45).
4. *Plastic:* These are similar in design to the rubber but are made of plastic.

Advantages of metal airways:

a. They are easily cleaned and sterilized by boiling.
b. They are permanent, and not damaged by ordinary wear.
c. They are inserted and removed readily in event of spasticity of muscles of the jaw.

to the lips, tongue, pharynx, or teeth.

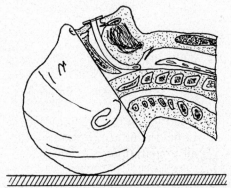

Fig. 44. Oral pharyngeal airway in situ. Note that the airway does not extend beyond the hypopharynx.

Disadvantages of metal airways:

a. They may cause trauma to the lips, tongue, pharynx, or teeth.

Advantages of rubber airways:

a. The possibility of trauma is minimized when used.

Disadvantages of rubber airways:

a. They often acquire obnoxious odors which are difficult to eliminate from the rubber.
b. They are difficult to insert or remove in patients whose jaws are tightly clamped because of spasticity of muscles.

c. They are not permanent; rubber deteriorates.

d. They are not conveniently sterilized by boiling.

Advantages of plastic airways

a. Disposable

b. Inexpensive.

c. Easily cleansed.

Comment

Airways are available in many sizes. The proper size must be selected for the individual patient.

Procedure for Insertion of Oropharyngeal Airways	*Reasons*
1. Select an airway of the proper size for the subject and place it within ready reach of the right hand.	Airways of improper size either may not adequately support relaxed structures or they may extend too far into the hypopharnyx. Obstruction may result in either case.
2. Turn off ether or other anesthestic gases (oxygen at metabolic rate may continue to flow).	The concentration of the drug in the inhaler may become excessive if gases or vapors continue to flow during the manipulation.
3. Unstrap the mask, but continue to hold it firmly to the face until all preparations are complete.	The patient should breathe room air for as short an interval as possible to prevent lightening of anesthesia and return of the pharyngeal reflex.
4. Close the obturator and lift the mask from the face.	The obturator prevents loss of the mixture of gas from inhaler. Anesthesia may thus be resumed without forming a new mixture.
5. Grasp the airway in the right hand and hold it in a horizontal position so that pharyngeal end rests on the lip (Fig. 46).	The airway is thus placed in a position for a rotary motion which is necessary to easily slip the tube into the pharynx.
6. Push lower jaw foward, insert a tongue blade or thumb to hold the tongue against floor of the mouth.	The tongue is thus prevented from falling back into the pharynx and causing obstruction.
7. Swing the curved portion of the airway into the pharynx using a rotary motion (Fig. 46).	The airway follows the curvature of the palate and slips into the pharynx without causing the tongue to drop into the pharynx.
8. Replace the mask on the face and open obturator.	The patient should resume breathing the anesthetic mixture as soon

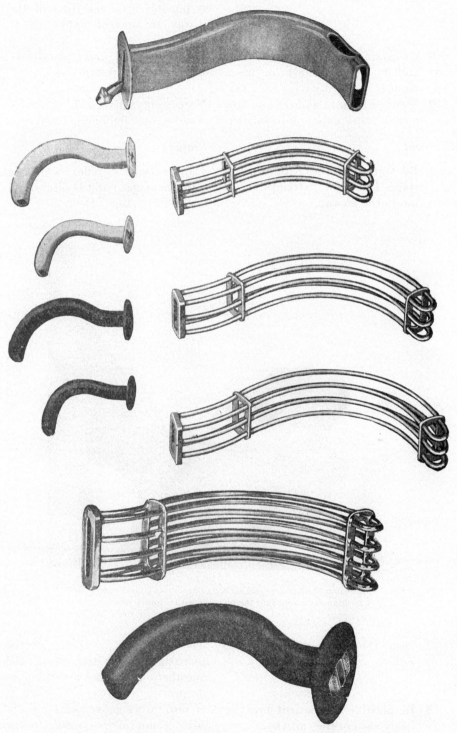

FIG. 45. Various designs of oropharyngeal airways commonly employed for inhalation anesthesia. (Courtesy of Richard Foregger, Ph.D.)

9. Ascertain that the airway is clear and fasten the mask in usual manner.

The improperly inserted airway often increases obstruction.

as possible after insertion of the airway to prevent lightening of anesthesia.

10. Secure a snug fit and resume flow of gases and vapors into inhaler.

More agent is invariably necessary because some lightening occurs.

Comment

1. Be sure that the patient is in stage III before attempting to insert the airway.

Reasons

The pharyngeal reflex which is active in stages I and II disappears in plane 1 of stage III.

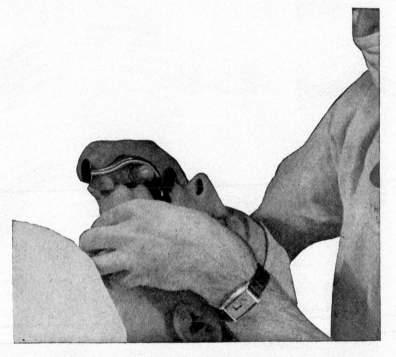

FIG. 46. Insertion of oropharyngeal airway. The airway is held in a horizontal position and swept into the pharynx with a rotary motion.

2. Delay the introduction of airways as long as possible.

The possibility of return of the pharyngeal reflex decreases as the anesthetic progresses and becomes deeper.

3 Be positive the patient breathes freely after the airway is inserted.

If respiratory movements are absent or not in proportion to the tidal exchange, it is because:

a. Patient became "too light" and pharyngeal reflex returns and the breath is held due to reflex stimulation. Remove airway immediately or emesis may follow.

b. The airway is not inserted correctly because the tongue is folded in the pharynx and is causing obstruction. (Fig. 47). Remove or replace it properly.

4. Arrange flange of airways so that it rests over the lips.

Laceration or other trauma to soft tissues may result if this is not done.

5. Never attempt to insert an airway by holding it in a vertical position.

Obstruction may result from folding of the tongue in the posterior pharynx.

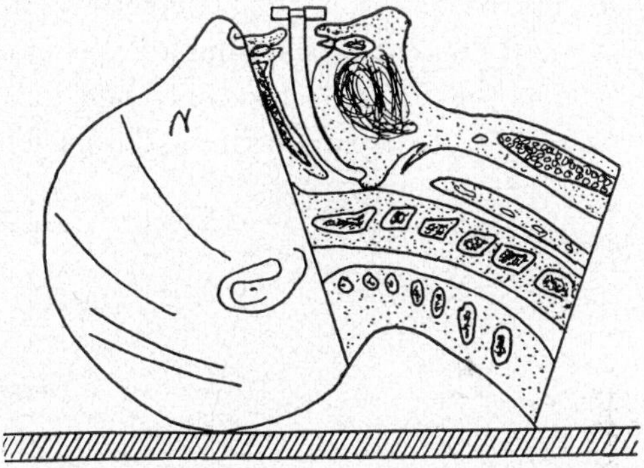

FIG. 47. Improper use of oropharyngeal airways may result in complete obstruction to respiration. The tongue is relaxed and has dropped into the pharynx. The airway is too small to relieve the obstruction.

6. Be positive the flange of the airway is completely covered by the mask.

A leak occurs if any overlapping is present.

7. Never use an airway to pry the jaws apart in the event of spasticity of muscles.

The teeth may be damaged. If necessary, insert the thumb or index finger at side of the mouth behind molar teeth and exert force there.

8. Remove airways which have become filled with mucus or secretions.

Mucus causes obstruction to respiration.

9. Never begin an anesthetic without having an airway of proper size within immediate reach.

Respiratory failure or obstruction may occur at the most unexpected times even in apparently simple cases.

NASOPHARYNGEAL AIRWAYS

Description: Nasopharyngeal airways consist of soft rubber catheters which extend from the nostrils to nasopharynx and act as pathways for respired gases (Fig. 49).

Features of Nasal Airways (Figs. 48 and 49):

1. They are composed of thin walled latex plastic or gum rubber tubing.
2. Their diameters vary from 26–32 French.

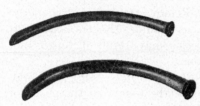

FIG. 48. Nasal pharyngeal airway. Note the funnel shaped slip joint to prevent the catheter from sliding into the nasopharynx.

3. The pharyngeal end is beveled laterally.
4. The nasal end is cut transversely and a safety pin is inserted through it to prevent its slipping all the way into the nose.
5. The length is usually one inch in addition to the distance from the tragus of the ear to tip of the patient's nostril.

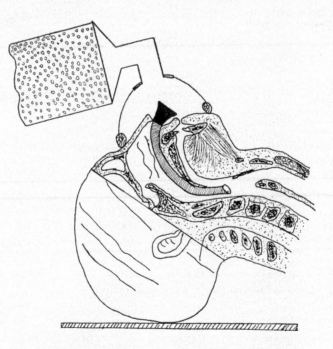

FIG. 49. Nasal airway in place. The airway must pass beyond the palate and support the tongue and other relaxed structures.

Advantages of nasal airways:

1. They may be employed when oral airways are difficult or impossible to introduce.

Disadvantages:

1. They are easily kinked or pinched by anatomical distortions.
2. They cause trauma to nasal mucous membranes which may be followed by epistaxis.
3. The lumen of the tube may not provide an adequate airway for the total tidal volume of the patient.

Procedure for insertion of nasopharyngeal airway:

1. Select a catheter of suitable size. The diameter should be slightly larger than the opening of the nostril.
2. Insert the safety pin transversely through the nasal end.
3. Lubricate the beveled end generously with lubricant for a distance of approximately one inch.
4. Insert the entire length of the tube into either nostril.

Comment

1. Do not force the catheter into the nostril.
2. Be positive that a satisfactory exchange is obtained.

Reasons

The use of force invariably results in trauma and epistaxis.
If catheters are too long and inserted too far, they may pass into the oesophagus and cause obstruction.

Care of Airways

1. Cleanse airway by threading its lumen with a ribbon of moistened gauze attached to a wire. If oily lubricant has been used, a second strip moistened with ether should be passed through it to remove it.
2. Wash with soap and water and rinse thoroughly.
3. Boil metal airways for 10 minutes. Immerse rubber tubes in alcohol (70%) for 30 minutes.
4. Rinse, dry, and thread with a dry gauze ribbon. The ribbon may remain in place until airway is to be used.

Tracheal Airways

Description: Tracheal airways are tubes composed of rubber, silk, or flexible metal. They pass into the trachea either through the oropharynx or nasopharynx and provide unimpeded pathways for respired gases. When directly connected to inhalers or insufflators, the anesthetic gases are introduced into the trachea.

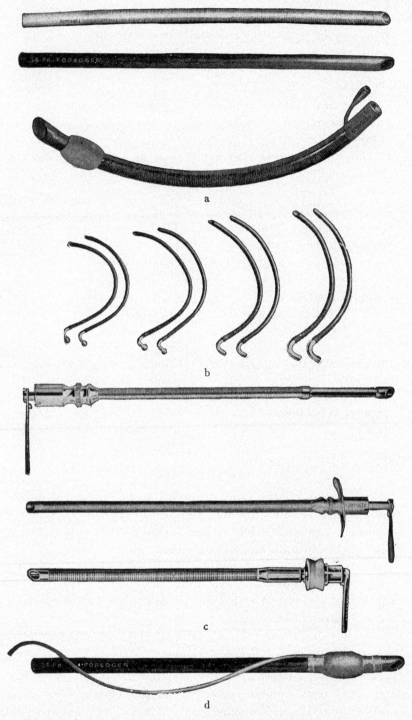

FIG. 50. Orotracheal and nasotracheal airways: (a) Latex or "a node" tubes, with metal spiral embedded in its wall. (b) Plain rubber or Magill nasotracheal tubes. (c) Metal (Woodbridge) tubes with stylet. (d) Silk woven catheters. (Courtesy of Richard Foregger, Ph.D.)

Types: Two types of tracheal airways are available: oral and nasal (Fig. 50).

   1. *Oral:* A variety of oral tubes is available. All accomplish the same purpose:

      a. Anode: This type is composed of latex rubber and has a metal spiral incorporated in its wall. The spiral acts as a support and prevents kinking or collapse.

      b. Plain rubber: This type is made from soft rubber tubing possessing sufficient rigidity to prevent collapse under ordinary circumstances.

      c. Silk: This type is woven from silk and coated with plastic so that it is semi-rigid and leak proof.

      d. Metal: This type (Woodbridge) is composed of flexible metal tubing possessing rigidity to prevent kinking. The surface may be protected by a rubber dam sheath (penrose drain) to render it leak-proof.

      e. Plastic. These are composed of soft pliable plastic.

   2. *Nasal:* Nasotracheal catheters are of one type (Magill). They are composed of soft thin-walled rubber or plastic tubing with a smooth exterior and a beveled tracheal end (similar to nasopharyngeal tubes).

Characteristics of Tracheal Airways:

   1. *Shape: Orotracheal* catheters are either straight or possess a slight curvature.

      Nasotracheal catheters usually possess a curvature of a circle whose radius is approximately 25–30 cms. The catheter should be soft but sufficiently rigid to maintain the curved form.

   2. *Length:* Catheters are usually supplied in lengths of 26–28 cms. The distance the catheter is introduced varies for each individual. The distance may be roughly estimated by placing the catheter along the anterior surface of the neck from the suprasternal notch to the tip of the chin.

   3. *Size:* The bore of tracheal catheters is expressed in terms of "French." Sizes vary from 28 to 40F for adults and 18 to 30F for children. The lumen should be as wide as possible but the wall should be as thin as permissible without risking danger of collapse.

      Diameter of catheters according to:

Age	Size
0–1 yr	8–18 F.
1–5 yr.	15–24 F.
6–15 yr.	24–36 F.
adults	28–40 F.

Uses of Intratracheal Airways:

   1. For conduction of intratracheal anesthesia for operations about the head, neck, mouth, or pharynx.

2. For a patient who is in the prone or other inaccessible position.
3. For relieving respiratory obstructions which are not readily corrected by oropharyngeal or nasopharyngeal airways.
4. For maintaining positive pressure for intrathoracic and other types of surgery in which positive pressure is required.
5. For maintaining a patent airway in extremely obese patients or other subjects in whom this is accomplished with difficulty.
6. For operations in which there is a possibility of aspiration of foreign particles or fluids (intestinal obstruction).
7. For upper abdominal or other types of surgery accompanied by reflex laryngeal spasm (Brewer-Luckhardt reflex).
8. For controlled and other methods of artificial respiration.

Advantages of the Intratracheal Airway:

1. It insures a completely patent and unobstructed airway when properly employed.
2. It allows a seal to be secured between the catheter and the tracheal wall which prevents vomitus, secretions, or blood from passing into the respiratory tract.
3. It allows the use of positive pressure when connected to a closed inhaler.
4. It facilitates the aspiration of mucus, blood, and other secretions from the respiratory tract.
5. It prevents or relieves laryngeal spasm.

Disadvantages:

1. The catheter acts as a foreign body in the respiratory tract and often causes irritation or initiates coughing or other reflexes.
2. The lubricant necessary to facilitate the introduction of the catheter into the trachea may be undesirable.
3. The wall of the catheter decreases the area of the tracheal lumen and causes partial obstruction, particularly in children and infants.
4. Anesthesia of a deeper plane than is ordinarily required for the operation is necessary to obtund the cough reflex in the trachea. (Second plane or deeper anesthesia is required to abolish the cough reflex in the trachea.)
5. Trauma to the pharynx or larynx or injury to teeth and other structures may be caused while introducing catheters or during laryngoscopy.
6. The bacterial flora from the nasopharynx is introduced into the trachea and bronchi, particularly if the nasal route is employed.
7. The coughing or straining during light anesthesia causes increased venous pressure which may be detrimental to patients. (Debilitated patients or patients having cardiovascular disease.)

8. Anatomical distortions in nose or nasopharynx may cause obstruction of the catheter when the nasal route is employed.
9. The dead space in mouth and pharynx is diminished. Respiration simulating Cheynes-Stokes may follow.

Complications During Intubation:

1. The catheter may become kinked, pinched, or obstructed by secretions from the tracheobronchial tree.
2. The catheter may be inadvertently introduced into the oesophagus instead of the trachea.
3. The teeth, tongue, or mucous membranes may be injured by the laryngoscope, catheter, or stylet.
4. The patient may bite upon the catheter if one does not insert a "bite block" before removing the laryngoscope.
5. Apnea may follow insertion of the catheter from reflex coughing or bronchiospasm.
6. The catheter may be inserted beyond the bifurcation of the trachea into a bronchus.
7. Tracheitis, laryngitis, or pharyngitis may result from repeated attempts at intubation or if intubation is attempted during light anesthesia.
8. Epistaxis may occur when the nasal route is employed.
9. The catheter may slip out of the trachea during anesthesia if it is not held securely or is not anchored to face.

INTRATRACHEAL ANESTHESIA

Definition: Intratracheal anesthesia is inhalation anesthesia conducted when an intratracheal catheter is in situ.

Techniques: The subject is anesthetized with a major anesthetic agent by the open, semi-closed, or closed technique. Orotracheal or nasotracheal intubation is performed and the anesthesia is resumed and maintained in one of the following manners.

1. The mask is replaced over the nose and mouth and the anesthesia is maintained by the open, semiopen, or closed technique. The catheter merely acts as an airway.
2. The catheter is connected to a semi-closed or closed inhaler and the gases are introduced directly into the trachea.
3. A catheter connected to an insufflation apparatus is threaded into the lumen of the tracheal catheter and the anesthesia is continued by insufflation.

Instruments Used for Intubation

Laryngoscope

Definition: A laryngoscope is an endoscope employed for visualizing the larynx and trachea. It consists of a *handle* to which is attached a *blade* for support of the tongue and epiglottis. An electric light bulb located at the end is the source of illumination.

Numerous types of laryngoscopes are available, but they may all be resolved into two main groups or types:

Types: U Type: In this type the handle is parallel to the blade and may be held either horizontally or vertically (Jackson). This type is less frequently employed for anesthesia.

L Type: The handle is at right angles to the blade and may be held

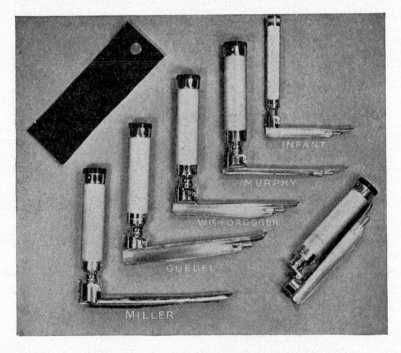

Fig. 51. The (L) type of laryngoscope commonly employed for intratracheal anesthesia. The blade and beak have been modified to suit the needs of various clinicians. (Courtesy of Richard Foregger, Ph.D.)

vertically (Flagg, Guedel). This type is the most popular for anesthesia (Fig. 51).

Macintosh—oropharyngoscope: This consists of a curved tongue blade attached to a handle containing a battery. A bulb at the beak illuminates the hypopharynx. The blade supports the tongue and exposes the larynx without touching the epiglottis (Fig. 52).

Sizes: Most laryngoscopes for anesthesia (L type) are provided with interchangeable blades of different sizes. One is for infants, one is for children, and one for adults.

Features:

1. The handle is cylindrical in shape and contains a low voltage battery

as a source of electric current for the bulb. A rheostat may be present at the end of the handle to vary the intensity of the light.

2. The blade is sturdy, detachable and has the following features:
   a. It is provided with a semi-circular groove whose concavity faces the right. This groove acts as a path for visualizing the larynx.
   b. It has a beak at its end for lifting the epiglottis.

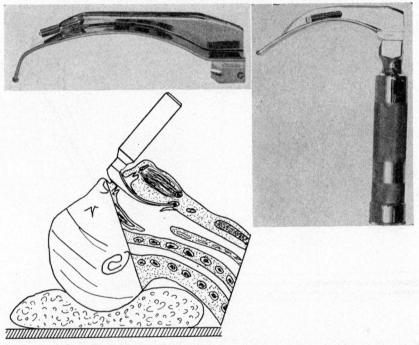

FIG. 52. A. The Macintosh Laryngoscope (actually an oropharyngoscope), consists of an illuminated tongue blade. Blades are detachable and are available in various sizes. B. Cross section showing position occupied by the blade in the hypopharynx. Note the beak does not touch the epiglottis, but is anterior to it and that exposure and visualization of the larynx is obtained by upward traction and displacement of the base of the tongue anteriorly.

Stylets

Definition: Stylets are rods composed of semi-flexible metal or plastic which fit into the lumen of soft intratracheal catheters and provide them with body and rigidity (Fig. 53).

Features: Stylets should have the following features:

1. They should be blunt at either end to prevent trauma to the operator's hand or to the larynx.
2. They should possess sufficient resilience so that they do not bend or buckle.
3. They should be provided with a stop which fits over the end of the catheter and slides up and down to vary the length of the part of the stylet which fits into the catheter (usually a cork is employed).

Slip Joints

Definition: Slip joints are short lengths of metal, hard rubber, or plastic tubing employed to connect intratracheal catheters to inhalers.

Types: Funnel type: Usually employed for nasal airways when the open
technique of anesthesia is used (Fig. 49).

Elbow type: Usually employed for nasal airways when the closed technique is used (Fig. 60).

Straight sleeve type: Employed for oral or nasal catheters when the
closed system is used (Fig. 53).

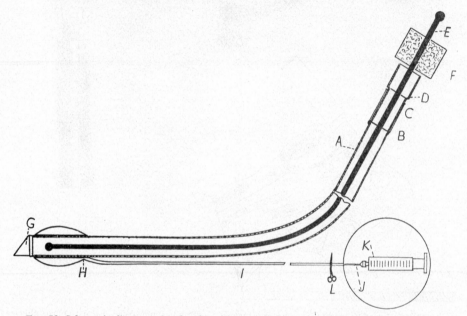

Fig. 53. Schematic diagram of a closed oral intratracheal assembly. The (A) latex catheter has
a wire spiral embedded in its wall to prevent kinking and collapse. The spiral ends at (B) so that section (C) of the catheter may accommodate the (D) metal slip joint. Note that the slip joint is introduced as far as the spiral, otherwise kinking occurs at this point. Note that the internal diameter of
the slip joint is the same as that of the catheter. The (E) stylet composed of stout semirigid metal is
knobbed at either end and fitted with a (F) rubber stopper guard. The end of the stylet rests several
centimeters from the (G) beveled silk woven tip. (H) The inflatable cuff composed of thin latex rubber
is provided with (I) a small catheter attached to a (K) 10 cc. syringe fitted with a (J) short needle
(L) A clamp is used to pinch catheter when the cuff is inflated.

Features: Slip joints should have the following features:
1. They should have a bore as wide as that of the catheter to which they
   are attached.
2. They should slip in and out of adapters easily.
3. They should form a leakproof union with adapters.

Cuffs

Definition: Cuffs are balloons composed of latex rubber designed to encircle
orotracheal catheters at the tracheal end. When inflated with air, they
produce a seal between the tracheal wall and the catheter (Fig. 53).

Features: Cuffs possess the following features:

1. They are one to two inches in length.
2. They are connected to a long thin catheter which is used to inflate them with air.
3. They encircle the catheter snugly or are built in the wall.

Insertion of Orotracheal Airways

Description: Under deep anesthesia the larynx is exposed by means of a laryngoscope. A catheter of suitable size is then inserted into the trachea.

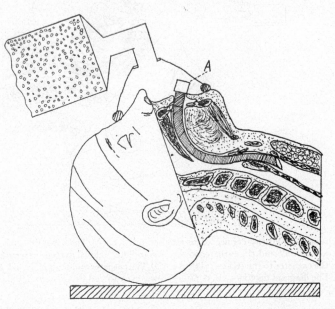

Fig. 54. Intratracheal anesthesia by the open oral technique is accomplished by introducing an orotracheal catheter by means of direct laryngoscopy, replacing the inhaler, and resuming anesthesia in the usual manner. No cuff is necessary. The catheter is secured by strapping the (A) metal adapter to the face with adhesive. The circle filter, the semi-closed inhaler, open masks, or insufflation technique may likewise be employed instead of the to and fro inhaler as shown above.

Types:

1. *Open oral:* In these intubations no seal exists between the catheter and the tracheal wall. The mask is replaced after the tube is introduced. Open masks, insufflators, semi-closed or closed inhalers may be employed to maintain the anesthesia (Fig. 54).
2. *Closed oral:* In these intubations, the catheter fits snugly into the trachea, is sealed by an inflatable cuff, which fits between the tube and the tracheal wall, or is sealed off from the pharynx by packing with strips of gauze. It is then connected to a closed rebreathing system for maintenance of anesthesia (Fig. 55).

Material:

1. Three tracheal catheters. One is of the size judged necessary for the patient, one is smaller and one is larger.
2. A semi-rigid stylet. This gives rigidity and body to soft flexible catheters (Fig. 53).
3. Petrolatum (vaseline) or similar lubricant for the stylet and catheter.
4. A suction apparatus equipped with a metal curved tip.

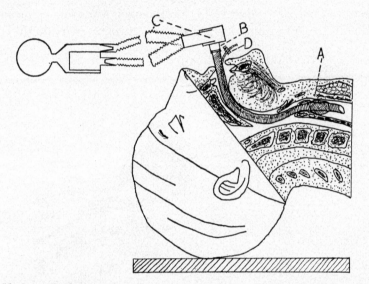

Fig. 55. Orotracheal airway connected to a closed inhaler. (A) The inflatable cuff allows a seal between the tracheal wall and the catheter so that a completely closed system is secured. (B) A slip joint connects the catheter to the (C) metal sleeve. (D) The catheter and the pinch cock communicate with the cuff. The diagram depicts a circle filter. However, a to and fro inhaler may be used equally well.

5. Urinary catheter which easily passes into the tracheal catheter. This should be fitted to a glass connecting tip for attachment to the suction tubing.
6. A pillow, approximately 3″ thick, to elevate the head.
7. Adhesive cut in strips 5/8″×8″. This is necessary to anchor the catheter to the skin of the face.
8. Two gauze packs 2″×12″ with rings for packing pharynx, or an inflatable rubber cuff for each catheter (Fig. 53).
9. Gauze pad to protect teeth, or a strip of adhesive 1″×1½″ folded in two, lengthwise.
10. A mouth prop (bite block). This may be made by wrapping a strip of adhesive around a partly-used roller bandage (approximately 5/8″×2″).
11. One pinch clamp or small artery forceps to pinch the tube leading to the cuff if a cuff is employed.

12. One 10 cc. syringe to inflate the cuff if a cuff is employed.

Preparation of Materials	*Reasons*
1. Arrange an instrument stand or tray on the righthand side of the operating table so that it is within ready reach of the anesthetist.	The "setup" should be on the right side because the right hand remains free for picking up instruments and other manipulations.
2. Spread the tray with a sterile towel and place equipment, all sterilized, upon it.	All objects which pass into the pharynx or trachea should be sterilized.
3. Lubricate the end of the catheter with sterile vaseline on a sterile sponge for a distance of 3″ to 4″.	If the entire catheter is lubricated, it is difficult to handle and hold during manipulations.
4. Bend the stylet to form a curve whose radius is approximately 28″ and lubricate generously the entire length of the stylet with vaseline.	It will be difficult to withdraw the stylet from the catheter if it is not well lubricated.
5. Adjust stylet into the catheter so that the tip rests approximately 1/2″ from its end (Fig. 53).	If the end of the stylet protrudes from the catheter, it may cause trauma to the vocal cords.
6. Moisten packs, if they are employed, with physiological saline or liquid petrolatum and express excess liquid.	Dry packs may cause irritation to mucous membranes of the pharynx.
7. Ascertain that the laryngoscope is correctly assembled, and that the battery and light are in working order.	The laryngoscope may become disassembled during manipulation if not properly put together.

Procedure	*Reasons*
1. Deeply anesthetize the patient with a major anesthetic drug, such as ether, cyclopropane, or halothane. Inject 40 mgm succinyl choline I.V.	Complete relaxation of muscles of neck with flaccidity of the jaw and abolition of pharyngeal reflex are necessary for successful intubation. The pillow elevates the head to the proper angle and causes relaxation of the anterior muscles of the neck (Fig. 56).
2. Place the pillow under the occiput so that it rests under the shoulders for a short distance. Arrange the head so that it is in the midline of the long axis of the body (Fig. 57).	
3. Extend the head by applying traction to the lower jaw so that the chin points directly towards ceiling.	Traction stretches the structures of the neck and elevates the trachea and epiglottis.

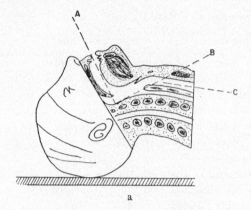

a

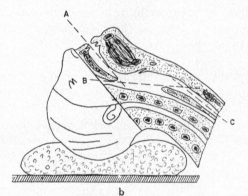

b

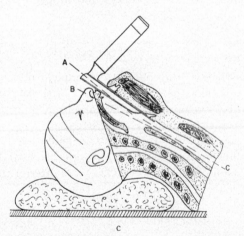

c

FIG. 56. The effects of elevating and hyperextending the head upon the improving the exposure of the larynx for endotracheal intubation. A. The relationship of the axes of the mouth, hypopharynx and trachea to each other under ordinary circumstances with the supine position with head unsupported. B. Elevation and hyperextension bring all three axes into an almost straight line. C. The forward traction upon and elevation of the structures in pharynx further hyperextend the head and bring all three axes into line so that the larynx may be fully exposed.

4. Hyperventilate by manually compressing and relaxing the breathing bag for approximately thirty seconds. Use oxygen-rich mixture or pure oxygen.

The apnea results from removal of carbon dioxide. The patient does not breathe and becomes "light" during intubation.

5. Close obturator, remove the mask from face, and withdraw pharyngeal airway.

Loss of mixture from inhaler should be prevented to facilitate reanesthetization.

6. Apply gauze protector to the upper incisor teeth.

Roughening or other damage from the laryngoscope occurs more frequently to the upper teeth.

7. Grasp the lighted laryngoscope in the left hand. Place the thumb into the right side of mouth and displace lower jaw forward.

The right hand remains free for insertion of catheter and other manipulations.

8. Insert the beak of the blade of laryngoscope into the right side of mouth at its angle. Gradually introduce it into the pharynx and, at the same time, displace the tongue as far to the left of the mouth as possible (Fig. 57).

The space to the right of the laryngoscope (the side to which the groove opens) is cleared and should remain free for passage of the tracheal catheter.

9. Gradually rotate the blade from a vertical to a horizontal position until the right anterior pillar is visualized. Then swing blade toward midline of the mouth.

The blade of the laryngoscope follows the curvature of the palate.

10. Hook right index finger over the upper teeth to make traction in a cephalad direction. At same time displace lower jaw with blade of the laryngoscope in a caudad direction (Fig. 57).

This maneuver allows the mouth to be opened widely. The blade of the laryngoscope is inserted so that pressure is avoided on the upper incisors.

11. Rotate blade more horizontally and continue to exert force on the lower jaw. This force should be a lifting of the handle in a direction toward the ceiling (Fig. 57).

A rotary force using the incisor teeth as a fulcrum for the laryngoscope should be avoided (Fig. 58).

12. As soon as the epiglottis is exposed, insert the beak of the blade beneath it and continue to lift upward on the handle of the laryngoscope, extending the head still more, if necessary. The larynx will then be seen.

The larynx is beneath and beyond the epiglottis and can only be visualized by lifting the epiglottis upward with the beak of the blade.

13. When the larynx is visible, determine the size of the catheter

If catheter is too large, spasms and trauma follow its attempted pas-

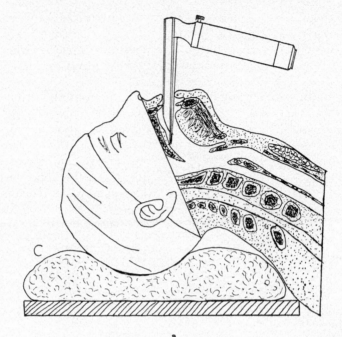

a

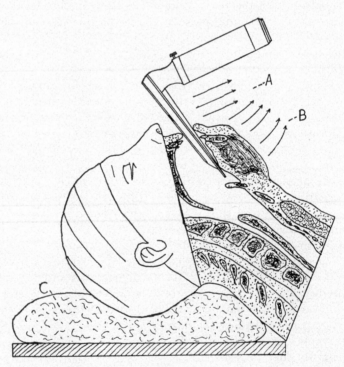

b

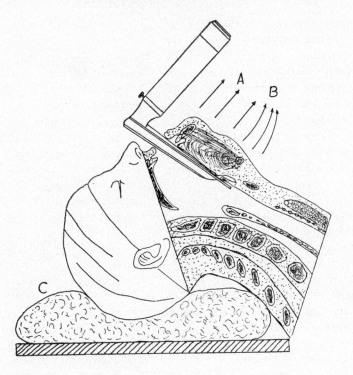

c

FIG. 57. Cross section showing introduction of the laryngoscope in performing laryngoscopy. Note the head is elevated by (C) a pillow.

(a) The blade is first introduced in a vertical manner at the right side of the mouth until the palate and posterior pharyngeal wall are visualized.

(b) The blade is rotated towards a horizontal position until the epiglottis is visualized. All force should be applied in the direction of the (A) and (B) arrows.

(c) The blade is introduced so that the beak elevates the epiglottis and pushes it up against the base of the tongue. Note that a lifting force is exerted upward (A) during laryngoscopy and the blade is away from the upper incisor teeth.

necessary for the patient (see table).	sage. A small one causes leakage or a partial obstruction to the airway if the closed system (cuff) is employed.
14. Quickly remove secretions from the pharynx by suctioning.	Remove secretions so that they will not pass into trachea and cause obstruction.
15. Grasp the stylet, together with the catheter, at its slip joint and hold them both in the right hand.	The stylet must be held so that it does not slide in or out of catheter.
16. Introduce the catheter into the mouth and pharynx along right side of laryngoscope blade and insert it a distance of 2–3 cms. into the trachea beyond the vocal	Long catheters may be introduced beyond the bifurcation of the trachea into a bronchus, particularly the right bronchus, if care is not exercised.

cords. Groove of blade must remain free for visualization of the intubation.

17. Partly withdraw laryngoscope but allow it to remain in mouth in vertical position to act as a "bite block."

If patient becomes "light" during the intubation, he may bite down on catheter, unless some protection remains between teeth.

18. Withdraw stylet, holding catheter with left hand, place bite block between teeth, and remove laryngoscope.

Patient may become "light" during intubation. Anesthesia should be resumed as soon as possible.

19. Connect the catheter to the inhaler if the closed orotracheal technique is employed or replace the mask if open orotracheal technique is contemplated.

The catheter merely replaces the oropharyngeal airway in the open oral method.

20. If secretions are present, remove these by using the suction. Then pack pharynx or inflate cuff if one is employed (Fig. 55).

This secures a seal which prevents a leak and loss of mixture around catheter.

21. Anchor catheter to the face with several strips of adhesive.

This prevents the catheter from slipping further into the trachea or from being accidentally jerked out of the mouth or nose.

Advantages of Orotracheal Airway:

1. Semi-rigid tubes or catheters may be employed to minimize the danger of compression or kinking.
2. Visualization of the larynx allows selection of catheters of proper bore and length and insures precision and elimination of guesswork in inserting the catheters.
3. It allows the use of a closed system with cuffs or packs.

Disadvantages:

1. Deep anesthesia is required for exposure of the larynx if a muscle relaxant is not used.
2. The possibility of causing trauma to the pharynx and trachea is ever present.

Comment

Reasons

1. Do not "rush" intubation. The patient must be deeply anesthetized (3rd plane of stage III) and completely relaxed before attempting intubation.

Patient becomes "light" during intubation due to inhalation of room air. Attempts at intubation during light anesthesia cause coughing, vagal reflexes, increased venous pressure, and other circulatory

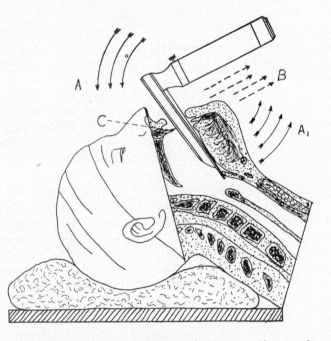

FIG. 58. Improper technique during laryngoscopy results in trauma. If a rotary force (A) and (A₁) is used to lift the epiglottis instead of (B), the (C) upper incisor teeth act as a fulcrum and are dislodged, loosened, or chipped.

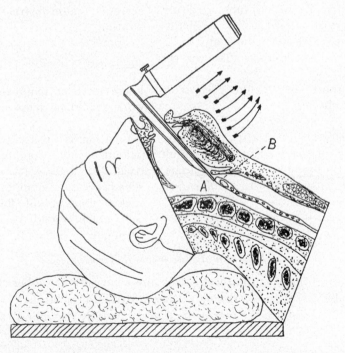

FIG. 59. The laryngoscope rests in the (A) esophagus causing obstruction of the (B) larynx. This may result from poor relaxation, introducing the blade too far, anatomical distortions, or failure to lift upward with the laryngoscope.

2. Always hold the catheter in the left hand at its point of emergence from the mouth during maintenance of anesthesia.

This avoids having catheter slip out of the larynx if head is suddenly moved by the operator.

3. Observe thorax closely for assymetrical respiratory movements, dyspnea, or labored respiration. Be positive that the respiratory effort is in proportion to the tidal exchange. Listen to both sides with a stethoscope.

Catheter may be in the right bronchus, thus occluding the left one. The right bronchus is more easily catheterized than the left because of its length and position.

4. Do not insert the laryngoscope too far into the pharynx. If larynx is not visualized, withdraw it partly until epiglottis is seen.

The beak of the blade may be passed beyond the larynx into the esophagus if the blade is long or the larynx is ventrally placed (Fig. 59). The force exerted may break, chip, or dislodge the teeth.

5. Do not tilt the blade of laryngoscope in such a manner that the incisor teeth act as a fulcrum (Fig. 58).

6. Hold the tongue against the floor of the mouth with the left thumb when packing pharynx with gauze.

This prevents the tongue from rolling back which might cause the frenulum to become torn.

7. Introduce a well-lubricated urinary catheter attached to a suction apparatus and remove any secretions which accumulate in the catheter.

Secretions cause obstruction to respiration.

8. Inspect teeth before performing intubation.

Loose teeth or removable dental work should be removed or protected.

9. Remember that attempts to save two or three minutes may result in the loss of fifteen and in trauma.

Intubation is unsuccessful if the patient is not properly anesthetized.

10. Be certain that the cuff is just below the vocal cords and not too far into the trachea.

This prevents accumulation of excessive amounts of fluid above cuff which would be aspirated when cuff is deflated.

Insertion of Nasotracheal Airways

Description: The patient is anesthetized and a curved soft rubber catheter of suitable size is passed through either nostril into the larynx. The intubation is accomplished either by laryngoscopy or by the "blind" technique.

Types:

1. *Open nasal:* In these intubations the catheter fits loosely in the trachea

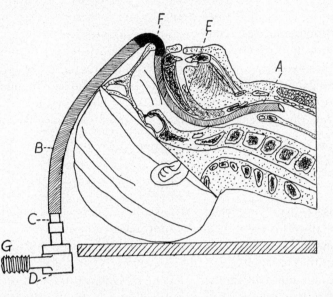

FIG. 60. (A) Closed nasotracheal airway connected to (G) the closed inhaler by means of (F) a metal elbow fitted to a (B) non-collapsible tube and (C) a sleeve and (D) a slip joint. (E) A gauze pack minimizes leakage of gases and absorbs secretions.

and no pack or cuff is employed. The mask is usually replaced after intubation and the anesthesia is continued in the usual manner.

2. *Closed nasal:* In these intubations, a seal is secured by a pack or snug fit existing between the catheter and the tracheal wall (large catheter). Anesthesia is continued by means of a closed or semi-closed inhaler connected directly to the catheter (Fig. 60).

Materials:

1. An assortment of tracheal (Magill) catheters. Prepare one which is larger and one which is smaller than the size necessary for the patient (see page 166 for sizes; Fig. 50).
2. Vaseline (sterile) or similar lubricant for the catheter.
3. Suction equipped with a metal curved tip and a catheter which easily slides into the tracheal catheter.

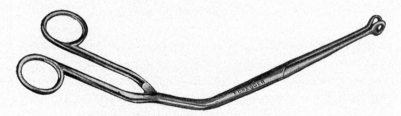

FIG. 61. Forceps for introducing nasotracheal airway into the trachea under direct vision. (Courtesy of Richard Foregger, Ph.D.)

4. Laryngoscope of Guedel, Flagg, or similar design.
5. Slip joints for the catheters and the adapter for the inhaler.
6. Pillow approximately three inches in thickness to elevate the head.
7. Adhesive strips 5/8″×8″ for anchoring catheter to the face.
8. Two gauze packs 2″ by 12″, moistened with saline or liquid petrolatum.
9. Gauze strip or square of adhesive folded lengthwise to protect teeth.
10. Intubation forceps for guiding the catheter into the larynx (Fig. 61).

Preparation of Materials: Follow directions given for insertion of orotracheal airways.

Procedure:

1. Anesthetize the patient, arrange head, pillow, etc., in the manner described for the insertion of orotracheal airways.
2. Examine each nostril and select the one without obstruction or deformities.
3. Extend and hold chin with left hand as for orotracheal intubations.
4. Grasp the catheter at its nasal end between thumb and index finger of the right hand. Allow the catheter to maintain its natural curve and hold it with the concavity upward.
5. Insert the catheter gently into the nostril and gradually thread it into the nasopharynx. Do not exert any force whatsoever while introducing it.
6. As soon as exhaled and inhaled gases pass through the catheter listen (with ear close to inlet of catheter) for the point of maximum intensity of respiration.
7. Halt its advance and at the point of maximum inspiration slip it into the trachea with a thrust.
8. Anchor catheter securely with adhesive and pack pharynx.
9. Connect the catheter to the inhaler or resume anesthesia by replacing the mask and using the catheter as an airway.

Signs of a Successful Intubation:

1. A sharp expulsive cough occurs which is followed by a change in uality of respiratory sounds to a lower pitch (under light anesthesia).
2. The thorax is easily inflated by cautious mouth to tube insufflation, otherwise a gurgling sound and bulging at epigastrium occurs.
3. Air returns through the catheter from the thoracic deflation when mouth to tube insufflation is practiced. The odor of the anesthetic drug employed is recognized if the catheter is in the trachea.
4. The breathing bag moves when the inhaler is connected and the thorax may be inflated when breathing bag is compressed.

Failures in "Blind" Intubations:

1. The catheter strikes the anterior commissure of the larynx (Fig. 62a).

Causes:

a. Hyperextension of the head.

b. Too great a curvature of the catheter.

Signs:

a. A feeling of resistance as the catheter is guided inward.

b. A whistling sound accompanying each phase of respiration.
   Correct this by flexing head, using a different catheter, or by guiding catheter into the larynx under direct vision.

2. The catheter enters the esophagus (Fig. 62b).

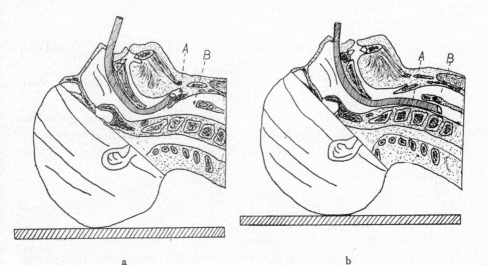

a   b

FIG. 62. (a) Nasotracheal airway improperly placed in (A) the anterior commissure instead of the (B) trachea. (b) Nasotracheal airway improperly placed in (A) the esophagus instead of (B) the treachea.

Causes:

a. The catheter is too soft or does not possess sufficient curvature.

b. The head is flexed too sharply.

Signs:

a. Disappearance of breath sounds as the catheter is advanced inward after a point of maximum intensity is reached.

b. A sucking sound with respiration due to movements of the esophagus with each phase of the respiration.
   Correct this by partially withdrawing the catheter, extending the head, and attempting it once again, or by changing the catheter.

3. Lateral displacement into right or left pyriform fossa.

Causes:

a. Abnormalities of the nasal septum or turbinates.

Signs:

a. A feeling of resistance as the catheter is inserted into the nostril.

b. The catheter may cause a bulge, or it may be felt passing laterally by the hand placed on outside of neck.

c. Breath sounds disappear as the catheter is advanced.

Correct this by withdrawing the catheter and rotating it slightly in the opposite direction. The point of the catheter rotates in the pharynx if the end is rotated. The thyroid cartilage may also be manipulated laterally to fit and guide catheter into the larynx.

Advantages of Nasotracheal Intubations:

1. The catheter may be introduced into the trachea without the aid of a laryngoscope.
2. The intubation may be accomplished either under light or deep anesthesia.
3. The technique may be employed when the mouth cannot be opened for oral surgery, or in circumstances in which the orotracheal route is not feasible, or when it has been attempted without success.

Disadvantages:

1. A completely closed system cannot be easily secured unless a special "flush wall" cuffed catheter is used.
2. The proper size of the catheter is difficult to determine.
3. Trauma to the mucous membranes frequently causes epistaxis, pharyngitis, and laryngitis.
4. Bacterial flora of the nose is introduced into the trachea.
5. Spurs and other abnormalities in the nasopharynx may cause pinching and obstruction of the catheter.
6. The catheter may become kinked in the pharynx or compressed by tight packing or flexion of the head, particularly in the prone position.
7. Suction catheters are not readily introduced into its lumen.
8. Intubation is not easily accomplished if respiratory movements are depressed.

Comment

1. Do not exert force if resistance is felt during introduction of the catheter. Attempt passage in the other nostril.

2. Always pack the pharynx with gauze if the catheter is connected to a closed inhaler.

Reasons

Adenoid tissue, spurs, and deformities may be present and cause trauma and epistaxis.

The pack acts as a seal and prevents loss of gases. It also absorbs blood and secretions in oropharyn-

3. Select as large a catheter as possible without risking injury to nares, pharynx, or larynx.

geal surgery.
Small catheters cause partial obstruction to respiration.

4. Always be positive that the tidal exchange is proportional to the respiratory effort.

Partial obstruction may be present due to distortion or compression of the catheter.

5. Do not attempt to force the catheter into the larynx if spasm is present.

The catheter will kink and bend upon itself. Wait until spasm "breaks."

6. Do not use any slip joint or connecting piece which has a diameter less than the catheter.

Narrow orifices cause obstruction to respiration.

7. Compress the opposite nostril with the free hand when listening for breath sounds.

This avoids confusion with the sound of respiration through it.

8. Do not attempt intubation with soft flaccid catheters which have lost their curvature and resilience.

Best results are obtained when the catheter employed is resilient and possesses a curvature conforming to the curvature of the nasopharyngeal fossa.

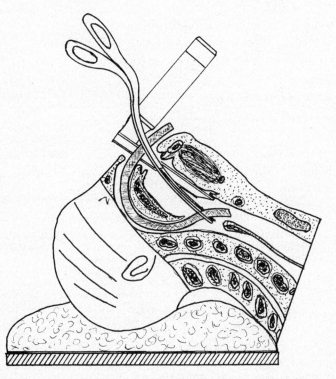

FIG. 63. Introducing nasopharyngeal airway by direct vision using the intubation forceps.

9. Use funnel-shaped slip joints for open nasal intratracheal anesthesia.

They prevent the catheter from slipping into the nose.

10. Intubation forceps should be employed merely to guide the catheter into the larynx.

Trauma to the larynx results if the forceps is introduced beyond the vestibule.

Nasotracheal Intubation by Direct Vision

If after several attempts, the catheter does not slip into the trachea, expose the larynx with the laryngoscope and introduce it with intubating forceps in the following manner:

1. Reanesthetize the patient if he is not sufficiently relaxed.
2. Inject succinylcholine 40 mgm. I.V. or other muscle relaxant.
3. Expose larynx as described for orotracheal intubation.
4. Advance the catheter gently into pharynx almost up to the larynx so that it rests in the midline.
5. Insert the forceps along the side of the groove of the laryngoscope on the right side.
6. Grasp the catheter with the forceps approximately one inch from the beveled end, place it in the vestibule of the larynx, and guide it inward (Fig. 63).
7. Withdraw forceps and laryngoscope.
8. Flex head on thorax and gently thrust catheter inward still further to insure freedom from kinking or obstruction.

Anesthetic Agents for Intratracheal Anesthesia

The anesthetic agent employed must produce relaxation of the neck muscles, flaccidity of the jaw, and abolition of the pharyngeal and laryngeal reflexes if intubation is to be successful. Intubation is simplified by using succinyl choline or other relaxant. Time is saved and trauma is averted. The utility of the various anesthetic agents may be summarized as follows:

	Utility	Advantages	Disadvantages
1. Ether	Most satisfactory and reliable. Recommended for beginners.	1. Glottis is relaxed. Cough reflex is abolished. 2. It is a respiratory stimulant. 3. It produces excellent relaxation. 4. Anesthesia lasts longer than with other agents, allowing sufficient time for intubation.	1. Induction may be prolonged and often difficult. Time consuming addition of a relaxant simplifies and saves time.
2. Cyclopropane	Very satisfactory but requires experience at in-	1. Induction is rapid, relatively simple, and	1. Recovery occurs quickly during intubation.

	duction and intubation. Succinyl choline facilitates procedures.	pleasant. 2. Relaxation is satisfactory with a relaxant.	2. Laryngeal spasm is frequent or easily provoked. Succinyl choline averts it. 3. Respiration is quiet.
3. *Halothane*	Satisfactory, but not recommended because of cardiac effects unless succinyl choline is used to keep anesthesia light.	1. Cough reflex is abolished. 2 Glottis is relaxed. 3. Induction is pleasant. 4. Duration of anesthesia allows sufficient time for intubation. None, except that induction is rapid.	1. It is a circulatory depressant. 2. The possibility of myocardial depression is always present. 3. The margin of safety is narrow—danger of overdosage.
4. *Vinyl Ether*	Not satisfactory.		1. Relaxation of muscles of neck and jaws is not satisfactory, even when a relaxant is used. 2. Anesthesia is evanescent and does not allow time for intubation.
5. *Ethyl Chloride*	Not satisfactory.	None, except that induction is rapid.	1. Relaxation of muscles of neck and jaws is not satisfactory. 2. Anesthesia is evanescent and does not allow time for intubation. 3. It is a circulatory depressant.
6. *Nitrous Oxide or Ethylene*	Not satisfactory unless administered with basal narcosis or heavy doses of premedication and in conjunction with topical anesthesia to the pharynx and larynx and with a muscle relaxant.	None, except that the induction period is short.	1. Intubation is difficult to perform without traumar without a relaxant. 2. It does not abolish cough reflex or relax muscles of neck or jaw. 3. Rapid recovery does not allow time for intubation.
7. *Ultra-short acting Barbiturates.* (Pentothal or Evipal or Surital)	Not satisfactory alone. (Spray nasopharynx and larynx with 4% cocaine prior to induction) and use muscle relaxant.	None, except that induction is simple and rapid.	1. Cough reflex is increased. Spasm of larynx is common. 2. Muscular relaxation is obtained with difficulty in robust subjects. 3. Respiration is depressed.
8. *Avertin*	Not satisfactory unless supplemented with gases or ether and muscle relaxant.	None when used alone.	1. It depresses respiration. 2. It does not completely abolish the laryngeal and pharyngeal reflexes. 3. It does not yield satisfactory relaxation of muscles of neck and jaws.
9. *Topical*	Suitable for patients with obstructive symptoms or for whom mask is difficult to apply.	Avoids obstruction.	1. Unpleasant to patient. 2. Relaxation secured with difficulty in non cooperative patients. 3. Gagging common since patients are awake.

Technical Complications During Intratracheal Anesthesia

1. *Absence of respiratory movements:*

Cause	Symptoms	Treatment
a. Overdosage	a. Signs of 4th plane or 4th stage anesthesia are present. b. The thorax is easily inflated when the breathing bag is compressed.	Deflate the breathing bag, fill with oxygen, and perform artificial respiration
b. Obstruction	a. The thorax is not readily inflated when the breathing bag is pressed. b. The respiratory effort is not in proportion to the tidal exchange (if partial).	Locate cause (see below)
c. Acarbia or hypocapnia	a. This usually follows hyperventilation. b. The thorax is easily inflated and deflated.	Allow apnea to persist until respiratory movements are resumed.
d. Reflex apnea due to excessive positive pressure or presence of the tube.	a. Breathing bag is over-distended. b. Signs of upper third stage anesthesia are usually apparent.	Deflate bag.
e. Light anesthesia.	a. Spasmodic expiratory efforts due to active cough reflex are present. b. Jaws are rigid.	a. Increase proportions of anesthetic agent. b. Gently increase the pressure by compressing the

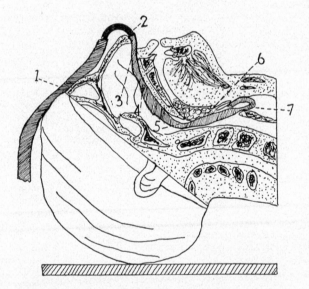

Fig. 64. Possible sites of obstruction in nasotracheal airway:

(1) Collapse of the extension tube.
(2) Undersized slip joints.
(3) Kink at the slip joint.
(4) Compression in the nasopharynx from anatomical distortions.
(5) Obstruction by secretions in the lumen.
(6) Compression from packs.
(7) Tube bent upon itself.

Cause	Symptoms	Treatment
	c. Swallowing movements are present.	bag.
f. Overdose of muscle relaxant.	a. Apnea.	a. Artificial respiration.

2. *Respiratory movements of the thorax are unimpeded, but movements of the breathing bag are absent:*

a. Catheter is in the esophagus instead of the trachea.	a. Expired gases pass through nose and mouth, none through the catheter.	a. Reanesthetize and replace catheter properly.
b. The obturator is closed.	a. The breathing bag cannot be compressed. b. No respiratory sounds are heard in the vicinity of the face. c. The anesthesia becomes lighter.	a. Open obturator and deepen the anesthesia.
c. The slip joint has become disconnected from the inhaler.	a. Respiratory sounds become audible about the mouth. b. Breathing bag may deflate quickly.	a. Replace and reanesthetize the patient.

3. *The breathing bag deflates rapidly, respiratory movements are unimpeded but shallow:*

a. The cuff is deflated or packs are ineffective. b. The catheter is pulled out of trachea.	a. Gas escapes from mouth and nose when bag is compressed.	a. Reinflate the cuff or repack the pharynx.
c. Presence of bronchopleural fistula or perforation in the trachea.	b. The bag is deflated when the bag is compressed, but no gas escapes from the inhaler or the nose and mouth.	b. Plug the fistula with sterile gauze if possible to minimize the leak.

4. *Bag becomes distended though flowmeters are functioning properly:*

a. A small catheter in a large trachea allows air to be drawn in around the vocal cords as they relax during inspiration. The air is forced into the inhaler as they become adducted during expiration.	a. This occurs in open oral or nasal technique. b. It usually occurs during light anesthesia c. Bag fills during expiration. Movement of bag is greater at expiration than at inspiration.	a. Replace the mask over face until patient is anesthetized. Pack pharynx or inflate cuff if closed technique is contemplated.

Causes of Obstruction During Intratracheal Anesthesia

1. The catheter is kinked at its slip joint, or in the nose, mouth, or larynx. Connecting tube from the slip joint to the adapter may be kinked.	a. A decreased volume of respired gases passes through the catheter. b. The respiratory effort is out of proportion to the tidal exchange. c. Signs of anoxemia or asphyxia, such as cyanosis, dilated pupils, hypertension, etc., are present.	a. Relieve the obstruction in the airway.
2. Patient bites on catheter because the anesthesia is light and mouth prop is faulty or the prop has inadvertently slipped out of the mouth.	a. Respired gases pass through the mouth and nose along the outside of the tube if it is of a smaller bore than the trachea.	a. Replace the mouth prop if jaws can be pried apart. Otherwise withdraw the catheter.

Anesthesia Techniques for Intubation

Intubation with Pentothal and Muscle Relaxant

Procedure:

1. Spray nose, pharynx or larynx with cocaine 4% or other desired local anesthetic solution.
2. Administer pentothal or other ultrashort acting intravenous anesthetic until patient is narcotized.
3. Inject 40–60 mgm. succinyl choline or equivalent dose of other muscle relaxant intravenously.
4. Introduce laryngoscope, expose larynx and pass catheter.
5. Connect tube to semi-closed apparatus and proceed with nitrous oxide or to closed apparatus and proceed with cyclopropane or other desired agent.

Intubation with Pentothal, Cyclopropane, and a Muscle Relaxant

Procedure:

1. Spray nose, pharynx or larynx with local anesthetic solution (optional).
2. Administer pentothal or other ultra short acting drug until basal narcosis is obtained.
3. Administer cyclopropane until patient is in 3rd plane.
4. Administer 40–60 mgm. succinyl choline or other muscle relaxant intravenously.
5. Hyperventilate, expose larynx, and intubate.
6. Connect apparatus and continue with cyclopropane or cyclopropane-ether.

Intubation with Pentothal, Nitrous Oxide-Ether and a Muscle Relaxant

1. Spray nose, pharynx and larynx with local anesthetic solution (optional).
2. Induce basal narcosis with pentothal, or other ultra short acting barbiturate.
3. Commence nitrous oxide as described under section on nitrous oxide.
4. Gradually add ether until plane 2 or 3 is reached.
5. Add 20–40 mgm. succinyl choline or other muscle relaxant intravenously.
6. Expose larynx and intubate.
7. Connect to closed system.
8. Maintain with oxygen ether.

Technique Using Indirect Laryngoscopy

Materials:

1. Nasal spray.
2. Cocaine 10% and 4%.
3. Jackson pledget holders (Pilling introducers).

4. Mirror for indirect laryngoscopy.
5. Head mirror or head lamp.
6. Nasopharyngeal syringe with long curved nozzle.

Procedure:

1. Anesthetize nose, palate, tongue and oropharynx by spraying with 4% cocaine.
2. Wrap pledget of cotton on Pilling introducer, soak with 10% cocaine and press dry.
3. Warm mirror and visualize each pyriform fossa. Spray each with 4% cocaine.
4. Introduce cotton pledget in each pyriform fossa and hold in contact for 5 minutes.
5. Remove, pledget holders and expose larynx.
6. Introduce 2 cc. 4% cocaine with syringe equipped with long curved nozzle into larynx.
7. Introduce intratracheal tube using curved stylet.

Transtracheal Anesthesia

Definition: Topical anesthesia of the larynx, trachea and bronchi obtained by injecting a local anesthetic solution into the trachea through the thyrocricoid membrane.

Anatomy: The thyrocricoid membrane may be identified by a dense triangular area of connective tissue between the thyroid and cricoid cartilages. This area may be pierced with a fine needle.

Materials:

a. 2 cc. syringe.
b. 4% cocaine, 2% pontocaine, or other topical anesthetic.
c. 23 gauge 1½ inch long needle.

Technique:

1. Position. Place the patient in the supine position with the head hyperextended.
2. Palpate the cricoid membrane between the thyroid (A, Fig. 65) and the cricoid (B) cartilages with the left forefinger.
3. Cleanse the skin over the trachea and apply a sterilizer.
4. Raise a wheal over the criocid membrane and introduce the needle with syringe attached containing solution in the midline (C, Fig. 65).
5. Advance needle perpendicular to the skin until lack of resistance is felt, at which time the point is within the trachea.
6. Instruct patient not to cough, swallow or talk.

7. Aspirate air to ascertain if the needle is in the trachea.
8. Quickly inject 2 cc. of solution and withdraw the needle.
9. Instruct the patient to cough in order to spread the solution throughout the trachea.

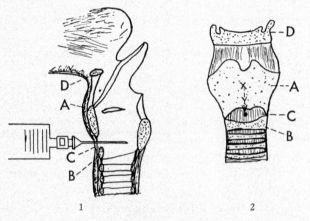

FIG. 65. 1. Cross section of larynx showing placement of needle in performing transcricoid instillation of local anesthetic drug. 2. Anterior view of larynx. (A) Thyroid cartilage. (B) Cricoid cartilage. (C) Thyrocricoid membrane. (D) Hyoid bone. (X) Point of injection in midline.

10. Spray the mouth and pharynx with a nebulizer with the same solution to obtain anesthesia of the epiglottis.

Comments

1. For bronchoscopy or endotracheal intubation perform the procedure with the patient sitting up.
2. Fix larynx with left hand if it tends to slip about.

Complications:

1. Possibility of fistulae cellulitis of the neck and thyroiditis.
2. Bleeding caused by using too large a needle.
3. Broken needle.

Pre-Anesthetic Intubation With Patient "Awake"

Description: The passage of an endotracheal catheter either nasally or orally before the patient is anesthetized.

Use:

1. In cases in which partial obstruction exists and complete obstruction during induction is feared.
2. In cases in which a mask cannot be applied to the face.
3. In cases in which the neck cannot be flexed because of fear of causing injury (fractured cervical vertebrae).
4. In cases in which avoidance of tracheotomy is imperative.

Materials:

   a. 4% Cocaine—(or 5% hexylcaine, 5% lidocaine (Xylocaine) or 0.5% pontocaine).

   b. Spray of Pilling type for laryngeal anesthesia.

   c. Endotracheal tubes, laryngoscopes, etc.

Procedure: Oral route:

1. Advise patient what is to be done and explain procedure. Advise he will not be able to talk but will be able to breathe freely after intubation.
2. Spray local anesthetic into nostrils and place patient in recumbent position. Have patient gargle and expectorate excess.
3. Next spray tongue, palate and oropharynx with local anesthetic in amounts not exceeding 1 cc. at each time.
4. With McIntosh or Guedal laryngoscope expose the hypopharynx. Spray hypopharynx and cords if they can be visualized.
5. Allow 3 or 4 minutes to elapse and attempt to visualize larynx. Spray again if cough reflex persists.
6. Expose larynx and introduce intratracheal catheter of proper size.
7. Add 1 cc. local anesthetic solution into tube if coughing persists.
8. As soon as "bucking" ceases induce anesthesia with pentothal, cyclopropane or other desired agent.

Procedure: Nasal route:

1. Proceed as above to anesthetize nasopharynx, oropharynx and trachea.
2. Introduce nasal tube into the most patent nostril and pass into hypopharynx noting point of maximum ventilation at expiration. Stop at this point.
3. Have patient inspire deeply.
4. Introduce catheter quickly during height of inspiration.

Comment

1. Transcricoid instillation may be used to anesthetize larynx and hypopharynx if desired. This obviates use of laryngoscope to anesthetize hypopharynx.
2. Do not administer barbiturates and then attempt intubation. Patient becomes disoriented and unmanageable and moves about because reflex activity is only partially obtunded.

Intratracheal Anesthesia Utilizing Tracheotomy

Procedure:

1. Select anode wire woven catheter same size or larger than tracheotomy cannula.

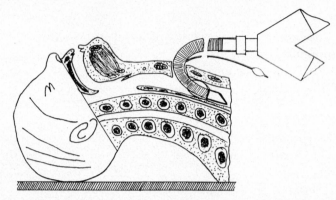

FIG. 66. The tracheotomy cannula may be replaced with a wire woven anode endotracheal tube with a cuff which is then connected to the anesthesia apparatus and anchored in position with adhesive. Anesthesia is then conducted in the usual manner using the semi-closed or closed system with whatever agent is desired.

2. Lubricate with local anesthetic ointment (Americaine, 2% Pontocaine, 1% Nupercaine, etc.).
3. Introduce gently into tracheotomy opening and guide beveled end into trachea (Fig. 66).
4. Pack area around tube with gauze.
5. Anchor tube to skin of neck with adhesive.
6. Connect adapter to filter.
7. Induce anesthesia with cyclopropane, or other desired agent.
8. When jaw is relaxed pack pharynx to prevent supra laryngeal leakage of mixture.

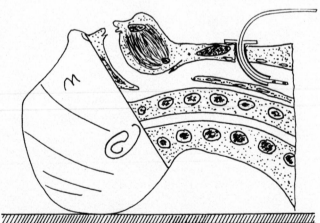

FIG. 67. Gases and vapors of volatile liquids may be insufflated directly into the tracheal cannula of a tracheotomized patient. The catheter, since it partly occludes the lumen of the cannula, may cause serious obstruction when the cannula fits snugly into the tracheotomy opening.

Alternate Methods

1. Adapters may be soldered to endotracheal slip joints and connection made directly to tracheotomy cannula.
2. Insufflation into the tracheotomy cannula with catheter may be used but is less desirable. Catheter partly occludes airway (Fig. 67).

Ayres Intratracheal Insufflation Technique

Definition: Insufflation of an anesthetic gas or vapor directly into the trachea using a nasal or oral intratracheal catheter connected to a Y piece at the slip joint.

Uses:

1. For oral or nasal surgery—particularly in infants and in situations in which connectors and slip joints interfere with the surgeon's movements if in the operative field.

Materials:

1. A metal Y connector whose internal diameter is the same or greater than the diameter of the endotracheal catheter.
2. A curved elbow which fits into the intratracheal tube.
3. Pieces of gum rubber approximately one inch in length to connect elbow to Y piece.
4. Piece of rubber several inches in length with several perforations along

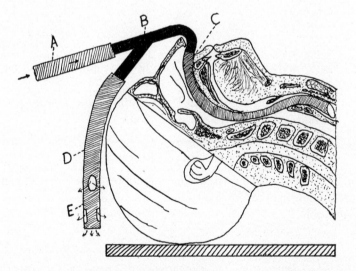

Fig. 68. An alternate method of insufflation nasoendotracheal anesthesia: Gases are delivered under slight positive pressure through (A) which is connected to the (B) "Y" piece which communicates with (C) the nasal tracheal airway. (D) Short exhalation and rebreathing tube open at the end. (E) Perforations are for the escape of exhaled and excess gases.

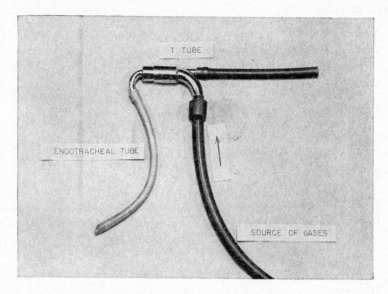

Fig. 69. The Ayres insufflation technique embodies the use of a Y tube, one limb of which is connected to the source of anesthetic mixture and the other to a short length of perforated tubing. The main limb is connected to the endotracheal tube. This technique is suitable for surgery of the head and neck in infants and children. (Courtesy C. R. Stephen, Elements of Pediatric Anesthesia. Springfield, Thomas, 1954. Fig. 8, p. 46.)

body which fits Y piece and has approximately same or larger internal diameter of the Y piece (Fig. 68, 69).

5. Insufflation apparatus.

Procedure:

1. Anesthetize subject (preferably with open drop ether) if ether is to be used.
2. Intubate and insert elbow into Y piece and connect to insufflation apparatus and continue with agent of choice.

Endobronchial Anesthesia

Definition: The introduction of a single catheter into one bronchus or a double lumen catheter into both main stem bronchi so that the lungs no longer communicate with each other. Anesthesia is then conducted into one or both bronchi as desired.

Indications for Endobronchial Anesthesia

1. For thoracic surgery to prevent drowning from excessive fluids or blood

2. To prevent contamination of the healthy lung by infected material when one is diseased.

Technique—Two Lung Endobronchial Anesthesia
Using a Carlen's Catheter

Materials:

1. A Carlen's double lumen catheter 13 mm. outside diameter for males and 11 mm. for females (Fig. 70).

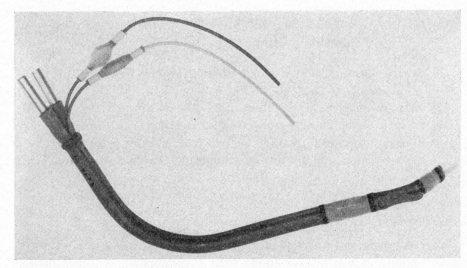

FIG. 70. The double lumen endotracheal catheter of Carlens permits isolation of the right bronchus from the left and prevents contaminated material from passing from one lung to the other.

2. 4% cocaine or other desired topical anesthetic.
3. A curved stylet, lubricated.
4. Laryngoscope of the Guedel or McIntosh type.
5. Double slip joint for intratracheal adapter.
6. Suction catheters which pass into the tube.

Procedure (With Local Anesthesia):

1. Anesthetize the pharynx, larynx and trachea topically. This is done by spraying the naso and oropharynx and by transcricoid instillation or by direct instillation into the larynx.
2. Arrange the patient in the sitting position.
3. Lubricate the catheter and tie the "carina hook" with a silk thread using a slip knot so that it is close to the tube and can be slipped into the trachea (Fig. 71).

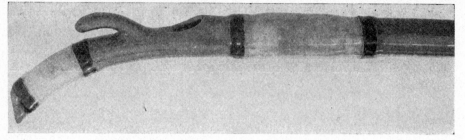

FIG. 71. The end of the Carlens catheter is shown.

4. Introduce lubricated curved metal stylet into tube.
5. Under direct vision introduce tube into larynx using slight rotary movement.
6. Gently release slip knot and push the catheter downward. It turns automatically to the left.
7. Withdraw the curved stylet.
8. As soon as the hook is engaged in carina inflate both cuffs (Fig. 72).
9. Replace mask over the tube for two lung anesthesia or connect to a circle filter with double adapter. Single adapter to desired bronchus is used for one lung anesthesia.
10. Commence anesthesia with cyclopropane or other desired agent.

Procedure (With General Anesthesia):

1. Prepare patient with topical anesthesia as above.
2. Commence general anesthesia with cyclopropane, or other desired agent.

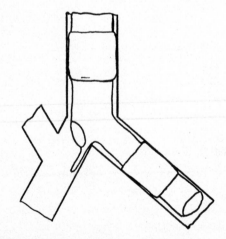

FIG. 72. Position of Carlens double lumen endobronchial catheter in the trachea and bronchi. The middle piece hooks over the carina and fixes the catheter in position. The catheter passes into the left. To prevent occlusion of the eparterial bronchus on the right side the catheter is cut short at the carina. The cuffs isolate the right lung from the left.

3. Administer muscle relaxant, such as syncurine (3–4 mgm.) or succinyl choline (20–40 mgm.). (See Part IV.)
4. Expose larynx with laryngoscope as for endotracheal intubation.
5. Introduce catheter as above.

Endobronchial Intubation Using Direct Vision

Definition: One lung anesthesia obtained by intubating the bronchus under direct vision employing bronchial tube or a catheter slipped over a bronchoscope.

Materials: Special Ruth-Bailey, Bonica, or other desired type endobronchial tube and bronchoscope (Fig. 73).

Prepare as Follows:

1. Apply Penrose tubing over the coil wire of the airway portion of the Ruth-Bailey bronchoscope or apply Bonica catheter over the bronchoscope.
2. Lubricate with anesthetic ointment.
3. Introduce the light carrier into the bronchoscope.

Procedure:

1. Anesthetize the patient in the usual manner using cyclopropane and a muscle relaxant or other desired anesthetic which has been preceded by topical anesthesia.
2. Expose the trachea with (McIntosh or Guedel) laryngoscope.
3. Introduce bronchoscope into the trachea.
4. Remove laryngoscope.
5. Advance bronchoscope into desired bronchus.
6. Insert bite block.
7. Remove and adjust light carrier and bronchoscope leaving airway portion of tube in bronchus.
8. Attach to anesthesia apparatus.
9. Inflate cuff.

Situations for Which Endobronchial Anesthesia Is Desirable

1. Tuberculosis with cavitation or secondary suppuration behind a bronchial stenosis.
2. Operations for bronchiectasis with copious secretions.
3. Purulent lung abscess or lung cysts.
4. Cases in which pulmonary bronchial hemorrhage is present or may occur.
5. Bronchopleural fistula.

Comment

1. The trachea is not cylindrical. Its antero posterior diameter is somewhat less than the transverse.
2. The distance from the gums to the bifurication is about 25 cms.
3. The trachea lies in the median plane as far as aortic arch after which it is deflected slightly to the right.

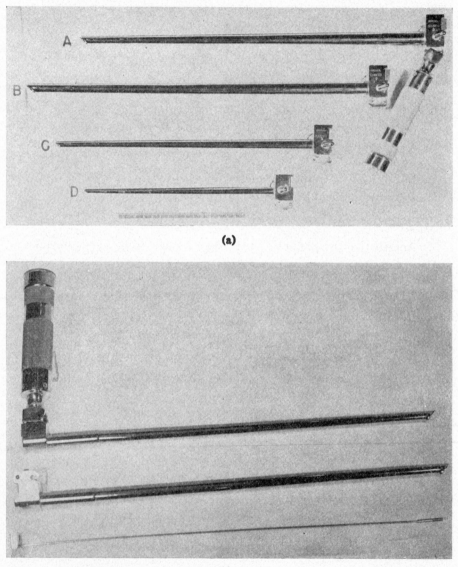

(a)

(b)

Fig. 73. Bronchoscopes used for introducing endotracheal catheters and for bronchoscopy for aspiration. (a) Davis bronchoscopes. (b) Tapered bronchoscopes for aspiration. (c) Infant bronchoscopes. (*See page 251 for (c).*)

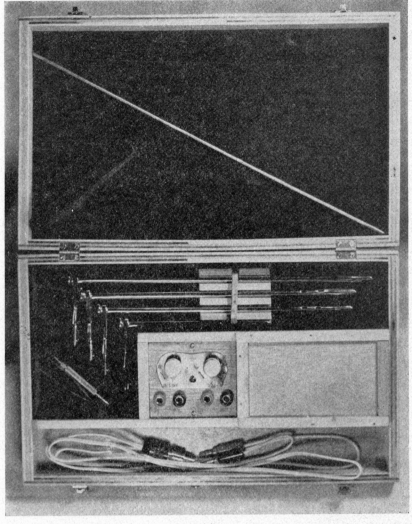

(c)

4. The opening of the right bronchus is equivalent to $\frac{2}{3}$ of the area of the terminal portion of the trachea. The carina thus is to left of midline.
5. The right bronchus deviates 25° from the median saggital plane, the left 45°.
6. The length of the right bronchus varies from 0.5 to 2.5 cms.
7. The eparterial bronchus on the right may be opposite the carina and may be blocked in one lung intubations.
8. The right bronchus is wider than the left.

Precautions:

1. Do not overinflate cuff. It may bulge over end and occlude lumen of tube.

2. Infiltrate hilum with procaine to obviate tracheobronchial reflexes.

3. Ausculate chest to ascertain whether or not ventilation is adequate on the intubated side in one lung intubations.

Advantages:

1. Prevents drowning of the patient in his own secretions when aspiration with an ordinary endotracheal tube does not prevent the secretions from the diseased lung passing into the healthy one.

2. Reduces the necessity for preoperative bronchoscopy.

3. Allows operations to be performed on a completely collapsed lung.

4. Prevents loss of anesthetic gas through a bronchopleura fistula.

5. Reduces incidence of contralateral atelectasis.

6. Decreases the number of aspirations during surgery as the functioning lung does not become "wet."

7. Permits the diseased lung to be deflated to provide greater operating space in the chest.

8. Permits lung to be inflated when lobar or intersegmental planes are developed.

9. Permits bronchus to be divided whenever this is suitable and left open until it is convenient to close it.

10. Relieves the necessity of applying clamp on the proximal part of the bronchus thus avoiding injury to the bronchial wall.

11. Permits removal of foreign material.

12. Permits inspection of the bronchus and aspiration through the opening in the open bronchus.

Disadvantages:

1. Necessitates the use of deep anesthesia.

2. Skill is required in bronchoscopic technique.

3. Possibility of trauma to the bronchus from the tube is present.

4. The cuff may be over-distended and obstruct the lumen of the bronchus.

5. The eparterial bronchus may be occluded on the intubated side.

6. The tube may become displaced during operation without notice of the anesthesiologist and asphyxia results.

7. The cuff may be partially deflated and permits passage of secretions around the tube.

8. The cuff must be deflated (in single catheter technique) when positive pressure is made to check if the bronchus is air-tight following ligation and severance.

9. Cross sectional area of trachea may be reduced unduly.

REFERENCES

Bonica, J., and Hall, W. Endobronchial Anesthesia. Anesthesiology, *12:* 344, 1951.
Bjork, O. V., Carlens, E. and Friberg, O. Endobronchial Anesthesia. Anesthesiology, *60:* 14, 1953.
Ruth, H. S., Grove, D. D. and Keown, K. K. Endobronchial Anesthesia. Anesthesiology, *9:* 422–429, 1948.

Insufflation Intratracheal Anesthesia

Principle: The patient is intubated by the nasal or oral route and a smaller catheter is passed through the tube to the bifurcation of the trachea. Ether-oxygen is conducted into the lungs through the smaller tube and the gases return through the larger one (Fig. 74).

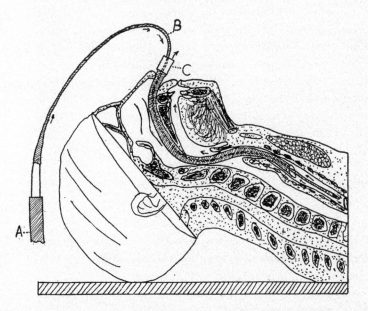

FIG. 74. Intratracheal insufflation anesthesia. (A) The delivery tube from source of anesthetic gases and vapors is connected to (B) the lubricated catheter which is threaded through (C) the naso-tracheal tube. The inner catheter protrudes beyond the bevel of the outer one and extends as far as the carina. Gases and vapors are delivered under a positive pressure not exceeding 25 mm. Hg. They return through the larger catheter or, between the tracheal wall and catheter and pass through the nose and mouth.

Materials:

1. An oral or nasal tracheal catheter.
2. The usual intubation equipment.
3. Catheter #18 F or smaller if a tracheal catheter of small bore is used.
4. Inhaler.
5. Insufflation apparatus for ether.

Technique:

1. Anesthetize and intubate the patient.
2. Attach catheter to insufflation apparatus consisting of an ether vaporizer and oxygen supply.
3. Commence the flow of ether vapor through catheter at pressure of 10–20 cms. H_2O.
4. Lubricate catheter well and introduce it into the trachea as far as its bifurcation.
5. Continue anesthesia in the usual manner.

Care of Catheters

1. Cleanse the lumen with soap and water. Use a test tube brush or a gauze ribbon to remove all foreign particles.
2. Remove the lubricant with ether. Adhesive should be soaked with ether before removal, otherwise rubber may be torn.
3. Rinse with soapy water, then water, and immerse in mercuric cyanide solution (1:1000) for an hour.
4. Rinse with water. Follow with 70% alcohol and dry and pack in sterile plastic sheaths.

Use and Care of Cuffs

Inflation:

1. Insert the short blunt needle into lumen of catheter leading to cuff.
2. Attach the 10 cc. dry syringe filled with air.
3. Inject air gently and slowly into the cuff until a resistance is felt on the plunger. Manually compress the breathing bag as the cuff is distended.
4. Clamp catheter when the gases no longer escape and the seal is complete. Remove syringe.

Cleaning:

1. Remove the cuff from the catheter and cleanse in the same manner described above for catheters.

Comment	Reasons
1. Do not over-inflate cuffs.	They may rupture and cause trauma to the trachea, initiate vagal reflexes, obstruct the end of the catheter, or denude the mucosa from the trachea.
2. Do not inflate the cuff during light anesthesia.	Distension of the cuff often elicits a violent cough reflex.

3. Do not use old non-elastic cuffs.

They are usually elongated and cover an excess area of the tracheal surface.

4. Do not use a cuff which possesses too thin a wall.

It may bulge over the end of the catheter and obstruct the lumen.

5. Do not use a cuff whose walls are too thick.

The pressure required to inflate the cuff may be so great that it compresses a soft intratracheal catheter.

6. Always test cuffs by inflating them and submerging in water. Fine bubbles will appear if a leak is present.

Small leaks are vexing and not easily detected.

7. Do not use cuffs which do not grip the catheter firmly.

The cuff may slip off the catheter during extubation.

General Comment Concerning Intratracheal Anesthesia

Reasons

1. Select the route of intubation which is most convenient to the surgeon and safest for the patient.

The catheter should not be in the operative field.

2. Select the route which promises to be the least traumatic.

Edentulate subjects or subjects with long, thin necks are more easily intubated by direct vision. Subjects with short necks are more easily intubated by the nasal route.

3. Intubate subjects with short, thick necks or with fragile or loose teeth by the nasal route.

The larynx is difficult to expose with the laryngoscope in these subjects but the nasal catheter by the "blind" technique slips in easily.

4. Avoid nasotracheal intubation in infants and children.

Adenoids and anatomical abnormalities are more common in children and interfere with the intubation.

5. Remember that the pharyngeal reflex, as well as the laryngeal reflex, is obtunded in debilitated subjects, patients in shock, etc.

This lack of activity facilitates intubation under light anesthesia, or without any anesthesia.

6. Remember that the pharyngeal reflex is hyperactive in subjects with pulmonary disease, in subjects with purulent discharge from the lungs, or in children.

Intubation is more difficult in these subjects because of this increased activity.

7. Select small catheters when the

Trauma is lessened. Gases pass in

open, oral, or nasal technique is employed.

and around catheter.

8. Use silk, metal, or anode tubes when the head is to be extended or flexed, or when patient is to be placed in any position other than on his back.

Soft catheters are easily kinked in these situations.

9. Use the closed endotracheal technique with an inflatable cuff or packs for oral surgery or when emesis or regurgitation is anticipated.

Aspiration of secretions is assured only by a closed system.

REFERENCES

Flagg, Paluel J. Intratracheal Inhalation Anesthesia in Practice. Arch. Otolaryngology 15: 844, June, 1932.

Gillespie, Noel A. Endotracheal Anesthesia. 2nd. Ed. University of Wisconsin Press, Madison, Wisconsin, 1948.

Magill, I. W. Technique of Endotracheal Anesthesia. Anesth. & Analg. 4: 164, July-August, 1931.

Waters, Ralph M., Rovenstine, E. A., and Guedel, Arthur E. Endotracheal Anesthesia and Its Historical Development. Anesth. & Analg., 12: 196, September–October, 1933.

PART III
COMPLICATIONS OF ANESTHESIA
COMPLICATIONS DURING GENERAL ANESTHESIA

Although many undesirable reactions and complications appear during general anesthesia, those of major importance may be divided into four groups: *respiratory, circulatory, neurological,* and *technical.*

RESPIRATORY COMPLICATIONS

Respiratory complications are the most vexing and frequent complications of anesthesia. If unrecognized and untreated, they ultimately lead to asphyxia. The following symptoms and complications are the most important.

ANOXIA

Definition: Interference with adequate oxygenation of tissues.

Causes:

1. A decreased oxygen tension in the inspired air.
2. Obstruction of the airway.
3. Impairment of pulmonary ventilation from:
   a. Overdosage of depressant drugs.
   b. Restraint of thoracic and diaphragmatic movements.
   c. Decrease in vital capacity by mechanical methods, such as pneumothorax.
   d. Alterations in permeability of pulmonary epithelium.
   e. Pulmonary edema.
4. Impairment of oxygen transport—carbon monoxide poisoning or circulatory disturbances.
5. Inability of tissues to utilize oxygen—cyanide and similar types of poisoning.

Sequelae:

1. None if immediate treatment is instituted and recovery follows.
2. Circulatory failure followed by a delay in treatment. In these instances death may be delayed for several hours or the patient may recover but may have signs and symptoms of cerebral damage.
3. Circulatory failure and death within a few minutes.

CYANOSIS

Definition: The bluish discoloration of the skin and mucous membrane due to an increase or excess of reduced hemoglobin in the blood.

Factors Influencing Its Appearance:

1. The quantity of reduced hemoglobin in the blood (usually 6 gms. per 100 cc. blood must be present).

2. The thickness of the skin—the thicker the skin the less intense the color.
3. The size and degree of dilatation of cutaneous vessels.
4. The degree of pigmentation of the skin.
5. Acuity of the observer.

Causes:

1. Decreased oxygen tension in the alveoli:
   a. Respiratory obstruction.
   b. Decreased partial pressure of oxygen in the inhaled mixture.
   c. Decreased ventilation from respiratory depression, respiratory failure, interference with respiratory movements, or diminished vital capacity.
2. Slowing of circulating blood through the capillaries from:
   a. Circulatory failure.
   b. Compression of a vessel or an extremity.

Comment	*Reasons*
1. Cyanosis is no index of depth of anesthesia.	It merely indicates the state of oxygenation of the blood.
2. Cyanosis may not appear in severe anemias.	The amount of reduced hemoglobin may not be sufficient for it to be visible through the skin.

HYPERPNEA DURING ANESTHESIA

Definition: An abnormally excessive rate or depth of respiration.

Causes:

1. Carbon dioxide excess (see hypercapnia).
2. Painful stimulation during light anesthesia.
3. Local stimulating action of the anesthetic drug used in conjunction with inhalation anesthesia.
4. Central disturbances—intracranial lesions.

APNEA DURING ANESTHESIA

Definition: A cessation of respiratory movements or ventilatory efforts.

Causes:

1. Hypocapnia from hyperventilation and raising the threshold of the respiratory center to carbon dioxide.
2. Reflex stimulation of pharynx, trachea, hilum, mesentery, etc.
3. Overdosage of central nervous system depressants.
4. Laryngeal or bronchial spasm.
5. Complete obstruction of the airway.
6. Neurological disturbances, particularly increased intracranial pressure, etc.

7. Circulatory failure (shock or cardiac arrest). (See overdosage, this chapter, for discussion and differential diagnosis.)
8. Overdistension of breathing bag.

HYPOPNEA DURING ANESTHESIA

Definition: Decreased tidal exchange without a notable decrease in respiratory rate.

Causes:

1. Depression of medullary centers due to drugs particularly nonvolatile central nervous system depressants.
2. Increased positive pressure in the inhalor—over distended bag.
3. Decrease in pulmonary ventilating surface such as is seen with pneumothorax mediastinal shift during chest surgery or atelectasis.
4. Cessation of painful stimulation during light anesthesia.
5. Lightening of anesthesia or discontinuing administration of drugs which cause exaggerated breathing (ether).
6. Obstructed airway.
7. Awkward positions interfering with proper ventilation.
8. Carbon dioxide excess which has persisted to point of causing depression of medullary centers.

Management:

1. Remove obstruction or other cause of interference with ventilation.
2. Increase oxygen tension in inhaler.
3. Reduce pressure in inhaler so that bag is partially deflated.

BRADYPNEA

Definition: Slow rate of respiration with or without a decrease in minute volume exchange. Tidal volume may increase to compensate for decrease in rate.

Causes:

1. Depression by narcotics (morphine, dilaudid, etc.).
2. Severe anoxia, terminal phase.
3. Central lesions which cause increased intracranial pressure.
4. Peripheral or central circulatory failure.

Management:

1. Be certain airway is patent and oxygenation is adequate.
2. Augment or control respiration when ventilation is not adequate.
3. Administer nalorphine (Nalline) if due to narcotics.
4. Reduce intracranial pressure if due to central lesions.
5. Administer circulatory stimulants, blood or fluids if due to failure of circulation.

POLYPNEA

Definition: An increase in both depth and rate of respiration.

Causes:

1. Anoxia—in early precrisis phases due to deficient oxygen tension in inspired mixture.
2. Local stimulating action of volatile drugs (ether, ethyl chloride, etc.).
3. Painful stimulation during light anesthesia or stimulation of hyper-responsive areas.
4. Carbon dioxide excess approaching peak of stimulation.
5. Central lesions causing derangement of respiratory center.

Management:

1. Increase oxygen tension in inhalor if due to anoxia.
2. Check carbon dioxide absorber, mask size or other sources of dead space which permits rebreathing.
3. Deepen anesthesia if due to stimulation or use procaine block in hyperresponsive areas.
4. Shift to non-stimulating agents such as cyclopropane or pentothal nitrous oxide, and use controlled respiration.

TACHYPNEA

Definition: An excessive rate of respiration.

Causes:

1. Local stimulating action of volatile drugs (ether, ethyl chloride, etc.) but especially trichlorethylene (trilene).
2. Painful stimulation during light anesthesia or stimulation of hyper-responsive agents.
3. Central disturbances due to neurological lesions.
4. Anoxia due to inadequate oxygenation of inhaled mixture.
5. Undersized endotracheal airways.

Management:

1. Oxygenate well.
2. Inspect absorber, valves, tubing, etc.
3. Eliminate or decrease size of dead space in masks, connectors, etc.
4. Deepen anesthesia if light when sensitive structures are manipulated (rectum, perineum, penis, vulva, periosteum, etc.).
5. Reduce intracranial pressure in central lesions by proper neurological measures recommended for the cause.

HYPERPNEA DURING ANESTHESIA

Definition: An abnormally excessive depth of respiration resulting in an increased minute volume exchange.

Causes:

1. Carbon dioxide excess (see hypercapnia).
2. Painful stimulation during light anesthesia or stimulation of a hyperesponsive area.
3. Local stimulating action of the anesthetic drug (ether, etc.) used in conjunction with inhalation anesthesia.
4. Central disturbances—intracranial lesions.
5. Cause undetermined.

Management:

1. Check absorbent and replace with fresh if any doubt exists concerning freshness.
2. Close main valves on carbon dioxide cylinders if present on apparatus.
3. Change mask to smaller one if possible to eliminate rebreathing as much as possible.
4. Deepen anesthesia if light and manipulations are painful.
5. Change to cyclopropane or pentothal-nitrous oxide or ethylene if due to ether or other volatile liquid.
6. Reduce intracranial pressure by proper neurosurgical measures if due to neurological lesion.
7. Curarize and control respiration if above fail and respiratory movements interfere with operation.

PERIODIC BREATHING

Definition: A progressive increase in depth of respiration which reaches a peak and gradually recedes which recurs at regular intervals which appears during general anesthesia.

Causes:

1. Marked or long standing depression of respiratory center due to non-volatile drugs (barbiturates).
2. Decrease in volume of anatomical dead space (during intratracheal anesthesia) causes more abrupt mixing of tidal air with alveolar air.
3. Central lesions cause medullary compression and inactivate respiratory center.

Management:

1. Augment breathing if due to depression by drugs.
2. Use analeptics if due to medullary depression caused by drugs.

3. Increase dead space in intratracheal anesthesia.
4. Reduce intracranial pressure by dehydration or neurosurgical measures if due to central lesions.

IRREGULAR BREATHING

Causes:

1. Central nervous system diseases which cause increased intracranial pressure and affect respiratory center.
2. Intermittent partial obstruction.
3. Second stage anesthesia.
4. Reflex due to stimulation of peritoneum, pleura, viscera, periosteum, rectum, genitalia and other hyperesponsive areas.

Management:

1. Be certain airway is not obstructed.
2. Remove stimulus to hypersensitive structures by procaine block.
3. Determine and remove cause if due to central lesion.

DIFFICULT BREATHING DURING ANESTHESIA

Definition: Difficult, labored, or gasping respiration. Inspiration, expiration or both phases of respiration may be abnormal. Tracheal tug may be present.

Causes:

1. Partial obstruction in the respiratory tract (see obstruction).
2. Difficult position, particularly prone, head down supine or lateral.
3. External force inhibiting thoracic movements.
4. Decreased vital capacity due to disease of lung (atelectasis or fibrosis).
5. Hypercapnia, particularly when sustained for a long time and high concentrations of carbon dioxide accumulates in the inhaler.
6. Chronic sub-oxygenation.
7. Pneumothorax or other factors decreasing ventilating surface or minute volume exchange.
8. Biochemical disturbances due to anoxia or carbon dioxide excess.
9. Faulty apparatus causing obstruction, particularly on inspirations.
10. Atelectasis developing during anesthesia.
11. High spinal anesthesia involving intercostal muscles.
12. Central derangements due to neurologic disease.
13. Fourth plane anesthesia.

Management:

1. Establish airway. Intubate if necessary to improve ventilation.
2. Assist or use controlled respiration to provide adequate ventilation.

3. Restore to position which eliminates interference with respiration.
4. Introduce needle and water trap if due to pneumothorax.

DYSPNEA

Definition: Sensation of suffocation or inability to breathe of which patient complains. Occurs during regional anesthesia while patient is conscious.

Causes:

1. Spinal is high involving intercostal muscles.
2. Prodromal response to overdosage of local anesthetic.
3. Psychogenic factors ensuing from apprehension.
4. Aggravation of pre-existing cardiac or pulmonary disease.

Management:

1. Sedate with intravenous narcotic or basal narcotic doses of barbiturate if due to apprehension.
2. Administer oxygen and assist breathing if due to high spinal.
3. Adjust position, administer oxygen and narcotics if due to cardiac and pulmonary disease.

COUGHING DURING ANESTHESIA

Causes:

1. Artificial airways or laryngoscopes stimulate reflex activity in the pharynx, larynx, or trachea when introduced in second stage or during basal narcosis with non-volatile drugs or in subjects with hyperactive cough reflexes.
2. Mucous and other secretions which have accumulated in the pharynx pass into the larynx and trachea and stimulate tracheal reflexes.
3. Strong concentration of ether or other irritating volatile agent suddenly introduced into the inhaler (this elicits a cough even when the patient is in surgical anesthesia).
4. Manipulation of the wall of a bronchus, hilum of a lung, or trachea in thracic or neck surgery.
5. Hyperactive cough reflex. Common in suppurative diseases of lung.

Management:

1. Avoid placement of airways in second stage anesthesia or during basal narcosis.
2. Suction secretions thoroughly—administer additional anticholinergic drug if dose has been inadequate.
3. Use topical anesthesia prior to intubation and coat airways with rapid acting anesthetic ointments (Americaine—20% benzocaine ointment).
4. Instill 1–2 cc. 4% cocaine into intratracheal tubes if due to tube.

5. Reduce concentration of volatile agent or change to non-irritating type agents if cough persists.
6. Block hyperesponsive area with procaine (hilum) or topically with cocaine.
7. Curarize and control breathing if due to hyperactive cough reflex which does not respond to addition of topical anesthetic agents and deepening of anesthesia.
8. Readjust position of endotracheal tube by withdrawing slightly.

SIGHING

Definition: Sudden deep inspirations appearing at irregular intervals without apparent cause during anesthesia.

Causes:

1. Light anesthesia accompanied by CO_2 excess or anoxia: usually preceded by excitement or crying during induction. Common during ether anesthesia in children.
2. Reexpansion of atelectatic areas of the lung due to surface tension effects in the alveoli.

Prophylaxis:

1. Premedicate patient well.
2. Avoid obstruction during induction of anesthesia.
3. Avoid secretions.

"BUCKING"

Definition: Spasmodic inspiratory and expiratory gasps due to stimulation of tracheal and bronchial reflexes. Usually occurs during thoracic surgery or intubation.

Causes:

1. Hilar, tracheal, bronchial or pleural stimulation in thoracic surgery.
2. Lightening of anesthesia when endotracheal tube is in place.
3. Stimulation due to airways, catheters, and bronchoscopes during light anesthesia.
4. Flooding of tracheobronchial tree by secretions, blood or pus, particularly if spasmogenic (thiobarbiturates) agents are used.
5. Traction of diaphragm or manipulation of pericardium, pleura and other structures in or about the thorax.
6. Intratracheal catheter is in a bronchus.
7. Subject cannot tolerate agent (ether) due to extremely active tracheobronchial reflexes.

Management:

1. Clear airway of all secretions by suctioning.
2. Use topical anesthesia prior to placement of airways.
3. Supplement topical anesthesia by instillation of cocaine 2 cc.—4% into intratracheal tube.
4. Obtund or block noxious stimuli arising from thoracic structures. Use procaine block if possible or anticholinergic agent intravenously.
5. Curarize and use controlled respiration if persistent and due to hyperresponsive reflexes.

SNEEZING

Causes:

1. Inhalation of irritating vapors (high concentrations of ether) during hypnosis with non-volatile drugs.
2. Stimulation of the cornea during eye surgery performed with basal narcosis induced with ultra short acting barbiturates.

Management:

1. Use topical anesthesia for occular surgery requiring stimulation of cornea.

HICCOUGHS

Definition: Abrupt periodic contraction of diaphragm. Usually impedes and annoys surgeon.

Characteristics:

1. Usually occurs during upper abdominal surgery particularly in stomach.
2. Occurs under both general or regional anesthesia. Common with pentothal and regional anesthesia.
3. During general anesthesia associated with inadequate ventilation—obstruction or CO_2 retention.

Causes:

1. Stimulation of phrenic nerve by pinching with clamps, or traction on areas supplied by nerve.
2. Hypoventilation with carbon dioxide accumulation particularly in electrolyte imbalance.
3. Distended or dilated stomach.
4. Infections and traumatic conditions in area of diaphragm.
5. Undetermined.

Treatment:

1. Improve airway and hyperventilate patient to remove excess CO_2.

2. Seek and remove or block possible offending stimuli to phrenic or vagus nerves.
3. Decompress stomach.
4. Change agents, particularly those which cause CO_2 retention.
5. Instill cocaine (1 cc. 4%) or other topical anesthetic into intratracheal tube.
6. Administer a muscle relaxant and control respiration if spasms interfere with surgery and other measures fail.

Comment   *Reason*

1. Do not use carbon dioxide.   This may aggravate rather than remove cause.

NOISY RESPIRATION

Causes: Vibrations in the respiratory passages as the tidal air passes through narrowed orifices, over secretions, over relaxed tissues, etc. It is a symptom of respiratory obstruction or inadequate pulmonary ventilation (see obstruction, laryngeal spasm, hypercapnia).

HYPERCAPNIA

Definition: The presence of carbon dioxide in excess in the blood resulting in stimulation of respiration.

Symptoms:

1. Hypertension with no change or a slight increase in pulse rate (this is an almost constant symptom).
2. Hyperpnea: this is followed by depression of respiration and gasping type of respiratory activity.
3. Twitching of muscles, followed by convulsions, usually generalized if the accumulation is excessive.
4. Increase in depth of narcosis.
5. Cardiac arrhythmias.
6. Phonation, crowing, wheezing, and other forms of noisy respiration.

Causes:

1. Soda lime is exhausted.
2. The "dead space" in mask, adapters, and other attachments is out of proportion to the tidal volume and causes excessive rebreathing.
3. Carbon dioxide supply from the flowmeter is not turned off.
4. Exhalation valves on inhaler or shunts on filters are defective so that carbon dioxide returns to the mask.
5. Carbon dioxide cylinder may be attached to a yoke intended for another gas.
6. Oxygen or other gases may be contaminated with carbon dioxide.

Sequelae: If carbon dioxide is allowed to accumulate in the inhaler, the point of stimulation is passed and the phase of depression follows. Toxic effects manifested by dyspnea, circulatory changes, and neuromuscular phenomena appear.

Excess Mucus Secretion

Source: Mucus is secreted by the salivary and mucous glands of the pharynx, larynx, and trachea.

Causes:

1. Premedication of atropine or scopolamine omitted, insufficient, or not administered at the proper time.
2. Concentration of anesthetic drugs is high.
3. Drug may stimulate mucous glands to activity (ethers).
4. Anoxia or excitement during induction period.
5. Administration of parasympathetic stimulating drugs or sympathetic depressants during surgery.
6. Use of iodides (thyroidectomy).

Treatment:

1. Lower head of patient in order to allow secretions to gravitate into the nasopharynx.
2. Apply suction, using metal suction tip or catheter.
3. Resort to bronchoscopy in severe cases.
4. Supplement atropine with additional drug intravenously.
5. Change agent if due to drug.

Pulmonary Edema During Anesthesia

Definition: Transudation of fluid from the capillaries of the pulmonary circulatory system into the alveoli.

Causes:

1. Increased pulmonary venous pressure from:
   a. Cardiac failure, selection of improper agent or technique, change in posture (Trendelenburg).
   b. Excessive amounts of intravenous fluids.
2. Protracted or excessive negative pressure in the alveoli (obstruction to inspiration from spasm of the larynx, defective apparatus, small airways, etc.).
3. Alteration of permeability of epithelium or endothelium (toxic agents such as nitric oxide—impurity of nitrous oxide, aspiration of vomitus).
4. Central lesions.

Symptoms:

1. Noisy respiration.
2. Dyspnea, cyanosis, and other signs of respiratory obstruction.

3. Frothy blood tinged fluid in trachea and lungs.
4. Increased venous pressure.

Treatment:

1. Locate cause and remedy it.
2. Administer oxygen under pressure (5 to 15 cms. H_2O pressure) by mask.
3. Reduce pulmonary venous pressure by phlebotomy or dehydration.
4. Suction secretions from respiratory tract.
5. Incline patient with "head up and feet down."
6. Increase peripheral venous stasis by applying tourniquets to each arm and leg.
7. Administer atropine gr. 1/150–1/100.
8. Digitalize patient if due to cardiac failure.
9. Induce hypotension with ganglionic blocking agent to reduce blood in lungs by pooling in periphery.
10. Inhalation of alcohol to reduce surface tension (Part IX).
11. Administer bronchodilators such as aminophylline.

OBSTRUCTION OF THE AIRWAY

Definition of Airway: The pathway for the inspired and expired gases extending from the nostrils to the alveolar membrane.

Importance of Patent Airway: The most common and pernicious complication of inhalation and other forms of anesthesia is the obstruction of the airway. This condition leads to anoxemia, carbon dioxide retention, and inability to anesthetize the patient because the drug does not readily pass into the lungs.

Causes of an Obstructed Airway	*Comment*
1. Relaxation of tissues.	The muscles of the neck, tongue, or pharynx are relaxed and block the passageway. The epiglottis sags in front of the glottis.
2. Spasm of larynx.	The spasm may be partial or complete (see laryngeal spasm).
3. Foreign body.	Vomitus, clots, artificial teeth, etc., may lodge in the respiratory tract.
4. Secretions.	Mucus, saliva, or purulent material from abscesses accumulate in the respiratory tract and interfere with the passage of gases.
5. Anatomical defects.	Tumors, enlarged tonsils, polyps, stenosis, collapse of the trachea, and edema of the larynx interfere with adequate exchange.

6. Faulty artificial airways.	These may be of improper size or improperly inserted, kinked, or plugged with secretions.
7. Bronchospasm.	This is due to vagal stimulation, asthma, or other causes.
8. Defective apparatus.	Stiff valves, narrow apertures in joints or tubes, or adapters, wet or fine mesh soda lime, long tubes, or empty breathing bag, cause partial obstruction.
9. Unsatisfactory posture.	The prone or Trendelenburg positions, hyperflexion or hyperextension of the head often interferes with adequate exchange.
10. Inhibition of thoracic movements.	This often results when assistants lean on the chest or straps, bandages, or casts are too tight.

Symptoms of Obstruction	*Comments*
1. Noisy respiration.	Manifested by crowing, snoring, or wheezing either during the inspiratory or expiratory phase of respiration.
2. Labored respiration	Occurs in partial obstruction. The tidal volume is not in proportion to respiratory effort. This is characterized by an exaggerated motion of the thorax and only a slight motion of the breathing bag.
3. Elevation of blood pressure.	Usually due to CO_2 excess, anoxia, or both.
4. Rapid pulse.	Bradycardia in severe obstruction. Arrhythmias may also be prevalent.
5. Cyanosis.	Noted particularly in severe or prolonged obstruction.

Maintenance of Patent Airway During Anesthesia:

1. Extend the head so that the chin points directly toward the ceiling (Fig. 75). Support head on a small pillow.
2. Insert an artificial airway; assists in support of pharyngeal airway if manual support is ineffective.
3. Remove mucus or other secretions by use of suction.
4. Remove or correct external factors which interfere with respiratory movements, such as poor position.

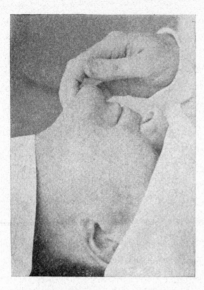

FIG. 75. Manner of maintaining a free airway in anesthetized or comatose subjects. The chin must be extended upward so that structures in the neck are elevated.

Results of Acute Complete Obstruction: Asphyxia, circulatory and respiratory failure follow unless treatment is instituted promptly. Post anesthetic circulatory, respiratory, or central nervous system derangements may follow if treatment is delayed.

Results of Continued Partial Obstruction:

1. Circulatory changes manifested by tachycardia, rise in blood pressure, bounding pulse, etc.
2. Respiratory disturbances, manifested by gasping type of respiration, cyanosis, mucus formation, dyspnea.
3. Pulmonary edema, if obstruction is principally inspiratory.
4. Pathological changes in the central nervous system, particularly in the cortical cells and various centers.

Comment

1. Noisy respiration is obstructed respiration and should never be tolerated.
2. Obstructed respiration may often be noiseless, particularly if respiration is depressed.
3. Any anesthetic procedure which removes the anesthetist from the airway so that he no longer has control over it is not a safe procedure (example—intravenous anesthesia in operations about face or head, when head is inaccessible to anesthetist).
4. The maintenance of a free, unobstructed airway is the most important duty of an anesthetist.

MANAGEMENT OF OVERDOSAGE OF INHALATION ANESTHETIC DRUGS

Definition: Overdosage occurs when the concentration of the anesthetic drug in the nervous system becomes sufficient to depress the vital centers in the medulla. The respiratory center is the first of these centers to be depressed by the currently employed inhalation anesthetic agents. It is then no longer capable of sending out rhythmical impulses.

Symptoms:

1. Absence of respiratory movements of the thorax and diaphragm.
2. Pulse palpable at first, but quickly disappears if the apnea persists and treatment is delayed.
3. Blood pressure falls rapidly and is often not obtainable.

4. Appearance of cyanosis with some agents, but not necessarily all (cyclopropane).
5. Complete depression of nervous system. The depression is manifested by absent reflexes and complete relaxation of tissues. Pupils are usually dilated and do not react to light.
6. Thorax is easily inflated if airway is patent.

Treatment:
1. Discard all anesthetic mixture from the inhaler and replace with oxygen.
2. Institute artificial respiration immediately.
3. Remove excess anesthetic drug from lungs.

Differentiate from:
1. "Breath-holding": This is frequently observed in stages I or II, but not in stage III. Associated *characteristics* are:
   a. Voluntary or semi-voluntary action.
   b. Normal or increased muscle tone.
   c. Exhibition of swallowing movements by patient.
   d. Presence of "lid lag" and other eye reflexes.
2 Medullary depression: This may be due to depression from premedication, other non-volatile drugs, cyclopropane following relief of anoxia, hyperventilation (not always easy to diagnose). *Characteristics* are:
   a. No abolition of reflexes (laryngeal and other reflexes present).
   b. Normal muscle tone.
   c. Light anesthesia indicated by eye signs.
   d. Normal or elevated blood pressure.
3. Laryngeal spasm: This may be due to a variety of causes (page 223). *Characteristics* are:
   a. Eye signs, those of light anesthesia.
   b. Difficult insufflation of thorax (does not inflate at all in complete spasm).
   c. Wheezing or crowing on inflation and deflation of thorax.
   d. Elevation of blood pressure.
   e. Slow, bounding pulse.
4. Hypopnea. This follows either voluntary (during induction) or manually induced hyperventilation. The addition of carbon dioxide restores respiratory rhythm. *Characteristics* are:
   a. Color of skin, usually remains normal (no cyanosis appears).
   b. Quality and rate of pulse unchanged.
   c. Blood pressure unchanged or lowered slightly.
   d. Reflexes of eye active during light anesthesia—tissues not relaxed.
5. Reflex apnea: This is due to reflexes caused by stimulation of various structures. Commonly encountered *reflexes* are:
   a. Pharyngeal—the apnea usually occurs when the patient passes from

stage III to stage II, particularly when an oropharyngeal or oro-nasal airway is in place. *Characteristics* are:

1. Swallowing—this is soon followed by retching if the airway is not removed.
2. Eye signs—those of light anesthesia.
3. Relaxation of muscles—incomplete.

b. Laryngeal—the apnea usually occurs when an intratracheal airway or other foreign body is inserted during light anesthesia. *Characteristics* are:

1. Eye reflexes, indicate light anesthesia.
2. Expiratory apnea usually present, opposing attempts at insufflation.
3. Possible presence of swallowing movements.
4. Incomplete relaxation of muscles.

c. Traction—an apnea usually accompanies stimulation and traction of the mesentery, celiac plexus, gallbladder, pelvic organs, pleura, hila of the lungs, bronchi, esophagus, rectum, and other viscera inervated by the autonomic nervous system. General *characteristics* are:

1. Abrupt onset—immediately follows stimulation of visceral structures and persists as long as stimulation is continued.
2. Accompanied by laryngeal spasm.
3. Light anesthesia indicated by eye reflexes and signs.
4. Inflation and deflation of thorax frequently accompanied by phonation.

d. Periosteal—similar to traction reflexes in most regards.

e. Carotid body—anoxia acts upon carotid body to reflexly stimulate respiration. The stimulation is removed by relief of anoxemia and temporary apnea results. The apnea lasts a brief interval—15–20 seconds, as a rule. The *characteristics* are:

1. Dilated pupils return to normal—other eye signs become active.
2. Cyanosis, if present, quickly disappears.
3. Blood pressure is elevated, pulse is slow.

f. Hering-Breuer—apnea is caused by forceful mechanical overdistension of the alveoli. *Characteristics* are:

1. Well-maintained circulation.
2. Eye reflexes active—indicate surgical planes of anesthesia.

6. Complete obstruction of the airway:

a. Thorax cannot be inflated or is inflated only with difficulty.
b. Pupils dilated from anoxia.
c. Cyanosis usually present.
d. Blood pressure elevated, pulse slowed at first.
e. Immediate relief by inserting airway change of position, suctioning of secretions, etc.

7. Circulatory failure (sudden cardiac arrest) respiratory failure is secondary to circulatory failure. *Characteristics* are:
   a. Absence of pulse, blood pressure, and heart sounds.
   b. Complete relaxation of tissues.
   c. Blue or grey cyanosis—not relieved by artificial respiration.
   d. Eyeballs fixed, pupils in mid-dilatation, do not react to light.
   e. Vocal cords relaxed and thorax is easily inflated.
8. Depression of the medullary centers from other than anesthetic drugs. Apnea of this type is usually caused by an increase in intracranial pressure, cerebral hemorrhage, neoplasms, or abscesses, etc. *Characteristics* are:
   a. Accompanies cerebrospinal surgery.
   b. Circulation usually well-maintained if effective artificial respiration is practiced.
   c. Signs such as unequal pupils, nystagmus, spasticity, and exaggerated reflexes revealed by neurological examination.

Comments	*Reasons*
1. If in doubt concerning the etiology, treat any apnea as though an overdose of the drug has been administered.	The circulation may fail in overdosage if artificial respiration is not instituted immediately.
2. Institute artificial respiration immediately. Do not waste time administering analeptic drugs.	Only ventilation of the lungs can remove the excess drug from the alveoli and supply the needed oxygen to the blood.
3. In performing artificial respiration, empty the mixture from the inhaler after every three or four inflations of the breathing bag and replenish with pure oxygen.	The anesthetic drug in the alveoli must be removed from the inhaler to allow elimination of the drug from the alveoli.
4. Resume anesthesia when normal respiration has been established.	The patient may "recover" from narcosis, particularly if anesthesia has been in progress only a short interval.
5. Do not become panic stricken and frantically compress thorax at random when apnea occurs.	Such movements are useless and usually serve to force valuable oxygen from thorax, particularly if spasm of the larynx is present.

MANAGEMENT OF LARYNGOSPASM

Definition: Laryngeal spasm is a spasm of the adductor muscles of the vocal cords which causes a partial or complete obstruction to the natural airway. The spasm may be *complete* or *partial*.

Symptoms: Partial spasm: Wheezing, crowing, grunting, phonation, and similar noises accompanying inspiration and expiration. The vocal cords are only partially approximated.

Complete spasm: Apnea and inability to inflate the thorax. The vocal cords are completely approximated.

Causes:

1. Secretions in the larynx. Mucus, blood, vomitus, and other secretions on the vocal cords initiate the spasm. This is perhaps the most frequent cause.
2. Irritations of the membranes of the larynx. High concentrations of anesthetic drugs, particularly ether, cause spasms. Soda lime dust, particularly in the to and fro canister, is caustic in action and irritates mucous membranes.
3. Mechanical stimulation. Trauma from airways, laryngoscopes, suction tips, and other foreign bodies also cause spasm. This is most frequent after attempted intubations.
4. Carbon dioxide excess. See hypercapnia.
5. Reflex stimulation. Traction on the gallbladder, stomach, spleen, mesentery, and trachea, rectal dilatation, vaginal, perineal, and periosteal stimulation cause adductor spasm of cords and jerky respiration.
6. Autonomic nervous system effects. Parasympathetic stimulation or sympathetic depression from drugs. Cyclopropane and pentothal are most common offenders.
7. Anoxia. Spasm of all muscles including those of the vocal cords frequently accompanies mild anoxemia.

Treatment: Incomplete Spasm:

1. Increase the oxygen in the inhaler.
2. Aspirate secretions from the pharynx using metal suction tip.
3. Insert an artificial (pharyngeal) airway if one is not already in place.
4. Inflate the inhaler with oxygen so that a positive pressure of approximately 10 cm. H_2O is attained.
5. Inspect or replace soda lime or check patency of exhalation valve to rule out carbon dioxide excess.
6. Insert an intratracheal catheter if these measures do not readily relieve the obstruction.
7. Use succinyl choline to facilitate intubation.

Treatment: Complete Spasm:

1. Attempt to inflate the thorax with mask and bag using positive pressure. A small amount of oxygen frequently relieves the anoxia and causes the spasm to "break." Compression of thorax may cause slight abduction of cords to facilitate this.
2. Perform intratracheal intubation.
3. Administer succinyl choline intravenously (30–50 mgm.). For infants

use 1.0 mgm. per lb. intramuscularly. Have in readiness and administer as soon as signs of spasm appear before it is complete and patient becomes anoxic.

REFERENCES

Batten, Charles T., and Courville, Cyril B. Mental Disturbances Following Nitrous Oxide Anesthesia. Anesthesiology, *1:* 263, November, 1940.

Beecher, H. K., Bennett, S. H., and Bassett, D. L. Circulatory Effects of Increased Pressure in the Airways. Anesthesiology, *4:* 612. November, 1943.

Best, C. H., and Taylor, N. B. Physiological Basis of Medical Practice. Pp. 479–604. Williams and Wilkins, Baltimore, 1940.

Burstein, C. L. Apnea During Anesthesia. Anesthesiology, *2:* 530, 1941.

Burstein, C. L., and Rovenstine, E. A. Apnea During Anesthesia. Am. J. Surg., *43:* 26, January, 1939.

Iglaurer, S. Relation of Respiratory Passages to Anesthesia. Anesthesiology, *3:* 195, March, 1942.

Reid, L. C., and Brace, D. E. Reflexes from the Mouth, Trachea, and Esophagus which Stimulate Respiration. Anesthesiology, *4:* 345, July, 1943.

Waters, R. M. Carbon Dioxide Absorption from Anesthetic Atmospheres. Proc. Royal Soc. Med., *30:* 1, November, 1936.

Waters, R. M. Bronchopneumonia. Anesthesiology, *1:* 136, 1940.

CIRCULATORY COMPLICATIONS

Circulatory complications during anesthesia are manifested by alterations in the rate and character of the pulse, an elevation or depression of the blood pressure, and changes in pulse pressure. Circulatory changes are intimately connected with respiratory and neurological complications. Commonly encountered circulatory complications and their symptoms are:

TACHYCARDIA

Definition: A rapid pulse rate.

Causes:

1. Excitement during induction of anesthesia.
2. Blood loss, shock, or trauma during surgery.
3. Atropine used for premedication (particularly in children).
4. Effect of anesthetic drugs upon the conducting tissue of the heart. A shift of the pacemaker and arrhythmias result. (cyclopropane)
5. Effect of sympatheticomimetic amines used in conjunction with anesthesia.
6. Hyperthyroidism.
7. Sympathomimetic effects of anesthetic drugs.

BRADYCARDIA

Definition: A slow pulse rate.

Causes:

1. Sinus bradycardia.
2. Asphyxia or anoxemia accompanying respiratory failure.

3. Increased irritability of conducting tissues of the heart with shift of the pacemaker to the auriculo-ventricular node or to the ventricle.
4. Epinephrine used in conjunction with anesthetic drugs which increase cardiac irritability.
5. Vagal stimulation in thoracic and other types of surgery in which the vagus nerves are exposed.
6. Development of heart block in cardiac patients.
7. Myocardial depression from cardiotoxic drugs (chloroform, local anesthesia).
8. Sympathetic depression with vagal predominance (spinal anesthesia).
9. Succinyl choline intravenously (infants and children).

ARRHYTHMIAS DURING ANESTHESIA

An arrhythmia is a disturbance of the normal rhythm of the heart. The types of arrhythmias which occur during anesthesia vary considerably. Many can be diagnosed by palpation of the pulse; others require the use of the electrocardiograph.

Causes:

1. Respiratory depression resulting in anoxia or carbon dioxide excess.
2. Effects of epinephrine and other vasopressors used in conjunction with anesthetic drugs.
3. Increase in cardiac irritability caused by the anesthetic drugs. Chloroform, cyclopropane, ethyl chloride may cause them. Less frequently other agents are responsible.
4. Autonomic effects due to stimulation of structures such as the carotid sinus, aortic plexus, hilum of the lungs, trachea, bronchi, etc.
5. Deep anesthesia from the anesthetic agent, particularly cyclopropane or chloroform.
6. Effects of the anesthetic and the surgical procedure upon pre-existing cardiac disease.
7. Direct stimulation of the heart during intrathoracic manipulation.
8. Electrolyte disturbances such as excess or deficiency in potassium ion.

Diagnosis:

Most arrhythmias during anesthesia can be diagnosed by palpating the pulse, but some can be detected only by use of the electrocardiograph.

Treatment:

1. If due to deep anesthesia add oxygen to lighten it and rule out anoxia.
2. Inspect the carbon dioxide absorber to rule out carbon dioxide excess.
3. Shift to another anesthetic agent if due to the agent and persists.
4. Cease offending stimulation if due to surgical manipulation or block area with procaine.

5. Investigate electrolyte balance.
6. Use drugs which reduce cardiac irritability such as procaine, procaine amide or quinidine intravenously or apply procaine to surface.

Comment: Most arrhythmias during anesthesia can be diagnosed by palpation of the pulse, but some can be detected only by use of the electrocardiograph.

HYPOTENSION WITH DECREASED PULSE PRESSURE AND TACHYCARDIA (Fig. 76)

Causes:

1. Shock from trauma, hemorrhage, toxemia, etc.
2. Deep anesthesia or overdosage.

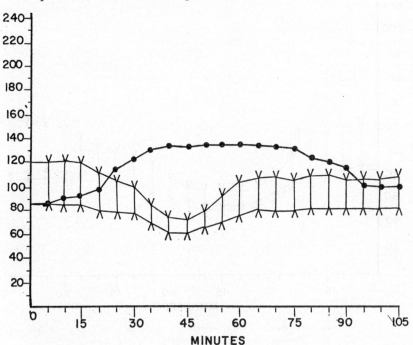

FIG. 76. Hypotension accompanied by tachycardia and decreased pulse pressure. (Traumatic shock, hemorrhage, etc.)

3. Cardiac failure from decompensation, coronary infarction, and other diseases of the heart.
4. Ganglionic blocking agents used in conjunction with anesthesia.

Management:

1. Lighten anesthesia or discard inhaled mixture completely and replace with oxygen.
2. Administer plasma volume expanders and blood if due to shock.
3. Treat for cardiac failure if due to this cause.
4. Use vasopressor if due to ganglionic blockade (Neosynephrine norephrine, etc.).

HYPOTENSION WITH DECREASED PULSE PRESSURE AND BRADYCARDIA (Fig. 77)

Causes:

1. Anoxia with deep anesthesia.
2. Spinal anesthesia.
3. Reflex stimulation due to traction on viscera, mesentery, or other structures.
4. Local anesthetic drug toxicity during general anesthesia.

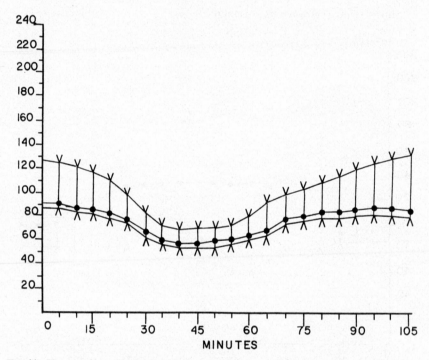

FIG. 77. Hypotension accompanied by a relatively slow pulse or bradycarpia and decrease in pulse pressure. (Anoxia, primary shock, heart block, etc.)

5. Transfusion reaction due to incompatible blood.
6. Over premedication.
7. Awkward position or positional changes.
8. Sympatholytic drugs (phenothiazines) used in conjunction with anesthesia.

Treatment:

1. 100% oxygen by mask if due to anoxia.
2. Ephedrine 25 mgm. I.V. or similar acting vasopressor if due to reflex activity, spinal anesthesia or over-premedication.
3. Procaine block of pathways from site of offending stimulus.

HYPERTENSION WITH SLIGHT OR NO CHANGE IN
PULSE RATE (Fig. 78)

Causes:

1. Carbon dioxide excess.

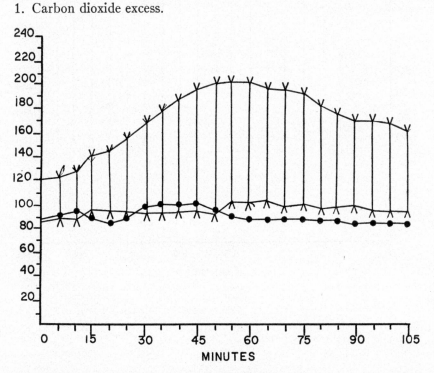

FIG. 78. Hypertension accompanied by relatively little change in pulse rate. CO_2 excess.

2. Cyclopropane anesthesia.
3. Bad posture during anesthesia.
4. Inadequate ventilation due to depressant drugs.
5. Intracranial lesions.
6. Stimulation during light anesthesia.

Treatment:

1. Assist or control respirations to remove excess carbon dioxide.
2. Correct defective posture.
3. Deepen anesthesia if light.

HYPERTENSION WITH INCREASE IN PULSE PRESSURE
AND TACHYCARDIA (Fig. 79)

Causes:

1. Anoxia, asphyxia.
2. Use of epinephrine and related drugs.

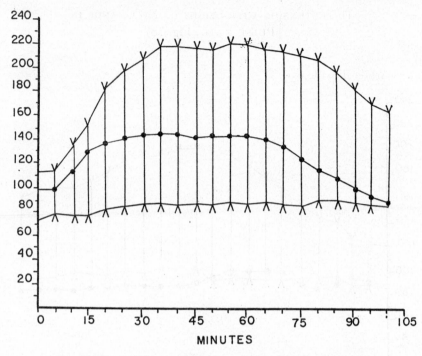

Fig. 79. Hypertension accompanied by tachycardia. (Thyrotoxicosis excitement during induction, etc.)

3. Cyclopropane anesthesia.
4. Thyrotoxicosis.
5. Prolonged excitement period.
6. Water intoxication (transurethral resections).
7. Oxytoxic drugs during special anesthesia during Caesarean sections.

Treatment:

1. Oxygenate patient.
2. Lighten anesthesia if deep.
3. Change agents if due to cyclopropane and lightening does not correct.
4. Discontinue surgery if tachycardia is unmanageable and severe (thyro-toxicosis).

HYPERTENSION WITH INCREASE IN PULSE PRESSURE AND BRADYCARDIA (Fig. 80)

Causes:

1. Increase in intracranial pressure.
2. Cyclopropane anesthesia.
3. Anoxia accompanying anesthesia.

Treatment:

1. Ventilate patient if (due to anoxia) with adequate oxygen.

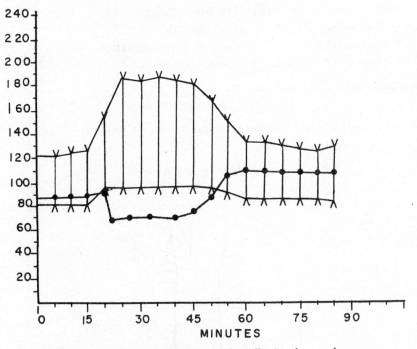

Fig. 80. Hypertension accompanied by bradycardia. Anoxia or cyclopropane
anesthesia with respiratory depression.

2. Lighten anesthesia.
3. Correct cause of increased intracranial pressure.

CARDIAC ARREST AND MASSAGE

Definition: Resumption of the circulation by massaging a heart which has
ceased to effectively propel blood through the vascular bed.

Purpose:

1 To reinstate the heart beat to its normal state.
2. To prevent the tissues, particularly those of the central nervous system, from being deprived of oxygenated blood and nutritive substance.

Types of Cardiac Arrest:

1. Asystole or complete stoppage.
2. Feeble cardiac contractions which are not detectable.
3. Ventricular fibrillation.

Causes of Cardiac Arrest on Operating Table:

1. Anoxia or asphyxia.
2. Overdosage of anesthetic drugs.
3. Respiratory acidosis due to hypoventilation.

4. Increased cardiac irritability from thyrotoxicosis or drugs such as cyclopropane, chloroform, ethyl chloride.
5. Vagovagal reflexes in presence of hypoventilation.
6. Hypovolemia due to blood loss.

Diagnosis (with Chest Closed):

1. Absence of heart sounds.
2. Absence of pulsation in the major vessels (if abdomen is open or artery is exposed).

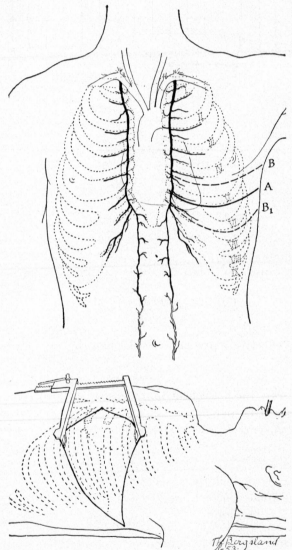

FIG. 81. To expose the heart the chest wall is incised on the left side between the fourth and fifth ribs from the parasternal area to the midaxillary line and the ribs spread apart. Care is taken to avoid the internal mammary vessels. (Courtesy Robert Hosler, Cardiac Resuscitation. Springfield, Thomas, 1954.)

3. Absence of pulsation in the retinal vessels.
4. Absence of capillary refill.

Treatment for Asystole:

A. Materials—(a) Scalpel
             (b) Rib spreader
B. Procedure
    1. Ventilate the lungs with 100% oxygen using any effective method of artificial respiration which is immediately available.
    2 Perform cardiac massage as follows:
        (a) Quickly prepare the skin with an adequate sterilizer. (Omit if material is not immediately available.)
        (b) Incise the chest in the fourth left interspace from sternum to posterior axillary line. Divide fourth and fifth costal cartilages and spread the ribs apart (Fig. 81).
        (c) Grasp the heart in the cup shaped right hand and compress as rapidly as possible or until the arterial pressure is raised to 60 to 80 mm. Hg. (about 60× per minute) (FIG. 84A).
        (d) Every fifth beat compress the aorta beyond the coronary vessels in order to increase coronary blood flow.

Comment	*Reason*
1. Maintain a rate as close to 60 as possible or one sufficient to yield a palpable pulse and audible blood pressure.	A more rapid rate is difficult to maintain. Too slow a rate results in ineffective circulation.
2. Have an assistant "scrub in."	One operator easily tires, particularly in protracted cases.
3. Do not waste time establishing a diagnosis with stethoscope or E.K.G.	It is best to err on the side of opening chest and finding a beating heart than to delay and have a decerebrate patient.
4. Institute an arterial transfusion if blood pressure is not maintained at 60 mm. Hg. or more.	The coronary arteries are perfused and an effective head of pressure is maintained to nourish tissues.
5. Use gentleness in compressing the heart.	The myocardium may be traumatized. Perforation may occur.
6. Inject 5 cc. calcium chloride (10%) solution into the right auricle if ventricles are atonic.	Calcium chloride increases tone of cardiac muscle.
7. Do not use epinephrine in the presence of drugs which increase myocardial irritability, such as cyclopropane, chloroform or ethyl chloride.	Asystole may be converted to fibrillation which is more difficult to treat.
8. Inject only 1/4 cc. of 1–1000	This confines the stimulus, me-

solution of epinephrine, when used, into the right auricle.

9. Do not be misled by the E.K.G. in making a diagnosis.

10. Open the pericardium if massage is difficult.

11. Do not extend the incision too close to the sternum.

chanical or chemical to the part of the heart in which fibrillation is of lesser importance or consequence. A current may still be generated by the heart and a tracing obtained even though the heart is not effectively propelling blood.

The heart may be grasped more effectively if the pericardium is open.

The internal mammary vessels may be cut. Bleeding may occur after resuscitation.

Management of Ventricular Fibrillation

Ventricular fibrillation is characterized by absence of signs of cardiac activity, no pulse and no blood pressure. Although it appears to come on abruptly four pre-ventricular fibrillation stages are recognized, as follows:

Stage   I. The undulatory stage which lasts from one to two seconds.

Stage   II. Convulsive incoordination which lasts from 15 to 40 seconds. Contractions are more frequent and involves smaller areas of the ventricular muscles.

Stage III. A tremulous incoordination which lasts from two to three minutes. The surface of the muscle is broken up into independently contracting areas of a never increasing size which are in a phase with each other. The ventricles appeared to be tremulous.

Stage IV. Final stage. Atonic fibrillation develops when anoxia of the cardiac muscle weakens its contractile force. This stage usually occurs 2 to 5 minutes following the first stage and is marked by weak contractions of wavelets. Object is to defibrillate individual isolated areas into larger ones by repeated electrical shocks then stop entire fibrillation with a final shock.

Treatment of Fibrillation:

A. Materials—(a) Defibrillator
            (b) Scalpel and rib spreader

B. Procedure
   1. Open chest in same manner described for asystole.
   2. Massage the heart in same manner as for asystole for 30 to 60 seconds with compression of the aorta distal to the coronaries to provide blood to the myocardium.
   3. Apply each electrode of the defibrillator to each side of the heart. (Use 60 cycle 110 volt current with a resistance sufficient to allow an average of 1 to $1\frac{1}{2}$ amperes to pass through the heart) (Fig. 82, 83).

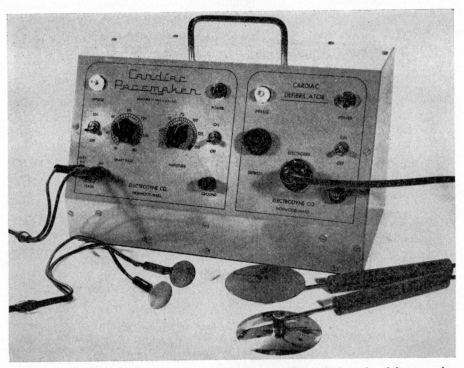

FIG. 82. Combination cardiac pacemaker and defibrillator. The small electrodes of the pacemaker are applied to the chest wall to send rhythmic electrical impulses into the heart to re-establish normal rythm. The broad electrodes of the defibrillator are applied directly to the surface of the heart when ventricular fibrillation has occurred. (Courtesy Electrodyne Company.)

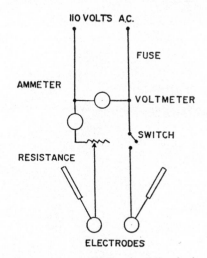

FIG. 83. Wiring diagram of defibrillator using 110 volt alternating current.

4. Shock the heart for 1/10 of a second at one to two second intervals until fibrillation disappears. The heart will then be in asystole. Three to 7 shocks are usually necessary.
5. Manipulate as for asystole.

Comment	*Reason*
1. Do not use epinephrine in the face of ventricular fibrillation.	Cardiac irritability is present. The drug further enhances it.
2. Cold isotonic saline solution at 0°C. may be poured over the heart during the period of electric shock.	Cold reduces cardiac irritability. May be used if defibrillator is not available.
3. Inject 5 cc. 10% calcium chloride into myocardium if it is atonic Inject 100 mgm sodium bicarbonate (1%) to combat acidosis of myocardium.	Calcium chloride increases the tone of the heart muscle.
4. Do not use digitalis or related glucosides.	It is felt that they increase myocardial irritability.
5. Do not attempt defibrillation with drugs.	No drug is satisfactory to defibrillate the heart.
6. Expect skeletal muscles to contract with each shock.	The current spreads throughout the body.
7. Apply procaine 1% to the surface of heart or into pericardium when marked irritability exists.	Procaine decreases cardiac irritability.

Adjunctive Therapy to Cardiac Resuscitation

1. Aspirate the pharynx, trachea and bronchi to maintain a free airway.
2. Administer antibiotics to reduce the incidence of pulmonary and wound infection.
3. Turn patient frequently in post recovery period to avoid hypostatic congestion.
4. Maintain adequate fluid balance, checking both blood volume and hematocrit.
5. Maintain artificial or assisted respiration if apnea or ineffective respiration is present.

Prognosis of Cardiac Resuscitation

1. Variable—depends upon the time therapy is instituted after arrest and the nature of the disease present. The sooner the heart is resuscitated the more likely it is to revive.
2. Patients developing arrest who have chronic illness are revived more easily than those who have acute infections.
3. Hearts of individuals with chronic tuberculosis are revived more easily than those of subjects with other diseases.
4. Hearts of children are more responsive than those of adults.

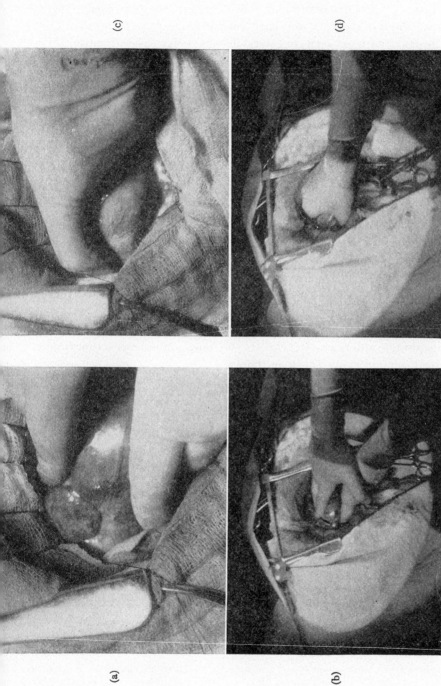

Fig. 84A. When attempting to re-establish the beat the heart is held between the palms of the hands and compressed rhythmically 80 times per minute or as rapidly as necessary to maintain an adequate head of blood pressure. The fingers of the left hand surround the left ventricle and the thumb lies across the right ventricle (c, d). When two hands are used the flat of each hand is placed over each ventricle flushing and compression is made towards the intra-ventricular septum (a, b). (Courtesy Robert Hosler, Cardiac Resuscitation, Springfield, Thomas, 1954.)

5. Hearts of patients with heart disease respond with greater difficulty than those of patients who have normal hearts.
6. Hearts of patients with congenital defects revive easier than those who have organic disease.
7. Hearts of patients with chronic emphysema revive more easily than those who have normal pulmonary function.
8. Spontaneous respiratory activity appears within 5 to 30 minutes after regular rhythm and blood pressure are restored.
9. Chances of recovery are good if period of circulatory stasis does not exceed one minute.
10. Anesthesia increases the resistance to anoxia probably by depressing cellular activity and reducing CO_2 output and O_2 demand.
11. Recovery is more common after asystole than fibrillation.

Performing Cardiac Massage With the Chest Closed When the Abdomen is Open

Purpose: To massage the heart without opening the thorax.

1. Introduce gloved hand to the left upper quadrant behind the diaphragm lateral to the liver.
2. Compress the heart against anterior chest wall by compressing the diaphragm anteriorly. Repeat 30 to 60 times a minute with thorax open. If fibrillation is present open thorax.

Comment:

1. This is a substitute and is not as effective as opening the thorax but may be used as temporary expedient until chest is opened.
2. This maneuver cannot be used for ventricular fibrillation.
3. This is ineffective for giving intracardiac injections of various drugs.
4. If hiatus hernia is present, maintain massage through it.
5. Maintain massage until heart no longer shows any evidence of contracting in cases of failure to respond.

Cardiac Arrest Closed Chest Compression Method

Principle

External cardiac massage is based upon the principle that the thoracic cage has enough resilience so that the heart may be compressed between the sternum and the vertebral column when an external force is applied over the sternum at the xyphoid (Fig. 84B).

Technique

1. Place patient in the supine position on a hard, flat surface. If the patient is on a bed place him on the floor or place a board under his back.
2. Stand in comfortable position at side of patient. (If necessary mount the adjacent bed or chair to be comfortable and at the right height.)

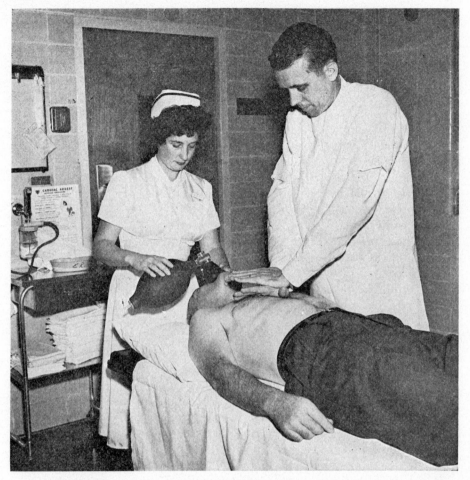

Fig. 84B. Technique of external cardiac massage and artificial respiration with the Ambu resuscitator. (Courtesy Corbin-Farnsworth.)

3. Place both hands on the sternum so that the heel of one hand is over the lower sternum. The second hand is placed over the first.

4. Exert the body weight over lower sternum by leaning forward with sufficient force so that thorax is compressed $\frac{1}{2}$–2″. Maintain the pressure for $\frac{1}{2}$ second and then let up abruptly to release it.
Repeat at a rate of 50 to 60 times per minute.

5. Simultaneously have a second person establish ventilation by mouth to mouth breathing or other immediately available means. In the operating room use bag, mask and airway at first and intubate at a convenient time if necessary.

6. Have an assistant palpate the pulse, observe size of pupils and attempt to read blood pressure to ascertain that compression is establishing an effective circulation.

7. Pause every 2–3 minutes to observe if spontaneous heart action has occurred. If so watch to see that it is sustained.

Comments	Reasons
1. Do not exert pressure on the rib cage or the epigastrium.	The heart is less effectively compressed and the ribs are easily fractured by this maneuver.
2. Place patient in head down supine (Trendelenburg) position.	Increases cerebral blood flow and guards against respiration.
3. Continue closed massage for one minute. If pulse and blood pressure are not felt during this time, open chest and perform internal massage.	Effective compression is not obtained in all cases in which the procedure is attempted.
4. Do not rely on compression of the chest to obtain adequate ventilation.	The exchange obtained by this method seldom exceeds a 50 cc. tidal volume.
5. Do not waste time making diagnosis by auscultation, E.K.G., etc.	Every second is precious.
6. Request an assistant to make observations, such as pulse, pupil size, etc.	The operator's activity should be confined solely to compressing the chest.
7. Observe the size of the pupil frequently.	Dilated pupils indicates the perfusion of the tissues is inadequate.
8. Use and E.K.G. to determine the nature of the arrest whether it is fibrillation or asystole.	Asystole responds to massage. A defibrillator is required for fibrillation.
9. If operator is alone compress chest five times and insufflate mouth to mouth once and repeat the cycle.	Cardiac resuscitation is useless without pulmonary ventilation.

External Ventricular Defibrillation

Materials

1. An external defibrillator operating on a 60 cycle, 110 volt AC current equipped with a transformer which permits the alternating current to be varied (5 amperes at 400 to 900 volts) and 2 three inch electrodes which can be weighted and applied firmly to the chest (Fig. 84C and 84D).
2. Conductive jelly.

Technique

1. Plug defibrillator into the electrical outlet.
2. Coat electrodes with conductive jelly.
3. Verify and establish the diagnosis of ventricular fibrillation with the

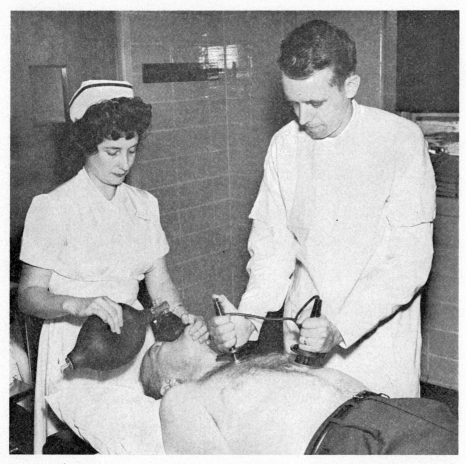

Fig. 84C. External ventricular defibrillation. (Courtesy Corbin-Farnsworth.)

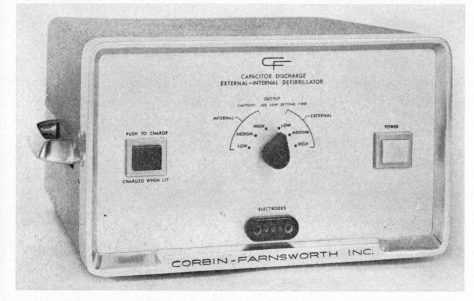

Fig. 84D. External ventricular defibrillator power unit. (Courtesy Corbin Farnsworth.)

E.K.G. Maintain external massage and artificial respiration constantly while this is being done.

4. Apply one electrode firmly over the cardiac apex and the other over sternal notch at the sternal clavicular junction.
5. Apply one shock of 440 volts for $\frac{1}{4}$ second. If ineffective repeat using 3 shocks in rapid succession.
6. If fibrillation continues, administer epinephrine 5 cc. of 1 to 1000 diluted in 10 cc. saline intravenously and increase the voltage to 880 volts and shock again for $\frac{1}{4}$ second.

Comment

1. Maintain cardiac compression until shock is applied. All persons should remove hands from patient while shocks are applied.
2. Maintain artificial respiration continuously. Only an unoxygenated myocardium defibrillates.
3. Maintain cardiac compression after defibrillation until a pulse of good volume is obtained and an adequate blood pressure develops. The E.K.G. pattern may appear normal yet the heart beat is ineffective to propel adequate amounts of blood.
4. If direct current defibrillator is available, it is preferable.

REFERENCES

Best, C. H., and Taylor, N. B. Physiological Basis of Medical Practice. Pp. 169–250 Williams and Wilkins, Baltimore, 7th Ed., 1961.
Elkin D. C. Diagnosis and Treatment of Wounds of the Heart, J.A.M.A., *111:* 1759, November, 1938.
Kavenhoven, J. R., Jude, G. G.: Closed Cardiac Massage, J.A.M.A. *173:* 1064–67, (July) 1960.
Thienes, C. H., Greely, P. O., and Guedel, A. E. Cardiac Arrhythmias under Cyclopropane Anesthesia. Anesthesiology, *2:* 611, November, 1941.

NEUROLOGICAL COMPLICATIONS

Neurological complications are the result of some undue stimulation of the nervous system. Disturbances of the autonomic nervous system are usually manifested by changes in the circulatory and respiratory systems and are therefore described under those headings. Disturbances of the central nervous system are manifested by increased muscular activity, rigidity, and convulsions.

CONVULSIONS UNDER ANESTHESIA

Definition: Convulsions are involuntary muscle contractions. They are manifestations of increased irritability of cortical and other cells which control motor function.

Causes:

1. Asphyxia from any cause.
2. Hypercapnia.
3. Awkward positions—lithotomy, lateral, prone, kidney, etc., caused by pressure or stretching of nerves.
4. Overdosage of local anesthetic drugs used in conjunction with anesthesia (see regional anesthesia).
5. Stimulation of motor centers by such anesthetic drugs as evipal and vinethene.
6. Preexisting pathological changes in the nervous system not related to anesthesia (brain tumor, epilepsy, meningitis).
7. Idiopathic—cause not determined. Often called "ether convulsions."
8. Tetany from hyperventilation.

Convulsions Due to Asphyxia

Features:

1. They accompany obvious asphyxia with its attendant signs and symptoms, such as cyanosis, sweating, bradycardia, etc.
2. Convulsions are spasmodic, begin in the small muscles as twitchings, but gradually involve the larger muscles.
3. Are obtunded by anesthesia.

Treatment:

1. Reestablish the airway and relieve anoxemia immediately.
2. Administer ultra-short-acting barbiturates, such as evipal or pentothal, intravenously if convulsions persist.
3. Reduce body temperature if elevated by use of ice mattress.

Convulsions Due to Carbon Dioxide Excess

Features:

1. They accompany rebreathing or the inhalation of high concentrations of carbon dioxide (15% or more).
2. Small muscles begin to twitch at first and gradually activity spreads to larger muscles.

Treatment:

1. Administer oxygen by means of a small mask or nasal catheter.
2. Eliminate all rebreathing.
3. Confirm the identity of all gases on the machine.
4. Use anticonvulsants (pentothal, surital) to control if they do not disappear.

Idiopathic (Ether) Convulsions

Causes: Their etiology remains unknown. Many theories regarding their possible cause have been advanced. Among the most prominent are:

Hypercapnia
Alkalosis
Acidosis
Hypocalcemia
Disturbed carbohydrate metabolism
Neurotoxin liberated during anesthesia
Impure air or oxygen
Overdose of atropine
Overoxygenation

Features:

1. They most frequently are seen in youthful patients or children receiving ether.
2. They accompany "toxic" or septic conditions.
3. They occur under deep anesthesia and are not relieved by lightening or deepening anesthesia.
4. They occur with ether anesthesia but can occur with other agents.
5. They are often accompanied by an elevation of body temperature.
6. They are more frequent when environment is hot.
7. They become worse as anesthesia deepens.
8. They are not related to impurities in ether.
9. They are generalized and not confined to any one part of the body.
10. They develop after the anesthesia has been established for 20 or 30 minutes.

Treatment:

1. Discontinue anesthetic agent and discard inhaler.
2. Reestablish the airway if it is not patent. Intubate if necessary.
3. Administer an ultra-short-acting barbiturate slowly in amounts sufficient to control them.
4. Administer alkalizing solutions (such as sodium lactate) intravenously.
5. Administer oxygen by catheter or semi-closed mask.
6. Cool body with alcohol sponges or fan or by use of tepid water bath.
7. Administer calcium salts intravenously. (1.0 gm. calcium gluconate).

Sequelae:

1. If convulsions persist untreated, the patient ultimately succumbs from asphyxia and circulatory failure. Hyperthermia supervenes. (Temperature varies from 105°F. to 110°F.)
2. If convulsions are controlled early and effective treatment is instituted, the patient may recover.

Comment	*Reasons*
1. Avoid any device which allows rebreathing or the accumulation of excess carbon dioxide in the inhaler.	Recent data suggest hypercapnia as one of the factors predisposing to convulsions.
2. Do not employ inhalers for the administration of oxygen during the treatment. Use nasal catheter or nonrebreathing semi closed inhaler.	The amount of carbon dioxide rebreathed in a small mask may disturb the biochemical mechanism involved.
3. Cool body with current of air and alcohol sponges or immerse in tepid water.	Excessively high body temperature contributes to the nervous system damage.
4. Empty breathing bag frequently if artificial respiration becomes necessary.	Complete removal of all carbon dioxide in the inspired air is necessary.

Convulsions Due to Vinyl Ether

Causes:

Drug stimulates motor centers in spinal cord or brain.

Features:

1. Occur in unpremedicated subjects more often than medicated.
2. Occur in children more often than adults.
3. Occur during induction period of anesthesia.
4. Occur in deep, prolonged anesthesia.
5. Disappear when drug is discontinued.
6. Not related to impurities in drug or to anoxia.

Treatment:

1. Discontinue drug—disappear as anesthesia lightens.
2. Administer barbiturates intravenously (pentothal) if they persist.

Localized Convulsions Due to Traction and Posture

Causes:

Nerves placed on stretch or irritated by physical factors.

Features:

1. Are localized in one part of body—usually lower.
2. Occur when patient is in awkward position—lithotomy, lateral, etc.
3. Disappear with change in posture.

Convulsions Due to Local Anesthetic Drugs

See Part VI, Regional Anesthesia.

EMERGENCE DELERIUM

Definition: Delerium, excitement and struggling during recovery phase of anesthesia.

Causes:

1. Second stage anesthesia on recovery from slowly eliminated agents (ether).
2. Emergence from gas anesthesia which was combined with basal narcosis with non-analgesic drugs such as barbiturates, avertin, scopolamine.
3. Anoxia due to reduced vital capacity (after pneumonectomy, atelectasis, pneumothorax, etc.).
4. Inadequate ventilation due to partial obstruction—secretions, laryngeal edema, compression of trachea due to hematomas, etc.
5. Carbon dioxide excess following use of drugs which cause its retention —cyclopropane, pentothal.
6. Rapid recovery from quickly eliminated anesthetic administered without premedication with narcotics (cyclopropane alone).
7. Chronic alcohol addict recovering from anesthesia.

Treatment:

1. If due to pain in presence of non-analgesic basal narcotic—administer a narcotic such as morphine, Demerol or dilaudid and so on intravenously.
2. If due to inadequate ventilation administer oxygen. Morphine may also be required. Use small doses.

GENERALIZED SHIVERING AT EMERGENCE

Causes:

1. Patient recovering in cold environment. Apply blankets and remove to warmer environment.
2. Pyrogenic reaction due to fluid administered when patient was under anesthesia. Temperature rises after chill—Apply blankets and sedate.
3. Emergence after pentothal—Hyperventilate and sedate with phenobarbital parenterally.

HYPERTHERMIA

Description: An elevation of body temperature above normal which may appear during operation or immediately postoperatively.

Causes: During Operation

1. Warm external environment.

2. Drugs which cause diminished sweating—atropine.
3. Aggravation of a pre-existing fever.
4. Heat added from closed system (To and Fro).
5. As a symptom of ether convulsions.

Post Anesthesia

1. Aggravation of fever from systemic disease.
2. Pyrogenic reaction caused by intravenous fluids.
3. After intentional hypothermia—temperature over-shoots mark on warming.
4. After deep anesthesia in which subnormal temperature occurs—over-shoots mark while recovering.
5. Drugs which inhibit heat loss—atropine etc.
6. Central damage from anoxia or CO_2 excess.
7. Heat stroke, postoperative.
8. Thyroid crisis.
9. Dehydration.

Treatment:

1. External cooling with ice pack, alcohol or ice blanket.

Comment

1. The heat regulatory center is inactivated by nervous system depressants. The patient tends to assume the temperature of the external environment.
2. Reduce temperature to several degrees above normal. Then proceed gradually otherwise mark will be overshot.

REFERENCE

Cassels, W. H., Becker, T. J., and Seevers, M. H. Convulsions During Anesthesia Anesthesiology, *1:* 56, July, 1940.

SWEATING DURING ANESTHESIA

Causes:

1. Warm external environment or excessive coverings over the patient.
2. Suboxygenation from obstruction, spasm, etc., during anesthesia, particularly ether.
3. Administration of drugs which stimulate the sympathetic nervous system.

TECHNICAL COMPLICATIONS

Technical complications arise from faulty or defective apparatus or improper manipulation of the equipment. They usually result in inability to maintain a constant level of anesthesia, hypercapnia, or anoxia.

Common technical difficulties encountered are:

EXCESS ACCUMULATION OF GAS IN THE INHALER

Symptoms:

1. Overdistension of the breathing bag.
2. Interference with satisfactory respiratory movements.

Causes:

1. The metabolic flow of oxygen is above body requirements.
2. The seats of pin valves are worn and leak.
3. The emergency oxygen valve is open slightly.
4. Air is drawn in around the intratracheal catheter during inhalation and exhaled into the inhaler (see intratracheal anesthesia).

LEAKS IN THE INHALER

Leaks in the semi-closed or closed system, whether large or small, should not be tolerated because they:

1. Prevent the maintenance of constant level of anesthesia.
2. Cause a costly loss of gases.
3. Increase the fire hazard.
4. Render the apparatus useless as an inhaler for artificial respiration in event of emergency or for positive pressure.

Sources of Leaks in Closed Inhalers:

1. Mask:
   a. It usually does not fit the face properly (see fitting masks, page 111).
   b. It is not fastened properly.
   c. Slip joints are loose.
2. Exhalation valve:
   a. The spring is defective.
   b. The valve is open.
3. Canister:
   a. The seams are ruptured from careless handling.
   b. Washers and other connections are worn or missing.
   c. It is overfilled with soda lime and not tightly sealed.
4. Rebreathing bags:
   a. Punctures and tears occur from fingernails or sharp instruments.
   b. The rubber is worn.
5. Rubber tubes: (Circle filters):
   a. The joints at the filters or at the masks are loose from wear.

  b. Holes are present in tubing.
6. Valves:
  a. Joints around valves are loose (circle filter).
  b. Valves are loose and worn or stiff.
7. Ether vaporizers:
  a. Jars are broken or loose or chipped about the lip.
  b. The vent on the dropper type is not closed.
8. Flow meters:
  a. The top is not screwed tightly on the hydraulic meters.
  b. The valve for replacing water may be open.
9. Delivery tube:
  a. The tube is old and worn.
  b. The tube is oversized and does not fit on sleeves.
  c. The tube is perforated.

Comment:

The majority of the leaks during anesthesia occur about the face piece.

Emesis During Anesthesia

Definition: The sudden expulsion of gastric contents through the esophagus into the pharynx. The act is partly voluntary and partly involuntary.

Causes of Emesis:

1. During the induction period (stages I and II):
  a. Difficult or prolonged induction from improper premedication, incorrect selection of agent or incorrect technique of administration.
  b. Full stomach from recently ingested food or liquids.
  c. The artificial airway is inserted into the pharynx prematurely and (in stages I and II) stimulates vomiting.
  d. Effect of opium alkaloids used for premedication upon the vomiting center.
2. During the maintenance of anesthesia:
  a. The patient, through carelessness of the anesthetist, or because of technical difficulties, passes from stage III to stage II and the artificial airway or mucus in the pharynx reflexly initiates vomiting.
3. During the recovery period:
  a. Central effect of drug acts on medulla and stimulates the vomiting center.
  b. Anoxia, regardless of the cause, is usually followed by vomiting.
  c. Artificial airway or secretions initiate vomiting when the pharyngeal reflex returns.
  d. Surgical manipulations (handling of intestines, and stomach traction on the gallbladder) may be responsible.

Treatment

1. Lower the head either over the edge of the table or place the patient in the Trendelenburg position.
2. Apply suction to the pharynx using metal pharyngeal suction tip (Fig. 85).

Reasons

The vomitus gravitates into the nasopharynx to minimize the possibility of aspiration into the larynx.

This aids in rapid removal of solid particles and liquids. Metal tip still permits suctioning should the patient bite.

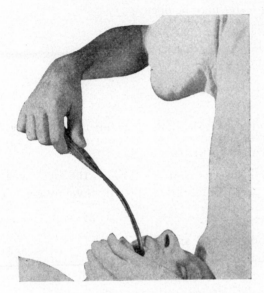

Fig. 85. The management of emesis, regurgitation, or hypersecretion is accomplished by lowering the head and aspiration by means of a metal pharyngeal tip attached to a suction apparatus.

Prophylaxis

1. Attempt as rapid an induction as possible—the zone of irritability of the vomiting center is passed quickly.
2. Administer adequate premedication to patient at the proper time.
3. Remove the artificial airway before the patient recovers from surgical anesthesia.
4. Withhold food and liquids by mouth for six to eight hours in patients scheduled for elective surgery.
5. Observe the patient carefully during maintenance phase of anes-

Reasons

The vomiting center is depressed in stage III, plane 1.

This assures a smooth and rapid induction and minimizes anoxia due to obstruction or spasm.

Stimulation of the pharynx and reflex vomiting are avoided.

Patients tend to evacuate contents of a full stomach when they are recovering from anesthesia.

Retching, particularly if an airway is in the pharynx, follows lighten-

thesia and avoid passing from
stage III to stage II.

6. Omit opium alkaloids for premedication if a known idiosyncrasy to these drugs exists.

ing of anesthesia.

Certain opium alkaloids excite the
vomiting center.

Dangers of Emesis:

1. The acid nature of gastric contents causes them to be highly irritating
to the laryngeal mucosa. Spasm and obstruction result.

2. Solid particles are aspirated into the respiratory tract. Acute asphyxia
and immediate death, bronchopneumonia (common), atelectasis of one
or more lobes, or peripheral circulatory failure, are the usual sequelae
of such accidents.

Comment

1. Remember that nausea and emesis and its sequelae may accompany or follow any type of anesthesia, whether inhalation, intravenous, rectal, or regional.

2. Be prepared for emesis in patients known to have full stom-
achs.

3. Remember that a patient may
vomit food even though he has
been fasting.

4. **Remember that asphyxia from
aspiration is a frequent cause of
sudden death on the operating
table.**

Reasons

The initiation of the vomiting reflex is of central origin and occurs
when non-volatile as well as volatile anesthetic drugs are employed.

The vomiting reflex is easily excited when the stomach is full.

The emptying time of the stomach
is usually retarded in the preoperative period in many subjects, possibly the result of psychic stimulation.

There is no effective treatment for
this accident when it occurs.

*A suction apparatus should be available in every operating room for the exclu-
sive use of the anesthetist.*

Management of Regurgitation During Anesthesia

Definition: The sudden expulsion of gastric or intestinal contents into the oropharynx during surgical anesthesia. The act is purely involuntary and
occurs during the surgical stage of anesthesia. Regurgitation differs from
emesis in that emesis is a partly voluntary act which occurs in stage II
of anesthesia.

Causes of Regurgitation:

1. Relaxation of the cardiac sphincter releases the contents of a dilated
stomach into the esophagus.

2. Manipulation of upper gastrointestinal tract forces fluid or solid materials into the pharynx. This is frequently a complication of pyloric or high intestinal obstruction, gastric hemorrhage, or dilatation.

Treatment: The same as for emesis.

Prophylaxis:

1. Insert a stomach tube and decompress the stomach before induction of anesthesia in all patients undergoing gastric surgery or suspected of having intestinal obstruction.
2. Allow the stomach tube to remain in place and allow continuous drainage during anesthesia.
3. Anesthetize patients undergoing gastric surgery as quickly as possible and insert an orotracheal catheter equipped with inflatable cuff to seal trachea from pharynx. Awake intubation may also be used.

Sequelae:

1. The patient usually drowns in his own secretions unless suction is applied quickly.
2. "Aspiration" pneumonia may follow if patient survives the sudden circulatory failure and the asphyxia which result from this accident.
3. Severe laryngeal spasm results which may cause acute asphyxia.

FIRES AND EXPLOSIONS

Definition:

1. A *fire* results when a combustible substance presents a small area of its total bulk to oxygen and oxidation occurs at a limited zone. Example, ether in a beaker burns.
2. An *explosion* results when an inflammable gas or vapor intimately mixed with air or oxygen becomes ignited. Combustion occurs so rapidly that the products of oxidation form almost instantly and expand with destructive violence.

Drugs Which Are Inflammable:

1) Ether   2) Vinethene   3) Ethyl chloride
4) Ethylene   5) Cyclopropane

Any of the above in the gaseous or vapor form mixed with nitrous oxide, air, or oxygen form explosive mixtures.

Drugs or Gases Which Are Non-Inflammable:

1) Nitrogen   2) Carbon dioxide   3) Helium   4) Oxygen
5) Chloroform   6) Trichlorethylene   7) Nitrous oxide
8) Halothane Methoxyflurane

Sources of Ignition in the Operating Rooms:

1. *Flames:* pipes, cigars, cigarettes, alcohol, gas lamps, etc.

2. *Electrical Equipment:* motors, heaters, x-ray equipment, cauteries, switches, endoscopes, lamps, etc.
3. *Static Electricity:* friction from blankets, rubber goods, clothing, personnel moving about room, tearing of adhesive, shuffling of feet, etc.
4. *Clicking Together of Metal Parts:* slip joints, sleeves, etc.
5. *Spontaneous Combustion:* impure anesthetic agents.

Precautions Pertaining to Selection of Agents:

1. Do not use cyclopropane, ethylene, ether, or vinethene when the cautery, electrosurgical unit, electric saw, portable x-ray or fluoroscope is used in any operating room.
2. Do not use inflammable gases or vapors in wards or other divisions of the hospital not protected by sparkproof electrical equipment, conductive flooring, and proper humidification.
3. Employ the closed system with carbon dioxide absorption wherever possible.

Precautions Pertaining to Operating Room Personnel	*Reasons*
1. Do not allow operating room personnel to wear shoes with combined rubber soles and heels. All shoes should be tested for conductivity periodically (Fig. 88).	Such individuals may acquire electrostatic charges. A spark may result if they touch the anesthetist, machine, or other apparatus which is positively charged.
2. Do not allow operating room personnel to wear silk, rayon, nylon, or woolen garments.	Such garments favor the accumulation of electrostatic charges.
3. Do not allow smoking in the operating room suite.	The temperature of open flames is above the ignition temperature of anesthetic mixtures.
4. Do not allow visitors, nurses, or doctors to touch the anesthetist or the anesthesia apparatus at any time while surgery is in progress.	They may have acquired an electrical charge opposite to that of the field. A spark results when the potential is equalized.
5. Do not unroll or tear adhesive in the vicinity of an anesthesia apparatus.	The friction causes an electrostatic discharge and formation of sparks.
6. Do not use non-sparkproof plugs or electrical connections unless placed five feet from floor.	A spark results in the switch when the electrical circuit is opened or closed.
7. Do not use lamps with open sockets in the operating room.	A spark results in the socket switch when the light is turned on or off.
8. Do not use ether for cleaning purposes.	Ether vapor is inflammable and may be ignited by friction.
9. Avoid using nonconductive rub-	The covering prevents the static

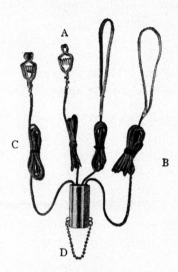

Fig. 86. The Horton intercoupler.

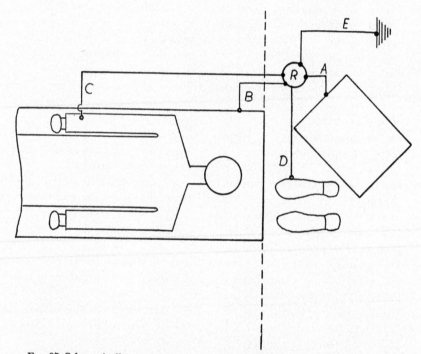

Fig. 87. Schematic diagram of the "hook up" of the intercoupler: (R) is a resistance of one megohm connected to the various leads. Lead (A) is connected to the machine (B) to the operating table; the wrist band of lead (C) is wrapped around the wrist of the patient, (D) is wrapped around the left wrist of the anesthetist, and (E) is clipped to the ground.

ber pads or pillows. If they must be used, cover them with a sheet, and do not remove cover during operation.

10. Do not use pails, buckets, and other mobile metal equipment which are not protected by rubber guards.

electricity which results from friction.

The protection prevents the formation of sparks by the striking of metal on metal.

Precautions To Be Observed by Anesthetists

Reasons

1. Do not move about the room and break contact with the patient.

A difference in electrical potential between the anesthetist and the patient may develop.

2. Install an intercoupler (Fig. 86) on all cases in which ether, cyclopropane, ethylene, or other inflammable gases or vapors are employed in room with nonconductive floor.

This device allows an equalization of potentials between each unit of the anesthetic field.

3. Maintain a relative humidity above 65% in the operating room.

A high relative humidity aids in dissipation of electrostatic charges and minimizes the tendency toward explosions.

4. Do not use electrical equipment which is not of sparkproof design.

The operation of motors is accompanied by the formation of sparks.

5. Be certain that all stretchers, stools, tables, etc., have bronze drag chains in contact with the floor.

Bronze is an excellent conductor of electricity and does not produce sparks when it strikes tile or metallic substances.

6. Use conductive rubber wherever possible.

"Ordinary" rubber is a poor conductor of electricity and favors the accumulation of electrostatic charges in the inhaler.

7. Do not cover anesthesia machines with drapes or sheets while they are idle.

An electrostatic charge may accumulate and cause a spark when the drape brushes over the apparatus when it is removed.

8. Do not jerk connections or slip joints apart during anesthesia.

Sparks may form when metal pieces strike each other.

9. Moisten the breathing bag and rubber tubes before commencing anesthesia. Rinse after anesthesia is ended.

Moisture aids in dissipation and neutralization of electrostatic charges.

10. Use *pure drugs* at all times.

Impure gases and vapors may have a lower flash point than the pure products.

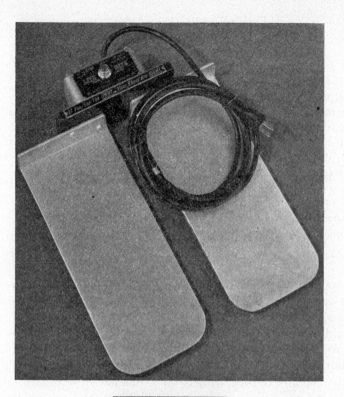

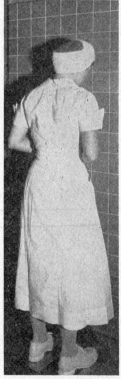

Fig. 88. Ohmeter for determining conductivity of shoes of operating room personnel. The instrument operates on ordinary 110 volt alternating current. When the resistance of the shoes exceeds one megohm the light does not show and the shoes are not considered safe. (Courtesy W. E. Anderson Co., Kansas City, Mo.).

11. Never lubricate any valve or gauge used on high pressure cylinders with oil or grease.

High pressure atomizes grease and forms an explosive mixture.

12. Always secure as snug a fit as possible at the mask to avoid leaks.

Escaping vapors are easily ignited.

13. Do not commence to flow inflammable gases from supply source into apparatus unless the mask is secure on the patient's face.

This prevents the escape of inflammable mixtures into the room.

14. Always close reducing valves when opening the main valve of a high pressure cylinder.

The high pressure may suddenly be transmitted to the inhaler if the valve of any high pressure cylinder is opened without first closing the reducing valve.

15. Protect all upright cylinders from toppling over. Use stand or support. Cap large ones.

Valve may break off and the contents which are under high pressure escape with explosive violence.

16. Turn off the flow of all gases and inflammable vapors when inserting airways. Close obturator on the mask.

Precautions to prevent the escape of inflammable mixtures into the room should be taken at all times.

17. Do not remove the breathing bag from the inhaler during anesthesia.

A difference in potential may develop and cause a spark to form when bag is replaced.

18. Use cotton blankets to cover the patient while he is in the operating room.

Wool is an excellent electrostatic generator and loses its charge to the air only if the relative humidity is very high (80–95%).

The Intercoupler

Description: The intercoupler is an electrical unit composed of a resistance of one megohm (one million ohms) connected to five leads which act as conductors. The resistance acts as a central connecting pair for the leads, is insulated, and is contained in a metal cylinder. One lead is attached to a hook which acts as a hanger for the device. The other four leads are insulated wires approximately six feet long, two of which terminate as clips and two as wristbands (Fig. 87). The intercoupler is used when nonconductive flooring is not available in the operating room.

Purpose: The intercoupler allows equalization of the electrical potential between the patient, anesthetist, anesthesia apparatus, and operating table. It thus prevents the occurrence of electrostatic sparks between members of the electrically connected group (Fig. 86).

To Connect:

1. Fasten one clip to an unpainted portion beneath the operating table.

2. Allow one clip to rest on the floor or fasten to the lead to the ground.
3. Encircle one band to patient's wrist (use wrist of arm used for blood pressure cuff).
4. Encircle one band around left wrist (anesthetist's).
5. Suspend the cylindrical portion on anesthesia machine by the hook provided for the purpose.

Care of Intercoupler

Reasons

1. Arrange wires in such a manner that they do not become tangled or caught in castors of machines, table, or in feet of operating room personnel.

If the leads are torn from the resistance, the unit is rendered useless.

2. Disconnect all leads immediately after the operation is completed and wind wires into a compact bundle.

The unit is often damaged when the machine is pulled away from the table, or the wires become hopelessly tangled.

Comment

Reasons

1. *Remember* that the unit is theoretically sound but does not supersede conductive flooring in efficiency.

The instrument should be employed routinely in suites with no conductive floors.

2. *Always* wear the band on the left (anesthetist's) wrist.

The right hand should thus remain free for charting and other duties.

3. *Remember* that if a member of the coupled field comes into contact with power lines, shocks are minimized.

A resistance of one megohm is sufficiently small to prevent discharges of large amounts of current.

4. *Remember* that although the lead for the ground need not be connected, it is preferable to do so.

Bodies outside the protected field which come into contact with the field usually have the same potential as the ground.

5. *Remember* that the resistance between any two terminals is unaffected by any connection to the other terminals.

A resistance of one megohm exists between any two terminals.

6. *Remember* that a spark may occur between objects in the interconnected field and objects outside the field.

A resistance of one megohm allows the potential to be equalized in one-thousandth of one second, this allows sufficient time for a spark to form under these circumstances.

TESTING HUMIDITY IN OPERATING ROOM

Principle: The wet and dry bulb thermometer combination is used (Fig. 89). The wet bulb is surrounded by a wick immersed in water. Evaporation cools the wet one. Differences in temperature are interpolated on the scale and relative humidity is read off in percent.

Procedure or Use:
1. Fill container with water at room temperature.
2. Allow wick to soak well and wet bulb to cool (5 min.).

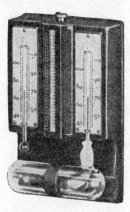

FIG. 89. The wet-dry bulb thermometer used for determining humidity in operating room.

3. Read both temperatures and subtract wet from dry.
4. Turn scale on top of instrument until figure representing difference between two readings comes into view.
5. Read down marginal scale to the figure corresponding to temperature of *dry* bulb. Figure opposite is relative humidity in percent.

WET TOWEL INTERCOUPLING

Principle: The patient, anesthetist, operating table and anesthetic apparatus are interconnected with wet towels.

Uses: In situations in which high resistance flooring is present in an operating location and a Horton intercoupler is not available.

Materials: Three moistened towels with excess water squeezed out of them.

Procedure:
1. Drape one end of towel over the bare shoulder of the patient and tuck the other end between the pad and the table.
2. Drape one end of second towel over base of operating table over caster or expanding metal part and other end on floor.
3. Drape third towel over base of anesthetic machine and other end on floor towards table.
4. Anesthetist places one foot in each towel.

Comment
    Both towels on floor may touch each other and anesthetist may then make contact with one foot.

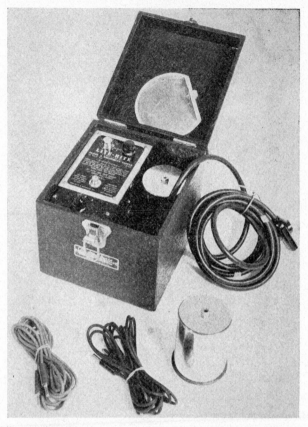

FIG. 90. The "megger" used to determine resistances of equipment in operating rooms and conductivity of floors. The circular weights are placed three feet apart on the conductive floor. Floors having resistance of more than half a megohm or less than 25,000 ohms are not acceptable. (Courtesy W. E. Anderson Co., Kansas City, Mo.).

REFERENCES

Greene, B. A. The Hazard of Fire and Explosion. Anesthesiology, 2: 144, March, 1941.
Adriani J.: Chemistry and Physics of Anesthesia, Chap. 26. Springfield, Thomas, 1962.

CARE OF PATIENT AT TERMINATION OF ANESTHESIA

The period following the discontinuance of anesthesia and before the complete recovery occurs is often the most critical and the one in which accidents are frequent.

The following precautions should be followed to prevent and minimize accidents:

Routine While Patient Is in Operating Room	*Reasons*
1. Remove the mask from the face and turn patient's head to one side.	This allows secretions to readily pass from the mouth in event of retching or emesis.

2. Remove the headband from beneath the occiput.

It may be soiled in the event emesis occurs.

3. Remove secretions by suction using a metal curved pharyngeal suction tip.

Secretions may cause laryngeal spasm, tracheal or bronchial obstruction, or initiate retching and vomiting during the recovery period.

4. Remove the artificial airway as soon as the patient reacts from anesthesia and the pharyngeal or laryngeal reflex returns.

Its presence may initiate retching and vomiting by pharyngeal stimulation.

5. Remove secretions, mucus, and wipe secretions from the face and mouth.

Irritation to the skin occurs if they are not removed.

6. Disconnect the intercoupler and fold neatly.

The leads may be broken off when the machine is rolled away from operating table.

7. Transfer patient to the stretcher and place him in the position desired by the surgeon.

The apparatus is usually removed in the operating room.

8. Unfasten and remove restraints from legs and wrists.

An unconscious patient is easily injured if attempts are made to lift him while he is in restraints.

9. Remove the cuff of the sphygonomanometer and the stethoscope and fold neatly.

The airway is the anesthetist's responsibility at all times, and he must observe it continuously during the recovery period.

10. Place a towel, airway, and tongue depresser alongside the patient's head.

Be prepared to combat obstruction and emesis en route to patient's room.

11. Stand at the "head end" of the stretcher and proceed to the patient's room. Support the chin to maintain a free airway (Fig. 75, page 270).

The anesthetist's responsibility ends only when the patient is no longer in danger of asphyxia, or circulatory or respiratory failure.

Routine in Halls and Elevator

Reasons

1. Cover patient with a blanket (woolen blanket not to be put on in operating room).

Movements of the blanket may create electrostatic charge which is dangerous if inflammable gases have been employed.

2. Carefully observe respiration and the airway. Reinsert pharyngeal airway if necessary.

Patients frequently lapse into deep sleep following emergence from anesthesia and develop respiratory obstruction.

Routine on Ward or in Patient's Room

1. Request attendants to close doors and windows.
2. Place patient in bed in position desired by surgeon.
3. Note character and rate of the pulse and record the blood pressure on the chart.
4. Place patient in the custody of a nurse or other responsible attendant as soon as he recovers and his reflexes return.

Reasons

Drafts and chilling may predispose to respiratory complications.
The position should be one that insures free airway at all times.
Circulatory depression frequently occurs after termination of anesthesia and changes in position.
All unconscious subjects should be observed continuously to avoid respiratory obstruction, aspiration, and other anesthetic accidents common in the recovery period.

Routine Following Cyclopropane, Nitrous Oxide, Ethylene, or Vinethene Anesthesia

1. Continue anesthesia up to moment of application of dressing.

2. Remove mask and empty inhaler. Proceed as listed under general directions and perform duties which apply to this type of anesthesia.

Reasons

Elimination of these agents is rapid and undesired premature recovery from anesthesia and restlessness of patient occurs.
Accumulation of inflammable mixtures in the inhaler is undesirable.

Routine Following Intratracheal Anesthesia

1. Remove packs or deflate cuff, and loosen any adhesive which anchors the catheter to the skin.
2. Apply suction to the pharynx using a curved metal tip. If necessary, expose hypopharynx with laryngoscope to completely remove secretions.
3. Remove the "bite block" and replace it with an oropharyngeal airway.

4. Disconnect intratracheal catheter from inhaler and allow patient to recover by breathing air.
5. Attach a lubricated 14 or 16 French, or other catheter of appropriate size, to the suction,

Reasons

The catheter should be free so that it may be removed instantly when desired.
Remove secretions completely to prevent laryngeal spasm.

This prevents obstruction which may follow removal of catheter. It also acts to prevent patient's biting on catheter.
Aspiration of pharynx is more easily accomplished if the patient remains anesthetized.
Remove secretions from the trachea and tracheal catheter as completely as possible.

pinch and pass it into the tracheal tube.

6. Replace mask on the inhaler, have it in readiness for administration of oxygen or resuscitation in event of complications.

7. Withdraw the catheter from the trachea when the laryngeal reflex returns or the patient coughs.

Spasm of the larynx or obstruction of airway may follow withdrawal of catheter and the inhaler will be required immediately.

The possibility of respiratory obstruction from relaxation of tissues is lessened if muscles of pharynx and tongue regain tone.

8. Apply suction to the pharynx again after removal of the tracheal catheter.

If secretions in the catheter are not completely removed, they pass into pharynx as catheter is withdrawn

Care of Patient in "Shock"
at End of Operation

Reasons

1. Adjust shoulder braces and place the patient in the Trendelenburg position if surgeon desires it.

This improves circulatory status of medullary centers.

2. Adjust inhaler, administer pure oxygen by semi-closed system at 6 liters per minute.

Inhalation of oxygen may be beneficial in peripheral circulatory failure.

3. Turn on filter to remove carbon dioxide.

Carbon dioxide is undesirable because it produces hyperpnea and may contribute further to circulatory changes.

4. Remove anesthetic drug by allowing exhalation valve to remain open.

Rebreathing of exhaled gases may keep patient anesthetized even though the concentration is low.

5. Do not remove restraints from knees.

Patient may become restless or delirious.

6. Do not remove sphygmomanometer until patient is ready to be returned to his bed.

Blood pressure readings should be taken frequently.

7. Maintain fluids, a free airway, and provide warmth.

The patient should not be returned to his room until the circulation assumes a satisfactory status.

Comment and General Precautions

Reasons

1. **At the termination of operations about the neck or face, do not remove patient to his bed until he recovers completely from anesthesia. Remove to recovery room if such a unit is available.**

Edema, tight bandages, secretions, etc., may cause obstruction or laryngeal spasm if patient is not observed closely.

2. **Never allow a patient having an artificial airway in situ to remain unattended.**

Stimulation of the pharynx by the airway may induce spasm, retching, or vomiting which may be unnoticed and cause asphyxia.

3. Do not remove the patient from the operating room if he commences to vomit or retch.

Suction the pharynx and allow the patient to remain in operating room until the episode is over.

4. Do not disassemble inhaler until patient is out of operating room.

Complications frequently occur at termination of anesthesia which require immediate use of an inhaler.

5. **Remain with the patient from the moment anesthesia is induced until he is safely in bed and can be left in custody of a responsible person.**

Obstruction, vomiting, or spasm, are so frequent and develop so quickly that even a moment's relaxation of vigilance may be fatal.

6. Allow the head to hang over the end of the stretcher if the patient vomits en route to bed. Use suction freely on arrival in patient's room.

This prevents aspiration of foreign material or fluid into respiratory tract by allowing it to gravitate into the nasopharynx where it is less harmful.

7. **Never allow a patient's arms or legs, hands, or feet to dangle over side of operating table or stretcher.**

Injury to limbs, paralysis of radial nerve or brachial plexus from pressure or traction may occur during transit.

8. Close main valves on cylinders on machine before leaving operating room.

Attendants may jar cylinders loose while cleaning room and cause contained gases to escape.

9. Take blood pressure reading on stretcher after patient has been lifted from operating table in cases in which blood pressure has been labile.

Hypotension may occur if vasomotor system is unable to compensate when the patient is moved.

PART IV

BASAL NARCOSIS AND ANALGESIA BY INTRAVASCULAR INJECTION

Principle: An aqueous solution of a central nervous system depressant is injected directly into the vascular system. The method is suitable for water soluble drugs. It is used most extensively for non-volatile drugs. The drug is administered by the intermittent, fractional or by the continuous infusion (drip) technique.

Available Drugs:

Ether: Ether is shaken with physiological saline, the excess removed, and the aqueous solution injected. This is rarely employed because ether is only moderately soluble in water and the volume of solution necessary to maintain surgical anesthesia therefore would be too great.

Paraldehyde: This drug is useful for hypnosis but not satisfactory for surgical anesthesia. The dose and duration of anesthesia are variable and not easily estimated.

Alcohol: Ethyl alcohol is mixed with distilled water and 5% dextrose and infused for analgesia.

Tribromethanol: The action and duration of this agent are variable and it is rarely used.

Narcotics: These are suitable for analgesia, basal hypnosis, or as a supplemental agent for inhalation or other types of anesthesia. Morphine, dihydromorphinone (dilaudid), meperidine (demerol), methadon, nisentil are the most commonly employed drugs.

Barbiturates: Short-acting barbiturates are used for sedation and as anticonvulsants. Sodium amytal, pentobarbital, and secobarbital are the most useful of this group.

Ultra-short-acting barbiturates are used for anesthesia. Thiopentobarbital (pentothal) surital, kemithal and evipal are the most commonly employed and popular in this group. They also are prepared in aqueous solutions of their sodium salt. Barbiturates are not analgesic to any extent and can only be used for basal narcosis.

Steroid compounds: Viadril is currently used for basal narcosis.

Local anesthetics: These are diluted and administered for premedication, analgesia and for vasodilatation.

Methods of Administration:

1. *Intravenous:* This is the most accessible and commonly employed route. The following sites listed in the order of frequency of use are utilized for the injection:

    a. Median basilic vein and other veins in antecubital fossa.

    b. Veins of the plexus on dorsum of the hand.

    c. Internal saphenous at inner aspect of the ankle, or the lateral marginal vein at the ankle.

    d. Veins of plexus on dorsum of the foot.

    e. Internal and external jugular veins.

2. *Intramedullary:* Fluids may be injected into the marrow cavities of the large bones. Absorption is as rapid and effective as if given by vein. The sternum is preferred as the site of injection in adults. Long bones are used in children.

3. *Intra-arterial:* This route is dangerous. Arterial spasm may occur which may be followed by gangrene of an extremity particularly when a terminal artery is used.

TECHNIQUE OF VENIPUNCTURE

1. Expose the arm well above the cubital fossa. Prepare the skin with ether or 70% alcohol.

2. Raise an intradermal wheal using a 26 or 27 gauge needle over the selected vein, using a 0.5% or 1% procaine solution as the anesthetic agent.

3. Shift wheal to side of vein by retracting the skin laterally.

4. Apply the tourniquet close to site of venipuncture to fix the vein (a blood pressure cuff may be used).

5. Insert an 18 or 19 gauge needle through the wheal at the side of the vein into the tissue surrounding the vein.

6. Relax the tension on the skin and allow the needle and wheal to shift back over vein.

7. Puncture the vein and hold needle so that bevel is parallel to wall of vein.

8. Release tourniquet.

Comment

1. The extremity may be wrapped with hot packs to cause veins to become prominent if they are difficult to visualize.

2. Local anesthesia is optional and may be omitted.

REFERENCE

Lundy, John, and Adams, Charles. Intravenous Anesthesia. Anesthesiology, *1:* 145, 1940.

TECHNIQUE FOR STERNAL PUNCTURE

Materials:

1. Hypodermic needle and syringe.

2. Special sternal needle (1.5 mm.$\times$30 mm. with a stylet).

3. Procaine (0.5% or 1% solution).

Procedure:

1. Locate the manubrium of the sternum.
2. Prepare the skin thoroughly with the desired antiseptic.
3. Raise an intradermal wheal several centimeters caudad to the center of the manubrium.
4. Infiltrate deeper structures over and including the periosteum.
5. Insert the sternal needle in a cephalad direction inclining the needle at an angle approximately 20° to 30° to the skin and pierce the bone.

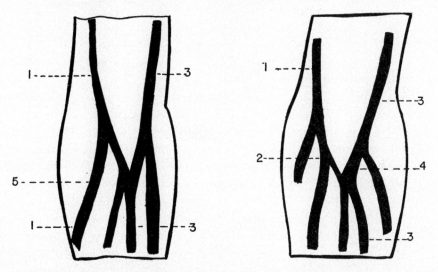

FIG. 91. Two common arrangements of the veins of the left cubital fossa. In the obese the veins are deeply subcutaneous and not visible or palpable. 1. Basilic. 2. Median basilic. 3. Cephalic. 4. Median cephalic. 5. Median cubital.

6. Attach syringe and aspirate when needle pierces bone and is felt to pass into marrow. (Blood is drawn into the syringe if the needle is in marrow cavity.)
7. Clear needle by injecting several cc.'s of physiological saline solution.
8. Inject desired fluid in the same manner and with the same precautions used for an intravenous injection.

Precautions:

1. Do not proceed with the injection unless marrow contents are aspirated.
2. Do not employ the technique in the face of local infections of the thorax, sternum, or septicemia.
3. Be positive that the needle has not pierced the lower plate of the sternum and has passed into the mediastinum.

REFERENCE

Papper, E. M. The Bone Marrow Route for Injecting Fluids and Drugs Into the General Circulation. Anesthesiology, *3:* 307, 1942.

INTRAVENOUS SODIUM PENTOTHAL (THIOPENTAL)

Description: Basal narcosis (profound hypnosis with amnesia) obtained by the administration of the ultra-short-acting barbiturate pentothal (sodium thiopentobarbital). Rapid loss of consciousness occurs. Consciousness returns within a few minutes after termination of the injection but may be followed by a variable period of somnolence. Reflexes are not completely abolished. Not satisfactory as a surgical anesthetic when used alone. Always used in conjunction with a drug which possesses analgesic properties.

Uses:

1. For brief minor procedures which require no marked degree of pain relief (without supporting drug).
2. For procedures in which general anesthesia is required in which the cautery or electrosurgical unit is employed (with nitrous oxide).
3. For narcointerrogation and narcoanalysis.
4. For basal narcosis to facilitate induction and maintenance of inhalation anesthesia. (In conjunction with nitrous oxide, ethylene, ether, cyclopropane and the muscle relaxants.)
5. As a hypnotic and sedative with local or spinal anesthesia.
6. For the relief of convulsive states produced by stimulating drugs (local anesthetics) or following increased irritability of the central nervous system (tetanus, rabies etc.).

Dosage: Average dose is 1 gm. (15 gr.) in 40 cc. of distilled water or physiological saline solution ($2\frac{1}{2}\%$). Dosage varies with the patient.

Preparation: The patient is prepared in the same manner and same principles and precautions are observed as for other types of general anesthesia.

Premedication	*Reason*
1. Atropine, hyoscyamine or scopolamine gr. 1/150 to 1/100, one hour prior to anesthesia.	This is necessary because it antagonizes vagal effects and minimizes secretions.
2. Morphine, gr. 1/6 to 1/4, one hour prior to anesthesia.	This may be omitted because it tends to enhance the respiratory depression characteristic of pentothal. It is analgesic and reduces the amount of pentothal used.

Materials:

1. Ampules of drug.
2. Sterile distilled water or physiological saline.
3. Syringe 20, 30 or 50 cc. size equipped with a Luer lock for the needle or an adapter to fit a three way stopcock.

4. 19 or 20 gauge needle.
5. Syringe holder (Fig. 92).
6. Arm board.
7. Tourniquet.
8. Krieslman resuscitator or other suitable device for artificial respiration.
9. Artificial airway of proper size.
10. Suitable skin sterilizer and sponges.
11. Infusion of saline or 5% dextrose in distilled water and administration set.
12. Three way stopcock.
13. Towel or strap for fastening arm to the board.

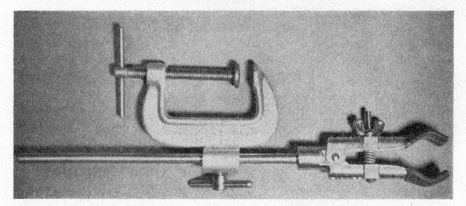

FIG. 92. Simple syringe holder for intravenous administration
of hypnotic and anesthetic drugs.

Note: The drug is usually packed in ampules containing either one gram or half gram. Larger packages are available for bulk preparation of drug.

Procedure:

1. Arrange the cuff of the sphygmomanometer to the arm with the less suitable veins.
2. Strap the arm with the most suitable veins to the board which has been placed in a convenient position. Fasten the palm of the hand upward to the board. If veins of arm are inaccessible, use those of foot.
3. Explain to the patient details of the procedure to obtain his confidence.
4. Prepare the skin, select the vein, apply tourniquet, and perform venipuncture as described in foregoing section. Commence infusion or introduce needle attached to syringe in vein (Fig. 93).
5. Fasten syringe holder to arm board and connect adapter to three way stopcock and to infusion if infusion is used.
6. Inject 5–10 drops of drug to test for intolerance. Wait several minutes.
7. Inject the drug slowly, but do not exceed 2 cc. in the first fifteen sec-

onds. Stop and wait (patient will be narcotized in 30–40 seconds). Repeat, if anesthesia does not ensue, repeat using same amount of solution at same rate.

8. Support the chin to insure a patent airway as soon as consciousness is lost.

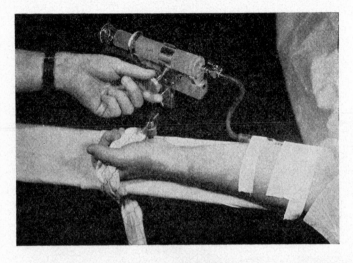

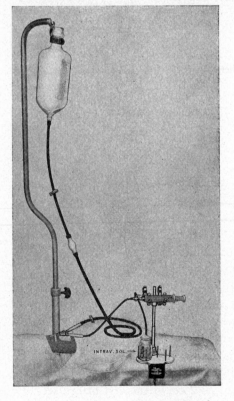

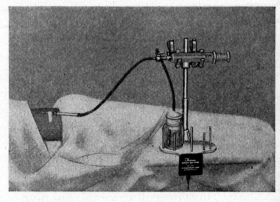

Fig. 93. Administration of pentothal using various types of syringe holders.

9. Administer fractions of 1/2 to 1 cc. of solution from time to time as the responses of the patient demands. This can be judged only from the reactions of patient to the stimuli of surgery and the response to the drug. Pause at least thirty seconds between fractions.

10. Proceed with nitrous oxide, ethylene or cyclopropane.

Signs of Anesthesia:

No reliable signs of pentothal anesthesia exist. The stages and planes applicable to inhalation anesthesia cannot be used as guides to anesthesia with the barbiturates. Slow administration of barbiturates results in various zones of "reactivity" which have been likened to planes of anesthesia. However, rapid and repeated administration results in a telescoping of these "stages." The anesthetist must attempt to maintain the patient between the zones of decreased reflexed activity and respiratory and circulatory failure.

Complications	*Reasons*
1. Respiratory failure.	This is usually due to an overdosage or to the use of large quantities of drugs over long periods of time.
2. Hypotension.	This is due to depression of the vasomotor and hypothalamic centers from the initial or too large a dose.
3. Laryngeal spasm.	This is caused by spasmogenic qualities of thiobarbiturates. Mucus, blood, and other secretions or any instrumentation of the pharynx and larynx in respiratory tract may initiate the spasm.
4. Coughing and sneezing.	The laryngeal and pharyngeal reflexes are not abolished by the drug. Stimulation of the cornea (eye surgery) may cause sneezing.
5. Slough at site of injection.	This is due to extravascular injection of the solution. Solutions of the sodium salts of barbiturates are alkaline (pH 9 to 10) and cause damage to tissues in event of seepage.
6. Phlebothrombosis.	The alkalinity of the solution causes damage to the vessel wall.
7. Arteriospasm.	This is caused by accidental intra arterial injection. Gangrene of the extremity may follow the spasm.

8. Prolonged somnolence.

Ultra-short-acting barbiturates are only partially detoxified immediately. Degradation products accumulate in the tissues and cause hypnosis if large amounts are given.

9. Twitchings of muscles.

Cause not determined. May be due to hypothermia, CO_2 excess, or cold environment or degradation products from detoxification of drug.

Advantages:

1. Induction of basal narcosis is simple, rapid, and accompanied by amnesia which is pleasant to the patient.
2. Basal narcosis may be induced in the patient's room as indicated.
3. A minimum of apparatus is required.
4. Post-anesthetic emesis is reduced (if the patient has been fasting).
5. It does not stimulate the production of secretions in the respiratory tract.
6. It causes no irritation to the mucous membranes of the respiratory tract.
7. Recovery is prompt in vigorous subjects if minimal doses are employed.

Disadvantages:

1. The basal narcosis is noncontrollable. Once the drug is in a vein, and overdosage has occurred, it cannot be retrieved, and one must wait until it is detoxified.
2. All reflexes are not abolished, particularly those of the larynx and pharynx, and laryngeal spasm may develop.
3. It cannot be used as the sole agent because it is not analgesic and causes anesthesia by inducing a severe depression.
4. The necessary effective dose is difficult to estimate because of differences in susceptibility of individuals to barbiturates.
5. A severe respiratory depression may ensue. The sensitivity of the respiratory center to carbon dioxide decreases progressively.
6. It is spasmogenic giving rise to severe laryngeal and bronchial spasm.
7. The muscular relaxation is not satisfactory, unless general anesthetics or muscle relaxants are also used.

Contra-Indications

1. Aged subjects with manifestations of degenerative changes.

Detoxification may be delayed.

2. Diseases of the heart with decompensation.

Objectionable primarily from deleterious effects it may have on respiration. Small doses permissible.

3. Hypotension due to contracted blood volume and other causes.

The vasomotor center is depressed by the drug and the hypotension may be enhanced. Drug is slowly detoxified in shock states.

4. Chronic diseases of the respiratory tract complicated by a decrease in vital capacity.

The drug depresses respiration. Hypoventilation may follow.

5. Acute or chronic obstruction of the respiratory tract (edema of the glottis, Ludwig's angina, etc.).

Obstruction from spasm may further affect the respiratory difficulty. Asphyxia may result when voluntary efforts to maintain airway patent are removed.

6. Anemia, regardless of the cause.

May be hazardous if respiratory depression occurs because oxygen carrying power of the blood is reduced.

7. Patients, who have sepsis, or who are cachetic or comatose.

The drug may be detoxified so slowly in these subjects that a marked respiratory or circulatory depression or prolonged somnolence occurs.

8. As a sole agent for operations in the pharynx, larynx, or bronchi, particularly if secretions are abundant.

Laryngeal spasm may develop because pharyngeal and laryngeal reflexes are not abolished.

9. Acidosis from any cause.

Respiratory depression may enhance acidosis by causing a retention of carbon dioxide in the tissues.

10. Diseases of the liver and kidney.

Acidosis may complicate these diseases. Detoxifying powers of the tissues may be poor and prolonged narcosis may follow.

11. As a sole agent for operations of undetermined length.

Large amounts of the drug may be necessary to complete the operation. This causes a marked depression of respiration and circution from cumulative effects.

12. As a sole agent for "major" operations and those requiring muscle relaxation.

Pentothal does not produce satisfactory muscle relaxation if used alone.

Precautions

Reasons

1. The limit should be approximately one gram of the drug for an adult.

The drug is promptly removed and stored in the adipose tissues. Prolonged narcosis results because it accumulates and is detoxified slowly.

2. Do not use artificial airways if basal narcosis is uncomplicated by obstruction.

Reflexes in the pharynx and trachea are not abolished and retching or spasm of larynx may result.

3. Do not inject the drug before the tourniquet is released.

Overdosage may occur if the drug is injected with tourniquet tightened and subsequently released.

4. Be positive that the drug is completely dissolved and that the solution is clear before performing venipuncture.

Undissolved particles act as foreign bodies in the solution and may cause "reactions."

5. Administer pure oxygen and assist respiration if cyanosis appears or if respiratory movements are shallow.

Anoxemia due to the respiratory depression is thus avoided.

6. Inject the solution slowly. Do not inject more than 6 cc. of a 2 1/2% solution at one time at the onset.

Overdosage can be avoided by fractionation and grading the dose.

7. Draw back as little blood as possible into the syringe (when an infusion is not used).

The blood proteins precipitate in the solution and the cells are hemolized. Large volumes of blood tend to dilute the total volume of solution making it difficult to judge dosage accurately.

8. From time to time ascertain whether or not the needle is in the vein and still patent by pulling on the plunger slightly if an infusion is not used.

This should be done to avoid sloughs by extravascular injection and to prevent clotting in the needle during the maintenance of anesthesia.

9. Clear blood from the needle by injecting a small amount of solution through it from time to time.

Clotting of the blood in needle invariably occurs unless this is done.

10. Do not add analeptic drugs to the solution of the barbiturate.

Have such drugs in readiness in event of emergency. Analeptic drugs antagonize the barbiturate action and defeat the purpose of the drug.

11. Administer fractional maintenance doses only when the patient responds to stimuli.

Pain is indicated by increased amplitude of respiration, phonation, or reflex action.

12. Do not employ for surgical anesthesia for office practice or for ambulatory patients.

Ataxia may appear and persist for several hours in recovery period. Resuscitative equipment and aid of assistants is usually not available in the office.

13. Withdraw the needle and reinsert it into another vein if patient

This usually indicates extravascular injection. Inject 1% procaine

complains of pain while injecting the drug during the induction.

14. Do not apply the tourniquet too tightly.

into the area. This causes vasodilatation and averts sloughing. The compression may cause arterial pulsation to disappear and intraarterial injection may accidently result if artery is mistaken for vein.

15. Do not induce anesthesia by this technique unless artificial airways and an inhaler for artificial respiration are available for instant use.

The uncontrollable nature of this type of anesthesia renders it extremely hazardous unless precautions for treating overdosage are available.

16. Do not use intravenous anesthesia for operations in which the anesthetist must be removed from absolute control of the airway.

The airway should be under the control of the anesthetist at all times. Use an endotracheal tube and topical anesthesia under such circumstances.

17. Do not administer pentothal to patients who have recently partaken of food or fluid.

Emesis frequently follows during recovery period. The gastric contents may cause a severe spasm of the larynx.

18. Do not use thiobarbiturates or short-acting barbiturates when suppurative diseases of the lungs are present.

Secretions may initiate laryngeal and bronchial spasm.

19. Use an infusion of saline or 5% dextrose in distilled water in conjunction with barbiturate narcosis of undetermined length.

Technical difficulties due to maintaining vein patent are averted.

20. Do not use solutions which have been standing for several days.

Barbiturates are not stable. Potency may have been lost.

REFERENCES

Adriani, John. Pharmacology of Anesthetic Drugs. 4th Ed. Pp. 72–88. Charles C Thomas, Springfield, Ill., 1960.

Adams, R. C. Intravenous Anesthesia—Apparatus and Methods of Administration. Proc. Staff Meet., Mayo Clin., *16:* 519, 1941.

Ruth, H. S., Tovell, R. and Others. Pentothal Sodium. J.A.M.A., *113:* 1864, 1939.

Thomas, George J. Clinical and Laboratory Observations on Intravenous Anesthesia. Anesth. and Analg., *17:* 163–168, 1948.

INTRAVENOUS SODIUM SURITAL (THIOSECOBARBITAL)

Description: Sodium surital is an ultra short-acting thiobarbiturate whose pharmacological actions are essentially similar to pentothal. The technique for administration and precautions are identical to those outlined for sodium pentothal. The drug is the sulphur (thio) counterpart of secobarbital (Seconal).

Variations in Technique:

1. Dose—one gram for an adult of average size and weight 150–175 lbs.
2. Strength—usually a $2\frac{1}{2}\%$ solution is necessary for successful anesthesia.
3. Rate of injection—1 to 3 cc. slowly 1/2 to 1 cc. in 10 seconds for the induction. The remainder at intervals determined by the reflex activity of the patient.
4. The drug is not used alone but is combined with nitrous oxide, ethylene, cyclopropane. The muscle relaxants may be added if relaxation is required.

INTRAVENOUS SODIUM EVIPAL (HEXOBARBITAL)

Description: Sodium evipal is an ultra-short-acting barbiturate of the N-methyl type whose pharmacological actions, from a clinical standpoint, are essentially similar to pentothal.

The technique of injection and precautions are identical to those for sodium pentothal except in the following details.

Variations in Technique:

Dose: One gram for an adult of average size and weight (150–175 lbs.).

Strength: Usually a 5% to 10% solution is necessary for adequate basal narcosis.

Rate of Injection: One to three cc. slowly (1/2–1 cc. in 10 seconds) for the induction, the remainder at intervals determined by the reflex activity of the patient.

INTRAVENOUS METHOHEXITAL (BREVITAL)

Description

Methohexital is an N-methyl barbiturate (dl-methyl allyl, methyl 2-pentynyl barbituric acid) prepared in the form of a sodium salt. It is an ultra short acting barbiturate similar to hexobarbital (Evipal) but more potent and more rapid acting.

Uses

Same as thiopental for:
1. Induction of general anesthesia.
2. As sole agent for minor surgical procedures.
3. As a basal for general anesthesia.

Procedure

1. Prepare a 1% solution by dissolving $\frac{1}{2}$ gram in 50 cc. water.
2. Inject 7–100 mgm. (7–10 cc.).

3. Maintain by fractional doses ranging from 20–40 mgm. (2–4 cc.) at intervals governed by signs of reflex activity.

Comment

1. Methohexital differs from thiopental in being more potent and requiring less total dosage.
2. Do not exceed ½ gram in patients with ordinary tolerance.

Differences from Thiopental

1. A N-methyl barbiturate. Neuromuscular phenomena such as twitchings are more frequent.
2. Less uptake by fat necessitating smaller doses but constant fractionation to maintain even level level of unconsciousness.
3. Induction equally as rapid as with thiopental but recovery more rapid.

Complications

1. Muscle twitchings.
2. Excitation, sneezing, coughing, hiccuping.
3. Laryngospasm.
4. Respiratory depression.
5. Post-anesthetic shivering.

Contraindications

1. Same as for thiopental.
2. Does not cause muscle relaxation.

Methohexital by Continuous Drip

Prepare .2% solution and use in similar manner as thiopental by the drip technique.

REFERENCE

Adriani, John. The Pharmacology of Anesthetic Drugs. 2nd Ed., p. 86. Springfield, Thomas, 1960.

SEDATION AND HYPNOSIS—WITH ULTRA SHORT-ACTING BARBITURATES (DRIP TECHNIQUE)

Principle: A dilute solution of pentothal, surital, or evipal is allowed to infuse intravenously at a rate to maintain hypnosis and sedation.

Uses:

1. For sedation and as adjunct to intravenous anesthesia.
2. For narcointerrogation (crime investigation) and narcoanalysis (psychiatry).
3. For management of convulsive states.

Materials: Same as described for pentothal. In addition 1000 cc. 5% dextrose in distilled water.

Preparation of Patient: Administer anticholinergic drug—atropine or scopolamine.

Procedure:

1. Dissolve 2 gm. pentothal, surital or evipal in 1000 cc. solution.
2. Perform venipuncture and perform sensitivity test by allowing few drops of solution to drip and then clamping tube and waiting several minutes.
3. Commence drip rapidly until patient is unconscious and slow down to maintain narcosis at desired levels.

NARCOINTERROGATION USING PENTOTHAL
(TRUTH SERUM)

Purpose: Narcointerrogation is performed on subject for the purpose of securing information for legal and other purposes. The subject is not a patient in the acceptable sense of the word but should be treated and managed as though he is.

Procedure:

1. Secure proper signed permission with witnesses.
2. Perform test in an operating room where all appliances of an emergency and resuscitative nature are available.
3. Have patient fasting.
4. Premedicate with atropine or scopolamine.
5. Narcotize as described above, using drip technique and pentothal, surital or evipal. Allow patient to lose consciousness. Allow to return to semi-narcotized state at level where conversation is coherent but he obviously is sleepy.

Comment	*Reason*
1. Allow patient to pass into narcotized state and return to semi-narcotized state before beginning interrogation.	Amnesia is not fully developed unless this is done.
2. Restrain patient's legs, arms may be left free.	Patient may roll off bed or table in narcotized state or upon emergence.
3. Allow only authorized persons to be present and interrogate subject.	Medicolegal complications may arise if this is not done.
4. Do not administer drug too rapidly.	Patient passes into deep sleep and does not respond to questioning.
5. Do not exceed 1–1 1/2 grams of pentothal.	If given intermittently the dilute solution permits 2–3 hours interro-

6. Have facilities for urination available.

Polyuria follows use of infusion of glucose and distilled water.

7. Provide a place for recovery of patient after procedure.

Are usually ataxic and drowsy for several hours later.

8. Fasten arm on a board.

Patient moves about and dislodges needle if this is not done.

9. Be prepared to cope with nausea, spasm, apnea and hypotension.

These complications are as apt to occur in this as any other procedure.

10. Administer benzedrine or caffeine (1/2 gram I.M.) when procedure is over.

These act as cortical stimulants and help wake patient up.

BASAL NARCOSIS USING SHORT-ACTING BARBITURATES

Description: A deep hypnosis induced by the intravenous or intramuscular injection of secobarbital (seconal), pentobarbital (nembutal) amobarbital (amytal).

Uses:

1. To "steal" patients who are uncooperative, apprehensive, excitable.
2. For basal narcosis preliminary to general anesthesia.
3. For sedation during regional anesthesia (spinal, etc.).
4. As anti-convulsants.
5. As premedication when intravenous ultra-short-acting barbiturates cannot be used.

Preparations: Seconal dissolved in polyethylene glycol. Pentobarbital in propylene glycol—10%. Amobarbital in water.

Procedure: Seconal, pentobarbital or amobarbital:

1. Slowly administer the selected solution undiluted intravenously in divided doses of 50 mgm. each at 3–5 min. intervals preferably into the infusion tubing until 100–150 mgm. of any of the three drugs has been given stopping if less is required.

Comment

Reason

1. Do not administer more than 150 mgm. at any one time.

Respiratory depression and overdosage may result.

2. Do not give continuously in fractions (like pentothal).

Overdosage results. Drug is not stored in lipoids like pentothal, but passes directly into brain.

3. Allow time for effect to be established (Fig. 94).

Latent period varies from 3–5 minutes for seconal and longer for other drugs.

4. Do not expect profound hypnosis similar to pentothal.

These drugs are not as potent as the thiobarbiturates.

5. Do not use for surgical anesthesia (as when spinal "wears off").   Barbiturates are non-analgesic and do not abolish pain.

6. Supplement with morphine or pentothal if maximum has been given and hypnosis is wearing off.   These drugs fortify the barbiturate which is in tissues and enhances effect.

7. Do not use same dose routinely for everyone.   Remember doses of barbiturates are variable from person to person. Always administer in fractions for this reason.

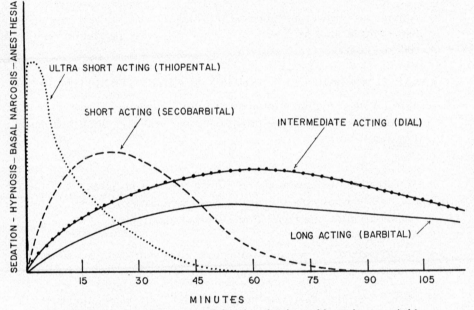

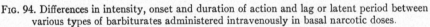

Fig. 94. Differences in intensity, onset and duration of action and lag or latent period between various types of barbiturates administered intravenously in basal narcotic doses.

INTRAVENOUS PARALDEHYDE

Description: Basal narcosis of several minutes' duration followed by a variable period of hypnosis induced by injecting intravenous paraldehyde.

Uses:

1. To rapidly sedate disoriented, unruly subjects (patients with delerium tremens etc.).
2. To control convulsions.

Dosage: Four to five cc. for an adult of average size and weight (150–175 lbs.).

Technique: Inject the pure drug slowly (1 cc. per 30–40 seconds) into suitable vein. Precautions and technique are essentially the same as mentioned above for sodium pentothal.

Contra-Indications:

1. Debilitated, cachetic, or anemic patients.

2. The presence of acute or chronic diseases of the respiratory tract.
3. Acidosis from any cause.
4. Diseases of the liver and kidneys.

INTRAVENOUS ETHER

Description: The administration of ethyl ether in saline by the intravenous route.

Uses:

1. For vasodilatation.
2. For bronchial dilatation (in spasmogenic states).
3. As a fortifying agent for analgesia with basal narcosis.

Procedure:

1. Add ether from freshly opened can to normal saline—about 6 cc. per 100 cc. solution.
2. Shake and siphon off excess floating on surface.
3. Commence drip of solution as rapidly as patient tolerates 80–120 drops per minute.

Objections:

1. Excitement and disorientation common.
2. Large volume of solution required to obtain anesthesia.
3. Coughing, salivation common unless anti-cholinergic drug is used.
4. Hemolysis and hematuria common.
5. Phlebitis may occur.

Comment

1. The ether is excreted by the lungs.
2. Analgesia and hypnosis cannot be obtained by use of ether alone—use basal narcosis.

INTRAVENOUS ETHYL ALCOHOL

Description: The intravenous administration of dilute solutions of ethyl alcohol preoperatively or postoperatively.

Uses:

1. For analgesia, preoperatively or postoperatively.
2. As a source of energy for parenteral feeding.
3. As a vasodilating agent (for the relief of spinal headache, angina pectoris, etc.).
4. As an aid in detoxifying methyl alcohol in poisoning.

Materials:

1. Intravenous set with 18–20 gauge needle.
2. 1000 cc. 5% alcohol in 5% dextrose in distilled water.

Procedure:

1. Perform venipuncture.
2. Commence flow of alcohol solution, giving initial dose of 50 to 200 cc. within 10 to 15 minutes.
3. Adjust the drip to 40 to 80 drops per minute, to suit needs of patient.

Comment

1. Reduce flow if restlessness and signs of inebriation appear.
2. Administer one liter in 3 to 6 hours.
3. Limit total to not more than 3 liters in 24 hours.

Advantages:

1. Does not depress respiration.
2. Does not depress the heart.
3. Acts as a vasodilator.

Disadvantages:

1. Analgesic qualities of alcohol questionable.
2. Patient must be watched closely.
3. Sclerosis of the veins may occur.
4. Cold solutions may initiate pain and discomfort along the course of the veins.
5. Rapid administration may cause inebriation in some patients.
6. Not all patients respond favorably—excitement and little or no analgesia results.

INTRAVENOUS HYDROXYDIONE (VIADRIL)

Principle: Analgesia and basal narcosis induced by injection of the sodium salt of the non-endocrine sterol, Viadril.

Uses:

1. For basal narcosis in conjunction with nitrous oxide, ethylene, cyclopropane, ether and other anesthetics.
2. To supplement spinal anesthesia which is "wearing off."
3. For minor procedures in which analgesia is desired.

Preparation: Same as that for basal narcosis with other intravenous agents.

Premedication: A narcotic (morphine or meperidine) and anticholinergic drug in usual dosages.

Materials:

1. Same arrangement and materials used for pentothal using infusion of 5% glucose in distilled water or saline, 1 gm. ampule of drug.

Procedure:

1. Dissolve the sterol in distilled water to make a 1½ or 2% solution.
2. Introduce in fractions of 1/8–1/4 gm. over 5–10 minute period until 1.0–1.5 grams have been administered and patient is asleep.
3. Commence nitrous oxide or other selected anesthetic.

Characteristics of Drug:

1. Not satisfactory as a sole agent.
2. Onset of action gradual requiring 10–15 minutes for establishment of basal narcosis.
3. Appears to potentiate other analgesics and anesthetics—not satisfactory if used alone except for superficial procedures.
4. Rapid awakening after discontinuance of nitrous oxide or other rapidly eliminated anesthetic.
5. Easily soluble in water to form an alkaline solution (pH 7–8).
6. Single dose sufficient for many hours. Fractionation not required once initial dose is administered.
7. Respiratory depression uncommon.
8. Laryngeal spasm does not occur. Airway tolerated after establishment of narcosis.
9. Nausea and vomiting uncommon in postoperative period.
10. Allows basal narcosis for long operations.
11. Does not disturb cardiac rhythm.
12. Patient may be intubated.

Disadvantages:

1. Phlebitis and thrombosis occur particularly when administered directly into vein without infusion.
2. Tachypnea frequent. Rates as high as 60 noted.
3. Nausea may occur if rapidly injected.
4. Transient hypotension occurs upon injection.
5. Muscle relaxation not always adequate if used alone.
6. Appears to be more effective in older than younger subjects.
7. Long latent or lag period before effects are established.
8. Increases in the pulse rate common.

Comment

1. The average dose appears to be 1 to 1½ gm.
2. The hypotension responds to vasopressors.

3. Muscle relaxation may be augmented by use of succinyl choline.
4. "Lightening" may be overcome by additional narcotic intravenously (meperidine 15 mgm.) instead of the sterol.

NARCOTICS BY THE INTRAVENOUS ROUTE

Definition: Analgesia and sedation induced by injection of narcotics intravenously. Opium alkaloids and their derivatives or synthetic analgesics may be used.

Uses:

1. For rapid premedication for emergency surgery.
2. As a supplemental agent to regional anesthesia.
3. To quickly obtain analgesia for severe pain, from colic, spasm, etc.
4. For sedation and analgesia for endoscopy and other minor procedures.

Dose: The amount required varies with the individual, his age, general state, metabolic rate, and other factors. When morphine is used the average dose is 1/6 to 1/4 gr. The range may be 1/8 to 1/2 gr. Use 1/2 to 2/3 of that which would be used if the subcutaneous route were employed. For other drugs see Table IV.

Technique (Direct injection):

1. Dissolve or dilute the desired dose in normal physiological saline so that each cubic centimeter contains 1/8 gr. of morphine sulphate or equivalent of other narcotic.
2. Draw the solution into a hypodermic syringe attached to a $1\frac{1}{2}$ or 2″ 26-gauge needle and inject it at approximately 1 cc. per minute.

Comment	*Reason*
1. Do not inject the drug rapidly.	Dizziness, tinnitus, or nausea, hypotension and even apnea may result. Cease injection momentarily and proceed at a slower rate if these symptoms appear.
2. Allow a period of ten minutes to elapse prior to induction of anesthesia if the drug is administered for pre-anesthetic medication.	The peak effect is established within 10–15 minutes.
3. Mix narcotic with anticholinergic drug if used for premedication. One part scopolamine hydrobromide to 25 of morphine sulphate or equivalent dose of other narcotic may be combined to enhance effects of the sedative.	The drugs are compatible. The anticholinergic drug is necessary for parasympathetic blockade to prevent secretions from forming and to prevent bradycardia and cardiac irregularities.

4. For direct injection use a longer needle than ordinary hypodermic needle. — The hypodermic needle does not easily enter a vein if less than 1″ long.
5. Inject drug into infusion tubing if a vein has been cannulated. — The saline or other solution acts as the diluent.
6. Do not use in the presence of hepatic or renal disease. — These subjects are sensitive to narcotics.

INTRAVENOUS PROCAINE

Description: The infusion of dilute procaine hydrochloride solution so that the blood concentration is maintained below the subtoxic level. Beneficial effects are supposed to be due to vasodilatation and analgesia.

Uses:

1. For analgesia for minor brief procedures such as removal of dressings, debridements, or first stage of labor.
2. For relief of intractable itching (jaundice).
3. For relief of allergic states—serum sickness, chronic asthma, urticaria, etc.
4. For relief of vasospastic states.
5. To reduce myocardial irritability in thoracic surgery.

Materials:

1. Sterile procaine crystals (1 gm.).
2. Sterile 5% dextrose in distilled water.
3. Dispensing set for infusion.
4. Blood pressure apparatus.

Procedure:

1. Dissolve the procaine in 1000 cc. of dextrose in distilled water.
2. Arrange infusion so that bottle is approximately $3\frac{1}{2}$ to 4 ft. above arm level.
3. Perform venipuncture in the usual manner for infusion and allow solution to drip at the rate of 2 cc. per minute for several minutes.
4. Increase rate to 3 or 4 cc. per minute depending upon the therapeutic response of the patient (tinnitus, diplopia, tremors).

Contra-Indications:

1. Circulatory depression, shock, hypotension etc.
2. Liver or renal disease.
3. Hyperirritable states of nervous system.

Precautions:

1. Perform skin and intranasal tests with the solution before starting infusion if possibility of intolerance to drug exists (Part VI).

2. Do not exceed flow of 4 cc. per minute (1 gm. in 1 hr.)
3. Decrease rate of infusion if dizziness, tremors, excitement or other symptoms of central nervous system stimulation appear.
4. Watch blood pressure and pulse. Procaine is a circulatory depressant.

Comment

1. The procedure is of doubtful value.

REFERENCES

Betlach, C. J. The Intravenous Use of Dilaudid for Analgesia. Anesthesiology, *2:* 171, 1941.
Graubard, H. Intravenous Procaine. Charles C Thomas, Springfield, Ill., 1950.
Presman, David, and Schotz, S. A Critical Analysis of the Intravenous Use of Morphine. Anesthesiology, *4:* 53, 1943.

MUSCLE RELAXANTS AS ADJUNCTS TO ANESTHESIA

Purpose: To cause muscle relaxation by inhibiting transmission of nerve impulses at the myoneural substance of skeletal muscle by the use of blocking agents. The muscle relaxants are non-anesthetic and must therefore be used in combination with anesthetic or analgesic agents. They act by:
1. Preventing the nicotinic action of acetyl choline.
2. Causing persistent depolarization of the membrane at the myoneural junction.

Uses:

1. To obtain relaxation in resistant subjects during cyclopropane or ether anesthesia.
2. To obtain relaxation when light anesthesia is required and deep anesthesia is contraindicated.
3. To obtain relaxation with agents not ordinarily capable of yielding it such as nitrous oxide, ethylene, or pentothal.
4. To obtain relaxation for laryngoscopy and intubations. Used in conjunction with inhalation and local anesthesia for this purpose.
5. As a supplement to spinal or other regional block which is "wearing off" in conjunction with inhalation anesthesia.
6. To control convulsions or muscle spasms during anesthesia.
7. To cause apnea for thoracic surgery or other techniques in which apnea is indicated.

Available Drugs: Curare and a variety of synthetic muscle relaxants are available as adjuncts to anesthesia. Curare is available as an aqueous solution of the mixture of the purified alkaloids. The standard preparation contains 20 units of curare per cc. The purified alkaloid, tubocurarine, which is the active principle, is preferred. The newer drugs are listed in Table VIII.

TABLE VIII

MUSCLE RELAXANTS

Drug	Curare	Tubocurarine	Dimethyl Tubocurarine	Benzoquinonium	Gallamine	Decamethonium	Succinyl Choline
Proprietary name	Intocostrin		Metubine Mecostrin	Mytolon	Flaxedil	Syncurine, C10	Anectine, Succostrin
Onset I.V.-min.	1½-2	1½-2	1½-2	2½-3	1½-2	2-3½	½-1
Peak effect—min.	5	5	5	6-10	2½-6	5	1-2
Duration—min.	25	25	20	15	15	5-12	3
Dose per 70 kgs.—154 lbs.	60-100 units 3-5 cc.	9-15 mgm.	3-16 mgm.	9-15 mgm.	60-80 mgm.	3-4 mgm.	20-40 mgm.
Repeat Dose	⅓ initial	⅓ initial	⅓ initial	⅓	⅓ initial	Tachyphylaxis. Do not use	Use infusion. Approx. 4 mgm. per min.
Dose with Ether	⅓ as much	⅓ as much	⅓ as much	⅓ as much	⅓ as much	No reduction	No reduction
Dose with Cyclopropane	No reduction	No reduction	No reduction	No reduction	No reduction	No reduction	No reduction
Dose with Pentothal, Surital or Evipal	No reduction*	No reduction	No reduction	No reduction	No reduction	No reduction	No reduction
Antagonist	Edrophonium (Tensilon) 5-10 mgm. Neostigmine	Edrophonium (Tensilon) 5-10 mgm. Neostigmine	Edrophonium (Tensilon) 5-10 mgm. Neostigmine	Edrophonium (Tensilon) 5-10 mgm. Neostigmine	Edrophonium (Tensilon) 5-10 mgm. Neostigmine	None available	None Blood transfusion

* Baird's solution 1 cc. (100 units) curare added to 19 cc. 2.5% pentothal contains 5 units per cc.

Dosage: Average size adults tolerate 80–100 units or approximately 0.5 unit per lb. of body weight. Dose varies with the individual and with the anesthetic agent employed and degree of relaxation required.

Procedure Using Curare:

1. Anesthetize the patient with the desired anesthetic agent in the usual manner with the usual premedication.
2. Introduce the estimated quantity of drug into a vein or infusion tube when the skin incision is made. Administer the drug in divided doses of 20 units each allowing 3 minutes between injections.
3. Intubate patient.

Duration: Relaxation of muscles is established within 3 or 4 minutes. Under anesthesia action remains apparent for 30–45 minutes.

Precautions

1. Edrophonium (Tensilon), 5–10 mgm. intravenously should be available to overcome overdosage.

   This drug antagonizes the curare action by retarding destruction of acetyl choline at the nerve endings and by displacing the curare.

2. Intubate the patient and be prepared to do controlled or assisted respiration.

   Complete paralysis of muscles of respiration may follow administration. Hypoventilation common.

3. Take body weight into consideration in estimating dose.

   Large doses may cause death by circulatory failure even though adequate pulmonary ventilation is maintained.

4. Administer drug in divided doses.

   Overdosage is averted thereby.

5. Decrease dose to one-third of average dose when used with ether.

   Ether possesses a curare-like action. Overdosage may result.

6. Use one-third to one-half the initial dose when repeating the drug.

   A cumulative action occurs when the drug is repeated.

7. Do not mix drug with pentothal solutions when using the combination.

   A precipitate forms due to incompatability.

8. Do not use drug intramuscularly for anesthesia.

   Absorption rate is too slow; onset of action is 15 minutes by this route.

9. Do not use without an anesthetic or analgesic drug.

   Curare does not possess any pain relieving properties.

10. Do not use in the presence of renal insufficiency.

    A depressant effect follows due to slow excretion.

11. Watch circulatory system closely.

    A hypotension may follow extreme relaxation.

12. Do not administer to point of apnea.	Large doses may depress centrally.
13. Watch patient closely in postoperative period.	Recurarization may occur due to redistribution of drug.
14. Do not use in dehydrated patients.	These appear to be more sensitive to effects of the drug due to electrolyte imbalance such as hypohalemia.
15. Do not use when acidosis or hypopotassemia is present.	These patients manifest an unusual sensitivity to the drug.
16. Do not use when a bronchial spasm exists or is easily induced (asthma).	Curare and tubocurarine induce a histamine like action.

SUCCINYL CHOLINE (DRIP METHOD)

Principle: Succinyl choline (Anectine, Sucostrin) is rapidly hydrolized by cholinesterase. Its action is brief—several minutes at the most. For sustained effect it must be administered by a continuous drip intravenously.

Uses:

1. To obtain relaxation with general anesthetic agents.
2. To obtain relaxation for electro shock therapy.

Procedure:

1. Add sufficient stock solution of succinyl choline chloride or iodide to normal saline or 5% dextrose in distilled water so that solution has 1 mgm. of drug per cc.
2. Induce anesthesia with desired agent.
3. Permit succinyl choline to pass rapidly into blood stream until 20 mgm. have been given, then pinch tubing.
4. Allow 1–2 minutes to elapse and note effect of this initial dose Add additional 10 mgm. fractions until desired relaxation is obtained.
5. Resume administration at rate required to maintain desired degree of relaxation.

Comment	*Reason*
1. The iodide contains less of the active principle than the chloride.	Iodine has a higher molecular weight than chlorine.
2. Exercise care in administration to cachetic, chronically ill individuals.	The serum cholinesterase may be low in these individuals.
3. Always assure an adequate airway by using an endotracheal tube.	Apnea results. May be sustained in exceptional cases.
4. Use fresh whole blood to overcome prolonged apnea.	Whole blood adds cholinesterase to patients blood.
5. Label bottle conspicuously.	Avoid error. Infusion may be left on after operation.

6. Remember muscle relaxants are not analgesic.   Administer analgesic and hypnotic drugs concomitantly.

Advantages:

1. It is short-acting. The action can be reversed at will.
2. By-products of detoxification are normally found in body (choline and succinic acid).
3. Hydrolized by pseudo-cholinesterase which is found in serum.
4. May be "titrated" to obtain relaxation as desired.
5. Autonomic effects negligible.
6. Does not possess histamine-like action and cause bronchial spasm.
7. Does not ordinarily depress nervous system.

Disadvantages:

1. In some individuals an apnea may result (central depression).
2. No antidote available which is wholly satisfactory.
3. It must be infused for sustained effect.

REFERENCES

Adriani, J. Pharmacology of Anesthetic Drugs. 4th Ed. Pp. 120–135. Charles C Thomas, Springfield, Ill., 1960.
Cullen, S. C. Clinical and Laboratory Observations on the Use of Curare During Inhalation Anesthesia. Anesthesiology, *5:* 166–173, 1944.
Foldes, F. Muscle Relaxants. Charles C Thomas, Springfield, Ill., 1956.
Griffith, H. R., and Johnson, G. E. Use of Curare in General Anesthesia. Anesthesiology, *3:* 418–420, 1942.

INTRAMUSCULAR SECONAL (SECOBARBITAL)

Uses: For premedication in infants and children.

Dose: 3/4–1 mgm. per pound of body weight—1 hour prior to anesthesia in conjunction with anticholinergic drugs.

COMBINATIONS OF MUSCLE RELAXANTS AND THIO-BARBITURATES PENTOTHAL—CURARE—(DRUGS SEPARATE)

Principle: Hypnosis is obtained by the use of the barbiturate and a muscle relaxant. Nitrous oxide is added for analgesia.

Materials:

1. Infusion set.
2. Syringe holder.
3. Three way stopcock.
4. Syringes for pentothal (30–50 cc.).
5. Syringe for relaxant (10 cc.)
6. Airway, resuscitator, Tensilon and other items as above.

Procedure:

1. Commence infusion with saline or 5% dextrose in distilled water.
2. Connect 3 way stopcock and pentothal syringe with infusion.
3. Pinch off infusion tubing and narcotize patient with pentothal (use technique described previously).
4. Add muscle relaxant into infusion tubing in divided doses.
5. Intubate and control or assist respiration.
6. Start nitrous oxide (see table for percentage composition of gas and flow.
7. Add pentothal or curare as each is needed.

PENTOTHAL CURARE MIXTURE (BAIRD'S SOLUTION)

Procedure:

1. Mix 1 cc. "strong" curare (100 units) with 19 cc. 2.5% pentothal. One cc. = 5 units curare.
2. Administer solution slowly until patient is narcotized and relaxed.
3. Intubate and maintain anesthesia by adding fractions are required.

Comment

1. Do not use the more dilute solution of curare—precipitation results.
2. Substitute tubocurarine (3 mgm. per 20 units) for curare if desired.

VARIATIONS FOR ABOVE

Surital, or evipal may be substituted for the barbiturate, and syncurine, flaxedil or mytolon or methyl tubocurarine may be used for the relaxant. (see table for dosage).

PENTOTHAL-SUCCINYL CHOLINE

Procedure:

1. Commence infusion with 3-way stopcock, etc. as described above.
2. Connect 3 way stopcock to syringe containing $2\frac{1}{2}$% pentothal.
3. Mix solution of saline containing 1. mgm. succinyl choline per cc. and connect to stopcock.
4. Narcotize patient with pentothal.
5. Clear pentothal from tubing and needle with infusion fluid to prevent precipitation.
6. Commence succinyl choline allowing 20 mgm. to flow in rapidly.
7. Intubate patient (use topical anesthesia).
8. Alternate pentothal and succinyl choline allowing the succinyl choline to drip at rate necessary to maintain relaxation.
9. Assist or control breathing.

PENTOTHAL-SUCCINYL CHOLINE-NITROUS OXIDE

Procedure:

1. Induce and maintain anesthesia as above carrying patient to apnea and continue to drip succinyl choline maintaining apnea.
2. Control respiration manually or by machine (Part VII).

Comment

1. Procedure hazardous because overconcentration of succinyl choline may result.
2. Procedure not controllable—patient may "wake up" from pentothal and remember events or painful stimulation during operation.

DEMEROL (MEPERIDINE)—PENTOTHAL SUCCINYL CHOLINE DRIP

Principle: Demerol in dilute solution is administered alternately with pentothal in dilute solution.

Procedure:

1. Prepare solution of demerol 0.5 mgm. per cc. in 5% dextrose in distilled water or in saline.
2. Prepare pentothal 1 gm. in 1000 cc. 5% dextrose in distilled water.
3. Prepare succinyl choline 1 mgm. per cc. in saline.
4. Cannulate vein using 3 way stopcock.
5. Administer scopolamine gr. 1/100 I.V. prior to anesthesia.
6. Connect solutions to stopcock.
7. Administer 75–100 mgm. demerol slowly over 5–10 minutes (at rate of 30–40 drops per minute.
8. Administer pentothal to point of loss of consciousness. Administer succinyl choline as needed.
9. Allow demerol to drip as needed. Determine requirements according to respiratory rate of patient and by reflex activity.
10. Add pentothal as required to maintain narcosis. Supplement with nitrous oxide (see table for flow and percentage composition).

REFERENCE

Ausherman, H., Nowill, W. K. and Stephen, C. R. Controlled Analgesia with Continuous Drip Meperidine. Exhibit, A.M.A., June, 1955.

PART V

RECTAL ANESTHESIA

Definition: Anesthesia, analgesia, or amnesia, produced by the rectal instillation of anesthetic or hypnotic drugs.

Available Drugs:

1. *Tribromethanol:* This drug dissolved in amylene hydrate is known as *avertin.* An aqueous solution of avertin is the most commonly employed and most useful agent.
2. *Trichlorethanol:* This drug is similar to tribromethanol and is used for the same purposes, in the same manner.
3. *Paraldehyde:* This drug is frequently employed in oil or in an aqueous solution to produce sedation or basal narcosis.
4. *Ether:* A mixture of ether in oil is used for analgesia.
5. *Barbiturates:* The most useful of this group of drugs are the short-acting-derivatives. They produce an intense, deep hypnosis.

Comment

1. Drugs instilled into the rectum in the form of an enema pass into the colon. The ileocecal valve is not patent. Little absorption occurs from the small intestine, unless the valve is patent.
2. Drugs absorbed from the intestines are carried by the portal system to the liver where they may be modified or stored.
3. The capacity of the rectum varies from one individual to the next but averages between 150 and 200 cc.
4. Rectally administered drugs do not produce complete anesthesia but rather a partial anesthesia or "basal narcosis." Reflexes arising from pain stimuli are rarely abolished by certain non-volatile drugs used for basal narcosis so that supplemental anesthesia is required.

BASAL NARCOSIS WITH AVERTIN

Definition: A deep hypnosis produced by the rectal instillation of an aqueous solution of tribromethanol dissolved in amylene hydrate (avertin fluid).

Description of the drug: Tribromethanol is a solid crystalline substance which is very soluble in amylene hydrate. Avertin is a clear colorless liquid with a camphor-like odor, consisting of one gram of tribromethanol dissolved in one-half gram of amylene hydrate, which equals one cubic centimeter. Therefore, each cubic centimeter of fluid contains 1000 milligrams of tribromethanol.

Uses	*Reasons*
1. For "psychic sedation" in appre-	The drug may be administered to

343

hensive patients (hyperthyroidism, psychoses, neuroses, etc.).

2. To control hyperirritable states of the central nervous system, such as convulsions, tetanus, and similar excitabilities.

3. To relieve "status asthmaticus."

4. For intracranial surgery.

a patient in his bed as a premedicating agent.

The drug is a depressant of the central nervous system, particularly the cerebral cortex.

Tribromethanol causes relaxation of the bronchi.

Tribromethanol causes a lowering of intracranial pressure.

Cubic centimeters of avertin fluid per kilo and per pound of body weight. Use 33 cc. for each cc. of drug to make a 3% solution.

Mgm. Per Kilo.	Cc. Per Kilo.	Cc. Per Lb.
60	0.060	0.0270
65	0.065	0.0295
70	0.070	0.0315
75	0.075	0.0339
80	0.080	0.0360
85	0.085	0.0380
90	0.090	0.0405
95	0.095	0.0427
100	0.100	0.0450
105	0.105	0.0472
110	0.110	0.0493
115	0.115	0.0517
120	0.120	0.0540

Dosage:

Adult—60–80 mgm. per kilogram of body weight in a 3% aqueous solution at 37°–40°C. (100–104°F.) by rectum.

Children—80–100 mgm. per kilogram of body weight in same concentration.

1. The maximum amount under ordinary circumstances should not exceed 8 cc. for females and 10 cc. for males.

2. Increase the dose if the metabolic rate is above normal to 80–100 milligrams per kilogram.

Premedication and Preparation

1. *Morphine*—1/6 to 1/4 gr. one hour before the administration of avertin.

2. *Atropine* or *scopolamine*—1/150 to 1/100 gr. one hour before the

Comment

This drug is omitted by some anesthetists because avertin depresses the respiratory center and the depression from the combination of the two drugs may be severe.

These drugs are used to decrease secretions which may be produced

administration of avertin.

by supplemental inhalation anesthetic drugs.

3. Prescribe a cleansing enema four to five hours or more before time of the operation.

Absorption of the drug will not be satisfactory unless the colon and rectum are evacuated.

4. Weigh patient well in advance of the operation.

The weight of the patient is necessary to calculate the amount of the drug required.

Materials (Fig. 95.)

1. A 25 or 100 cc. container of avertin.
2. A thermometer to measure the temperature of the solution.

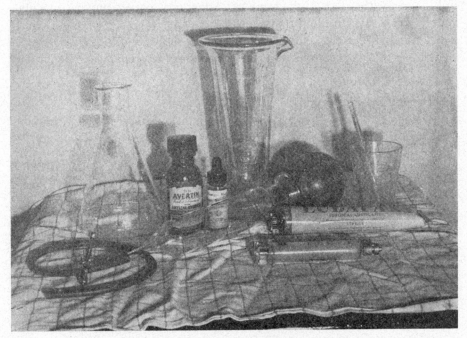

Fig. 95. Assembly for rectal administration of avertin.

3. A rectal catheter, size 16 to 20 French.
4. A glass funnel with stem which fits into the mouth of the rectal catheter.
5. A thin-walled glass flask (preferably a pyrex, Erlenmeyer flask, of 500 cc. capacity).
6. A thermos bottle—500 cc. capacity.
7. A 10 cc. graduated syringe.
8. A 500 cc. graduate.
9. A vial of Congo red indicator (1/1000 aqueous solution).
10. An eye dropper for the Congo red indicator.
11. A pharyngeal airway.

12. A tongue depressor.
13. A sphygmomanometer (the aneroid type is preferred).
14. An ampule of metrazol (1 cc. of 10% solution).
15. A sterile hypodermic syringe and needle for the analeptic.
16. Lubricant for the catheter.
17. A pinch clamp or artery forceps for the catheter.
18. A tray on which utensils for mixing and instilling the drug should be kept.

Calculations of the Required Volume of Drug:

The weight of patient in pounds multiplied by the factor .00045, the result multiplied by the dose (milligrams per kilogram), equals number of cubic centimeters of avertin fluid required.

The number of cubic centimeters of avertin fluid multiplied by 33 equals the number of cubic centimeters of water necessary to prepare a 3% solution.

Example:

Patient's weight is 154 pounds.
Dosage requested by physician is 80 mgm. of tribromethanol per kilogram of body weight.
154 pounds $\times$ .00045 equals .0693.
.0693 $\times$ 80 equals 5.54 cc. avertin fluid.
5.5 $\times$ 33.0 equals 181 cc. water necessary for a 3% solution.

Procedure: Begin preparation of the solution at least 45 minutes before the time of operation. The solution may be prepared in the anesthesia room.

1. Measure the calculated amount of distilled water in the graduate and place it in the thin-walled flask.
2. Warm the water to 103 or 104° F., or 39 to 40° C., by holding the flask in a stream of hot tap water. Use the thermometer.
3. Aspirate the calculated volume of avertin into the 10 cc. calibrated syringe and add it to the warmed water in the flask.
4. Add several drops of Congo red solution to the entire solution—the color should remain red. A blue color indicates that the solution contains an acid and, therefore, decomposition has occurred.
5. Shake mixture until all the avertin is dissolved and no globules are visible at the bottom of the flask.
6. Warm the interior of thermos bottle with hot water and transfer the solution to it.
7. Proceed to the patient's room with the stretcher, an attendant, the prepared solution, and the necessary implements to complete the instillation.
8. Screen the bed, apply the sphygmomanometer, and record the blood pressure, pulse, and respiration.

9. Arrange a draw sheet beneath the patient so he may be removed from the bed when narcotized.

10. Request the patient to turn on his left side and insert the well-lubricated catheter into the rectum for approximately six inches.

11. Attach the funnel to the catheter and instill the entire amount of solution into the rectum as quickly as it will flow by the aid of gravity.

12. Clamp the catheter. Do not remove it from the rectum.

13. Strap the buttocks together with two strips of adhesive which extend from the lateral aspects of the thighs. This prevents expulsion of the catheter and solution.

14. Replace patient in supine position and allow him to remain undisturbed until narcosis ensues.

15. As soon as the patient is narcotized (about 15 minutes), lift him onto the stretcher and remove him from his room to the anesthesia room.

16. Proceed with the supplemental anesthesia selected for the particular case. The following techniques are usually employed:

    a. Nitrous oxide or ethylene with oxygen. If relaxation is desired, ether may be added or a muscle relaxant may be used.

    b. Cyclopropane with a muscle relaxant

    c. Ether, open drop.

    d. Nerve blocks, infiltration or topical anesthesia.

    Supplemental anesthesia is induced and maintained in the same manner as anesthesia without avertin. Many of the signs of anesthesia are obscured by avertin and depth of anesthesia is judged with difficulty.

CHARACTERISTICS OF AVERTIN NARCOSIS

Onset: Consciousness is lost within 5 to 10 minutes. Narcosis is well-established in 30 minutes.

Duration: Narcosis may last anywhere from 1 1/2 to 2 1/2 hours. The duration is variable and unpredictable.

Depth: The stages and planes used as guides during inhalation anesthesia are not applicable to avertin narcosis because:

1. Superficial reflexes are not abolished. Painful stimuli tend to rouse the patient. The drug is not an analgesic.

2. Pharnyngeal and laryngeal stimulation cause gagging.

3. Oculomotor, pupillary, and lid reflexes are abolished as soon as narcosis is established and remain obtunded.

Advantages of Avertin:

1. Patient may be narcotized in his room and taken to the operating room in an unconscious state. Apprehension is avoided.

2. The onset of narcosis is rapid and recovery is gradual. The pre-anesthetic and post-anesthetic periods are clouded by amnesia.

3. Excitement during induction is uncommon.
4. There is a decrease in metabolic rate and reduced reflex irritability.

Disadvantages	*Reasons*
1. The depth of narcosis is uncontrollable.	Once the drug is administered it cannot be retrieved even when the rectum is emptied. One must rely upon the mechanism of detoxification for elimination from the tissues.
2. The dose is difficult to estimate accurately.	Susceptibility to the drug varies between different individuals.
3. The superficial reflexes are not completely abolished. The narcosis must be supplemented by inhalation or regional anesthesia in order to abolish all reflexes.	Pathways from periphery to cortex are not completely blocked during narcosis as with some agents.
4. The duration of the narcosis varies and is not predictable (usually $1\frac{1}{2}$ to $2\frac{1}{2}$ hours).	It is influenced by the rate of absorption, elimination, and metabolic state of the subject which are variable.
5. Narcosis is frequently induced in locations and in situations where oxygen and appliances for resuscitation are not instantly available.	The drug is usually administered in the patient's room.
6. The circulatory, respiratory, and other physiological functions are disturbed.	Profound pharmacological changes are common.
7. Excitement during emergence is occasionally observed.	Usually it is precipitated by stimulation, particularly by pain.

Contra-Indications	*Reasons*
1. Acute or chronic infections of the respiratory tract.	Secretions may cause coughing or precipitate laryngeal spasm. The reflexes in the respiratory tract are obtunded but not completely abolished.
2. Diseases accompanied by a decrease in vital capacity.	A marked depression of respiration occurs due to medullary depression. It invariably occurs if large doses are employed.
3. Diseases of the heart—hypertension, hypotension, anemias, and other circulatory disturbances.	Hypotension, characterized by a fall in systolic pressure and a decrease in pulse pressure, is common. Respiratory depression may affect the circulation secondarily.

4. Nephritis and other diseases accompanied by renal insufficiency. The products of detoxification are eliminated by the kidneys.

5. Diseases of the liver or other conditions accompanied by hepatic insufficiency. Liver function is decreased during avertin narcosis. The drug is detoxified by the liver by conjugation with glycuronic acid.

6. Diabetes or acidosis from any cause. The carbon dioxide combining power is decreased by avertin. Carbon dioxide is retained due to the respiratory depression.

7. Diseases of or operations upon the rectum or colon. The solution may irritate the mucosa of the rectum or may not be entirely absorbed and interfere with the operation.

COMPLICATIONS

1. *Respiratory failure*—Caused by overdosage or asphyxia due to obstruction. Treat by:
   a. Artificial respiration.
   b. Analeptic drug, such as metrazol or bemegrid, intravenously.
   c. Empty the rectum by loosening the clamp on the catheter.
2. *Failure to obtain narcosis*
   a. Dose was underestimated or incorrectly calculated.
   b. The drug was not thoroughly dissolved.
   c. The solution was expelled around the catheter or the catheter was not left *in situ*.
   d. The cleansing enema was omitted or not satisfactory, or the avertin was administered too soon after the enema.
   e. The avertin was not added to the water.
   f. The patient is "resistant" to the drug.
3. *Circulatory failure*
   a. The drug was given to a patient with a circulatory deficiency.
   b. Overdosage—circulation fails secondary to respiration.
4. *Proctitis*—Follows the use of decomposed or overheated solutions of the drug.
5. *Prolonged drowsiness*—Usually due to:
   a. Overdosage or incorrectly calculated dose.
   b. The presence of hepatic or renal insufficiency or other disturbances which prevent normal detoxification.
   c. Use of the drug in aged individuals.
   d. The use of repeated successive doses of the drug.
   e. Prolonged use of supplemental agents such as ether.
   f. Use of another nonvolatile drug in conjunction with avertin.
6. *Skin rash*—This is uncommon but is possibly caused by elimination of compounds containing bromine which is derived from the avertin.

7. *Overdosage*—This is caused by:
   a. Careless preparation of solutions.
   b. Incorrect weight used for calculations.
   c. Calculations incorrect.
   d. Error in estimation of dose required for the particular patient.

Comment	*Reasons*
1. Remain with the patient from the moment of injection of drug until complete recovery has occurred.	Relaxation of pharyngeal structures and falling backward of the tongue cause asphyxia from respiratory obstruction.
2. Do not insert artificial airways into the pharynx unless absolutely necessary.	The pharyngeal and laryngeal reflexes are not abolished during avertin narcosis. Coughing or retching occurs unless supplemental anesthesia is employed.
3. Administer the solution at least 30 minutes before the scheduled time of operation.	Absorption of the drug and establishment of complete narcosis may require at least 30 minutes.
4. Use only freshly prepared solutions.	The drug is easily decomposed by light, heat, or air. Solutions which are allowed to stand any length of time become impure.
5. Avoid overheating the solution.	Irritating byproducts (hydrobromic acid and aldehydes) may form.
6. Maintain the solution at body temperature until it is injected.	Patients expel cold solutions. The solubility of the drug decreases as the temperature falls and the drug may precipitate from the solution.
7. Shake the solution well and be positive that the drug is completely dissolved.	Undissolved avertin sinks to the bottom of the flask when added to water and remains there after watery portion is drawn off. Underdosage results.
8. Always use distilled water to prepare avertin solution.	Tap water may contain minerals and salts which hasten deterioration of the drug.
9. Never use an old or deteriorated solution.	Proctitis or colitis may result.
10. Support the chin constantly to maintain an unobstructed airway.	Obstruction to respiration may easily result from the relaxation of the tongue and muscles of the neck.
11. Always apply restraints to the patient on the stretcher when en route to operating room. Observe	The patient may not be completely narcotized and suffer injury should restlessness or excitement ensue.

similar precautions when patient is on the table during the pre-operative period in the operating room.

12. Record blood pressure, pulse, and respiratory rate every *five minutes* after the patient is narcotized.

Circulatory and respiratory depression may develop rapidly in some circumstances.

13. Reexamine the calculations if more than 8 cc. of avertin fluid are required. There is possibility of an error.

Maximum dose should not exceed 10 cc. unless patient is large.

14. Do not attempt to use avertin alone for complete anesthesia. Always use supplemental agents.

Pathways from periphery to the cortex are not completely blocked. Other drugs are necessary to assist in abolishing reflexes.

15. Do not administer repeated successive doses of avertin except in instances of sustained stimulation (tetanus, convulsions, etc.).

The drug may accumulate in tissues due to slow detoxification and cause prolonged, sustained depression.

16. Store avertin in a cool place.

Heat, light, and oxygen hasten the decomposition of the drug.

17. Remember that amylene hydrate possesses mild narcotic properties.

The drug is a tertiary amyl alcohol.

"Stealing" a Patient with Avertin

Definition: The administration of avertin to a patient without his being aware of the fact that he is to be narcotized and undergo surgery.

Uses: For performing operations upon extremely apprehensive patients. The procedure was widely employed for preparation of patients with thyrotoxicosis.

Procedure:

1. Weigh patient several days before the operation and estimate the volume of avertin solution which will be required.
2. Administer an enema consisting of a volume of physiological saline equivalent to the volume of avertin solution. Add several drops of Congo red to the saline and instill by the same technique as described for avertin.
3. Remove the catheter after several hours.
4. Repeat the instillation of saline for two or three days before the operation at approximately the same time of day the operation is to be performed.
5. Substitute the solution of avertin for the saline on the scheduled day of operation.

Comment

1. Administer the saline solution in exactly the same manner as the avertin.
2. Select one individual to administer all the enemas and caution him not to vary the technique at any time.
3. Do not administer the premedication until patient is narcotized by the avertin.
4. Do not apply the sphygmomanometer until the patient is narcotized.
5. Instruct nurses and attendants not to discuss the procedure or mention details of surgery to the patient.
6. Instruct nurses, operating room attendants, and others not to enter patient's room until narcosis is established.
7. Do not transfer the patient to the stretcher until narcosis is established.

REFERENCES

Adriani, John. Pharmacology of Anesthetic Drugs. 3rd Ed. Page 57. Charles C Thomas, Springfield, Ill., 1955.
Council of Pharmacy and Chemistry, Report, J.A.M.A., *109:* 953, 1937.
Waters, R. M., and Muehlberger, C. W. Avertin, Arch. Surg., *21:* 887, 1930.

BASAL NARCOSIS WITH TRICHLORETHANOL

Definition: A deep hypnosis produced by the rectal administration of an aqueous solution of trichlorethanol.

Uses: Same as for avertin.

Description: Trichlorethanol is a clear, colorless liquid possessing an ethereal odor. No amylene hydrate is required as a solvent because the drug is a liquid.

Cost: Relatively inexpensive. The manufacture of the drug is not restricted by patent, as is avertin.

Dose: For adults, 100–125 mgm. per kilogram. The specific gravity of the drug is 1.550. Therefore, 1 cc. equals 1,550 milligrams of drug.

Calculations of Required Volume of Drug:

The weight of the patient in pounds multiplied by .00045, multiplied by milligrams per kilogram, divided by 1.55 equals the number of cubic centimeters of trichlorethanol fluid required.

The number of cubic centimeters of trichlorethanol multiplied by 33 equals the number of cubic centimeters of water required to make a 3% solution.

Example: Patient's weight is 154 pounds.

Dosage requested by physician is 100 mgm. per kilogram of body weight. 154×0.00045 equals .0693.

.0693×100, divided by 1.55 equals 4.60 cc. trichlorethanol fluid required. 4.6×33.0 equals 151.8 cc. water necessary to make approximately a 3% solution.

Premedication: Same as for avertin.

Materials: Same as for avertin.

Procedure: Prepare and administer the solution in the same manner as avertin.

Advantages: Its advantages over other drugs are the same as for avertin. It is superior to avertin in the following ways:

1. It is less expensive.
2. It is somewhat more stable.
3. It does not require amylene hydrate or other solvents as a vehicle.

Disadvantages: Its disadvantages over other drugs are the same as for avertin. It is inferior to avertin in the following ways:

1. It is less potent.
2. Its response and duration of action are more variable.
3. It causes a more pronounced respiratory depression.
4. Its dose is judged with more difficulty and the results are more variable.
5. The duration of hypnosis is shorter.

Comment

1. The chemical configurations for tribromethanol and trichlorethanol are the same, save that the halogen atoms differ.
2. The solution should be mixed, warmed, tested, and administered in the same manner as avertin.

REFERENCES

Adriani, John. Pharmacology of Anesthetic Drugs. 3rd Ed. P. 58. Charles C Thomas, Springfield, Ill., 1955.

Case, E. H. Present Status of Trichlorethanol. Anesthesiology, *4:* 523, September, 1943.

Molitor, H., and Robinson, H. Pharmacological Properties of Trichlorethanol. Anesth. and Analg., *17:* 258, September, 1938.

Wood, D. A. Avertin: An Appreciation and Comparison. Anesth. and Analg., *17:* 252, September, 1938.

PARALDEHYDE

Definition: Analgesia and hypnosis produced by the rectal instillation of aqueous or oily solutions of paraldehyde.

Uses:

1. For sedation in apprehensive subjects. The drug is employed, particularly for chronic alcoholic addicts and psychopathic subjects.
2. For analgesia in obstetrics.
3. For basal narcosis in inhalation anesthesia.

Cost: A relatively inexpensive drug.

Description: A colorless, mobile, slightly water-soluble liquid, with a pungent, fruity, penetrating odor.

Dose: 1.0 to 1.5 cc. per 10 pounds of body weight.

Materials:

1. Paraldehyde (U.S.P.).

2. Benzyl alcohol (N.N.R.).
3. A rectal instillation set similar to that employed for avertin.

Premedication: Morphine, gr. 1/6 to 1/4, 3/4 to 1 hour previous to instillation. Atropine or scopolamine, gr. 1/150 to 1/100, 3/4 to 1 hour previous to instillation.

Technique:

1. Measure required volume of paraldehyde and add to it 1.5 cc of benzyl alcohol. Use the lower limit dosage for obese, extremely old or young subjects. Mix well. Follow the routine described under avertin for the instillation.
2. Allow solution to flow by gravity into the rectum. It should flow as rapidly as possible.
3. Follow with 30 cc. of physiological saline to rinse out the catheter tube and dissipate the drug in rectum and colon.
4. Clamp the catheter and follow directions described for avertin.
5. Repeat dose when necessary.

Advantages: It is a non-toxic drug in hypnotic doses.

Disadvantages:

1. It is partly eliminated through the lungs and causes irritation and salivation.
2. It possesses a clinging odor which persists for several days in the vicinity of the patient.
3. It is irritating to the mucous membranes of the rectum and colon.
4. Its dose is estimated with difficulty because susceptibility varies between individuals.
5. Its depth and duration of narcosis are non-controllable.

Contra-Indications:

1. Chronic infections of respiratory tract or any disease in which the vital capacity is decreased.
2. Diabetes or acidosis from any cause.
3. Diseases of the kidney or liver.
4. Diseases of the colon or rectum.

Comment

1. Observe the usual precautions for rectal anesthesia with avertin.
2. Do not omit the benzyl alcohol. It acts as a local anesthetic and prevents irritation to the rectal mucosa.

REFERENCE

Kane, H. F., and Roth, G. B. Combined Oral and Rectal Administration of Paraldehyde for the Relief of Labor Pains. Anesth. and Analg., *19:* 282, September, 1940.

ETHER IN OIL RECTALLY ADMINISTERED

Definition: Analgesia, or anesthesia, depending upon dose and state of subject, produced by the rectal instillation of ethyl ether in oil.

Uses:

1. For analgesia or anesthesia for surgery (superficial operations).
2. For analgesia in obstetrics.
3. For relief of "status asthmaticus."

Cost: The ether-oil technique is inexpensive.

Materials: The utensils and instruments listed for avertin are satisfactory for ether and oil.

1. Ether (U.S.P. for anesthesia).
2. Olive, cottonseed, or other bland vegetable oil.
3. Rectal catheter, 16–20 French.
4. A glass funnel approximately 2 inches in diameter with a stem which fits into catheter.
5. One graduated syringe (10 cc.) to measure ether and oil.
6. A pharyngeal airway and tongue depressor.
7. A clamp for the catheter.
8. Anesthesia apparatus with inhaler for resuscitation and rebreathing.

Dosage for Adults:

1. 3/4 to 1 cc. ether per pound of body weight. The usual preparations consist of a mixture of 50 to 65% ether in bland oil (1 cc. ether:1 cc. oil to 1 cc. ether:1/2 cc. oil).
2. Use the lower limit of the dose except for obese, large subjects.
3. Do not exceed 160 cc. ether, regardless of the weight of the patient.

Premedication:

1. Paraldehyde, 7.5 cc. to 15 cc. in an equal volume of oil by rectum, one hour prior to administration of ether (use technique described below for premedication).
2. Morphine sulphate, gr. 1/6 to 1/4   ⎰one hour prior to adminis-
   Atropine or scopolamine, 1/150 to 1/100⎰tration of ether.
3. Cleansing enema 3 to 4 hours prior to instillation (as for avertin).

Procedure: Follow the routine described for avertin:

1. Instill the mixture 20 minutes before hypnosis is desired.
2. Place patient in Sim's position or on left side.
3. Lubricate the anus and surrounding skin with vaseline to prevent irritation.

4. Insert the catheter approximately six inches into the rectum.
5. Allow the solution to flow into the rectum by gravity as rapidly as possible.
6. Clamp but allow the catheter to remain in place. Strap buttocks (as for avertin) to prevent expulsion of the solution.
7. Return the patient to the supine position and observe the airway closely and insert the artificial airway if necessary.
8. Attach the inhaler arranged for rebreathing, fill with oxygen, and allow the patient to rebreathe the exhaled ether.

Signs of Anesthesia: These are exactly the same as for ether anesthesia by inhalation.

Advantages: The analgesic effects of ether can be utilized to better advantage by this method than by inhalation.

Disadvantages:

1. The depth of anesthesia is non-controllable. Once the drug is administered, it is difficult to retrieve.
2. The dosage cannot be estimated accurately. Instillation may have to be repeated or supplemented. Inhalation or other forms of anesthesia may be required.
3. The duration of action is unpredictable. It varies with size and metabolic state of the patient.
4. It possesses the same pharmacological disadvantages as ether by inhalation.
5. The greater part of it must be eliminated by the lungs.
6. Excitement and salivation are common during induction or recovery.

Contra-Indications: These are the same as for ether by inhalation.

Complications:

1. Overdosage—this is characterized by respiratory failure as with ether by inhalation.
2. Proctitis—this is due to the irritating action of ether upon the mucosa.
3. Respiratory obstruction—this is due to relaxation and obstruction of the airway, as in inhalation anesthesia.
4. Excitement—this is caused by ineffective premedication, insufficient ether, or slow absorption.
5. Salivation—this results because the belladonna alkaloid is ineffective or has been omitted.
6. Failure to obtain narcosis—this results because the solution is expelled or there has been underdosage.

Comment	Reasons
1. Do not warm the solution.	Ether is highly volatile and passes off.
2. Prepare the solution at the time of injection.	This precludes the possibility of irritation from decomposed ether.
3. Do not omit premedication.	Salivation, mucus formation, and excitement are common without it.
4. Always have an inhaler available for instant use.	Overdosage may readily occur in such an uncontrollable technique.
5. Employ the 65% solution for rapid induction and more intense narcosis.	The absorption of ether is retarded by the oil.

ETHER OIL IN OBSTETRICS

Premedication: Pentobarbital, three grains orally at onset of pain.

Dosage:

Ether, 60 cc. (2 oz.)
Paraldehyde, 7.5 cc. (0.25 oz.).
Olive oil, 120 cc. (4 oz.).

Technique: Same as above.

Comment

1. Be sure catheter passes beyond presenting part of fetus.
2. Repeat every several hours if necessary.
3. Supplement by inhalation anesthesia if necessary.

REFERENCES

Gwathmey, J. T. *Ether-Oil Anesthesia.* Lancet, 2: 1756–1758, December, 1913.
Gwathmey, J. T. Obstetrical Analgesia. Surg. Gyn. Obs., *51:* 190, August, 1930.

RECTAL PENTOTHAL

Definition: Basal narcosis by the rectal instillation of an aqueous solution of sodium pentothal.

Uses:

1. As a preliminary to surgical anesthesia for children and other subjects in whom intravenous administration of drugs is not feasible.
2. To control convulsive states.
3. To perform diagnostic and non-painful minor procedures such as X-ray examinations, endoscopic examinations, etc.

Materials:

1. Large syringe (20–30 cc.) of the bulb type or one with long nipple.
2. Rectal catheter of desired size (14–18F.) which attaches to syringe.
3. Lubricant.
4. 2 strips of adhesive for strapping buttocks together.
5. Clamp or artery forceps for catheter.
6. Pentothal for rectal use.
7. Distilled water or normal saline.

Preparation of Patient:

1. Cleanse colon with a saline enema at least 6 hours before induction time (night before preferable).
2. Administer scopolamine, hyoscyamine or atropine in proper dosage (see premedication).

Dosage:

a. Heavy basal narcosis—1 gm. for each 50 lbs. of body weight.
b. Light basal narcosis—1 gm. per 75 lbs. body weight.
c. Hypnosis—1 gm. per 100 lbs. body weight.

Procedure:

1. Dissolve pentothal in water warmed about body temperature to make a 10% solution. Draw into syringe.
2. Attach catheter to syringe and lubricate tip.
3. Turn patient on left side and insert catheter 4 or 5 inches into the rectum.
4. Instill solution as fast as patient tolerates it.
5. Draw small amount of saline or water into syringe and force into catheter to wash out solution remaining in catheter into rectum.
6. Clamp catheter and remove syringe.
7. Strap buttocks together to help retain catheter in place.

Onset of Action:

1. Within 5 minutes. Peak attained in 15 minutes.

Duration:

1. About one hour.

Advantages:

1. Does not irritate the mucosa.
2. Precipitation due to cooling does not occur (with avertin it does).
3. Duration of basal narcosis longer than by intravenous route.

4. May be administered at bedside.
5. Induces amnesia and hypnosis without excitement.
6. Reduces post-anesthetic nausea and vomiting.
7. Permits use of drug when intravenous route is not feasible.
8. May be used in infants and children.

Disadvantages:

1. May cause respiratory depression.
2. Response variable due to variation in individual tolerance.
3. Laryngeal spasm may occur.
4. Patient rouses when stimulated unduly.

Contra-Indications:

1. Conditions characterized by respiratory depression, dyspnea, pulmonary insufficiency or obstruction.
2. Suppurative diseases of the respiratory tract with secretions. Spasm results.
3. Cardiac diseases with decompensation.
4. Hypotensive states particularly if due to reduced blood volume.
5. Renal disease with insufficiency.
6. Dehydration with electrolyte disturbances.
7. Anemia of sufficient degree to reduce oxygen carrying power of blood.
8. Inflammatory diseases of the rectum.
9. As a sole anesthetic agent for procedures in which painful stimulation occurs.
10. Debilitated subjects and subjects in older age groups.

Comment	*Reason*
1. Follow precautions listed under avertin.	Basic principles of rectal anesthesia are same for all drugs.
2. Omit enema if time of administration is less than 5–6 hours prior to anesthesia.	Stasis of fluid dilutes solution and inhibits proper absorption of drug.
3. Use saline for enema.	Soap irritates mucosa. Fluid may be retained for sometime after enema.
4. Do not exceed a total of three grams.	Overdosage may occur.
5. Have ephedrine, metrazol or picrotoxin available.	These are effective in combating respiratory and circulatory depression.
6. Do not introduce artificial airways unless absolutely necessary during basal narcosis.	Laryngeal spasm may result.

7. Reduce dose for states characterized by low metabolic rate.

Such patients are less tolerant to non-volatile drugs.

8. Omit narcotics for premedication in children.

Resiratory depression may occur.

9. Non-sterile tap water may be used to prepare solution.

Satisfactory if distilled water is not available.

10. Administer only to fasting patients.

Vomiting and aspiration may occur if patient has full stomach.

11. Although more concentrated solutions are preferred solutions as dilute as 2% may be used.

Large volume is chief objection to dilute solution.

RECTAL EVIPAL

Follow same procedure as that described for rectal pentothal using same dose and concentration.

RECTAL SURITAL

Follow same procedure as that described for rectal pentothal using same dose and concentration.

RECTAL METHOHEXITAL (*Brevital*)

Follow same procedure as that described for rectal pentothal using half the dose and concentration.

PART VI

REGIONAL ANESTHESIA
GENERAL CONSIDERATIONS OF REGIONAL
ANESTHESIA

Definition:

Anesthesia produced by applying a drug at a point along the course of a nerve and abolishing conduction of afferent and efferent impulses through the segment affected.

Synonyms:

Conduction anesthesia; block anesthesia.

Types:

Regional anesthesia is subdivided into various types classified according to the site of application of the drug (Fig. 96).

1. *Spinal:* The spinal nerves are blocked at the anterior and posterior roots in the subarachnoid space (Fig. 96A).
2. *Epidural:* The spinal nerves are blocked in the epidural space (Fig. 96B) after acquiring a dural sheath.
3. *Paravertebral:* The spinal nerves are blocked as they emerge from the intervertebral foramina, or in the vicinity of the vertebrae (Fig. 96C).
4. *Nerve:* The somatic nerves are blocked at some point along their course to the periphery of the body before they divide into their terminal branches (Fig. 96D).
5. *Field:* The large terminal branches are blocked by injecting a wall of local anesthetic drug at the border of the area they supply just as they branch (Fig. 96E).
6. *Topical* ⎫ The nerve end-
7. *Infiltration* ⎬ ings are anesthetized by injecting

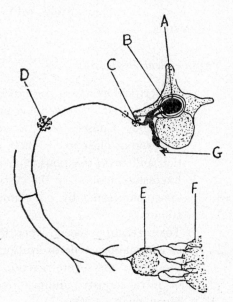

Fig. 96. Types of regional blocks. (A) Subarachnoid or spinal. (B) Epidural. (C) Paravertebral. (D) Nerve block. (E) Field block. (F) Infiltration. (G) Sympathetic block. Note that in field block the nerves are anesthetized as they divide into terminal branches. In infiltration, and topical the nerve endings are anesthetized.

or spreading the drug in the area they supply (Fig. 96F).

361

LOCAL ANESTHETIC DRUGS

Although numerous local anesthetic drugs have been prepared and are in use, all in current use possess certain common physical, chemical, and physiological properties. The most important of these may be summarized as follows:

Physical and Chemical Properties:

1. They are synthetic substances (except cocaine).
2. They are basic substances possessing complex molecular structures. The majority are amines. Most of them are esters.
3. They form salts with mineral and organic acids. The salts of hydrochloric acid are the most common. The salt is more stable and soluble in water than the free base. Aqueous solutions of salts are acid in reaction. (pH 6±)
4. The base is more soluble in oils and other lipoids. Aqueous solutions are alkaline. The free base is easily precipitated by alkalis from aqueous solutions of salts.
5. They are incompatible with salts of mercury, silver, and other metals.

Physiological Properties:

1. The critical effective concentration of a drug which penetrates a nerve is higher than the blood concentration which gives rise to toxic manifestations. Consequently, the drug must be localized in as small an area and as close to the nerve as possible to prevent systemic absorption and toxic reactions.
2. Excessive amounts in the systemic circulation give rise to toxic reactions manifested by circulatory collapse or central nervous system stimulation.
3. Toxic reactions occur when the rate of absorption exceeds the rate of elimination or detoxification. A large amount slowly absorbed may produce a less severe reaction than a small amount quickly absorbed or intravenously administered. The response obtained varies with blood levels.
4. Systemically small amounts are violent central nervous system stimulants or cardiac depressants; large amounts are profound central nervous system depressants and cause paralysis. Sedative drugs, particularly the barbiturates, antagonize the stimulation of the nervous system but do not protect the heart.
5. The duration of action, local tissue reactions, and effect upon various components of the nervous system vary with and are dependent upon

TABLE X

CURRENTLY EMPLOYED LOCAL ANESTHETIC DRUGS

Name	Synonym	Salt	Use				
			Spinal Block	Epidural Block	Nerve Block	Field Block and Infiltration	Topical
Procaine U.S.P.	Neocaine Novocaine	Hydro-chloride	Widely employed 50–150 mg.	Recom-mended 50 cc. 2%	Widely employed 50 cc. 2%	Widely employed 100 cc. 1%	Possesses no action
Cocaine U.S.P.		Hydro-chloride	Not employed	Not employed	Not employed	Not employed	Useful (with caution!) 4%
Pontocaine N.N.R.	Tetracaine U.S.P. Pantocaine	Hydro-chloride	Widely employed 5–20 mgm.	Employed 50 cc. 0.10%	Employed with caution 75 cc. 0.10%	Not employed 100 cc. of 0.1%	Useful (with caution!) 2%
Nupercaine N.N.R.	Percaine Dibucaine	Hydro-chloride	Widely employed 2½–15 mgm.	Not employed	Not recom-mended 0.1%	Not recom-mended 0.05–0.1%	Useful (with caution!)
Butyn U.S.P.	Butacaine	Sulphate	Not employed	Not employed	Not employed	Not employed	Useful 2%
Metycaine N.N.R.	Neothesine Piperocaine	Hydro-chloride	Widely employed 75–125 mgm.	Widely employed 50 cc. 1.5%	Widely employed 50 cc. 1.5%	Widely employed 75 cc. 1%	Useful 3%
Benzocaine U.S.P.	Anesthesin	Not employed	Ineffec-tive	Ineffec-tive	Ineffec-tive	Ineffective	Useful 20%
Benzyl Alcohol N.N.R.		None	Not useful	Not useful	Not useful	Not useful	Useful 4%
Monocaine		Formate	Recom-mended 50–100 mgm.	Useful 1.5%	Useful 1%	Useful 1%	Not employed
Nesacaine	Chlor-procaine		Useful 50–100 mgm.	Useful 50cc. 2%	Useful 50 cc. 2%	Useful 1% up to 100 cc.	Not employed
Apothesene N.N.R.		Hydro-chloride	Useful	Not employed	Useful 1%	Useful 0.5%	Not useful
Butescin		Picrate	Not employed	Not employed	Not employed	Not employed	Useful
Lidocaine N.N.R.	Xylocaine	Hydro-chloride	Not employed	2% 25–35 cc.	30 cc. 2%	50 cc. 1%	5%
Hexylcaine	Cyclaine	Hydro-chloride	20–50 mgm.	2% 25–35 cc.	30 cc. 2%	50 cc. 1%	5%
Perido-caine	Lucaine	Hydro-chloride	50–100		2%	1%	
Carbocaine	Mepi-vacaine	Hydro-chloride	50–100	25–50 cc. 2%	2%	1%	

the chemical nature of the drug. The properties vary from drug to drug.

6. Each possesses a latent period which varies with the chemical nature of the drug and the concentration. Time interval between moment of application of drug on nerve until blockade is completely established is greater for longer lasting drugs as a rule.
7. They are potentiated by proteins, potassium ion, xanthines and numerous other substances.
8. The action is reversible. The conduction in the nerve fibre is restored to normal when the drug is removed or eliminated.
9. They are detoxified by the liver. The more easily and quickly they are detoxified the less toxic the drug.
10. The effective concentration varies with the size of nerve fibre. Sensory fibres are smaller and affected before motor fibres. Stronger concentrations are necessary for penetration into sheathed and myelinated fibres.

The comparative toxicity and potency of local anesthetic drugs are difficult to establish because these factors not only vary from one species to the next, but also with the mode of administration, rate of administration, concentration employed, and rate of absorption within a given species.

Characteristics of a Suitable Anesthetic Drug:

1. Onset of action should be rapid, consuming not more than a few minutes.
2. Duration of action should allow sufficient time to complete the operation.
3. There should be freedom from local irritation to the nerves or tissues.
4. Systemic toxicity should be low.
5. The drug should be soluble in water.
6. The drug should be stable and boilable.
7. It should be compatible with vasoconstrictors and with components of tissue fluid.

Approximate values for toxicity and potency of some common drugs (cocaine = 1):

TABLE XI

Drug	Toxicity	Potency
Cocaine Hydrochloride	1	1
Procaine Hydrochloride	$\frac{1}{4}$	$\frac{1}{5}$
Metycaine Hydrochloride	$\frac{1}{4}$	$\frac{1}{4}$
Pontocaine Hydrochloride	3	2
Butyn Sulphate	$\frac{3}{4}$	$\frac{1}{4}$
Nupercaine Hydrochloride	3 to 5	$2\frac{1}{2}$

Use of Procaine in Regional Anesthesia

Procaine hydrochloride is the least toxic and most useful of all the local anesthetic drugs, and, therefore, the drug of choice. The duration of action averages approximately one hour. The hydrochloride is dissolved in aqueous physiological saline or distilled water.

TABLE XII

Concentration	Uses	Maximum Dose
0.5%	Infiltration, skin wheals, subcutaneous injection	200 cc.
1.0%	Infiltration, field blocks	100 cc.
2.0%	Nerve, epidural, and para-vertebral blocks	50 cc.
5.0%	Spinal anesthesia	2 cc.
10.0%	Spinal anesthesia	1.5 cc.

Comment:

1. Decrease the dose for debilitated, cachetic, or aged subjects.
2. Boil sterile physiological saline, add the desired weight of procaine hydrochloride crystals, and boil three minutes longer to prepare a sterilized solution of the drug.

TABLE XIII

COMPARATIVE DOSAGE OF LOCAL ANESTHETICS

	CC's of Drug Equivalent to 1 cc. Procaine			
Procaine Maximum Volume	2% 50 cc.	1% 100 cc.	.5% 200 cc.	.25% 400 cc.
Pontocaine	.15% 1 cc.	.1% 1 cc.	.05% 1 cc.	.02% 1 cc.
Metycaine	1.5% 1 cc.	.75% 1 cc.	.50% 1 cc.	.25% 1 cc.
Xylocaine	1% ½ to 1 cc.	.5% ½ to 1 cc.	.25% ½ to 1 cc.	.1% ½ to 1 cc.
Carbocaine	2% ¾–1 cc.	1% ¾–1 cc.	.5% ¾–1 cc.	.25% ¾–1 cc.
Cyclaine	2% ¾ cc.	1% ¾ cc.	.5% ¾ cc.	.25% ¾ cc.
Nesacaine	2% ¾ cc.	1% ¾ cc.	.5% ¾ cc.	.25% ¾ cc.

Use of Vasoconstrictor Drugs in Regional Anesthesia

Purpose:

1. To produce local vasoconstriction for the prevention of rapid absorption of local anesthetic drugs. Toxicity is decreased and the action is prolonged thereby.

2. To overcome hypotension caused by vasomotor disturbances resulting from regional anesthesia.

Drugs available: The sympathomimetic amines are the most useful vasopressor drugs. *For infiltration,* epinephrine and cobefrin are preferred. *For hypotension,* ephedrine, neosynephrine, epinephrine, oenethyl, methedrine, and methoxamine (vasoxyl) are employed.

Uses:

1. To prolong anesthesia:

Epinephrine: a stock solution, 1:1000 (U.S.P.), is added to the local anesthetic solution. The dilution employed varies from 1/10,000 to 1/100,000, depending upon the physiological status of the patient and the preference of the surgeon. Usually 1:100,000 is ample.

Cobefrin: 1/200 is diluted to 1/1000 to 1/10,000. Cobefrin is less pronounced in its action than epinephrine and produces less systemic disturbances.

2. To relieve hypotension: See spinal anesthesia.

Indications:

1. When injection of local anesthetic drug is made into highly vascular areas (scalp, genitalia, etc.).
2. When concentrated solutions of anesthetic drugs are employed.
3. When local anesthetic drugs of relatively high toxicity are employed.

Contra-Indications:

a. When hypertension or cardiac disease exists.
b. If the subject is emotionally disturbed (thyrotoxicosis).
c. For anesthesia of the extremities, particularly if peripheral vascular disease is present.
d. In obstetrics—labor may be delayed by use of epinephrine.
e. During combined local and inhalation anesthesia, particularly if cyclopropane, chloroform, or ethyl chloride are employed.

OVERDOSAGE OR TOXIC REACTION OF LOCAL ANESTHETIC DRUGS

Causes of Overdosage:

1. Accidental intravascular injection of a drug.
2. Injection of excessive quantities of the drug at one single time.
3. Injection of a concentrated stock solution through error.
4. Injection of a solution into highly vascular areas without the addition of vasoconstrictor substances.
5. Use of highly toxic drugs or drugs whose margin of safety is narrow.
6. Topical application of excessive quantities or concentrated solutions to mucous membranes.

7. Use of average quantities in subjects who are debilitated, cachetic, or otherwise possess an impaired detoxifying mechanism.

Types of Reactions:

Two types of systemic reactions from local anesthetic drugs are recognized: neurological or stimulating and circulatory or depressant types.

1. Neurological type

Cause: If local anesthetic drugs gain access to the systemic circulation, they cause intense stimulation of the nervous system. If the dose is large or stimulation is prolonged, depression follows. The reaction may be divided into an early or stimulating phase and a delayed or depressed phase. The most common symptoms are those which occur in the following physiological systems:

TABLE XIV

Phase	Central Nervous System	Circulatory System	Respiratory System
Early part of stimulating phase.	Excitement, apprehension, or other symptoms of emotional instability. Sudden headache. Nausea or vomiting Twitchings of small muscles, particularly of face, finger, etc.	Pulse varies, slowing of pulse more common than an increase Either an elevation or fall in blood pressure but a change does occur. Pallor of skin.	Increased respiratory rate and depth.
Advanced part of stimulation phase.	Convulsions.	An increase in both blood pressure and pulse rate.	Cyanosis, dyspnea, and rapid respiration.
Depressed phase.	Paralysis of muscles. Loss of reflexes. Unconsciousness.	Circulatory failure. No palpable pulse.	Respiratory failure. Ashen grey cyanosis.

Treatment:

1. Inhalation of oxygen. If respiratory movements have failed, inflate the thorax by use of the mask and bag or other suitable method of artificial respiration.
2. Inject a barbiturate intravenously. Any barbiturate is suitable, but an ultra-short-acting drug such as pentothal or evipal is preferred. Observe the following precautions:
   a. Inject very slowly but enough drug to control the convulsions.
   b. Start injection as soon as possible.
   c. Support the airway and administer oxygen or artificially respire the patient if respiratory failure ensues.

Prophylaxis:

1. Always administer a therapeutic dose of a barbiturate in addition to other premedication when contemplating the use of a local anesthetic drug.

2. Add epinephrine or some other suitable vasoconstrictor substance to solutions when anesthetizing vascular areas, such as the scalp, neck, perineum, etc.
3. Use the weakest effective solution of the selected drug.
4. Measure accurately all solutions or drugs employed.
5. Label stock solutions plainly or color them so that they are easily identified and not confused with dilute solutions.
6. Aspirate before injecting any solution.

Comment:

1. An assistant trained in anesthesia should observe and record blood pressure, pulse, and respiratory rate throughout all operations performed with regional anesthesia.
2. An apparatus for administration of oxygen and artificial respiration should always be instantly available for all patients receiving local anesthetic drugs.
3. A soluble barbiturate and sterile equipment for intravenous administration should be available for immediate use when any local anesthetic drug is used for any purpose.
4. Immediately terminate injection of any local anesthetic drug if any untoward symptoms appear.
5. Never diagnose an apprehension which appears during administration of local anesthetic drugs as "hysteria."

2. Circulatory or depressant type

Cause: The local anesthetic drug, even after the injection of minute amounts, produces syncope and circulatory failure by myocardial depression or vasodilatation or both. This reaction has frequently been termed an idiosyncrasy. However, it may occur after the use of therapeutic amounts of the agent. Two types may be differentiated, the immediate and the delayed. The symptoms are as follows:

Immediate type

1. Pallor.
2. Tachycardia, occasionally bradycardia or arrhythmia.
3. Sudden collapse characterized by hypotension and low pulse pressure.
4. Reaction on skin in area of injection.

Delayed

1. Progressive drowsiness.
2. Hypotension—feeble, slow pulse.

Treatment:

1. Prone position, lower head.

2. Artificial respiration with oxygen by any method which is instantly available.
3. Vasoconstrictors (ephedrine, epinephrine, neosynephrin, etc.) if hypotension is present.
4. Perform cardiac massage if asystole has occurred—without delay. Inject epinephrine into the right auricle (0.25 cc. 1/1000).

Prophylaxis

1. Never inject a local anesthetic drug into a patient who presents a history of sensitiveness or idiosyncrasy to a drug without investigating the claim.
2. Perform an intranasal test with the drug before it is employed.

Comment

1. Barbiturates are ineffective in the circulatory type of drug reaction.
2. Accidents frequently occur after injections of small amounts of drugs.
3. Onset is sudden and without warning. Treatment is usually ineffective, with disappointing results.
4. Local anesthetics depress cardiac tissue.
5. Reactions are more frequent in debilitated, cachetic and aged subjects.

SUBSTANCES USED TO PROLONG ANESTHESIA

Absolute Alcohol

Mode of Action:

Causes destruction of nerve tissue. Attacks smaller nerve fibers with greater ease than large resulting in greater sensory than motor loss in mixed nerve.

Dosage:

An area of necrosis 1 cm. in diameter results from injection of 5 cc. into soft tissues. Average dose 2 to 3 cc. for each nerve trunk to be injected. Absolute alcohol must be used from a dry syringe.

Duration:

One to six months or longer.

Objectionable Features:

a. Painful neuritis frequently follows its use.
b. Abstracts water from tissues and becomes diluted, producing an incomplete block.

c. Does not yield satisfactory block unless needle is in direct contact with nerve or ganglion to be blocked.

d. Results not satisfactory if injected after a block using aqueous solution of local anesthetic because of dilution factor.

e. Duration of block variable because nerve regenerates.

Benzyl Alcohol

Mode of Action:

Causes anesthesia and degeneration of nerve fibres. Usually combined with procaine, benzocaine and other local anesthetic drugs. Not ordinarily used alone.

Bromsalizol

Mode of Action:

Causes a blockade and some degeneration of nerve fibres by sclerosing action. Usually dispensed in a concentration of 4% in peanut oil.

Dosage:

Usually 5 cc. at each nerve trunk.

Duration of Action:

Several days to several weeks. Very variable.

Local Anesthetics in Oil

Bases of procaine, nupercaine, are prepared in oily solutions, combined with benzyl alcohol, anesthesin, phenol, etc.

Mode of Action:

Slow release of the agent into the tissue from oil which tends to withhold the drug. Yields prolonged effect. Also some nerve destruction.

Dosage:

Procaine 5 cc. 2%
Nupercaine 5 cc. 0.2%

Ammonium Sulphate

Mode of Action:

Not known.

Is alleged to cause a selective degeneration of C type of sensory fibre, which carries diffuse deep, dull pain impulses. This has never been verified.

Dosage:

Usually used in combination with the anesthetic solution. One cc. 10% sterile solution is combined with 1 cc. 2% procaine or other local anesthetic of equivalent strength. The volume used equals the volume of procaine contemplated to be used if block were performed without it.

Duration of Action:

Very variable. No effect in many cases. One day to six weeks duration may be expected. Causes no anesthesia, paresis or motor effects.

Phenol—6%

Mode of Action:

Like alcohol. Used in same volume and for same purpose. Causes neurolysis.

Dosage:

5 cc. per nerve trunk.

Duration of Action:

Like alcohol.

MATERIALS REQUIRED FOR NERVE AND FIELD BLOCKS AND FOR INFILTRATION ANESTHESIA (FIG. 97)

1. Two wheal needles ($\frac{1}{2}$ cm. long, of 24 or 25 gauge).
2. Ether and skin sterilizer, for preparing skin.
3. Sponge forceps and sponges for preparing skin.
4. Six sterile towels for draping operative field.
5. Four sterile towel clamps.
6. Ten cc. syringe for regional anesthesia equipped with a lock (Fig. 98).
7. Needles—10 cm. 20 gauge.
               8 cm. 22 gauge.
               5 cm. 20 or 22 gauge.
8. 0.5% procaine solution for skin wheals.
9. Procaine or other desired drug in necessary amount.
10. Sterile container, 250 cc. or 500 cc., preferably of glass or enamel, for reservoir for solution of local agent.
11. Epinephrine solution (1:1000 U.S.P.).
12. Physiological saline for drug which is to be diluted, or for testing needles.
13. Several squares of rubber (5 mm. $\times$ 5 mm.) cut from rubber tubing, which are to be used for markers (Fig. 102, page 323).
14. Gloves and powder.
15. Metal ruler (sterilized).
16. India ink or other marking substance which will not dissolve in ether or skin sterilizers.
17. Short-acting barbiturate and sterile apparatus for administering the same in the event of overdosage or toxic reactions.
18. Inhaler for artificial respiration.

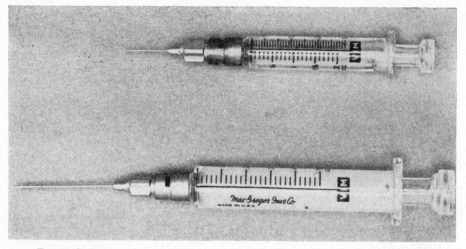

Fig. 97. Syringes used for regional anesthesia. The lock type of syringe is preferable for ease in handling and to avoid leakage about the hub of the needle.

Comment

1. Arrange the above instruments upon a tray approximately 12 inches by 18 or 20 inches. Wrap and have in readiness for use (Fig. 99).
2. The number of needles necessary varies with the type of block to be performed. Two of each are desirable if available.
3. Syringes and needles may be of any type, but those designed exclusively for regional anesthesia are preferred.

TESTING FOR SENSITIVITY TO A LOCAL ANESTHETIC DRUG

Object:

To determine whether or not the patient has an intolerance to the drug which is to be employed.

Materials for Skin Test:

1. Local anesthetic drug to be tested.
2. Wheal needle and a small syringe.
3. Physiological saline solution.
4. Seventy per cent alcohol.
5. Ether.
6. Sponges.

Procedure:

1. Cleanse skin on anterior surface of one of the forearms with ether and sterilize with alcohol.
2. Raise a small intradermal wheal approximately 5 mm. in diameter with saline solution.

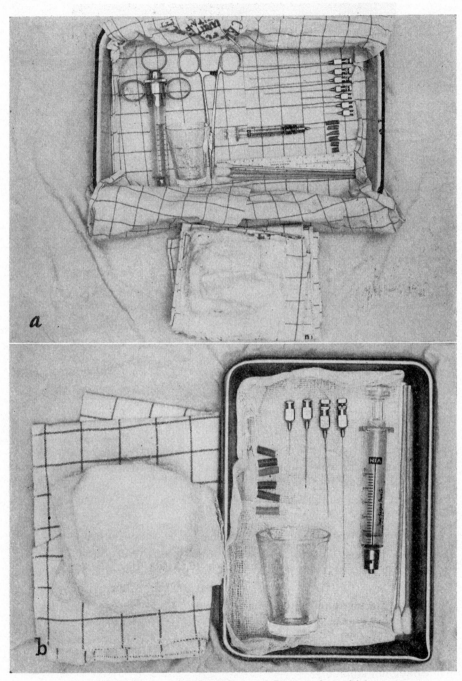

Fig. 98. Assembly for regional anesthesia. (a) Large set for multiple nerve blocks. (b) Small set to be used for single nerve blocks.

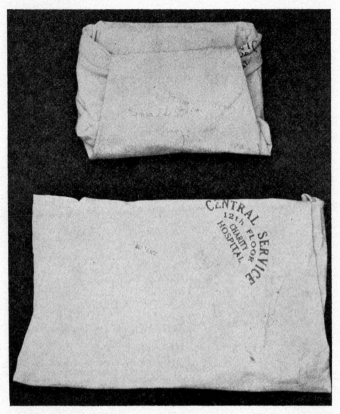

Fig. 99. Assembly wrapped and ready for use. The instruments are packed in a tray and wrapped and sterilized by autoclaving and kept in readiness for use.

3. Raise a similar wheal 3 or 4 cm. from this area using the local anesthetic drug to be tested.

Comment

1. After 5 minutes, if both wheals appear to be alike the test is negative; if the wheal produced by the drug is red and spreads over a wide area the test is most likely positive and the drug should not be employed.
2. A negative response is not assurance of tolerance, but merely indicates absence of allergic response.

INTRANASAL TEST

Materials:

1. Sphygmomanometer.
2. Several cubic centimeters of solution to be employed.

Procedure:

1. Apply sphygmomanometer to arm and record blood pressures at

3-minute intervals until stabilized. Have patient supine and comfortably placed.

2. Record pulse until stabilized.
3. Introduce one drop of the solution to be tested into the conjunctival sac. Wait 8 minutes and introduce one drop into one nostril with patient in supine position.
4. After three minutes introduce two drops into one nostril and note pulse and blood pressure.
5. After three minutes more introduce 4 drops into one nostril and note pulse and blood pressure. Double quantity at 3 minute intervals until volume becomes 1 cc.
6. Observe blood pressure and pulse every 3 minutes for next 15 minutes. Neither a slowing or acceleration of the pulse nor an elevation or depression of blood pressure should occur. Look for tremors, convulsions, signs of excitement and other manifestations of central nervous system stimulation.

Comment:

Sensitivity to drug will be manifest by significant lowering of blood pressure and alterations of pulse rate.

1. Intolerance is not an allergic type of response resulting from an allergen-antibody interaction. Signs and symptoms same as overdose.
2. The nasal test should always supplement the skin test.
3. The nasal test when positive indicates effects resulting from absorbing drug into blood and therefore is more logical and reliable. The skin test is of questionable value.

PREPARATION OF PATIENT

1. For nerve blocks for major surgical procedures:
   a. Withhold food.
   b. Morphine gr. ⅙—Scopolamine gr. ¹⁄₁₅₀—1½ hours prior to surgery.
   c. Seconal gr. 1½ or pentobarbital gr. 1½ or other short acting barbiturate in equivalent dose two hours prior to surgery.
2. For nerve blocks for minor surgical procedures:
   Seconal or other barbiturate, as above.
3. For diagnostic and therapeutic nerve blocks in ambulatory patients:
   a. If patient is ambulatory and block is simple no premedication is required.
   b. If patient is apprehensive a barbiturate, as above, may be necessary.
   c. Withhold food for at least four hours prior to the block.

REFERENCE

ADRIANI, JOHN. Anesthesia for minor surgery. S. Clin. North America, *31:*1507, Oct., 1951.

Conduct of Various Aspects of Regional Anesthesia

Comment

1. Always raise an intradermal wheal preliminary to the insertion of a needle through the skin.

Reason

The skin is the most sensitive structure through which the needle will pass.

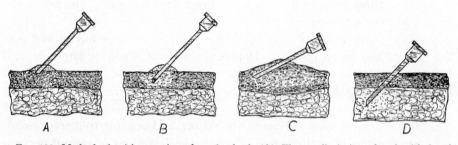

FIG. 100. Method of raising an intradermal wheal. (A) The needle is introduced with bevel down through a drop of procaine until it pierces the skin. (B) The needle is then rotated and enough of the drug injected *intradermally* to form a (C) blanched area with an orange peel appearance. Incorrect method of raising a wheal is shown in (D). The needle should not be introduced into the subcutaneous areas.

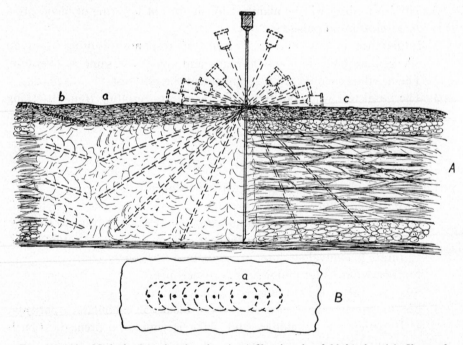

FIG. 101. (A) Method of performing fanwise infiltration for field blocks. (a) Shows the solution infiltrating the tissues as the needle is advanced. (b) Shows the overlapping of the solution from the injection made through the adjacent wheal so that a continuous wall of solution is thrown into the tissues. (c) Shows needle penetrating all layers of tissues.

(B) Method of raising a continuous intradermal wheal. The wheal is first raised at point *a*, the needle is then introduced at the periphery on each side and a succession of wheals is thus produced. The needle point should always be thrust into the anesthetized area after the first wheal is raised. A continuous intradermal wheal around a limb is known as a "garter band."

2. Always insert a needle in a direction normal to the skin.

3. Do not connect the syringe to the needle until the needle is properly placed, unless so specified.

The weight of syringe and leverage exerted obliterates sense of direction transmitted to fingers if only the needle is used.

4. Add the desired vasoconstrictor drugs to the local anesthetic solutions at the time the block is performed.

Vasoconstrictor drugs are amines and are easily decomposed if allowed to stand for any length of time.

5. Do not use discolored solutions of local anesthetic drugs.

Decomposition may have occurred and the drug may be ineffective or toxic.

6. Advance the needle gently as it approaches a bony landmark.

The periosteum is (very) sensitive and the patient may be disturbed from careless manipulations.

7. Always attempt aspiration by drawing back on plunger when the needle is placed in the desired location. Rotate the needle and repeat so as to aspirate in two planes. Withdraw and replace needle in the event blood is aspirated (Fig. 103).

This prevents intravascular injections of toxic amounts of the drug. The needle may be in a vessel and compressed against a bone thus not revealing blood on asperation unless it is rotated.

8. Watch patients during injection for signs and symptoms of toxic reactions. Injections should be terminated in the event reactions occur.

Treatment should be instituted immediately when prodromal signs appear. Do not wait until the severe toxic manifestations occur.

9. Always perform regional anesthesia under circumstances in which an anesthetic machine is available.

The machine is needed for oxygen, artificial respiration, or general anesthesia if the block fails.

10. Always have a soluble short-acting or ultra short-acting barbiturate available together with a sterile syringe and needle and sterile water when using any local anesthetic drug.

In the event toxic reactions occur the convulsions may be controlled by the intravenous administration of the sedative.

11. Always drape the operative site and maintain absolute sterility.

Prevent local infections and abscesses.

12. Avoid injections into highly vascular areas or in the region of vascular tissues such as hemangiomas.

Rapid absorption or intravascular injection of the local anesthetic may occur.

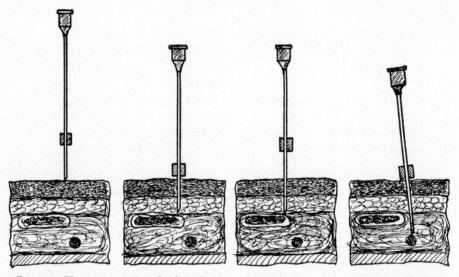

FIG. 102. The purpose of a depth marker for introducing a needle into tissues is shown. The marker consists of a piece of cork or rubber which can be moved the length of the shaft of the needle.

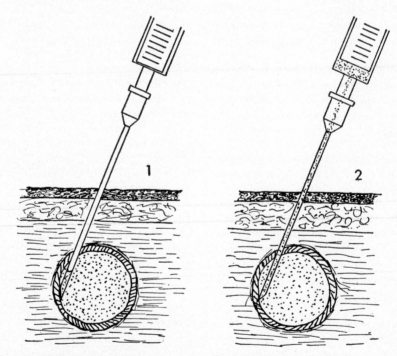

FIG. 103. After attempting aspiration, rotate needle 180° and attempt aspiration (2) again in event needle bevel had been impinged upon wall of vessel first time (1).

13. Test needles and syringes for patency by passing some solution through them.

Needles may be occluded by charred blood, oil, etc.

14. Do not overpremedicate patients.

Patients will be too drowsy to cooperate with anesthetist.

15. Do not omit premedication.

Drugs minimize toxic-reactions. Patients are apprehensive and uncooperative.

16. Always warm solutions to body temperature.

Onset of anesthesia is delayed or very slow when cold solutions are employed.

17. Omit vasoconstrictor drug from local anesthetic solutions in blocks on digits of hands or feet or when cardiovascular and peripheral vascular diseases are present.

Vasospasm may be enhanced and gangrene of extremity result. Drugs also cause systemic vascular disturbances.

18. Never introduce any needle entirely to the hilt or hub.

Needles frequently break at the junction of the hub and shaft and are thus difficult to retrieve.

19. Avoid piercing nerves or performing intraneural injection.

Neuritis may result from intraneural injection.

20. Reject blood stained solutions in the event blood is aspirated. Fill syringe with clear solution.

Proteins of blood may precipitate in solution.

21. Repeat the aspiration test frequently during injection of the drug.

The needle point may shift slightly during injection and pass into a vessel.

22. Always withdraw the needle as far as the subcutaneous tissues when changing its direction.

The needle may be bent or broken; direction is not changed if this is not practiced.

23. Always test the area of anesthesia with a blunt needle when the block is completed or before surgery is started.

The block may be repeated in event of failure before operative field is prepared.

24. Always use a marker as a guide to distance needle is introduced (Fig. 102).

Most nerve blocks are "blind" procedures which may result in damage to vital structures if carelessly performed.

SPINAL ANESTHESIA

GENERAL CONSIDERATIONS OF SPINAL ANESTHESIA

Definition:
Anesthesia produced by the injection of a solution of a local anesthetic drug into the subarachnoid space. A temporary paralysis of the sensory,

autonomic, and motor fibers in the anterior and posterior roots emanating from the area bathed by the drug results. Block is not caused by the drug's entering the cord proper.

Synonyms:

Subarachnoid block, spinal analgesia.

Types:

Spinal anesthesia may be divided into the following types: (a) single injection, and (b) continuous.

Extent:

1. "High Spinal"—anesthesia and analgesia extending above the costal margin accompanied by varying degrees of intercostal muscle paralysis.
2. "Medium Spinal" or "Spinal"—anesthesia and analgesia extending above the umbilicus but below the costal margin.
3. "Low Spinal"—anesthesia and analgesia not extending above the umbilicus.
4. "Saddle"—anesthesia and analgesia confined to the sacral segments only.

Uses:

1. For surgical anesthesia.
2. As an aid to diagnosis of diseases of the autonomic nervous system (megacolon, vasospastic diseases, etc.).

Drugs Employed:

Although many local anesthetic drugs have been employed with success, the following are currently popular for spinal anesthesia.
1. *Procaine.* Also called novocaine, neocaine. Yields one hour's anesthesia.
2. *Pontocaine.* Also called pantocaine, tetracaine (U.S.P.). Yields two hours' anesthesia.
3. *Nupercaine.* Also called percaine, dibucaine. Yields three hours' anesthesia.
4. *Metycaine.* (piperocaine U.S.P.) Also called neothesine. Yields one to 1½ hours' anesthesia.
5. *Monocaine.* (butethamine) Yields one hour's anesthesia.
6. *Lucaine.* (peridocaine) Yields ¾ hour's anesthesia.

Materials:

1. One skin wheal needle, 25 or 26 gauge, ½"-¾" long.
2. One spinal needle, 20 gauge, and one spinal needle, 22 gauge, rustless with 45° bevel.

3. One short needle, 19 or 20 gauge, approximately 1½"-2" long (Wassermann needle).
4. One syringe, 2 cc., equipped with a lock which fits the various needles in the set.
5. One syringe, 5 cc., also equipped with a lock which fits the various needles in the set.
6. One medicine glass, 2 oz. size, for mixing drugs or to act as a reservoir for procaine (optional).
7. One per cent procaine, 2 cc. sterile ampule, solution for infiltrating skin and interspinous space.
8. Several ampules of ephedrine sulphate solution (¾ gr., 50 mgm.), or other vasopressor substance.
9. One file for opening glass ampules.
10. Four sterile towels and towel clips (or special draping sheet with square opening, 6" by 6", in the center).
11. Skin sterilizer.

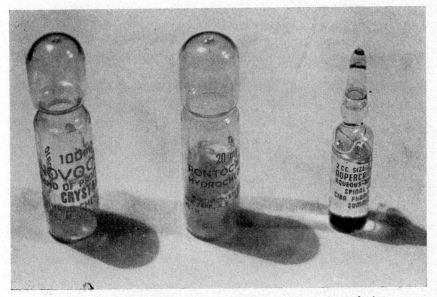

FIG. 104. Sealed ampules of local anesthetic drugs for spinal anesthesia.

12. Several gauze sponges and one sponge forceps for preparing skin.
13. One ampule of the selected drug (optional or varies with technique) (Fig. 104).
14. One introducer or Sise guide (Fig. 105).
15. Completely equipped anesthesia machine.
16. Pillow for supporting the head.
17. Sphygmomanometer.

Premedication:

1. Morphine, grs. 1/6 to 1/4, and scopolamine or atropine, grs. 1/150 to 1/100, subcutaneously, one hour prior to induction of anesthesia.

2. Intramuscular injection of ephedrine sulphate, 3/4 gr., in instances in which hypotension is anticipated (see below).

Reason:

In case the block fails and general anesthesia is necessary, the patient will be prepared for it. Act to sedate patient during operation.

Vasopressor drugs combat hypotension of spinal anesthesia more effectively than other drugs.

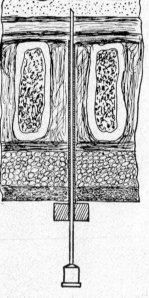

FIG. 105. The Sise guide is a trochar designed to facilitate spinal puncture and prevent contamination by having needle come into contact with the skin.

Preliminary Preparation:

1. Apply blood pressure apparatus to right arm.
2. Record preliminary reading of tension, pulse rate, and respiratory rate.

Position of Patient (Fig. 107):

1. Place the patient on his side (lateral prone) with head flexed toward knees and knees flexed on thighs. Use upright position for saddle or in obstetrical patients, have assistant hold patient.
2. Arrange the patient so that his back is at the edge of the operating table and perpendicular to the floor—upper shoulder should be level with iliac crest (Fig. 107).

Preparation of Hands:

1. Scrub hands with soap and water or detergent in the same manner as for surgical operation, for at least five minutes.
2. Wipe dry and apply sterile rubber gloves.

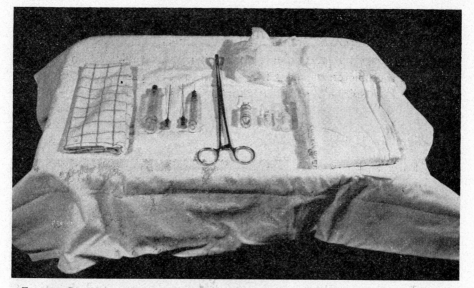

FIG. 106. Set up for spinal anesthesia. The entire set may be placed in a small tray three or four inches wide and six or eight inches long, enclosed in two thick wrappers and sterilized. The wrapper may be unfolded and spread over a flat tray providing a sterile set up. The sterilized ampules are not included but are added, at the time the set up is prepared.

Preparation of Skin for Puncture:

1. Open ampules of all drugs and test patency of needles and syringes by washing them out with saline solution.
2. Locate and mark selected intervertebral space.
3. Cleanse an area of skin with ether to remove skin lipoids.
4. Apply accepted skin sterilizer to skin. Wait for sterilizer to act (three minutes). Prepare a large area.
5. Remove excess sterilizer over site of puncture with a sponge.

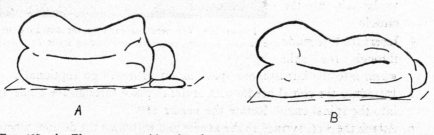

FIG. 107. A. *The correct position* for the patient in performing spinal punctures: The shoulder should be at the level of the iliac crest. The surface of the back should be perpendicular to the table. The patient should be placed with his back at the edge of the operating table with knees and thighs flexed and head flexed towards the knees.

B. *The incorrect position* in performing spinal puncture: The shoulder is thrown forward, the head is extended, the vertebral column is twisted.

Site of Lumbar Puncture:

1. For "High Spinal," 2nd or 3rd lumbar interspace, or any space below, if these are not accessible (an imaginary perpendicular line dropped from the iliac crest passes through 4th lumber space).
2. For "Low Spinal," 3rd and 4th lumbar interspace.

Procedure for Lumbar Puncture:

1. Raise a skin wheal over the selected site with procaine. Use the wheal needle and 2 cc. syringe for this purpose.
2. Change wheal needle to larger (Wassermann) needle and infiltrate deeper tissues between vertebral spines with procaine.
3. Draw ephedrine into 2 cc. syringe still attached to Wassermann needle and inject it into muscles lateral to vertebral column. Insert the needle through the wheal at a 45° angle to the skin into the muscle.

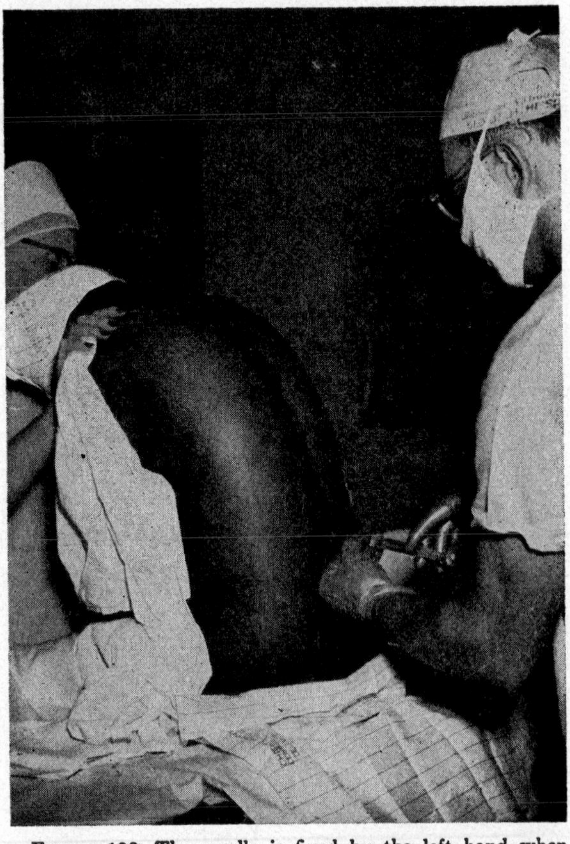

FIGURE 108. The needle is fixed by the left hand when attaching syringes, removing or replacing stylet or injecting solutions.

4. Insert the Sise guide through the skin wheal into the intraspinous space as far as it will go (optional).
5. Introduce the spinal needle with stylet in place through the guide and into the spinal canal. Rotate the needle 180°.
6. Attach the 5 cc. syringe to the needle and withdraw the desired amount of spinal fluid. Replace stylet.
7. Attach Wassermann needle, add fluid to the drug in the opened ampule, and draw the solution in and out of the ampule until all crystals are completely dissolved.

8. Draw dissolved drug into syringe, remove the stylet, and attach syringe to spinal needle.

9. Hold needle firmly with left hand and syringe in right. Draw back slightly on plunger and withdraw approximately 0.5 cc. of spinal fluid into syringe to determine whether or not there is a free flow of fluid and the needle is still well placed (Fig. 108).

10. Inject solution of drug at desired rate (see Individual techniques).

11. After injection again withdraw 0.5 cc. of fluid (to ascertain if needle is still in place).

12. Withdraw needle, cover puncture site with a sponge and place patient in desired position as quickly as possible.

13. Establish the desired level of anesthesia.

SUBARACHNOID PUNCTURE-INTERLAMINAR (SUBLAMINAR) APPROACH

Uses:

When puncture is not feasible by the midline or lateral approach.

Materials:

Standard spinal set containing 15 cm. 20 gauge needle.

Procedure:

1. Arrange patient in same manner as for classical technique (sitting or lying).

2. Raise wheal 1.5 to 2 cm. lateral to midline at 4th or 5th lumbar vertebrae.

3. Introduce needle 30-45° to surface of skin medially, cephalad, and anteriorly (Fig. 109).

4. As soon as bone is encountered initiate to and fro movement changing angle slightly and advancing until laminar hiatus is reached.

Comment:

1. The needle enters the subarachnoid space 1 cm. higher than the vertebra at which needle enters.

2. The course of the needle is determined by the slanting position of the lamina and not the position of the spinous process.

3. If done above L-2, cord may be injured. Cord ends at L2.

SUBARACHNOID PUNCTURE, LATERAL APPROACH

Uses:

When the puncture is not feasible by the midline approach.

Procedure:

1. Mark the center of the interspace with appropriate marker.

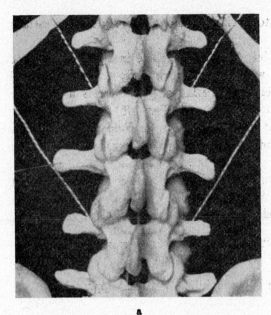

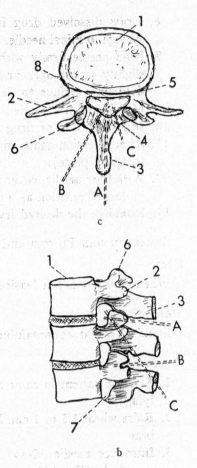

Fig. 109. (a) Dorsal view of lumbar vertebrae on mounted skeleton. (b) Lateral view of 1st., 2nd., and 3rd. lumbar vertebrae. (c) Top view of second lumbar vertebra. A. Position of needle in direct or classical approach for lumbar puncture. B. Lateral approach. C. Interlaminar approach. 1. Body of vertebra. 2. Transverse process. 3. Dorsal spine. 4. Lamina. 5. Pedicle. 6. Articular process. 7. Vertebral notch. 8. Spinal canal.

2. Raise the wheal 1.5 cms. from the midline opposite the center of the interspace.

3. Introduce needle (ordinary needle) through the wheal at angle of 25° to midline horizontally with no deviation caudad or cephalad.

4. Guide needle towards midline pointing towards the left thumbnail which is held there while procedure is being carried out.

5. As soon as resistance is encountered (as the needle approaches the ligamentum flavum) the needle is advanced slowly and carefully until it enters the subarachnoid space.

Comment:

1. The needle lies lateral to the supraspinous and intraspinous ligament.

2. When bony resistance is encountered it is due to the vertebral arch. The needle may be "worked" cephalad or caudad until the ligamentum flavum is encountered.

3. Flexion of the spine is not required.

4. The needle does not have to be directed either cephalad or caudad.
5. May be done in prone position.

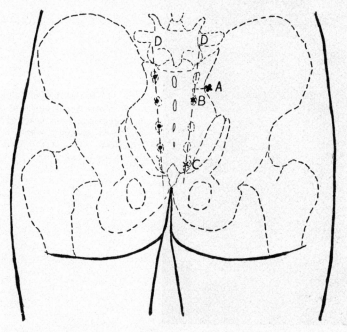

FIG. 109A. Landmarks for transacral blocks. (A) Posterior-superior iliac spines. (B) Sacral foramina. (C) Sacral cornua. (D) 5th lumbar vertebra.

LUMBOSACRAL SUBARACHNOID PUNCTURE

Definition

Subarachnoid puncture performed by passing a needle in the direction of the lumbosacral joint.

Purpose

1. For "low" spinal anesthesia or other intrathecal injections.
2. For withdrawing cerebrospinal fluid for diagnostic purposes.

Materials

Standard regional set containing a 12 cm. 20 gauge needle.

Technique

1. *Landmarks.*
   a. Posterior superior iliac spines. (A Fig. 109A)
   b. Second sacral foramina. (B Fig. 109A)
   c. Fifth lumbar vertebra (from Nerve Blocks. (A-109A, 109B)

2. *Position.* Place the patient in the prone position with pillow beneath the hips as for sacral block.

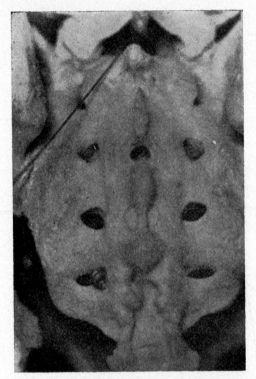

FIG. 109B. Method of inducing lumbosacral subarachnoid puncture. Note needle
in lumbosacral joint space. The needle is
introduced through a wheal raised over the
2nd sacral foramina and inclined towards
the 5th lumbar vertebra.

3. *Procedure.* Follow the same techniques described for transsacral block.

   a. Locate and mark the position of the posterior superior iliac spine on either right or left side, whichever is convenient.
   b. Raise an intradermal wheal 1 cm. medial and caudad to the point indicating the spine (second sacral) (Fig. 109B).
   c. Introduce the 12 cm. needle through the wheal in a medial and ceph-alad direction. Direct it so that there is an angle of 55° between it and the skin and it points toward the lumbosacral joint.
   d. Continue to advance it until it pierces the ligamentous layer. A sense of break of resistance is felt as the ligament is pierced.
   e. Rotate needle and aspirate gently to obtain cerebrospinal fluid.

Advantages

   1. Provides a useful method of subarachnoid puncture in cases of fusion of spine or other anatomical deformities.
   2. Allows a greater assurance of a "low spinal anesthesia" in poor risk subjects.
   3. The prone position is of greater comfort to patient.

Comment

   1. Note that the medial angle over which needle is advanced varies accord-ing to the width of the sacrum.

2. Always direct the needle so that it points to the midline and lumbosacral joint.

3. Withdraw fluid by aspiration if it does not flow freely.

4. Perform injection for spinal anesthesia in the same manner as if lumbar spaces were used as site of puncture.

REFERENCES

KERSHNER, D., and SHAPIRO, A. L.: Interlaminal spinal anesthesia. Am. J. Surg., *122:* 43-46, 1946.

SURKS, N. and WOOD, P.: Anesthesiology, *12:*241-243, March, 1951.

Control of Level and Intensity of Anesthesia:

The following six extrinsic factors may be varied to affect level and intensity of anesthesia. All these factors should be fixed for a given level of anesthesia.

1. *Volume of solution injected.* This is an important factor. The greater the volume of solution prepared with a given weight of drug the higher the level of anesthesia. Sensory anesthesia will be more diffuse and motor effects less intense. Duration of action slightly shorter. This

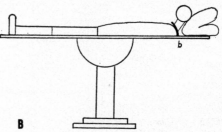

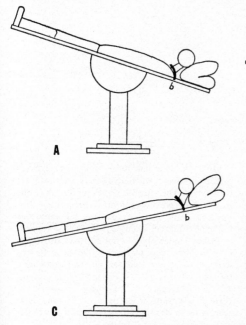

FIG. 110. Positions for establishing level of spinal anesthesia when hyperbaric solutions are employed. (A) Trendelenburg position necessary to secure level of anesthesia for upper abdominal surgery. Note the doubled pillow to sharply flex the neck and prevent ascent of drug into the cervical region. (B) Position to which patient is returned after level is established in (A) or is placed for anesthesia for lower abdominal surgery. (C) Position for "low" spinal. The drug gravitates caudad. Note that the shoulders are supported by (b) braces.

factor is best maintained constant by employing as small a volume of solution as possible.

2. *Rate of injection of fluid.* Rapid injection causes drug to ascend into higher levels of the spinal canal. Slow injection causes the drug to be deposited and localized at the site of puncture. A "Low Spinal" results.

3. *Specific gravity of the solution.* The specific gravity of spinal fluid averages 1.006 but ranges from 1.003 to 1.009.

   a. If specific gravity of the solution injected is greater than that of spinal fluid, the solution is termed *hyperbaric.* Such a solution tends to diffuse downward.

   b. If specific gravity of the solution approximates that of spinal fluid, the solution is termed *isobaric.* Diffusion of such a solution is not easy to control and may be upward and downward.

   c. If the specific gravity is less than that of spinal fluid, it is termed hypobaric. Such a solution tends to diffuse upward and bathes posterior roots when the patient is in the prone position.

4. *Position of patient after injection.* This factor depends upon the specific gravity of the solution employed. The object is to prevent the solution from diffusing cephalad into the cervical region.

   a. *Hyperbaric solutions* (Fig. 110). For low spinal anesthesia, the patient is placed in a flat or Fowler's (head up) position so that the solution gravitates caudad.

   For high spinal, the Trendelenburg position with head sharply flexed is employed.

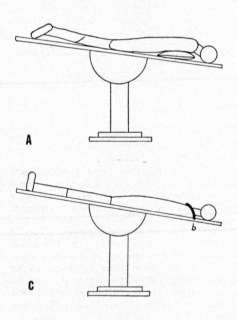
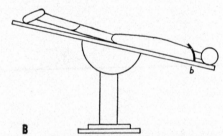

FIG. 111. Position for establishing level of spinal anesthesia when hypobaric solutions are employed. The prone position insures contact of drug with the dorsal sensory roots. (A) Position required to secure level of anesthesia for upper abdominal surgery. Note that a pillow is placed under the thorax so that the trunk is in a horizontal plane and the neck is well flexed to prevent passage of the drug into cervical region. (B) Position for abdominal and pelvic surgery. (C) Position to which the patient is turned from prone to supine after anesthesia is established. Note that the shoulders are supported by braces.

   b. *Isobaric solutions.* The flat position is employed. The level of anesthesia is difficult to control by varying the position.

   c. *Hypobaric solutions* (Fig. 111). The Trendelenburg position is employed to insure a caudad diffusion of the drug. Prone position is often necessary to affect the sensory roots (see nupercaine).

5. *Site of injection.* This factor has little influence upon the height of "high" spinal anesthesia. Injection at lower segments may result in high levels of anesthesia if the rate of injection is rapid or the position of the patient is modified after injection.

6. *Dose of drugs.* The greater the amount of drug, the higher the level and the greater the intensity of the paralysis. The duration of anesthesia is only slightly increased by increasing the dose (Figs. 124, 126).

The following intrinsic factors have no influence the level and intensity of anesthesia, and are not controllable. They must be taken into consideration in inducing anesthesia.

1. The length of the cord. The longer the cord the less intense the anesthesia a given dose of drug will produce.

2. The diameter of the cord. This factor plays only a minor role unless the subject is unusually large or small.

3. The subarachnoid volume. The greater the subarachnoid volume the greater the dilution and the less intense will be the anesthesia.

4. Curvatures of vertebral column. Variations in curvature of lumbar and thoracic portions of the vertebral column may cause pooling of the solution of the drug in thoracic or sacral areas depending upon the specific gravity of the solution and position of the patient after injection of the drug.

5. Variations in intraspinal pressure. Straining, coughing, deep breathing and labor pains in obstetrics cause changes in spinal fluid pressure which cause cephalad advancement of the drug beyond desired spinal segments.

Factors Influencing Duration of Anesthesia:

1. *Chemical nature of drug.* This is the most important factor which influences duration of anesthesia. Others are relatively insignificant.
    The average duration of the common drugs is as follows:
    Procaine, one hour
    Pontocaine, two hours
    Metycaine, 1½ hours
    Nupercaine, two to three hours.

2. *Dose of drug.* This influences duration to a certain extent, but not in proportion to increase. Large doses provide more intense and extensive anesthesia.

3. *Concentration of solution.* Concentrated solutions produce more intense anesthesia. An increase in duration occurs but not in proportion to the increase in dosage.

4. *Vasoconstrictors.* These prolong duration by retarding absorption Epinephrine is the most serviceable. See page 366.

Intensity of Anesthesia:

Intensity of anesthesia refers to the completeness of the block to the passages of impulses in a nerve by the drug. It depends upon the following two factors:

1. The size of the nerve fibers. Sensory and autonomic fibers are smaller than motor. Consequently they are more easily and quickly affected.
2. Concentration of drug in the solution. Dilute solutions affect the smaller nerve fibers more effectively than the large, and produce sensory anesthesia with partial or no motor loss when these fibers are exposed to a given concentration of drug.

Advantages of Spinal Anesthesia:	*Reasons:*
1. It provides excellent muscular relaxation.	The reflex arc is interrupted and the muscle is completely paralyzed.
2. It is accompanied by little disturbance of metabolic processes.	This applies if no hypotension accompanies the anesthesia.
3. It dispenses with the inhalation of irritating drugs.	Loss of consciousness, secretions, excitement, post-anesthetic nausea, and somnolence, as well as other disagreeable features of inhalation anesthesia, are absent.
4. It allows use of cautery and electrical appliances.	Most inhalation anesthetic drugs are inflammable.
5. It is inexpensive in comparison with some anesthetic agents and techniques of administration.	The quantity of drug required is one small initial dose.
6. May be administered by the operator.	The surgeon may serve as anesthetist when an anesthetist is not available.

Disadvantages of Spinal Anesthesia:	*Reasons:*
1. It is noncontrollable.	Once anesthesia has been instituted, it cannot be terminated or all deleterious effects combatted.
2. Its duration, although usually predictable, is always uncertain.	The operation may outlast anesthesia and supplementary anesthesia subjects the patient to the bad effects of two anesthetics.
3. The possibility of failure, or technical errors cannot be wholly excluded.	Technical difficulties occur even in most skilled hands.

4. It is often accompanied by motor paralysis at high levels.

This causes respiratory depression or failure from the resulting intercostal paralysis.

5. It is often accompanied by distressing circulatory changes.

Paralysis of the muscles and autonomic nervous system cause peripheral circulatory failure.

6. It is occasionally followed by postoperative neurological complications.

These may result from the effect of the drug on the cord, trauma from needle, infections, etc.

7. The patient remains conscious throughout the operation.

All patients are not co-operative—some are not suited for it. Patients become tired in long procedures.

8. The vagal pathways from the viscera are not blocked during abdominal surgery.

Retching, nausea, and vomiting follow traction on the viscera.

9. Impulses pass into cord above area of block.

Retrograde transmission along sympathetic chain can occur.

Complications of Spinal Anesthesia: Reasons and Treatment:

1. *Hypotension* (often called "spinal shock" or primary shock). The degree of shock depends upon the number of segments paralyzed. It is usually more pronounced in "high" spinal anesthesia.
2. *Characteristics of "spinal shock"*
    a. It occurs early during anesthesia. It is probably due to sudden relaxation of vascular bed.
    b. Systolic pressure falls. Due to decreased cardiac output (Fig. 112).
    c. Diastolic pressure is well maintained. If it falls, it falls slightly. It does not fall in proportion to systolic. The peripheral resistance is only slightly decreased. Venous and capillary stagnation occur.
    d. Pulse pressure is decreased. Due to decreased cardiac output.
    e. Circulation time is prolonged. Due to decreased cardiac output.
    f. Bradycardia is more frequently observed when ephedrine or other vasopressor drugs are not used. Possibly due to vagal predominance following sympathetic paralysis.
    g. The blood volume is not reduced, the vascular space is increased.
3. *Treatment.* Administer a vasopressor drug if the hypotension is severe. Administer the amount necessary to obtain the desired therapeutic effect. Any of the following is satisfactory.
    a. *Ephedrine*, gr. ¾ (50 mgm.), half intravenously, half intramuscularly.

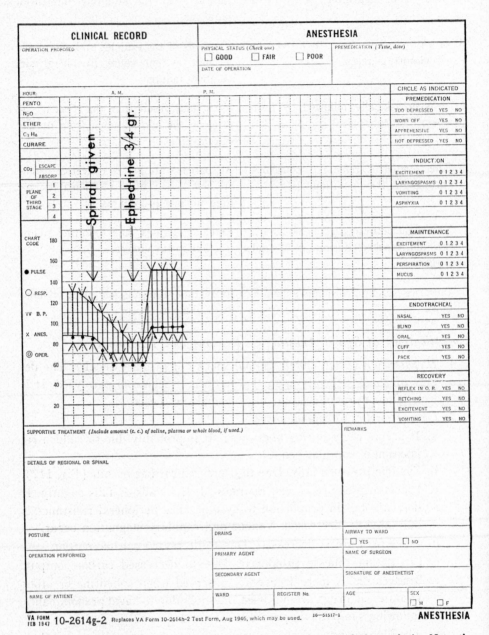

Fig. 112. Blood pressure pattern commonly observed during spinal anesthesia. Note the marked decrease in systolic blood pressure, the comparatively smaller decrease of the diastolic, the narrowed pulse pressure and the bradycardia. Note the prompt effect of the vasopressor.

b. *Neosynephrine*, gr. ¼ mgm. intravenously very slowly.

c. *Desoxyephedrine*, 10 mgm. Half intravenously, half intramuscularly.

d. *Vasoxyl*, 5-10 mgm. Half intravenously, half intramuscularly.

e. *Oenethyl*, 50-100 mgm. Half intravenously, half intramuscularly.

f. *Ephedrine*, gr. ¾ (50 mgm.); and pitressin, 5 units. Half slowly intravenously, and half intramuscularly.

4. *Respiratory failure.* The two most common causes are these:

a. Central depression resulting from cerebral anemia caused by the hypotension. This responds to artificial respiration and vasopressor drugs if treated immediately.

b. Paralysis of phrenic and intercostal nerves at the anterior roots in subarachnoid space due to cephalad migration of drug. This responds to artificial respiration with oxygen by insufflation with bag and mask until nerves regain function.

5. *Nausea and emesis.* This complication occurs during the anesthesia. There are five underlying causes.

a. Anemia of medulla accompanying hypotension. Heralded by yawning. Usually relieved by inhalation of 100% oxygen in conjunction with a vasopressor drug.

b. Traction on the mesentery and intra-abdominal organs. This causes impulses to reach the medulla via the vagi. Light anesthesia with cyclopropane, pentothal, nitrous oxide, or intravenous morphine should be given.

c. Diffusion of the drug into the medullary area. Use sedation.

d. Narcotics used for premedication.

e. Stimulation caused by vasopressors used to overcome hypotension.

Contra-Indications to Spinal Anesthesia

Reasons

1. *Cardiovascular diseases.*

a. Myocardial disease.

b. Hypertension, moderate or severe.

c. Hypotension from any cause (including shock).

d. Disturbances of cardiac rhythm.

e. Decompensation from any cause.

Circulatory depression is a prominent and common disturbance in spinal anesthesia. It is the result of physiological changes due to paralysis of central nervous system and paralysis of the sympathetic fibers. The relaxation of muscles and paralysis of intercostals interfere with the venous return to the heart.

2. *Neurological diseases.*

a. Degenerative diseases of the entire or any part of the nervous system.

b. Suppurative diseases of the nervous system.

Patient may ascribe symptoms of previously existing lesions to spinal anesthesia. Often of medicolegal importance.

3. Diseases of the respiratory system accompanied by a decrease in vital capacity.

Intercostal paralysis may decrease tidal exchange and further decrase vital capacity.

4. *Anemia.* The type matters little. The reduction in total hemoglobin is the important factor.

The oxygen-carrying power of the blood is reduced. Anoxia may occur in high spinal if intercostal paralysis is present.

5. *Reduction in blood volume.* Hemorrhage or operations which may be complicated by hemorrhages. Dehydration, shock.

Severe hypotension may ensue. The compensatory mechanisms which attempt to readjust the vascular system to normal are disturbed by spinal anesthesia.

6. *Diseases causing increased intra-abdominal pressure.* Distension, ascites, pregnancy, ovarian tumors, etc.

These conditions restrain diaphragmatic activity and prevent venous return to the heart contributing further to circulatory failure.

7. *Septicemia.*

The infecting organisms may be carried into the spinal canal by the needle.

8. *Infections about the vertebral column.*

The infective organisms may be carried into the spinal canal by the needle.

9. *Upper abdominal surgery.*

Circulatory disturbances occur frequently during "high spinal" anesthesia. The incidence of respiratory complications in the post-operative period is high if spinal anesthesia is employed for this type of surgery (10-12%).

10. *Anatomical disturbances of the vertebral column.*

The lumbar puncture may be impossible to perform under these circumstances.

11. *Psychically disturbed subjects.*

They are disturbed during the operation and become restless. Mentally unstable subjects may suffer "psychic trauma."

12. *Patients of advanced age.*

Cardiovascular changes are the rule rather than the exception. If hypotension is a complication, it does not respond readily to asopressor drugs or other therapy.

13. *Children.*

Circulatory system is more labile in children. The level of anesthesia is difficult to control. They are psychically unsuited for surgery in a conscious state.

Failures:

Incomplete or unsatisfactory anesthesias are due to inexperience or to errors in technique. The following are some of the more common causes of failure:

1. The needle possessed too long a bevel and thus rested partly in and partly out of the subarachnoid space (Fig. 113).

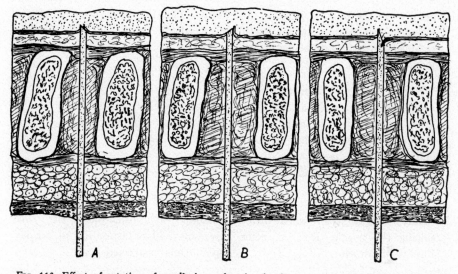

FIG. 113. Effect of rotation of needle in performing lumbar puncture. (A) Position of needle as it pierces the arachnoid. Note the flap of tissue in lumen which interferes with free flow of spinal fluid. (B) Needle rotated through an angle of 180°. Note that the lumen is cleared and a free flow of fluid is insured. (C) A long beveled needle used for spinal anesthesia. Note that the needle is partly in and partly out of the subarachnoid space. The drug will be partly if not almost entirely deposited in the extradural space.

2. The needle was not held with the left hand when solution was injected and its position was shifted by the pressure on the plunger of the syringe.
3. The patient moved suddenly after the puncture or during injection and caused the needle to shift its position.
4. The drug was old or decomposed from heat or other factors.
5. Some unknown intrinsic factor, such as resistance of the patient to the drug, tumors in the canal, or anatomical distortion, was present.
6. The operator neglected to add drug to the solution.
7. The solution was injected too slowly or too rapidly.

8. The patient was not placed in the correct position after injection.
9. There was a delay in placing the patient in the correct position after the drug was injected.

Comment	Reason
1. Never introduce a needle as far as the hub.	Needles may rust or become weakened at the junction of the hub and shaft and break at this point.
2. Warn the patient when the intradermal wheal is raised or the skin is cleansed.	The patient may be startled and move suddenly out of the arranged position if he is not warned of such maneuvers.
3. Always hold the needle with the left hand when the solution is being injected. Manipulate plunger with right hand when aspirating or injecting solutions.	The needle may shift if it is not held firmly. Failures result from shifting of the needle.
4. When attaching syringe to spinal needle to aspirate fluid or inject drug, hold it in the right hand. Grasp plunger with thumb and second finger and barrel with third, fourth, and fifth, and apply to the needle.	The barrel of the syringe and the plunger are both under control so that air is neither drawn in nor out and no solution is lost.
5. Always use a stylet when introducing the needle. Replace, after fluid is withdrawn.	Tissue or blood often blocks the lumen. Loss of fluid or aspiration of air into spinal canal is averted.
6. If lumbar puncture is unsuccessful in one interspace, attempt it in another.	"High spinal" anesthesia may be induced by injecting the drug at a lower level, and varying the technique correspondingly.
7. Do not barbotage (repeatedly withdraw and reinject solution).	The level of anesthesia is difficult to control, because the drug is spread over a considerable distance in the spinal canal.
8. Do not allow the patient to flex or extend his head or "strain" after drug has been injected.	The drug may diffuse into the upper thoracic or cervical region from the effects of the increased venous pressure which often results from straining.
9. Do not administer carbon dioxide with the oxygen in the event of	Carbon dioxide has no vasopressor effect during spinal anesthesia. Increased

hypotension, nausea, or vomiting.

respiratory volume may cause "pushing" during abdominal surgery.

10. Administer ephedrine or other vaso-pressors preoperatively only when hypotension is anticipated.

Not all patients develop hypotension during spinal anesthesia. Undesirable side effects may follow use of drug.

11. Place the patient in the desired position promptly after the drug is injected.

A delay may result in diffusion of the drug to undesired levels or in failure to secure the desired level.

12. Allow the patient to remain in bed after the anesthesia for a minimum of four hours. Use pillow to support the head.

This precaution is believed to avoid "spinal" headache.

13. Request an attendant to hold the patient in the desired position during the induction of anesthesia.

The patient may shift his position or make sudden movements during the lumbar puncture.

14. Always draw back on the plunger (aspirate) when injecting any local anesthetic drug into any tissue.

Avoid intravascular injection of the infiltrating agent.

15. Withdraw and cleanse needle if gross blood is obtained in attempting the puncture. Attempt puncture at another interspace.

The needle may be in an artery or vein.

16. Hold the needle at the hub when forcing solution in and out of the ampule (if syringe has no lock).

The needle may drop into the ampule and spoil solution by contamination

17. Strap legs and restrain wrists after anesthesia is induced.

The block may fail or "wear off" during the operation and general anesthesia will be needed in which case it is desirable to have the patient restrained.

18. Be positive the spinal fluid flows freely before injecting the drug.

A sluggish flow indicates needle is not properly placed in the subarachnoid space (Fig. 113).

19. Always determine the level of anesthesia at frequent intervals and record it according to the spinal segment involved (Th-1, Th-2, etc.).

In some techniques the height may shift during surgery.

20. Always have an anesthesia apparatus available for instant use, when conducting spinal anesthesia.

Failure to obtain prolonged or satisfactory anesthesia may require supplemental inhalation anesthesia. Respiration may fail and an inhaler may be necessary for artificial respiration.

21. Record blood pressure and pulse every two or three minutes during the first 15 minutes of anesthesia, and every five minutes during the remainder of the operation.

Circulatory collapse occurs most often in the period immediately after induction of anesthesia.

22. Watch respiration closely. Ask the patient to take a deep breath from time to time.

Respiratory failure may occur before circulatory failure if the drug ascends into the cervical region.

23. Never allow the patient to be unattended at any time during the course of anesthesia.

Changes in the patient's status occur quickly and unexpectedly and may result in a fatality.

24. Administer morphine or a barbiturate intravenously when the patient becomes restless in cases involving prolonged anesthesia (1/8-1/6 gr.).

The sedative minimizes restlessness which always accompanies long anesthesia in even the most unco-operative subjects.

25. Remember that the level of sensory anesthesia is not an index of the degree of motor paralysis.

Sensory nerves are more easily attacked by drugs and a higher level of sensory anesthesia than motor may result from diffusion.

26. Always record the exact moment of injection of the drug.

Reference to it may be necessary to determine whether or not it is safe to change the position of the patient during surgery.

27. Cover the patient's eyes during the operation (Fig. 114).

If the operating room lamps have a mirror or high polish patient may see surgery.

28. Minimize conversation between members of the surgical team during the operation and bear in mind the patient is conscious.

Conversation may have a disturbing psychic effect on the patient. Patient may hear comments concerning the malignant disease or details of operation which may upset him.

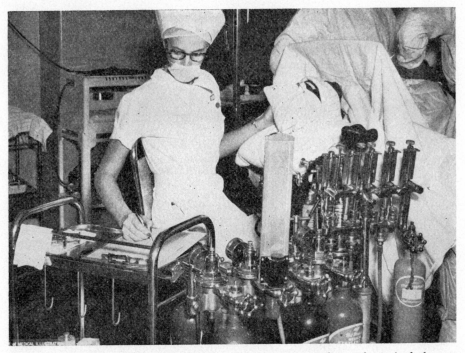

Fɪɢ. 114. A towel is placed over the eyes during the surgical procedure and a trained observer watches the patient during every moment of the procedure.

29. Always have a syringe and a vasopressor drug in readiness, particularly at onset of anesthesia. Have canula in a vein for immediate use if needed.

Onset of hypotension may be rapid in many instances and treatment must be instituted without delay.

30. Place the patient in the sitting position if the subject is obese or in instances of difficult lumbar puncture (Fig. 125, page 427).

The vertebrae are rendered more prominent and lumbar puncture is simplified in the upright position.

31. Remember that the onset of and disappearance of motor and sensory anesthesia are not simultaneous.

Each type of nerve fiber responds in a different manner to a given drug.

32. Use sealed, sterile, individual ampules of all drugs and solutions for intrathecal injection.

Withdrawal of drugs from multiple dose vials held from without sterile field may lead to contamination or infection.

33. Sterilize ampules by autoclaving for 20 minutes at 15 lbs. pressure.

Cold sterilization by submersion leads to contamination of solution through microscopic cracks.

POSTANESTHETIC COMPLICATIONS OF SPINAL ANESTHESIA

Headache:

This is the most vexsome and annoying complication encountered in the postanesthetic period.

1. *Cause.* Not definitely known. Believed to be due to:

   a. Leakage of spinal fluid from the puncture in dura. Loss of cushioning effect causes traction of brain on meninges and blood vessels.
   b. Sterile or chemical meningismus or meningitis.
   c. Excess accumulation of spinal fluid.

2. *Symptoms.* Throbbing, pulsating headache distributed over frontal or occipital area or behind eyes or over back of the neck, aggravated by changes in posture, particularly when shifting from recumbent to upright position, often accompanied by nausea, dizziness, tinnitus, etc.

3. *Onset.* Usually after first 24 hours after lumbar puncture; unusual immediately after puncture. May be delayed seven or eight days. More frequent in women than men and in apprehensive and emotional subjects.

4. *Duration.* Several days. May be prolonged for weeks or months.

5. *Contributory factors*

   a. Sex. More frequent in females than males.
   b. Type. More frequent in obstetrical patients and in "low spinal."
   c. Psyche. More frequent in intellectual type of patients.
   d. Drug. Of no notable significance. Occurs with all drugs.
   e. Volume of solution used of no consequence.

6. *Treatment.* Therapy is directed to (a) pain relief, (b) sedation, (c) correcting or removing cause.

   a. Place patient at rest. Changes in posture may aggravate and in certain cases cause nausea. Ice cap may be beneficial.
   b. Administer an analgesic—aspirin, codeine, demerol, etc. Start with milder analgesics and work upward, using narcotics only as a last resort.
   c. Sedation. Phenobarbital, gr. 1.0 q. 4 h. I.M.; seconal, gr. 1 to 3 at night. Also inhibits nausea.
   d. Replace spinal fluid or promote increased secretions.

(1) Intrathecal normal saline until spinal fluid pressure is restored to normal; usually once or twice affords relief.

(2) Intracaudal saline—30 cc.; usually one injection suffices; may be repeated.

(3) Peridural injection of saline—5 to 10 cc. daily, if necessary.

(4) Use of drugs (vasodilators or vasopressors) to promote secretion of spinal fluid. Nicotinic acid, octin, pitressin, adrenal cortical extract, ergotamine, caffeine, sodium benzoate intravenously, are tried but are of questionable value.

(5) Hypertonic saline 500 cc. 1.5% twice daily or hypertonic glucose 50 cc. 3 or 4 times daily.

(6) Mechanical methods of increasing spinal fluid pressure—tight abdominal binder.

7. *Prophylaxis*

a. Hydrate patient preoperatively with fluids.

b. Keep patient at rest first 24 hours.

c. Use small gauge needles to perform block (25 or 26 gauge) has been suggested.

d. Do not suggest or mention headaches to patient.

e. Skillful technique in performing lumbar puncture. Avoid repeated attempts at puncture.

f. Perform puncture with bevel of needle horizontal (suggested to avoid splitting the longitudinal fibres of the dura as little as possible). Of questionable importance.

Neuropathies:

A variety of neurological complications (usually unpredictable and unavoidable) may be encountered in the postanesthetic period. The etiology in certain instances is unknown. They are as follows:

1. *Palsies.* May affect any nerve, but usually affect the cranial nerves. Both sensory and motor changes may be encountered. The sixth nerve seems to be affected most frequently. Heralded by onset of diplopia several days to a week after the lumbar puncture. May last from several weeks to one year. Usually involves one nerve or its branches.

2. *Paraplegia.* Usually confined to the legs and trunk from the waist down.

   a. *Description.* Pathological changes described are variable. Myelitis, menigomyelitis, arachnoiditis, leptomeningitis, peridural abscess, etc., have been found. Inflammations are aseptic.

b. *Symptoms.* Paralysis and loss of sensation of lower half of body. Most frequently accompanied by urinary and fecal incontinence. Often referred to as "cauda equina syndrome."

c. *Onset.* Usually heralded by excruciating pain in lower half of body accompanied by shock-like state and often coma, and rapidly ensuing paralysis. Also, onset may be gradual in from one to several days after the spinal anesthetic. Characterized by progressive loss of sensation, paresis and loss of sphincter control.

d. *Probable causative factors*
   (1) Pre-existing neurological disease, such as cord tumors, myelitis, multiple sclerosis, combined degeneration of the cord, tabes, etc., which is aggravated by the procedure. This is most probable cause. Patient previously unaware of pre-existing symptoms. May notice them after and associate them with the spinal anesthesia.
   (2) *Trauma.* Due to performing the lumbar puncture above L-2.
   (3) *Technical error.* Inadvertant injection of wrong substance mistaken for the drug.
   (4) Idiosyncrasy or hypersensitive response to drug.
   (5) Use of concentrated solutions of local anesthetic drugs.
   (6) Contamination of drug by sclerosing agents (alcohol, phenol) used for sterilization of ampules.

e. *Incidence.* Very infrequent. Figures vary with clinics. Some report 1 in 100,000 or less.

f. *Treatment.* Entirely symptomatic. Analgesics for pain, physiotherapy, etc.

g. *Prognosis.* This is the most serious and feared and almost entirely unavoidable complication of spinal anesthesia. Unless symptoms begin to regress rapidly within several weeks the outlook is grave and damage is permanent.

h. *Prophylaxis*
   (1) Do not use spinal anesthesia when neurological diseases are present.
   (2) Do not use an excess of drug or concentrated solutions.
   (3) Check labels carefully. Do not use unlabeled ampules or ampules from which label has been lost.
   (4) Inspect ampules of all agents used closely for cracks and possible contamination. Add a dye (methylene blue) to the sterilizing fluid if ampules are submerged for sterilization.
   (5) Do not perform lumbar puncture above L-2.
   (6) Rinse all needles and syringes with distilled water before sterilizing. Do not use detergents for cleaning equipment.

Infections:

Peridural abscess, meningitis, myelitis, etc. These are usually due to infective organisms.

1. *Causes*

   a. Bacterial contamination of solutions, needles, catheters, gloves, drapes, or faulty aseptic technique.
   b. Performing lumbar puncture in presence of septicemia.
   c. The presence of infection about vertebral column at site of puncture.
   d. Coincidental presence of pre-existing infection.

2. *Treatment.* Isolate organism and administer appropriate chemotherapeutic agent or antibiotic.

Backache:

1. *Causes*

   a. Remaining for prolonged periods on operating table in relaxed state.
   b. Trauma from needle to periosteum or intraspinous ligaments.
   c. Trauma to intervertebral disk.
   d. Pre-existing orthopedic disturbance of spine or sacrum aggravated by surgery.
   e. Deep abscesses, hematomas, etc., due to faulty technique.

Urinary Retention:

Not related to spinal anesthesia. May occur with any type.

REFERENCES

ADRIANI, JOHN: Pharmacology of Anesthetic Drugs. 3rd Ed. Charles C Thomas, Springfield, Ill., 1953, pp. 47-51.
MAXON, L. H.: Spinal Anesthesia. Philadelphia, Lippincott. 1938.
SCHUMACHER, L. F. and EVERSOLE, U. H.: The techniques of spinal anesthesia. Anesthesiology, *3:*630-643, November, 1942.

SPINAL ANESTHESIA USING PROCAINE (HYPERBARIC)

Definition:

Anesthesia induced using procaine as the anesthetic agent. (Routine procedures described above are followed.)

Dose:

"Low spinal," 80 to 100 mgm.; *"medium spinal,"* 120 to 150 mgm.; *"high spinal,"* 150 to 200 mgm. Dosage depends upon the length of the cord (number of segments) and degree of motor and sensory anesthesia desired.

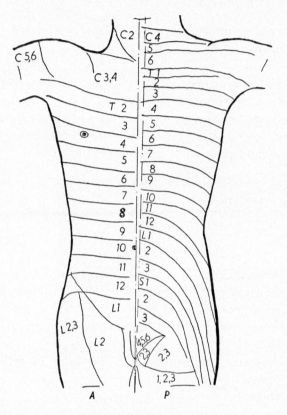

FIG. 115. Sensory distribution of the body
(A) Anterior. (P) Posterior.

Concentration:

For general use, a 5% solution. This is hyperbaric, or heavier than spinal fluid. A 2½% solution of procaine in distilled water is nearly isobaric.

For sensory anesthesia, a 3½% solution.

For intense anesthesia with marked relaxation, a 7½% solution.

Materials:

1. The standard spinal anesthesia set listed under *general considerations.*
2. An ampule of procaine hydrochloride crystals containing the desired weight of drug.
3. Ampule of epinephrine (1 mgm.) 1:1:000.

Procedure:

1. Prepare hands and drape patient in the routine manner described under *general considerations.* (page 379)
2. Perform lumbar puncture in routine manner with patient in lateral prone position as described under *general considerations.*

3. Apply syringe to the spinal needle and withdraw 2 cc. of spinal fluid for each 100 mgm. of procaine to be used (for 5% solution). Remove syringe and reinsert stylet. Or:

3a. Dissolve the drug in physiologic saline and have in readiness for injection as soon as puncture is complete.

4. Apply Wassermann needle to syringe and force spinal fluid in and out of ampule containing procaine crystals until they are dissolved. Add ½ cc. of epinephrine (0.5 mgm.).

5. Remove the stylet from needle, attach and lock syringe containing procaine solution to the hub with right hand. Hold needle with left hand.

6. Aspirate approximately 0.1 cc. of spinal fluid to ascertain needle is still properly placed. If a free flow is not obtained, readjust the needle.

7. Inject solution taking precautions mentioned under general directions. Use rate of 1.0 cc. per second for "high" spinal; 0.50 cc. per second for "low" spinal. When injection is complete, aspirate 0.1 cc. and reinject (to assure that needle has not been dislodged during manipulations).

8. Withdraw needle and turn patient to supine position. Operating table should be level. Support head on pillow.

Anesthesia:

1. *Onset.* Anesthesia is completely established within three minutes.
2. *Duration.* It usually averages one hour but ranges from three-quarters of an hour to one and one-half hours. With epinephrine it may last two hours.

Comment:

1. Remember that the level of anesthesia with procaine is attained by varying the rate of injection (diffusion) rather than by gravitation.
2. Use the upper limit of dose range and a rapid rate of injection to force drug high into canal in tall subjects.
3. Allow five minutes after injection before shifting to Trendelenburg position if this position is required.
4. Use a 3½% solution for diffuse sensory anesthesia without undue motor paralysis.
5. Employ a 7½% or 10% solution if marked relaxation is desired.
6. Employ the lower dosage range in debilitated or old subjects.

Prolongation of Anesthesia with Vasoconstrictors

Vasoconstrictor substances combined with the spinal anesthetic agent prolonged duration of anesthesia and intensify motor effects from 50-75%, depending upon the drug used. In order of efficiency are epinephrine, pitressin, arterenol, neosynephrine. Ephedrine is ineffective. The doses are as follows:

TABLE XV

	Epinephrine	Pitressin	Arterenol	Neosynephrine
Procaine—each 50 mgm.	¼ mgm.	5 units	.03 mgm.	1 mgm.
Pontocaine—each 5 mgm.	¼ mgm.	5 units	.03 mgm.	1 mgm.
Nupercaine—each 2½ mgm.	¼ mgm.	5 units	.03 mgm.	1 mgm.
Metycaine	¼ mgm.	5 units	.03 mgm.	1 mgm.

SPINAL ANESTHESIA USING PONTOCAINE AND GLUCOSE (HYPERBARIC)

Definition:

Prolonged anesthesia induced by employing a solution of pontocaine made hyperbaric by glucose.

Dose:

"Low Spinal"—5-10 mgm. (for perineal surgery).
"Medium Spinal"—12-15 mgm. (for lower abdominal surgery).
"High Spinal"—15-20 mgm. (for upper abdominal surgery).

Materials:

1. The standard spinal anesthesia set listed under *general considerations*.
2. Pontocaine hydrochloride crystals, two 10 mgm. or one 20 mgm. ampule. A 0.5% solution, crystals or microcrystals may be used.
3. Glucose (5% aqueous solution) 5 cc.
4. Shoulder braces for the operating table.
5. Epinephrine 1:1000—(1 cc.) ampule.

Procedure:

1. Record preanesthetic pulse and blood pressure and arrange patient in the lateral prone position as described under *general considerations*.
2. Dissolve pontocaine in 4 cc. glucose. Mix well by drawing pontocaine solution in and out of the ampule with the syringe. If solution is used mix equal portions with the glucose solution. Draw up the desired amount (1 cc. = 5 mgm. of drug) into the syringe. Add ¼ mgm. epinephrine (¼ cc.) for each 5 mgm. pontocaine.
3. Perform lumbar puncture in routine manner at desired level—L2 or 3 for "high spinal," L3 or 4 for "low spinal."
4. Inject solution at rate of 1 cc. per second for "high spinal," or at rate of 0.5 cc. per second for "low spinal."
5. Note and later record exact moment of injection of drug.
6. Immediately turn patient to the supine position and arrange as follows:

a. For a "high spinal" tilt table to a 10° Trendelenburg position for one to three or four minutes and follow the ascent of hypalgesia (not anesthesia) closely from moment to moment. When *hypalgesia* is established at the desired level, place the patient in the flat position (Fig. 110). This may require less than one minute but may take up to three or four minutes.

b. For "medium spinal" tilt the table to a 5° Trendelenburg position and allow the patient to remain in this position until desired level of hypalgesia is established. Then place in level position (Fig. 110).

c. For "low spinal," place in level position until hypalgesia extends to the desired level. Then place in 5° Fowler's position (Fig. 110).

Anesthesia:

1. *Onset.* Requires 5-10 minutes to become fully established.
2. *Duration.* Averages two hours but it may last from 1½ to four hours. Epinephrine increases duration 60 to 80%.

Comment	*Reason*
1. Test level of anesthesia frequently during the first five minutes. If it extends beyond the desired height, place the patient in 5° Fowler's position (Fig. 143).	The pontocaine solution is hyperbaric and gravitates cauded. Reversal of position causes drug to regress.
2. Flex the head sharply by supporting on thyroid rest or on a doubled pillow (Fig. 152).	This prevents the drug from ascending into the cervical region even though it reaches the upper thoracic segments.
3. Administer morphine and scopolamine or a barbiturate intravenously if the patient becomes restless during the anesthesia (gr. 1/8-1/6).	Prolonged surgery is tiring to patient and may cause discomfort even if anesthesia is satisfactory.
4. Induce anesthesia with patient lying on pathological side in nephrectomy or other types of surgery performed with patient on his side.	More intense anesthesia is obtained on that side because drug is hyperbaric and is deposited there.
5. Wait 10 minutes if Trendelenburg position is required. Otherwise, place patient in 10° Fowler's position for two minutes, then in desired inclination.	If the table is allowed to remain tilted, the drug diffuses cephalad.
6. Remember that the motor paralysis usually requires a longer interval to appear after injection than the sensory.	Motor fibers are the last to be affected by local anesthetic drugs.

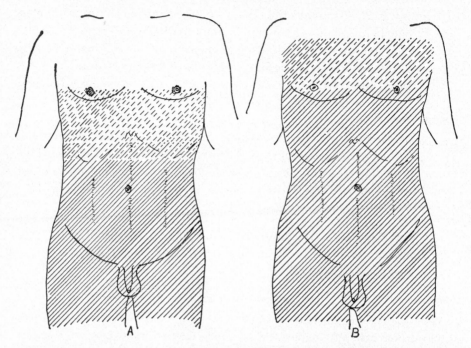

FIGURE 116. The ascent or "creeping" effect of long acting spinal anesthetic drugs. Solid lines indicate anesthesia; dotted lines, hypalgesia. (A) During induction. (B) After anesthesia is fully established. Note that hypalgesic areas in (A) have become anesthetic in (B) and that upper thoracic segments have become hypalgesic. To prevent creeping, following ascent of drug in spinal canal by studying the hypalgesic zones rather than the anesthetic.

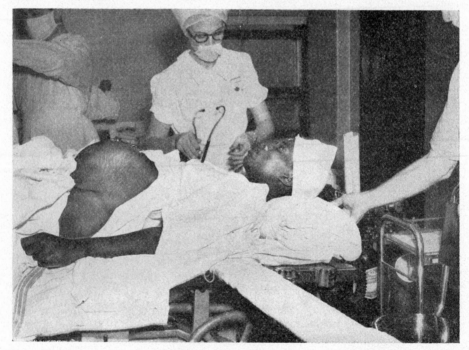

FIGURE 117. The head is sharply flexed and supported by a pillow immediately after injection of a hyperbaric solution to prevent cephalic migration of the drug.

7. Do not exceed 20 mgm. at any single injection.

Pontocaine is a highly toxic drug which could cause irreversible changes if used freely.

8. Test the level of *hypalgesia* and anesthesia from moment to moment throughout the early part of operation.

The anesthesia tends to "creep" beyond the initially established level. Hypalgesia precedes analgesia. It appears immediately. **(Fig. 116)**

9. Remember that complete anesthesia requires from 10 to 15 minutes to be fully established.

The onset of action is delayed when longer-acting anesthetic drugs are employed. Anesthesia follows hypalgesia.

REFERENCE

Sise, L. F.: Pontocaine-glucose solution for spinal anesthesia. S. Clin. North America, *15:* 1501-1511, December, 1935; *16:*1707-1711, December, 1936.

Spinal Anesthesia Using Procaine and Glucose (Hyperbaric)

Use procaine hydrochloride crystals in doses described under *Spinal Anesthesia Using Procaine* (p. 348). Mix with glucose 5% in saline or distilled water using 1 cc. for each 50 mgm. of procaine hydrochloride. Follow the technique described above for pontocaine with glucose. Epinephrine ¼ mgm. per 50 mgm. procaine may be added to prolong anesthesia.

Spinal Anesthesia Using Nupercaine (Hypobaric)

Definition:

Prolonged anesthesia produced by employing a solution of nupercaine and dilute sodium chloride.

Materials:

1. One standard spinal anesthesia set listed under *general considerations.*
2. One ampule (20 cc.) of a solution of nupercaine hydrochloride containing 1 mgm. in 1½ cc. of ½% saline (1/1500), known as Jones' solution (warm to 37° C.).
3. One syringe (20 cc.) with Luer lock.
4. Shoulder braces to support patient.
5. Pillow or thyroid rest.
6. One ampule 1:1000 epinephrine (1 cc.)

Dose:

"Low spinal," 8-12 cc. of 1:1500 solution.
"Medium spinal," 12-15 cc. of 1:1500 solution.
"High spinal," 15-18 cc. of 1/1500 solution.
Add ¼ mgm. epinephrine for each 5 mgm. nupercaine used.

Procedure:

1. Record preanesthetic blood pressure and pulse rate and arrange patient in a lateral prone position. Do not support head on a pillow.
2. Warm anesthetic solution to body temperature by placing the ampule in tepid water (50° C.).
3. Warm 20 cc. syringe by forcing tepid sterile physiological saline through it. Fill with desired volume of anesthetic solution.
4. Perform lumbar puncture in the usual manner using a 20 gauge needle. Remove 5 cc. of spinal fluid with the 5 cc. syringe and discard it.
5. Attach the syringe containing the drug and inject the drug at a rate of ½ cc. per second. *The rate should be constant from start to finish and not interrupted or changed.*
6. Turn patient immediately to the prone position (use shoulder braces) as soon as the injection is complete.
7. Immediately tilt table to a Trendelenburg position of 10°-15°.
8. Elevate the thyroid bar or place a pillow under the thorax so that the head is well flexed but thoracic portion of vertebral column is level or nearly level depending upon level of anesthesia desired (Fig. 111).
9. "Break" table and also tilt feet at same angle as head if shoulder braces are not available (Fig. 111).
10. Test the level of anesthesia with a sharp instrument every half minute during the first 10 minutes. At end of 10 minutes, straighten feet and place the patient in the supine position, but allow to remain in Trendelenburg position for an additional five minutes.

Anesthesia:

1. *Onset.* It requires 10 to 15 minutes.
2. *Duration.* It lasts from two and one-half to five hours, with an average duration of three hours. Epinephrine prolongs it 60-75%.

Comment	Reason
1. Maintain the head lower than the remainder of the body at all times during the establishment of anesthesia.	The solution is hypobaric and does not diffuse cephalad in this position.
2. Do not shift the patient into the supine position until at least 10 minutes have elapsed after injection of the drug.	Anesthesia is not established immediately when nupercaine is used. Longer lasting drugs require a longer time to be fixed.
3. Inject the solution at a constant rate,	"Patchy" anesthesia may result. The

neither too rapidly nor too slowly. Use a watch to gauge the rate of injection.

level may be too low or too high.

4. Do not exceed 20 cc. (15 mgm. of drug) of solution at any time.

Nupercaine is highly toxic and may injure tissues if excessive amounts are employed.

5. Use clean glassware at all times. Slightly acidify syringe before sterilization.

Nupercaine precipitates in alkaline solutions which have a pH as low as 7.1.

6. Do not use a needle of small bore in performing lumbar puncture.

A small bore interferes with the desired rate of injection.

7. Allow the patient to remain in prone position until level recedes if anesthesia should extend too far cephalad.

The drug diffuses upward and involves sensory roots to a greater extent than motor roots in the prone position. The intercostal muscles remain active.

8. Use lower limits of dosages for short subjects and upper limits for tall individuals.

More drug is required, when the cord is longer, to obtain satisfactory anesthesia.

REFERENCE

Jones, W. H.: Spinal analgesia, a new method and a new drug, Percaine. *Brit. J. Anes.*, 7:99-113, April, 1930.

Nupercaine-Glucose (Hyperbaric) Technique

Follow exactly the same technique described for pontocaine-glucose (page 351) using the following doses of a 1:200 buffered solution:

"High spinal," 10-15 mgm.
"Medium spinal," 7-10 mgm.
"Low spinal," 5-7 mgm.

Comment

1. Nupercaine not available in crystalline form.
2. For each 5 mgm. (1 cc.) use 1 cc. 10% glucose.

Supplementing Spinal Anesthesia

For incomplete block. Use an inhalation anesthetic—cyclopropane, ethylene-ether, nitrous oxide-ether, nitrous oxide-pentothal, evipal or surital, barbiturate with curare, if indicated.
For block which has failed. Same as above.
When operation outlasts block. Same as above.
For a satisfactory block, but the patient is apprehensive. Pentothal, surital

or evipal 1% by intravenous drip slowly; seconai 100-200 mgm. I.V.; pentobarbital 100-200 mgm. I.V.; morphine gr. ⅛ to ⅙ combined with scopolamine ½₀₀-¹⁄₁₀₀ I.V.

For nausea. Allow patient to inhale oxygen. If nausea persists, induce surgical anesthesia with cyclopropane, pentothal, nitrous oxide, or seconal, as above.

"One Legged" Spinal Anesthesia (Hyperbaric Technique)

Definition:

Anesthesia for one leg induced by subarachnoid block, using a hyperbaric solution.

Uses:

For operations on one extremity. Usually selected for "poor risk" patients.

Materials

1. Drug of choice—determined by duration desired (see below).
2. 10% glucose 1 cc.
3. Standard spinal set as in other forms of spinal anesthesia.
4. Operating table which can be tilted.

Dose of Drug:

Procaine 75 mgm.—dissolve in 1 cc. glucose 10%.
Pontocaine 5 mgm.—dissolve in 1 cc. glucose 10%.
Nupercaine 3½ mgm.—mix with 1 cc. glucose 10%.
Epinephrine ¼ mgm. added to any of above if prolonged anesthesia is desired.

Procedure:

1. Prepare solution. Check needle, syringe, etc., as for any spinal anesthetic technique.
2. Place patient in lateral recumbent position with diseased extremity *down*.
3. Incline table 20° head up, feet down.
4. Perform lumbar puncture in usual manner.
5. Inject solution as fast as gentle pressure on plunger permits.
6. Allow patient to remain on side for 10 minutes, after which time he is placed in the dorsal recumbent position.

Precautions:

1. Watch blood pressure, pulse and respiration in same manner as for other techniques of spinal anesthesia.
2. Allow patient to remain in tilted position for an additional five minutes.

CONTINUOUS SPINAL ANESTHESIA

Definition:

Anesthesia inducted by the ordinary technique but modified so that the spinal needle (or a flexible catheter) remains *in situ*. This is accomplished by the aid of an elevated special mattress provided with a recess for the

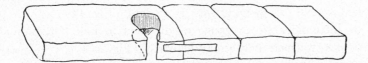

FIG. 118. Special mattress for continuous spinal anesthesia. Note the segmental arrangement which allows use of lithotomy and positions other than level on the table.

needle. Successive repeated doses of the drug are added from a syringe through a tube connected to the needle during the course of the operation.

Synonyms:

Repeated spinal, serial spinal or fractional spinal.

Uses:

For operations expected to last over one hour.

Materials:

1. One special mattress, 18″ × 6′ × 6″, with a recess approximately 8″ × 10″ in the region over which the lumbar vertebrae would lie when patient is in supine position (Fig. 118).
3. One two-way stopcock to fit the syringe and tube (Fig. 119).
4. One three-foot rubber tube with the adapter for syringe and needle.

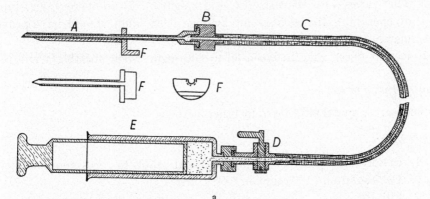

FIG. 119. Assembly of continuous spinal anesthesia. (A) Soft malleable silver needle. (B) Lock. (C) Thick walled rubber tubing. (D) Two-way stopcock. (E) 10 cc. syringe. (F) Top side and end views of the introducer.

This should possess hard walls, *3 mm. diameter*. (It must not bulge and fill up with an excess of solution (Fig. 119).)

5. One Wassermann needle (19 gauge or 20 gauge).
6. One hypodermic syringe and needle for wheals.
7. 1% procaine solution for wheal.
8. One medicine glass (2 oz.).
9. One flexible German silver needle (18 gauge) and one flexible German silver needle (20 gauge), 2½" to 4" long (Fig. 119).
10. One introducer (a 15 gauge needle filed in half longitudinally and cut to a two-inch length may be used) (Fig. 119).
11. Several ampules of 200 mgm. procaine hydrochloride crystals.
12. Physiological saline for preparation of solutions.
13. Skin sterilizer, towels, clamp, etc.
14. Several ampules of ephedrine sulphate, ¾ gr. (48 mgm.).
15. One holder or rest for the syringe.
16. Shoulder braces and wrist cuffs.

Premedication:

Patients become restless during long operations performed with spinal anesthesia. Therefore, sedation should be good. *Administer:* Morphine, gr. ⅙ to ¼, with scopolamine, gr. ¹⁄₁₅₀ to ¹⁄₁₀₀, one hour preoperatively, by hypodermic needle. Barbiturate—seconal, nembutal, or similar short-acting barbiturate in therapeutic doses, one hour before anesthesia. Ephedrine, intramuscularly, before anesthesia is induced (48 mgm.), if hypotension is anticipated. Repeat morphine during operation if surgery is prolonged. Intravenous short acting and ultra short acting barbiturates may be used.

Dose:

1. This varies with the age, sex, and height of the individual, and type of operation. Initial dose for average-sized adult should be approximately 150 mgm.
2. Repeat doses vary between 80 to 100 mgm. when anesthesia recedes.

Contra-Indications:

Same as for spinal anesthesia by other methods.

Technique:

1. Dissolve the procaine in physiological saline to form approximately a 3% solution (100 mgm. in 3 cc. saline).
2. Fill the 10 cc. syringe with this solution. Attach stopcock to the syringe and tube to stopcock. Open stopcock and fill tube with solution. When all air is forced out and tube is filled close stopcock. (This requires approximately 2 cc. of fluid.)

3. Place patient on side in usual position for lumbar puncture (the patient's back should face the opening in side of mattress).
4. Raise an intradermal wheal over interspace of L2 or L3 and anesthetize interspinous space with 1% procaine.
5. Insert the introducer into the interspinous space and prepare a tract for the needle.
6. Insert the malleable spinal needle through the path prepared by the introducer and perform the puncture as in other techniques.
7. Attach distal end of tube to spinal needle.
8. Turn patient on his back (flat) so that needle is in recess in mattress and touches nothing. Patient should make no effort to assist in turning. Assistants should turn patient.
9. Tilt table to 5° to 10° Trendelenburg position after shoulder braces are applied.
10. Open the stopcock and aspirate 1½ cc. of spinal fluid into tube. Reinject 3 cc. (1½ cc. of spinal fluid and 3 cc. of solution). Withdraw 1½ cc. more and reinject 3 cc. (barbotage). Withdraw 1½ cc. more and reinject 3 cc., giving a total of 150 mgm. of procaine.
11. Close the stopcock and fasten syringe securely with adhesive at the head of table on a rest.
12. At the end of 45 to 50 minutes, repeat the injection, using 80-100 mgms. Inject by the barbotage technique.

Advantages:

It allows the use of repeated doses of drugs of relatively low toxicity (such as procaine).

Disadvantages:

1. The needle may shift and technique may fail.
2. There is a possibility of central nervous system changes from repeated or prolonged use of the drug.
3. The mattress interferes with the convenience of the surgical team.
4. Considerable time is often consumed in executing the technique.

COMMENT

1. Watch the patient closely after each injection. Observe the level of anesthesia as well as circulation and respiration.
2. Remember that the onset of anesthesia is often delayed, sometimes as long as five minutes after the injection.
3. Control the hypotension which often follows each injection with intravenous ephedrine as in the "one dose" technique.
4. Use only soft silver needle for performing the puncture and always use an introducer.
5. Inspect all connections for leaks.

6. Administer morphine, gr. ⅙ to ⅛, and scopolamine, gr. ¼₅₀ to ½₀₀, intravenously if the patient becomes restless or complains of discomfort.

7. The successive doses required as the operation progresses are smaller than the initial dose.

8. Anticipate the point at which the anesthesia "wears off" and inject the next dose before it "wears off."

9. No definite limit is placed upon the number of successive doses which one can employ.

10. Do not allow the introducer to remain *in situ* under any circumstances.

REFERENCES

LEMMON, W. T.:* A method for continuous spinal anesthesia. Ann. Surg., *111*:141-145, January, 1940.

CONTINUOUS SPINAL ANESTHESIA—CATHETER TECHNIQUE

Materials:

1. Plastic catheter #4—30 to 60″ long with centimeter markings on the first 12 cms. (Fig. 121).
2. Tuohy needle with stylet (Fig. 121).
3. Wheal needle and syringe.
4. Rubber adapter to fit over free end of catheter (or the top of a 22 gauge needle).
5. Syringe to connect to adapter or needle top.
6. Adhesive.

Procedure:

1. Raise an intradermal wheal at the desired interspace and infiltrate the deep tissues.
2. Introduce 19 gauge needle into the subarachnoid space.
3. Slip larger needle over 19 gauge needle and introduce it until the ligamentum flavum is encountered. Avoid introducing it into the subarachnoid space (Fig. 121).
4. Withdraw 19 gauge needle entirely. Maintain grasp on larger needle during this maneuver.
5. Introduce the catheter through the needle and pass into the subarachnoid space for a distance of 4 cms. beyond end of the needle.
6. Remove the large needle without disturbing the catheter in place. Secure with adhesive over site of puncture.
7. Attach adapter and syringe to catheter and introduce drug in same manner as described above.

---

* Originated the technique.

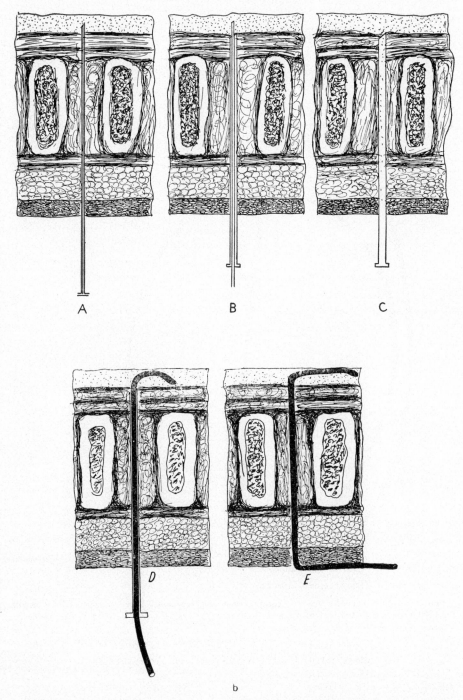

A B C

b

D E

Fig. 120. Assembly for continuous spinal anesthesia by catheter technique. (A) Special spinal needle (without flange) and stylet placed in the subarachnoid space. (B) Outer trochar introduced as far as the dura, stylet of inner needle out. (C) Inner needle removed. (D) Catheter introduced into subarachnoid space to replace inner trochar. (E) Outer trochar removed and the catheter properly placed.

COMMENT

1. Do not use old, worn or cracked catheters.
2. Sterilize catheters by immersing in bichloride of mercury or by gas sterilization.

REFERENCE

TUOHY, E. B.: Continuous spinal anesthesia. Its usefulness and technique involved. Anesthesiology, 5:142-148, March, 1944.

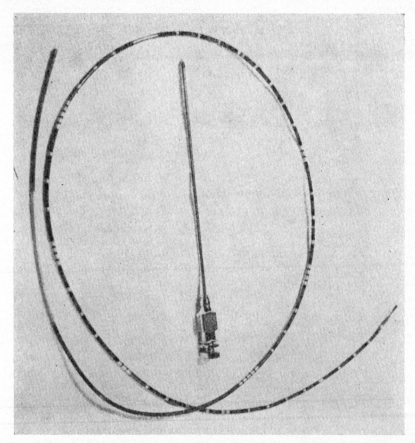

FIGURE 121. Catheter for use for continuous spinal anesthesia together with Tuohy needle. Plastic catheters may be used in place of the fine gauge ureteral catheter shown. The needle has a special point or tip known as the Huber point.

SEGMENTAL CONTINUOUS SPINAL ANESTHESIA

Description:

Continuous spinal anesthesia induced by introducing and threading the cephalad or caudad catheter in the subarachnoid space and localizing the block to several desired spinal segments.

Material:

1. Continuous spinal set.
2. Tuohy 16 gauge needle with Huber point.
3. Plastic catheter which is marked in centimeters.

Procedure:

1. Introduce spinal needle at L3 or L4 with bevel pointing laterally. Patient in lateral position.
2. Withdraw stylet and rotate needle to point cephalad or caudad, as desired.
3. Inject 5 mgm. pontocaine dissolved in 1 cc. 5% dextrose.
4. Introduce catheter and advance 15 to 35 cms. in the subarachnoid space beyond the point of needle depending upon distribution of anesthesia desired.
5. Withdraw needle as the catheter is introduced.
6. Attach needle to catheter and connect with stopcock and syringe.
7. Attempt aspiration of spinal fluid to ascertain if catheter is properly placed.
8. Wrap sterile piece of gauze 3 cm. or 4 cm. square around point of emergence of catheter to prevent contamination.
9. Turn patient in prone position and support head on pillow.

COMMENT

1. The catheter is inserted cephalad to one or two dermatomes below the desired level of anesthesia.
2. Never withdraw the catheter over the needle. It may become sheared or shaven.
3. Measure the desired distance from point of lumbar puncture to desired dermatomes before proceeding.
4. Inject 2-3 mgm. of solution at hourly intervals. The amount and frequency are determined by the height of anesthesia and reactions of patient.
5. For patients on side (kidney operations, etc.) or for injections in sacral area hypobaric solution of 1:1000 pontocaine may be used. Use "head down" position.
6. Procaine with glucose may be substituted for pontocaine. Dosage on milligram basis is 10 times as much.

REFERENCE

SAKLAD, M., DWYER, C. et al.: Anesthesiology, *8:*270-287, May, 1947.

Continuous Drip Continuous Spinal Anesthesia
(Arrowwood and Foldes)

Description:

Continuous spinal anesthesia induced by the techniques described above and maintained by connecting the indwelling catheter to a reservoir of procaine solution and allowing the solution to drip in continuously.

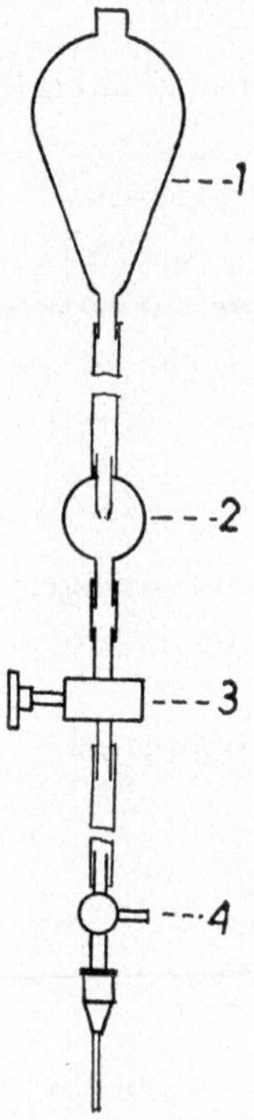

Materials:

1. Continuous spinal set described above.
2. Leveling bulb for solution 250 cc. capacity.
3. Procaine 0.5%.
4. Two-way stopcock.
5. Murphy drip.
6. Stand for drip.
7. Needle valve to regulate flow.
8. Stop watch.

Procedure:

1. Induce anesthesia injecting 6 cc. 2.5% procaine in 2.5% glucose in isotonic sodium chloride (150 mgm. procaine) (Fig. 122).
2. Place table in 5% Trendelenburg and establish anesthesia to desired level.
3. Suspend leveling flask containing .5% procaine 60-80 cms. above level of spinal needle.
4. Withdraw the procaine in the catheter in the connecting tube and other attachments. (The volume should be determined for a particular set-up before anesthesia is induced.)
5. Attach stopcock tube and tube from leveling bulb set up to the catheter.
6. Immediately replace fluid in catheter with 0.5% procaine from set-up.
7. Regulate valve to deliver the desired amount of procaine (usually eight drops per minute for upper abdominal surgery (on basis of 20 drops = 1 cc.).

Fig. 122. Assembly for "continuous drip" of continuous spinal anesthesia. (1) Leveling bulb. (2) Drip. (3) Needle valve for controlling the rate of flow. (4) Two-way stopcock. The stopcock fits into the needle or the adaptor to the continuous spinal catheter.

Comment

1. **Determine the volume of solution which will be contained in the** needle, catheter and adapters and mark it on the set-up.
2. **Calibrate the dropper in cubic centimeters per minute so that number of drops per cubic centimeter will be known for that particular dropper.**
3. **Test cutaneous levels of anesthesia at frequent intervals in order to** be assured that level has not receded.

4. Check the rate of flow dropping of procaine. It varies with the spinal fluid pressure.

DIFFERENTIAL SPINAL BLOCK (ARROWWOOD AND SARNOFF)

Description:

A subarachnoid block induced with dilute procaine solutions to obtain block of sudomotor, vasomotor, pin prick sensation while maintaining motor power, position, vibratory, touch and deep pressure sensations.

Uses:

For diagnostic and therapeutic purposes in which autonomic blockade is desired without loss of motor power.

Materials:

1. Same as for continuous drop spinal technique, described in preceding section.
2. .2% procaine solution.

Procedure:

1. Perform puncture at L3 or L4.
2. Introduce 15 to 18 cc. of 0.2% procaine solution.
3. Continue at rate of 0.6 cc. per minute as long as block is needed.

REFERENCES
SARNOFF, S. J. and ARROWWOOD, J. G.: J. Neurophysiol., *10:205-209*, 1947.
ARROWWOOD, J. G. and FOLDES, F.: Arch. Surg., *49:241-244*, 1944.

INTRASPINAL ALCOHOL

Description:

Production of anesthesia, usually permanent, of certain segments by the intrathecal injection of alcohol. Anesthesia is confined to the sensory fibers by using small volumes of alcohol.

Uses:

For the relief of intractable pain in malignant disease when all other forms of therapy have failed.

Materials:

1. Absolute alcohol sterilized to insure no contamination by spores.
2. Tuberculin syringe.
3. Standard spinal set.

Procedure:

1. Place patient in lateral prone position with afflicted side uppermost.
2. Perform lumbar puncture at site of spinal segments in which pain relief is sought.
3. Withdraw 2 or 3 cc. spinal fluid into a small syringe and discard.
4. Inject 0.5 cc. absolute alcohol into the subarachnoid space. Alcohol must be accurately measured and injected slowly (about 60 seconds).

5. Turn patient into the prone position and allow to remain at an angle of 5° Trendelenburg for approximately 30 minutes.

COMMENT

1. Alcohol is hypobaric and gravitates upward.
2. The stated quantity of alcohol is sufficient for only one or two spinal segments. Repeat injection in other areas if anesthesia does not cover desired area.
3. Motor paralysis may result if stated quantity of alcohol is exceeded.
4. Premedication, technique, preparations and precautions are same as for spinal anesthesia.

CHEMICAL ABLATION OF SPINAL CORD (WITH ALCOHOL)

Definition

The destruction of the lower portion of the spinal cord by alcohol in patients who have transection in lower thoracic or lumbar segments.

Purpose

To abolish the mass reflex which is characterized by pain, marked muscle spasm. Involuntary activity of muscles, twitchings, etc. in paraplegics.

Selection of Patient

1. To be performed only in patients with marked discomfort in whom injury to the cord is permanent and there is no hope of any regression of symptoms and who have fecal and urinary incontinence.

Materials

1. Set ordinarily used for spinal anesthesia.
2. Absolute alcohol (20 cc.)
3. Twenty cc. syringe attachable to 20 or 22 gauge spinal needle.
4. Shoulder braces.
5. Table which can be "broken" and tilted.

Procedure

(a) Preparation of patient.
    1. Omit breakfast.
    2. Premedicate with narcotic or barbiturate.
(b) Technique
    1. Arrange the patient on operating table as would be done for induction of spinal anesthesia but place in prone position. Have hips over break in operating table. Tilt table so that the head is below level of hips. Break so that legs are dependent.
    2. Maintaining positioning of patient, induce 22 or 20 gauge needle at L2 or L3 to perform lumbar puncture. Aspirate to obtain fluid since it does not issue spontaneously from the needle.
    3. Inject slowly over 3–5 minutes (with patient still in head down position) 10 cc. of the alcohol if distribution is to be between L5

and S5; 12 cc. if it is to be between L3 and S5; 15 cc. if it is to be between L1 and S5.

4. Introduce ½ cc. of saline to wash alcohol out of needle and withdraw needle.

Comment

1. Large volumes of alcohol in order to cause complete ablation of the cord.
2. Allow patients to remain in the prone position for 15 minutes. Then turn to the supine and maintain the head-down inclination.
3. Changing of position done by assistants and not aided by patients. Allow to remain in head-down, legs up position for 30 additional minutes.
4. Take control pressure. Record blood pressures frequently. Administer vasopressors if blood pressure falls.
5. Set up intravenous cannula before procedure is started for the administration of vasopressors in the event severe hypotension rapidly ensues.
6. 50 mgm. of procaine dissolved in 5 cc. of spinal fluid may be used for anesthetizing lower part of the body if desired. This may be administered 10–15 minutes before the block is commenced.

SADDLE AND MODIFIED SADDLE BLOCK ANESTHESIA

Definition:

A form of low spinal anesthesia confined exclusively to the perineal area (distribution of sacral nerves). By varying the technique the following distributions of anesthesia may be obtained (Fig. 124).

1. Perineal analgesia and relaxation of pelvic muscles and sphincter— no analgesia or paralysis of the extremities (true saddle) (Figs. 123, 124).

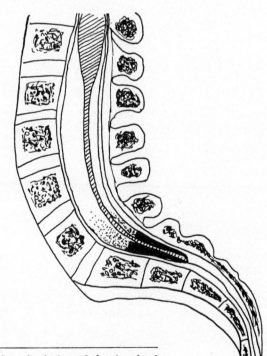

FIG. 123. Cross section of lower portion of spinal canal showing dural sac ending at S-2. When a hyperbaric solution is injected with the patient in the upright sitting position, the drug becomes localized in the conus after one minute and the sacral roots alone are affected. A true saddle block results.

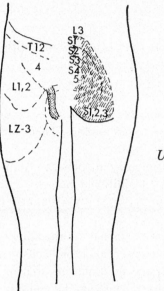

Fig. 124. Distribution of anesthesia in a true saddle block. Only the perineal areas are anesthetized.

2. Perineal analgesia and relaxation of pelvic floor with analgesia but no motor paralysis of the extremities (modified saddle) (Figs. 126, 127).

3. Sensory anesthesia and motor paralysis of the legs and perineum. No abdominal involvement (low spinal).

Uses:

1. *Saddle.* Rectal, urological, gynecological surgery involving perineum, rectum, scrotum, but not pelvic organs such as bladder, fundus of uterus, etc.

2. *Modified saddle.* Rectal, urological, gynecological surgery requiring lithotomy position.

3. *Low spinal.* Orthopedic, rectal, urological, and perineal surgery requiring loss of pain sensation in the fundus of the uterus, dome of the bladder and other pelvic structures.

Drug:

Procaine, metycaine, or monocaine for short procedures; pontocaine or nupercaine for long procedures. Dosage and concentration and duration of action are summarized in the following table:

TABLE XVI

Variations in Dosage, Volume of Solution and Timing Necessary to Obtain Saddle or Low Spinal Anesthesia with the Currently Employed Anesthetic Drugs

Drug	Preparation	Anesthesia in Saddle Area				Saddle Anesthesia Sensory of Extremities				Low Spinal, Motor and Sensory of Extremities			
		Dose (mg.)	Time Patient Sits Upright (sec.)	Duration of Anes. (hr.)	Glucose Solution (cc.)	Dose (mg.)	Time Patient Sits Upright (sec.)	Duration of Anes. (hr.)	Glucose Solution (cc.)	Dose (mg.)	Time Patient Remains Upright (sec.)	Duration of Anes. (hr.)	Glucose Solution (cc.)
Procaine	Crystals	50–75	35–40	$1\frac{1}{4}$–$1\frac{1}{2}$	1	75–100	15–20	$1\frac{1}{4}$–$1\frac{1}{2}$	1.5	100–125	0–5	$\frac{3}{4}$–1	2.0
Metycaine	10% solution	50–75	35–40	$1\frac{1}{2}$–$1\frac{3}{4}$	1	50– 75	15–20	$1\frac{1}{4}$–$1\frac{1}{2}$	1.5	75–100	0.5	1 –$1\frac{1}{2}$	2.0
Intracaine	Crystals	20–25	35–40	$1\frac{1}{4}$–$1\frac{1}{2}$	1	25– 30	15–20	$1\frac{1}{4}$–$1\frac{1}{2}$	1.5	30– 35	0–5	1 –$1\frac{1}{2}$	2.0
Monocaine	Crystals	35–50	35–40	$1\frac{1}{2}$–2	1	20– 75	20	$1\frac{1}{2}$–$1\frac{3}{4}$	1.5	75	0–5	$1\frac{1}{4}$–$1\frac{1}{2}$	2.0
Pontocaine	Crystals or powder	5	35–40	2 –$2\frac{1}{2}$	1	5– 8	20	2 –$2\frac{1}{2}$	1.5	8– 10	0.5	2 –$2\frac{1}{2}$	2.0
Nupercaine	0.5% solution	$2\frac{1}{2}$	40	$3\frac{1}{2}$–4	1	$2\frac{1}{2}$–5	20	$3\frac{1}{2}$–4	1.5	5	0–5	3 –$3\frac{1}{2}$	2.0

Materials:

1. Standard set for spinal anesthesia.
2. Drug desired for the contemplated procedure.
3. Glucose (10% in physiological saline or distilled water).

Procedure:

1. Dissolve or mix the drug (depending upon the **preparation selected**) with the necessary amount of glucose, draw into syringe and set aside

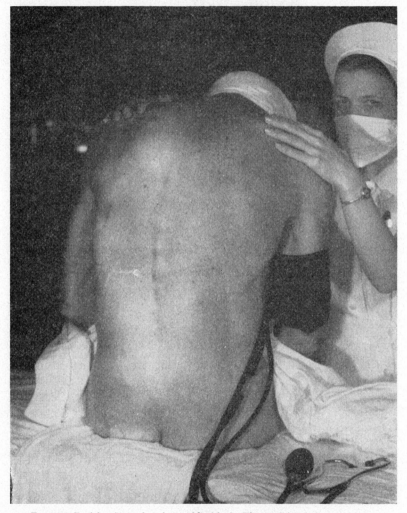

FIG. 125. Position in performing saddle block. The upright sitting position is mandatory for performing a saddle block.

until lumbar puncture is performed.

2. Place patient in upright sitting position with legs dangling over side

of the table, shoulders supported by an assistant. The patient should lean forward slightly (Fig. 125).

3. Perform lumbar puncture at L₄. L₃ may be used if L₄ is not accessible.

4. Attach syringe containing drug to needle, inject solution as rapidly as gentle pressure on the plunger permits.

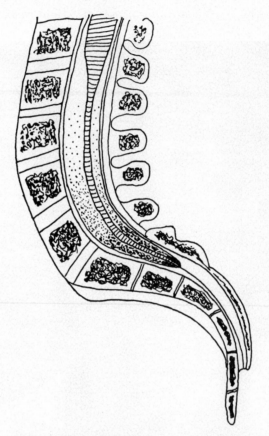

Fig. 126. Cross section of lower portion of spinal canal showing the dural sac ending at L-2. The time the patient sits upright is shortened to thirty-seconds or less. The drug diffuses into the lumbar segments and a block of varying intensity or modified saddle block results.

5. Withdraw needle. Allow patient to remain upright the necessary time (see table). Use a watch for timing.

6. Restore to the recumbent position. Place a pillow doubled upon itself under the head.

7. Place the table in Fowler's position at an angle of 5° for 5-10 minutes.

COMMENT

1. Timing and volumes of solution must be accurate.
2. Inject drug as rapidly as gentle pressure upon the syringe allows.

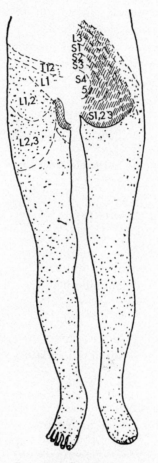

FIG. 127. Distribution of anesthesia in a modified saddle block. The shaded area represents true anesthesia. Hypalgesia and paresis are present in the dotted areas.

3. Identify the area affected by the zone of hypalgesia which immediately ensues. Anesthesia requires approximately five minutes to be completely established.

4. Do not change to lithotomy, Sims, Trendelenburg or other position for 10 minutes after the injection.

SADDLE BLOCK FOR OBSTETRICS USING NUPERCAINE

The technique is followed exactly as above with the following modifications.

1. Use 2½ mgms. nupercaine (or 5 mgm. pontocaine).
2. Use 1 cc. 10% glucose solution.
3. Allow patient to remain upright *30 seconds*.
4. Do not perform injection during a uterine contraction. The drug will be forced upward.

REFERENCES

ADRIANI, J. and ROMAN, D. A.: Saddle block anesthesia. Am. J. Surg., *71*:12-18, January, 1946.

PARMLEY, R. T. and ADRIANI, J.: Saddle block anesthesia in obstetrics using nupercaine. South. Med. J., *39*:191-195, March, 1946.

SADDLE BLOCK ANESTHESIA (HYPOBARIC TECHNIQUE)

Definition:

Saddle block anesthesia induced by using a hypobaric solution of a local anesthetic intrathecally and confining it to the sacral segments.

Indications:

For operations and diagnostic procedures requiring anesthesia of the saddle area in which the prone position is mandatory.

Materials:

1. Standard spinal anesthetic set.
2. Potent drug (pontocaine or nupercaine) which will yield a hypobaric solution in a small volume of distilled water.
3. Sterile distilled water.

Technique:

1. *Position*

    a. Place the patient in the prone position with the hips level with the "break" of the operating table.
    b. Place two pillows to support the lower part of the abdomen. This eliminates the lumbar curve.
    c. Incline the lower half of the table to an angle of 45 to 50° in order to separate spines of vertebrae.

    d. Lower the head of the table slightly to approximately 10°.

2. *Procedure*

    a. Prepare the skin.

    b. Raise a skin wheal and perform the interspinous injection with procaine at the 3rd and 4th lumbar interspace. Lateral route may be used.

    c. Perform lumbar puncture. Aspirate if spinal fluid does not flow freely.

    d. Turn the bevel of the needle caudad. As soon as spinal fluid is obtained lower the operating table to a 30° position.

    e. Inject solution (5 cc. of .010% pontocaine or 4 cc. of 0.75% nupercaine 1:1500) in a period of two to five seconds. Allow patient to remain in prone position with head down.

    f. Withdraw needle and remove pillows beneath the abdomen.

Anesthesia:

1. *Onset.* Five to 10 minutes.
2. *Duration.* Pontocaine 1½ to two hours; Nupercaine two to 2½ hours.
3. *Distribution.* Complete in saddle area. Hypalgesia and possibly paresis may be present in the extremities.

Complications:

Drug may spread to higher spinal segments and produce a greater extent of anesthesia than saddle distribution.

Comment

Lumbar puncture is not always feasible in prone position. In event of failure use lateral prone position with head down position of 15-20°. Place in the prone position, table tilted immediately after injection.

EPIDURAL ANESTHESIA

Definition: Anesthesia obtained by blocking the spinal nerves as they pass through the epidural space.

Synonym: Peridural anesthesia, extradural anesthesia.

Types: Two types are available according to the route used to obtain access to the epidural space:

    1. "Spinal" epidural or lumbar epidural. This is obtained by introducing a needle between the lumbar spines as for lumbar puncture.

2. Caudal anesthesia. This is obtained by introducing a needle through the sacrococcygeal membrane into the caudal canal.

"SPINAL" EPIDURAL ANESTHESIA

Definition: Anesthesia obtained by blocking the lumbar and thoracic spinal nerves in the epidural space.

Uses:

 Anesthetic: For operations upon the lower extremity and abdomen.
 Therapeutic: For relief of intractable pain.

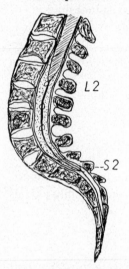

 Indications: In cases in which the analgesia of spinal anesthesia is desired, but in which spinal anesthesia is contraindicated.

 Anatomy: The epidural space extends from the coccyx to the foramen magnum. The dura, at the foramen splits into two layers, an external and an internal. The external layer covers the bony surfaces of the spinal canal and corresponds to the periosteum. The internal layer covers the cord and is actually the true dura. The space which lies between the two layers is epidural space. It is filled with fat and a plexus of veins. When the back is arched sharply, a negative pressure develops in the space. The cord ends at L 2, the dural sac at S 2 (Fig. 128).

FIG. 128. Cross section of lower portion of spinal column. Note spinal cord ending at (L 2) and dural sac at (S 2).

 Materials: Same as for spinal anesthesia, but in addition provide:

 1. One 20 cc. syringe which can be attached to a 19 G short bevel spinal needle.

 2. A container to act as reservoir for local anesthetic solution (100 cc.).

3. A glass connecting tip or observation tube which fits into the hub of spinal needle provided with a bore of small calibre 0.5 to 1 mm.

Dosage: Procaine hydrochloride 2% solution:

 a. 35 cc. for perineal and low pelvic surgery
 b. 45 cc. for lower abdominal surgery.
 c. 50 cc. for upper abdominal surgery.

Technique:

 1. *Position*
  a. Lateral prone as for spinal anesthesia. This is the preferred position.
  b. Upright sitting.
 2. *Landmarks:* 2nd or 3rd lumbar interspaces.

Procedure:

1. Prepare skin, raise an intradermal wheal, and anesthetize subcutaneous and interspinous tissues as for spinal anesthesia.
2. Introduce the 19 gauge needle (short beveled) until it is well engaged in the interspinous ligament.
3. Remove stylet and attach glass adapter to the needle. The capillary tube should previously be filled with procaine solution.
4. Request an assistant to arch back of patient well to accentuate the negative pressure in the epidural space.
5. Advance needle into epidural space (a snap is felt as needle passes through interspinous ligament). The fluid in glass adapter is sucked inward due to negative pressure if the needle is in the epidural space (Fig. 129). If fluid pours outward, it is in subarachnoid space.*
6. Attach 20 cc. syringe containing 10 cc. 2% procaine to the needle and attempt aspiration.
7. Rotate needle through an angle of 180° and aspirate once again.
8. If no spinal fluid or blood is obtained, inject 10 cc. of solution as rapidly as it flows (approximately 1 cc. per minute).
9. Disconnect syringe, replace stylet, but do not allow patient to shift position or remove needle.
10. Allow 5 minutes to elapse. Test lower extremity for motor paralysis and analgesia. If none exists and no other outward effects have appeared, it may be assumed needle is not in the subarachoid space and remainder of the drug may be safely injected.
11. Withdraw stylet, attach syringe, and attempt aspiration once again. Inject the remainder of the solution as rapidly as solution will pass into the epidural space.
12. Withdraw needle and place the subject in the supine position for abdominal surgery, Trendelenburg position (10°) for upper abdominal and Fowler's (5°) for pelvic surgery.

Anesthesia:

Onset: Usually appears within 10 minutes and is completed within fifteen to twenty minutes.

Distribution: Motor anesthesia and sympathetic paralysis is only partial. Sensory anesthesia of lower extremities and abdomen is complete. Analgesia as far as clavicles may ensue.

Duration: One and a half to two hours. The analgesia recedes gradually.

---

* The negative pressure in the epidural space is not a constant finding. Because of this Abajian has suggested attaching a small syringe containing 2 cc. of normal saline solution to the needle just as it approaches the ligamentum flavum and exerting pressure upon the plunger. The sense of resistance felt on the plunger as the needle passes the ligament immediately disappears as entry into the epidural space is made and the liquid then flows freely. The syringe is removed and the needle advanced cautiously until it is engaged in the epidural space.

Complications:

1. The needle may enter subarachnoid space and the total dose be inadvertently injected there. This is approximately 10 times the average dose for spinal anesthesia.
2. The needle may enter one of the intraspinal veins and an intravascular injection results.

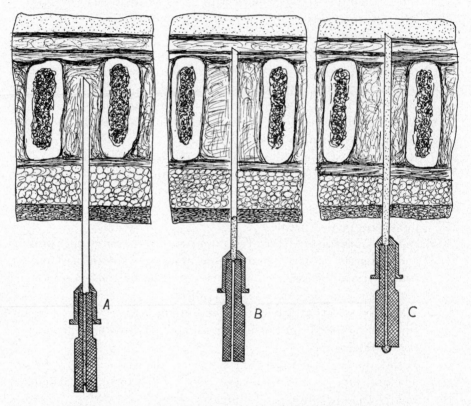

FIG. 129. Method of performing lumbar epidural block. (A) Needle and glass adapter. The capillary tube is filled with procaine solution. (B) Needle in epidural space. Note aspiration of fluid from the glass adapter into the needle and epidural space. This is caused by the negative pressure in the epidural space. (C) Needle in subarachnoid space. Flow of the spinal fluid indicates needle has been advanced too far.

3. Segmental (spotty) anesthesia may result.
4. Hypotension if motor paralysis is intense and widely distributed (as for spinal anesthesia).
5. Reaction due to hypersensitivity or rapid absorption of the drug.

Advantages:

1. Duration of action is prolonged compared to spinal anesthesia.
2. The drug diffuses from the epidural space along the course of the nerve and anesthesia comparable to paravertebral block results.

3. There is no contact between the bare nerve roots or cord and drug as in spinal anesthesia.
4. The drug cannot pass into the medullary region because the epidural space ends at the foramen magnum.
5. Headaches infrequent in comparison to spinal anesthesia.
6. Danger of meningitis or encephalitis or other neurological complications is minimized compared to spinal anesthesia.

Disadvantages:

1. The placement of the needle in the epidural space is difficult to verify. The danger of entering the subarachnoid space and depositing an overdose of local anesthetic drug is ever present.
2. Muscle relaxation is inadequate and unsatisfactory.
3. Level of analgesia is difficult to control and unpredictable.
4. Large quantities of drug are necessary to secure anesthesia (almost one gm. of procaine).
5. Drug may not penetrate each of the nerves concerned with similar facility or ease and anesthesia is incomplete or segmental.

Comment

1. Withdraw the needle and reinsert into different interspace if spinal fluid is obtained.
2. Treat hypotension in the same manner as that which accompanies spinal anesthesia.
3. Observe the same precautions described for lumbar puncture in introducing the needle.
4. Do not omit premedication particularly if patients are apprehensive.
5. Do not fail to administer a barbiturate preoperatively.
6. Always perform the puncture in the midline.
7. Always employ a needle with a short bevel.

8. Do not arch back until the needle enters the epidural space.
9. Always perform the puncture in the lumbar region.
10. Do not employ weak solutions of procaine (less than 2%).

Reasons

Spinal anesthesia may result if injection is attempted after puncturing the arachnoid.
The mechanism of its production is similar to that which accompanies spinal anesthesia.
The technique is essentially the same in both cases.

The intensity of anesthesia and analgesia is not profound and the patient may have some sensation.
This minimizes reactions to the local anesthetic drug.
Trauma to the meningeal vessels is avoided.
A long bevel may partially enter the subarachnoid space as well as epidural space.
This prevents dilatation of the veins in the space.
The epidural space is larger in this area.
The dura passes over the nerves as a sheath in the epidural space,

and the drug penetrates this with difficulty.

11. Insert stylet to clear the needle before solution is injected.

Some tissue may have entered the lumen while the needle was traversing the ligament.

Variations in Technique

1. Epinephrine (0.75 cc. of a 1:1000 solution) may be added to the procaine to prolong anesthesia. Its use may be accompanied by systemic disturbances from the sympathetic stimulation.
2. Pontocaine, 10 mgm. in 50 cc. of 2% procaine, may likewise be added to prolong anesthesia, but its use is accompanied with more danger.
3. Intracaine, 2% in saline, lidocaine 1% or metycaine 1 1/2% or pontocaine 0.1% or 2% carbocaine may be used instead of procaine.
4. 2% procaine or intracaine base in sweet almond oil may be employed for therapeutic purposes.

SEGMENTAL EPIDURAL ANALGESIA

Segmental epidural analgesia may be accomplished by introducing the needle in the lumbar or thoracic vertebral interspaces corresponding to the spinal segments desired and injecting 20 to 25 cc. of 2% procaine. Blocking of the desired pathways at these selected levels of the cord obviates filling the entire epidural space with drug and limits the extent of anesthesia (see Abajian, J., listed below).

CONTINUOUS EPIDURAL BLOCK

Materials

1. One 7.6 cms. 16 gauge Tuohy spinal needle.
2. One Tuohy adapter.
3. One 2 cm. 23 gauge Lok needle.
4. One 3.5 Bard ureteral x-ray catheter with stylet or one 90 cm. (3 ft.) plastic tubing with stylet.

Procedure

1. Locate and mark off 2nd lumbar interspace.
2. Raise skin wheal and infiltrate with 1% procaine.
3. Introduce 16 G Tuohy needle. (Face bevel cephalad for abdominal surgery; cauded for rectal) in same manner as for ordinary technique.
4. Introduce catheter or plastic tube with stylet in Tuohy needle holding needle with left hand and threading catheter with right.
5. Withdraw stylet $\frac{1}{4}''$ when catheter encounters curve of Tuohy needle and is no longer movable.
6. Measure off the distance catheter or tubing is to be introduced into epidural space on catheter.
7. Insert for the measured distance (about $2\frac{1}{2}$ or $3''$).

8. Withdraw Tuohy needle exerting constant pressure on tubing inward so it will not be dislodged and come out with needle.

9. Remove stylet.

10. Attach catheter adapter to catheter or 2 cm. 23 gauge Lok needle to plastic tube.

11. Introduce 3 cc. of local anesthetic solution at 1 cc. per 2 or 3 seconds.

12. Wait 5 minutes and test for spinal anesthesia in lower extremities.

13. Place piece of gauze over catheter or tubing over point of emergence from skin.

14. Place patient in supine position.

15. Add 7 to 12 cc. of procaine 2% (or other desired solution).

16. Test area for adequacy of anesthesia.

Comment

1. Do not attempt to withdraw tubing or catheter once it has passed point of needle. It will be sheared off by needle point if this is attempted.

2. Partially remove stylet for each cm. of advancement of catheter.

3. Perform puncture at L2. The widest portion of epidural space is at this point.

4. Perform block using same technique and precautions recommended for epidural block by the ordinary technique.

5. Repeat ⅔ of dose of drug when signs disappearing sensory loss become apparent.

REFERENCES

Abajian, J., Jr. Peridural Segmental Anesthesia with Intracaine. Anesthesiology, *4:* 372–384, July, 1943.

Odom, C. B. Epidural Anesthesia. Am. J. Surg., *34:* 547–558, December, 1936.

Odom, C. B. A Review of Pages' Epidural Anesthesia with a Report of 100 cases. New Orleans M. & S. J., *88:* 618–627, April, 1936.

Tovell, R. M., and Hinds, C. B. Abdominal Block with General Anesthesia for Upper Abdominal Surgery. J.A.M.A., *115:* 1690–1692, November 16, 1940.

CAUDAL ANESTHESIA

Definition: Caudal block is a block of the lumbosacral and coccygeal plexus obtained by depositing a solution of local anesthetic drug in the epidural space in the sacral canal. The nerves are bathed as they emerge from the dural sac.

Synonym: Caudal, peridural, or extradural block.

Uses:

1. *Anesthetic:*

   a. Urological operations (except those involving the dome and the sides of the bladder. This portion of the bladder is innervated by the vesical plexus, which arises from the hypogastric plexus).

   b. Rectal operations.

    c. Perineal operations (except those involving the clitoris and the
dorsal surface of the penis; their innervations are derived from the
hypogastric plexus).

    d. Obstetrics.

  2. *Therapeutic:*

    a. Relief of acute sciatica.

Anatomy: The sacrum is a wedge-shaped bone jointed by ligaments to either
side of the ilium (Fig. 130). The upper surface or apex is attached to the
coccyx. The sacrum is formed from five fused modified vertebrae. The
posterior surface of the sacrum is irregular, convex upward and backward and presents on two sides two rows of openings, each known as the

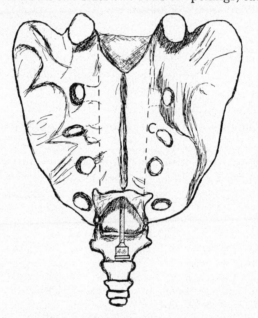

FIG. 130. Dorsum of the sacrum showing the
caudal needle in the sacral canal. Note that the
sacral hiatus lies between the sacral cornua and
that the needle is not introduced beyond the level
of the second sacral foramina (C).

posterior sacral foramina, through which the posterior primary divisions
of the sacral nerves pass to the region of the dorsum of the sacrum. The
first four foramina, about one cm. in diameter and almost parallel with
the midline, are inclined inward to follow the margin of the bone. A
spinous crest which is the remnant of the spinous process is present on
the midline from S_1 to S_4. The fifth spinous process is absent and leaves
an opening at the apex called the sacral hiatus which is "V" shaped. The
hiatus is bounded on either side by two prominences or sacral cornua
which are used to identify the hiatus. The anterior surface of the sacrum
is smooth, triangular, and concave and presents two rows of foramina,

the anterior sacral foramina through which the anterior primary divisions of the nerves pass. The anterior and posterior foramina face each other and communicate with a canal, lying within the sacrum called the sacral canal. The sacral hiatus which is the entrance to this canal, is covered by a thick membrane, the sacrococcygeal membrane. The dural sac, which encloses the filum terminale, ends at the level of the second sacral foramina. The second sacral foramina is approximately one cm. caudad and one cm. medial to the posterior superior iliac spine. The nerves involved during caudal block are those arising from (a) the sacral plexus. This is formed by L_4, L_5, S_1, S_2, and S_3 (the anterior primary divisions). From the anterior and posterior surface of this plexus numerous branches are given off, but the main portion of the plexus is continued as the sciatic nerve, (b) the pudenal nerve. This derives its branches from the anterior divisions of S_2, S_3, and S_4. (c) The coccygeal plexus. This derives its branches from the anterior divisions of S_4 and S_5 and the coccygeal nerve. The posterior primary divisions of these various nerves are also blocked in caudal block.

Materials:

1. In addition to the standard nerve block tray, the following materials are necessary:
2. One 18 or 19 gauge (10 cm.) semi-flexible needle.
3. One 10 cc. syringe which fits the needle. Select a type satisfactory for regional anesthesia.

Technique:

1. *Position:*
   a. Place the patient in the prone position with a pillow under the hips to elevate the sacrum. The operator should stand at the patient's left side. This position is preferred.
   b. In Sims or knee chest position for obstetrics.
2. *Landmarks:*
   a. *The coccyx:* This may be palpated in the gluteal cleft with the right index finger at the base of the vertebral column.
   b. *The sacro-coccygeal joint:* The depression felt at the joint corresponds to the sacral hiatus. It may be palpated by drawing the finger cephalad over the coccyx.
   c. *The sacral cornua:* These represent the inferior articular process of the fifth sacral vertebra. The cornua mark the lateral boundaries of the sacral hiatus.
   d. *The second sacral foramina:* Palpate the posterior superior iliac spine. Measure and mark a point on the skin one cm. caudad and one cm. medially. This point overlies the foramen.

3. *Procedure:*
  a. Locate and mark both sacral cornua and the second sacral foramina.
  b. Raise an intradermal wheal at a point midway between the cornua. This overlies the sacral hiatus.
  c. Inject 1/2 cc. of anesthetic solution into the subcutaneous tissues and the sacrococcygeal membrane.
  d. Locate and mark both second sacral foramina.
  e. Place the needle along the sacrum and mark off the distance between the foramina and the cornua.

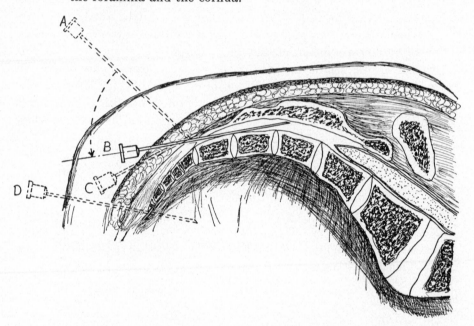

Fɪɢ. 131. Cross section of the sacrum during a caudal block. (A) Position of the needle while contacting the sacrococcygeal membrane. (B) Position after the needle has pierced the membrane and is entering the caudal canal. Note the needle lies in a plane almost parallel to the surface of the sacrum. (C) Incorrect placement of the needle when the hiatus is inaccessible or missed. The needle lies upon the surface of the sacrum. (D) The needle is shown in the pelvis. This occurs if the tip of the coccyx is mistaken for the sacrococcygeal joint. Note the position of the dural sac.

  f. Stretch the skin over the hiatus with the thumb and index finger of the left hand to facilitate puncture.
  g. Grasp the needle (with the stylet in place) with the thumb and index finger of the right hand and pierce the wheal so that an angle of 45° is made with the skin overlying the sacrum (Fig. 131).
  h. Advance the needle to the sacrococcygeal membrane which is encountered approximately 3/4 cm. from the skin surface.
  i. Swing the hub of the needle downward to an angle of approximately 20° to the surface of the sacrum (Fig. 131).
  j. Pierce the sacrococcygeal membrane and introduce the needle into the sacral canal, as far as the marker.

k. Withdraw the stylet, attach the syringe and attempt aspiration. Rotate needle and attempt aspiration once again. If no blood or spinal fluid is obtained, introduce 5 cc. of 2% procaine slowly into the canal. The solution should pass in freely with slight pressure on the plunger if the needle is in the canal. Place the hand upon the dorsum of the sacrum during the injection to note the appearance of tumefaction which indicates the needle is subcutaneous rather than in the canal.

l. Remove the syringe from the needle and replace the stylet. Watch closely for toxic reaction or the appearance of spinal anesthesia.

m. Allow five minutes to elapse and, if no untoward reaction appears, inject the remainder of the procaine solution (20 cc.) slowly into the canal. Aspiration should be done frequently during the injection.

n. Withdraw the needle from the canal, but not completely from the subcutaneous tissue. Divert it towards each cornua, first one side, then the other, and inject 1/2 cc. of solution into the fifth sacral foramen. This blocks the fifth sacral nerve which emerges beneath the cornua.

Anesthesia:

1. Onset gradually appears in 10 to 15 minutes.
2. *Distribution:*
   a. Complete anesthesia of the anal sphincter, structures about the anus, structures over the sacrum, vagina, labia majora and minora, the under surface of the penis, the scrotum, the bladder (except the dome), the urethra, the cervix, and th lower uterine segment. Partial anesthesia is obtained over the outer under surface of the foot and a band extending along the posterior aspect of the leg. Muscles of pelvic floor are relaxed.
3. *Duration:*
   a. From one to two hours.

Complications:

1. Intravascular injection: The peridural space in the sacral canal is lined with a rich plexus of veins anyone of which may be pierced by the needle.
2. Intraspinal injection. Spinal anesthesia results. This is caused by advancing the needle beyond the level of the second sacral foramina into the dural sac (Fig. 131).
3. Piercing of rectum: The needle is inserted through the anococcygeal ligament if incorrect landmarks are chosen (Fig. 131).
4. Subperiosteal injection. No anesthesia is obtained. The solution is injected with difficulty.

5. Local infections or peridural abscess. To prevent these, asepsis must be rigidly observed.
6. Broken needle in the caudal canal. Test all needles before performing the block.

Contra-Indications:

1. Distortion of the bony landmarks, by arthritis, old fractures, tuberculosis, neoplasms, etc.
2. The presence of local infection at the site of injection.
3. For emotionally unadjusted patients.
4. For prolonged operations.
5. Aspiration of blood or spinal fluid after introducing the needle in attempting block. Select another technique of anesthesia.

"High" Caudal Anesthesia

Definition: An epidural block produced by the injection of a large volume of local anesthetic solution into the caudal canal so that it diffuses into the lumbar or thoracic peridural space.

Uses:

1. For urological operations, such as on the dome of the bladder or of the suprapubic type.
2. For operative obstetrics.

Procedure: The procedure for "high caudal block" is similar to caudal block with the exception that a larger volume of fluid is necessary to force a sufficient amount of fluid to involve the nerves in lumbar or thoracic regions.

Technique:

1. Proceed exactly as described for caudal block. Insert the needle in usual manner, and inject 5 cc. of 2% procaine.
2. Allow 5 minutes to elapse as in caudal block.
3. Inject 50–60 cc. of 2% procaine instead of 25 or 30 and follow directions and precautions as for caudal block.

Comment on Caudal Block	*Reasons*
1. **Do not proceed with the block if spinal fluid or blood is aspirated into the syringe.**	The drug may pass into the subarachnoid space or into the vascular system.
2. Treat hypotension by means of ephedrine or other vasopressor in the same manner as hypotension in spinal anesthesia.	The mechanism producing it is similar to that caused by spinal anesthesia.

3. Remember that the drug leaves the peridural space by diffusion along the spinal nerves. | The drug does not diffuse through the dura.

4. **Always allow twenty minutes between completion of the block and scheduled time of operation.** | Satisfactory anesthesia is not complete in less than twenty minutes.

5. **Always rotate the needle and attempt aspiration twice.** | The needle tip may be in a vein and pressed to the bony surface. This prevents aspiration of blood and would be misleading if aspiration is attempted only once.

6. Place a gauze sponge in the intergluteal fissure in preparing the patient. | Antiseptic solutions employed to prepare the skin are prevented from spreading to anus and genitalia.

CAUSES OF FAILURE OF CAUDAL BLOCK

1. Inability to correctly introduce the needle into the sacral canal. This may be due to:
   a. Absence of reliable landmarks.
   b. Impermeability of sacrococcygeal membrane to the needle.
   c. Distortions of sacrum due to disease.
2. The solution employed is insufficient in volume or weak in strength.
3. The sacral canal is large and the volume of solution is not sufficient to fill it.
4. Bleeding within canal due to trauma to veins interferes with diffusion of the drug.
5. The injection was made into subcutaneous tissues or posterior aspect of sacrum because needle is not properly placed.
6. The injection was made into the pelvis because needle was inserted through sacrococcygeal ligament at tip of coccyx instead of at sacrococcygeal joint.
7. The neural sheaths are too dense or impermeable to the drug.
8. The dura may be adherent to the periosteum and does not allow the drug to pass into the lumbar epidural space. (The dura is frequently adherent at the lumbosacral joint.)

REFERENCES

Labat, Gaston. Regional Anesthesia. P. 496. Philadelphia, W. B. Saunders Co., 1922.

Lundy, J. S. A Method for Producing Block Anesthesia of the Sacral Nerves. Am. J. Surg., 4: 262–270, March, 1928.

Tuohy, Edward B. Regional Block Anesthesia for Operations on the Perineum, Anus, Genitalia and Lower Extremities. 2: 369–387, July, 1941.

"Continuous" Or Repeated Caudal Block

Definition: Caudal block, either high or low, which may be sustained over a long period of time by allowing the needle to remain *in situ* and repeating the injection of drug.

Uses:

1. *Obstetrics:* For relief of pain or labor and operative procedures.
2. *Urological or gynecological and rectal surgery:* For prolonged operations upon the perineum, rectum, or genitalia.

Materials: Same as for caudal by single injection, but in addition provide:

1. One three way stopcock (Luer) or one way valve (Fig. 132).
2. One length of thick walled rubber tubing 4 feet long, equipped with Luer lock hub which fits the caudal needle at one end and the stopcock or one way valve at the other.
3. One length of similar tubing 2 inches long equipped with adapter for attaching the syringe.
4. One wide mouth sterile glass receptacle of approximately 500 cc. capacity (preferably calibrated) (Fig. 132).
5. One rubber stopper with two perforations to fit the glass receptacle (Fig. 132).

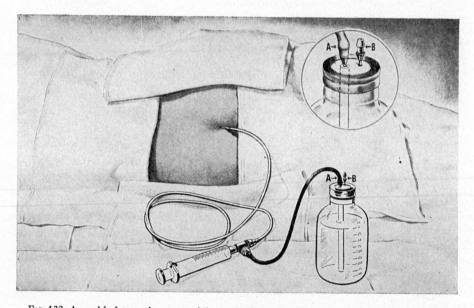

Fig. 132. Assembly for continuous caudal anesthesia. The needle is a special one made of malleable metal. Note knob near hub which acts as a guard. The tube connecting the needle with the valve and syringe must be at least four feet long and must have a thick wall because it will be subjected to considerable pressure. Soft rubber tubing is used for connecting the valve to the reservoir for the local anesthetic solution. (Courtesy Dr. Robert A. Hingson.)

6. One piece of glass tubing approximately 3/16″ in diameter, bent at right angles to fit the stopper and slide in the full length of the glass receptacle or a 15 gauge long aspirating canula with hose type connection (Fig. 132).

7. One 18″ length of rubber tubing to fit end of stopcock and glass receptacle (Fig. 132).

8. Gauze, or felt pad to protect needle.

9. Special 19 gauge malleable needle and stylet (Fig. 132).

10 One 10 cc. syringe with Luer lock.

Technique:

1. *Landmarks* are the same as for caudal block by single injection.
2. *Position* is the same as for caudal block by single injection.
3. *Procedure:*
   a. Arrange apparatus as shown in Fig. 132.
   b. Prepare patient as described for caudal block.
   c. Introduce special needle in same manner as described for caudal block.
   d. Remove stylet from needle, attach 2″ tubing to hub.
   e. Attach syringe and attempt aspiration as described in caudal block.
   f. Introduce 10 cc. 2% procaine or equivalent of other preferred drug, replace stylet and allow 5 minutes to elapse as in caudal block.
   g. Expel air from long tube by filling with solution and attach it to the hub of the needle.
   h. Attempt aspiration frequently during injection.
   i. Close stopcock, secure needle with adhesive after padding hub well with gauze or felt.
   j. Place patient in a comfortable position.
   k. Repeat the injection when the diminution of analgesia is becoming apparent. Successive doses should be introduced in the same manner and with the same care as the initial dose.

Anesthesia:

1. *Onset:* Same as in caudal block by single injection.
2. *Duration:* Same as in caudal block by single injection. Repeat as often as necessary using same volume as for initial injection.
3. *Extent:* May be high or low, depending upon need of individual cases. May be controlled by varying volume of fluid. 30 cc. for low (perineal); 45 cc. for medium (suprapubic) and 60 cc. 2% procaine for high (abdominal) anesthesia.

Advantages: Same as for caudal block by single injection, except that duration may be prolonged.

Complications:

1. These are the same as for caudal block, but the following additional objections are offered:
   a. Needle may break in canal.
   b. The needle may shift position and enter a vessel or the dura.
   c. Tissues may be injured from repeated or prolonged exposures to the local drug.
   d. Asepsis is not easily maintained and peridural or local abcesses form.
   e. A sense of fullness in sacrum or pain in legs may accompany injection of the drug. This soon passes away.

Contra-Indications: Same as for caudal block.

Remarks:

1. The anesthetist should attend the patient constantly. Repeated doses should be administered by a physician.
2. Individualize the dosage and frequency of injection.
3. Exercise the same precautions in subsequent injections as at the initial injection.
4. Repeat premedication if patient becomes apprehensive during surgery.
5. Cleanse skin in area of injection thoroughly to avoid infection.
6. Add epinephrine 0.75 cc. of a 1 to 1000 solution to each 50 cc. of the drug to prolong its action and inhibit absorption.

CONTINUOUS CAUDAL ANESTHESIA IN OBSTETRICS

Procedure: A "high" caudal block is performed in the manner described above, so that epidural anesthesia involving the lumbar segments (or higher) is induced to produce relief of pains of labor.

Advantages:

1. Complete relief of pain if the block is "high."
2. Uterine contractions are not abolished and labor continues.
3. Relaxation of muscles of pelvic floor is excellent and facilitates and quickens labor. Dilatation of the cervix is facilitated.
4. Respiratory and other functions of fetus are not depressed.
5. Patient is conscious and retains normal faculties.
6. Metabolic and other functions are not disturbed.

Disadvantages:

1. Unavoidable failures due to technical difficulties or anatomical distortions limit its use.
2. Bladder urge is lost and urine leaks with each uterine contraction.

3. Analgesia may mask ensuing complications, such as rupture of uterus.
4. Circulatory failure or depression may occur if anesthesia is intense.
5. Toxic reactions may occur from rapid absorption of the drug.
6. Labor is retarded if ascent of anesthesia extends beyond Th 10.
7. Greater incidence of instrumental deliveries.
8. Malpositions, particularly posterior presentations, do not correct themselves.

Contra-Indications:

1. Subjects in whom disproportion between size of fetus and canal exists.
2. Cases of placenta praevia.
3. The presence of deformities of spine or sacrum or other anatomical distortions.
4. The presence of local infection in vicinity of sacrum.
5. Versions and similar type of operative obstetrics.
6. Cases of hypotension.

Remarks:

1. Inject one full dose of the drug at time of delivery if the interval ensuing between it and previous injection is more than thirty minutes.
2. Disconnect the tube, replace stylet but leave needle in place during delivery. Inject another volume of drug if required.

REFERENCES

Edwards, Waldo B., and Hingson, Robert A. The Present Status of Continuous Cauda Analgesia in Obstetrics. Bulletin of the New York Academy of Medicine, *19:* 507 July, 1943.
Hingson, Robert A., and Edwards, Waldo B. Comprehensive Review of Continuous Caudal Analgesia for Anesthetists. Anesthesiology, *4:* 181, March, 1943.

ALTERNATE TECHNIQUE FOR CONTINUOUS CAUDAL ANESTHESIA

Description: A French ureteral or plastic catheter is inserted into the caudal canal instead of a malleable needle.

Materials: In addition to the materials described above supply:

1. One #5 ureteral or plastic catheter 30″ long.
2. One #13 gauge needle 8 cms. long which will accommodate catheter.
3. One needle #22 gauge or size to fit into ureteral catheter.

Technique:

1. Proceed as above and introduce 13 gauge needle into the caudal canal.
2. Thread the catheter into the needle if no blood or spinal fluid are obtained by aspiration.

3. Withdraw needle in such a manner that the catheter is not disturbed and remains in the caudal canal. Fasten securely with adhesive.
4. Insert the 22 gauge needle into the free end of the catheter, attach the syringe and inject procaine as described in the technique above.

TECHNIQUE USING DRUGS OTHER THAN PROCAINE

1. An equivalent volume of 1.5% metycaine may be substituted for procaine—duration 1 ½–2 hrs.
2. An equivalent volume of 0.10% pontocaine in physiological saline may be substituted for procaine—duration 2 ½–4 hrs.

REFERENCE

Adams, R. C., Lundy, J. S., and Seldon, T. H. A Technique for Continuous Caudal Anesthesia and Analgesia. Surgical Clinics North America, *23:* 1196, August, 1943.

PARAVERTEBRAL BLOCK ANESTHESIA

Definition: Anesthesia induced by distributing a solution of local anesthetic drug about the bodies of the vertebrae and infiltrating the nerve trunks as they emerge from the intervertebral foramina.

Types:

1. Cervical paravertebral block.
2. Thoracic paravertebral block (see below).
3. Lumbar paravertebral block (see below).
4. Transacral block.

Indications:

1. *Anesthetic:* For operations in areas innervated by the various nerve segments which are accessible for this type of block.
2. *Diagnostic:* To produce sympathetic block to differentiate diseases of autonomic nervous system from other conditions.
3. *Therapeutic:* To relieve vasospasm, neuritis, or other types of segmental pains.

Anatomy: See individual blocks that follow.

Materials: Standard regional set. This should include one needle for each nerve to be blocked.

Technique:

1. *Position:* Either of two positions may be employed:
   a. Place the patient in the lateral prone position lying on the side opposite to the one to be injected. Place a pillow beneath the loin to straighten vertebral column.

b. Place the patient in the prone position with pillow beneath thorax or abdomen depending upon the block to be performed.

2. *Landmarks:*
   a. Spines of the vertebrae.
   b. Transverse process of the vertebrae (or ribs in thoracic block).

3. *Procedure:* See individual blocks that follow.

CERVICAL PLEXUS BLOCK

Definition: Anesthesia obtained by blocking the cervical nerves as they emerge from the vertebral column.

Synonyms: Paravertebral cervical block.

Types:

1. Lateral approach (most common).
2. Posterior approach (employed when the lateral route is not practical).

Indications:

1. *Diagnostic:* For differentiation of neuralgias (hypoglossal) or for carotid sinus syndrome.
2. *Anesthetic:* For operations on the neck.

Anatomy: The anterior primary divisions of the first four cervical nerves emerge from the cervical intervertebral foramina, pass behind the vertebral arteries and then to the tip of the transverse processes of the vertebrae. The transverse processes of the cervical vertebrae have two tubercles, an anterior and a posterior. These tubercles lie from 1–2 cms. below the skin surface. As the nerves pass through the sulcus formed by the tubercles, they divide into an ascending and descending branch which connect with each other to form a series of loops known as the cervical plexus, the plexus which lies beneath the sterno-mastoid muscle. Each loop gives rise to two branches: a *superficial* which emerges at the posterior edge of the sterno-mastoid and supplies the skin and other superficial structures, and the *deep* which supplies the muscles and other deep structures of the neck.

Materials: Standard regional set. The set should be provided with two 8 cms needles (22 G) and six 5 cms. needles (22 G).

Lateral Approach

Technique:

1. *Position:* Place the patient in the supine position with the chin pointing upward (no pillow). The operator should stand on the side which is injected.

2. *Landmarks:*
   a. Condyle of the mandible of the jaw.
   b. Surface of the second lower molar tooth.
   c. Transverse processes of the cervical vertebrae.
3. *Procedure:*
   a. Palpate, bisect, and mark the point of bisection of the condyle of mandible of the jaw (A, Fig. 133).
   b. Draw a line through the condyle perpendicular to the operating table (B, Fig. 133).
   c. Draw a horizontal line perpendicular to the vertical one along the transverse processes of the vertebral column (C, Fig. 133).

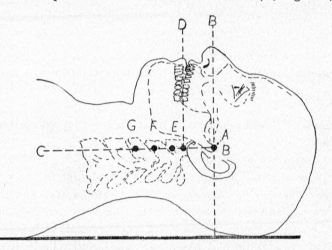

FIG. 133. Landmarks for cervical plexus block. (A) Condyle of mandible. (E), (F), (G), 2nd, 3rd and 4th cervical vertebrae respectively.

   d. Drop a second perpendicular line passing along the surface of second molar tooth. Mark the point on the skin where this line intersects the horizontal line (D, Fig. 133).
   e. Mark the skin one cm. below this point along the horizontal line (E. Fig. 80). This corresponds to the second cervical vertebrae. Mark skin also 2 1/2 cms. and 3 1/2 cms. below this first point. These points correspond to third and fourth cervical vertebrae. Four points are thus indicated (F, G, Fig. 133).
   f. After the landmarks are located, turn head to one side and raise intradermal wheals on the lower three marks on skin.
   g. Insert 5 cm. needle perpendicular to the skin. Set marker at 1 1/2 cms. and establish contact with the anterior tubercle of transverse process. Inject 5 cc. of 2% procaine at this site.
   h. Repeat the procedure on the points indicating the third and fourth cervical vertebrae. Establish contact with the anterior tubercle as

in the previous vertebrae. Inject 4 cc. of 2% procaine at these sites.

i. Inject 10–15 cc. of 1% procaine along posterior border of the sterno-mastoid muscle in subcutaneous tissues.

j. Repeat the injection on opposite side using exactly the same technique if a bilateral block is desired.

Anesthesia:

1. *Onset:* Usually within 5–10 minutes if procaine is employed.
2. *Distribution:* Lateral and anterior superficial and deep structures of neck Also the skin on posterior aspect of neck, occiput and a capelike distribution over the shoulders extending to the level of the second rib.
3. *Duration:* One hour, approximately.

Complications:

1. The carotid sheath may be pierced by prevertebral injections and signs of vascular compression ensue.
2. The carotid artery may be entered by the needle.
3. The needle may enter the spinal canal and even pierce the dura.
4. An intravenous injection may be performed. This area is highly vascular.

Precautions: Do not inject drug in front of the transverse process.

Contra-Indications:

1. Infections of the neck.
2. Tracheal obstruction.

Comment

1. The first cervical nerve is not anesthetized in this procedure.
2. The fourth cervical nerve is blocked but the motor power of the diaphragm remains intact or a paresis results. The diminished ventilation due to the paresis is compensated for by the increase in intercostal activity.
3. The transverse process of the cervical vertebrae is thin and the needle point easily slips from its surface.
4. The sympathetic nerves are also affected by the block and a Horner's syndrome frequently appears.
5. The lower cervical vertebrae become progressively superficial. The needles therefore need not be inserted as deeply in seeking their tubercles.

PARAVERTEBRAL BLOCK—THORACIC REGION

Definition: A block of the spinal nerves of the thoracic region accomplished by injection of a local anesthetic solution in the paravertebral area.

Indications:

1. *Diagnostic and therapeutic:* Coronary pain, causalgias, neuralgias of the intercostal nerves.
2. *Anesthetic:* For thoracic surgery or superficial operations on thorax. The block is employed in conjunction with cervical plexus or lumbar block. It is rarely employed alone.

Anatomy: Each of the twelve thoracic vertebra consists of a body, a spinous and two transverse processes. The latter articulate with the ribs. The spinous processes of the thoracic vertebrae are not natural landmarks for their homologous nerves or intervertebral spaces. The spinous processes increase in length and slope downward as they descend from the upper to the lower vertebrae. Therefore, the spine may point to the rib or interspace below the designated vertebrae. In the erect posture, with the arms lying along the side of the trunk, a line joining the spines of the scapulae passes through the third thoracic spine; a line joining the lower angles of the scapulae passes through the seventh thoracic spine. These landmarks are subject to displacement or variations of the scapulae. A line 5 cm. long drawn from a point along the twelfth rib perpendicular to the midline of the back will mark the spine of the twelfth thoracic vertebra. The spine of the seventh cervical vertebra is the most prominent in the upper part of the vertebral column.

Each thoracic nerve emerges from the intervertebral foramen and divides into an anterior and posterior primary division after having first given off the meningeal nerve to the dura and vertebrae. The posterior primary division supplies the muscles and skin of the back; the anterior gives off the ramus communicans to the sympathetic ganglion after which it passes into the paravertebral space. The thoracic nerves lie midway between the transverse processes of the two vertebrae as it emerges from the intervertebral foramen. The nerve passes toward the rib above it and enters the intercostal groove.

Technique:

1. *Position:* The patient may be placed in one of two positions:
   a. Lateral prone with patient lying on side opposite to one to be blocked (as for spinal anesthesia).
   b. Prone with pillow beneath thorax.
2. *Landmarks:*
   a. Spinous process of the thoracic vertebrae above the spinal nerve to be injected.

b. Transverse process of the same vertebrae or the rib attached to it depending upon the size of the vertebrae.

3. *Procedure:*

a. Draw a line 4 cm. from 'and parallel to the midline of the vertebral column (Fig. 134).'

b. Palpate the spinous processes of the vertebrae above the spinal nerves supplying the segmental areas to be blocked and mark their level on the line described in step a.

c. Raise intradermal wheals on a level with the desired spinous processes. Bear in mind that the corresponding rib may not be in direct line with the processes in the lower thoracic region.

d. Introduce an 8 cm. needle (with the marker set at approximately 2.5 cm. from the tip) in a direction perpendicular to the skin until rib is encountered.

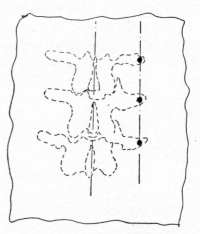

FIG. 134. Method of inducing paravertebral block. Wheals are raised over the transverse processes of the vertebrae at the level of the corresponding spines. The vertebrae are seen from the back.

e. Set the marker another 2.5 cm. upward on the shaft of the needle. Advance the needle at an angle 45° downward (caudad) so that it glances off the edge of the rib.

f. Withdraw the needle almost to the skin and reinsert it towards the lower edge of the rib.

g. Advance the needle one cm. into the space between the transverse processes and inject 5 cc. of 1% procaine. Repeat procedure on the opposite side if a bilateral block is desired.

Anesthesia:

1. *Onset:*

a. Usually within five minutes if procaine is employed.

2. *Distribution:*

a. 1st thoracic nerve is part of the brachial plexus.

b. 2nd
3rd heart and nipple and chest wall anteriorly.
4th level of the respective vertebrae posteriorly.
5th

c. 6th
7th anterior wall of abdomen above umbilicus.
8th level of the respective vertebrae posteriorly.
9th

    d. 10th region of umbilicus, level of respective vertebrae posteriorly.

    e. 11th

       12th area between umbilicus and pubis.

Complications:

1. The drug may be accidentally injected into the subarachnoid or epi-dural space.
2. The drug may be injected into an intercostal artery or vein.
3. The needle may pierce the pleura and the lung.

Precautions:

1. Always rely upon the marker when seeking the depth of a bony land-mark.
2. Always inject the drug slowly at first. Withdraw the needle if patient coughs or if blood, air, or spinal fluid is obtained.

Contra-Indications:

1. Infections in the area of injection.

Comment

1. Note that the cutaneous nerves overlap. Therefore, several segments must be anesthetized to obtain an effective block.
2. Remember that the anesthesia does not extend to the midline, but ends approximately an inch from it due to overlapping of filaments from the thoracic nerves on the opposite side.
3. Note that in the upper portion of the thorax, the cervical nerves over-lap into the area supplied by the first three of four thoracic segments. Therefore, the block must be supplemented by a cervical block or local infiltration.
4. Always test the field of anesthesia after the blocks are performed. Supplementary injection of an upper or lower segment, depending upon the case will be necessary if the area of anesthesia is not sufficiently extensive.
5. Do not introduce the needle beyond the distance designated by the marker.
6. Note that the ribs may lie as many as 5 cms. below the skin surface in obese or muscular subjects.

CERVICO-THORACIC SYMPATHETIC BLOCK (STELLATE GANGLION BLOCK)

Definition: A paravertebral block of the lowest portion of the cervical sympathetic chain.

Types:

1. Posterior approach: This is the least commonly employed route.
2. Anterior approach: This route is commonly employed.
3. Lateral approach ⎤ The subclavian vessels are too close to path of the
4. Superior approach ⎦ needle. These routes are not frequently employed.

Indications:

1. *Diagnostic:* Not important. Used to differentiate various types of vasospastic diseases, asthma, and cardiac diseases.
2. *Therapeutic:*
   a. To relieve vasospasm of upper extremity, head and face.
   b. To relieve "status asthmaticus."
   c. To relieve angina and other forms of cardiac pain.
   d. To relieve hyperhidrosis of the upper extremity.

Anatomy: The stellate ganglion, a fusion of the inferior cervical and first thoracic ganglia, is a mass approximately $2 \times 2 \times 0.5$ cms. which lies behind the vertebral artery in the space between the transverse process of the 7th cervical vertebra and the neck of the first rib. The apex of the right lung is in close relation to the ganglion on the right side but lies approximately 2 cm. lower on the left and therefore is not so close. The ganglion is in close relation to the junction of the subclavian artery, the inferior thyroid and the first intercostal artery. The central branches of the ganglion arise from the 7th and 8th cervical nerves. Peripheral connections are to the middle and superior cervical ganglia, cardiac plexus, cervical spinal nerves, to brain along vertebral arteries. Small branches may pass to recurrent laryngeal and phrenic nerves.

Materials: Standard regional set containing 10 cm. needles.

Technique: Posterior Approach:

1. *Position:*
   a. Place the patient in the prone position on his side with pillow under head or:
   b. Allow the patient to sit up over the edge of an operating table leaning forward with arms folded or resting on an elevated stand. The operator stands behind the patient.
2. *Landmarks:* Spine of 7th cervical vertebra and each vertebra above and below it.
3. *Procedure:*
   a. Palpate and mark the site of the spine of the 7th cervical vertebra.
   b. Raise an intradermal wheal along the transverse process of the 7th cervical vertebra 4.5 cms. from the midline.
   c. Introduce a 10 cm. needle perpendicularly through the wheal following the median sagittal plane and establish contact with the

transverse process. Introduce the needle approximately 5–6 cms. Use marker.

d. Withdraw needle slightly and reinsert in a caudad direction and medially towards body of vertebra so that it slips off the transverse process.

e. Incline the needle so that it forms an angle of 20–30° with the median sagittal plane. Insert until the body of first thoracic vertebra is encountered (a distance of 5–8 cms.).

f. Turn the needle so that bevel is in contact with the body of the vertebra.

g. Advance needle along the lateral aspect of the vertebra until contact with bone is lost.

h. Place a drop of procaine solution on the hub of the needle head and ask patient to breathe. If needle is in pleural space, bubbles will be observed.

i. Inject 5 cc. 2% or 10 cc. 1% procaine in divided doses over a period of several minutes.

j. Allow needle to remain in place if the procaine is to be followed by alcohol.

k. Inject 2–5 cc. of absolute alcohol (see page 369).

Anesthesia:

1. *Onset:* Five to 15 minutes if procaine is employed.
2. *Distribution:* If the block is successful, Horner's syndrome results. The following signs are noted:
   Miosis.
   Enopthalmos.
   Narrowed palpebral fissure.
   Hypoidrosis on face and arms of affected side.
   Increased skin temperature on affected side.
   Injection of conjunctiva.
3. *Duration:* Varies.

Complications:

1. The needle may pass into the pleural space especially on the right side and produce a pneumothorax.
2. The subarachnoid space may be entered and an intraspinal injection result.
3. The needle may enter a vessel and intravascular injection result.

Precautions:

1. Always attempt aspiration to obtain blood or spinal fluid.
2. Always perform test using drop of procaine solution in hub of needle to determine if needle is in pleura.

3. Always perform block with an assistant and in an operating room equipped for resuscitation and other emergency measures.

Comment

1. Withdraw needle and reinsert at a slightly different site if blood or spinal fluid is obtained.
2. Allow 15 minutes to elapse after the procaine block if therapeutic block with alcohol is being performed.
3. **Remember that stellate ganglion block is fraught with dangers and should be performed only by experienced individuals.**

Technique: Anterior Approach:

1. *Position:* Place the patient in the upright sitting position with his arms at his side. The operator should face the patient.
2. *Landmarks:*
   a. Midpoint of clavicle.
   b. Body of the seventh cervical vertebra.
3. *Procedure:*
   a. Locate and mark midpoint of clavicle on the skin overlying it.
   b. Raise an intradermal wheal 1 cm. medial to this mark and just above the upper border of the clavicle.
   c. Introduce an 8 or 10 cm. needle through the wheal in a horizontal direction at level of clavicle. Direct it posteriorly and medially at angle of 45° to skin for distance of 6 or 7 cms. until the body of first thoracic vertebra or the junction of 1st thoracic and 7th cervical vertebrae is encountered.
   d. Inject 5 cc. 2% or 10 cc. 1% procaine at the vertebrae.

Remarks: Precautions, anesthesia, and other factors are same as described under directions for the posterior approach.

ALTERNATE METHOD—ANTERIOR APPROACH*

Position of Patient:

1. Recumbent supine with head turned to side opposite to the injection.
2. Arm of side to be blocked at side.
3. Depress shoulder caudad.

Landmarks: (a) Sixth cervical transverse process. (b) Seventh cervical transverse process. This is identified by locating the 6th cervical first and measuring downwards 2 cms. from that point. (c) Midpoint of clavicle.

Procedure:

1. Raise a skin wheal 1 cm. above the midpoint of the clavicle.
2. Introduce an 8 cm. needle through the skin wheal at an angle of 45°

* Technique of Volpitto and Ritsteen.

with the saggital plane of the body. Direct it downward and medially towards the seventh cervical transverse process. At a depth of 5 or 6 cms. the tip of the transverse process of the 7th cervical or the neck of the first rib is encountered.

3. Withdraw needle slightly when contact with bone is made and reinsert directing it downward and inward. The needle is on the first rib. Contact with the first rib must be made.

4. Place needle once again on the neck of the first rib (or may it impinge upon the transverse process of the first dorsal vertebra).

5. Change position of hub of needle so that an angle of 80–90° is made with the saggital plane of the body.

6. Advance needle 1 or 2 cms. until it impinges upon bone. The needle will be within the fascial plane of the stellate ganglion.

7. Inject 5 cc. of 1% procaine at this site.

STELLATE GANGLION BLOCK—ANTERIOR TISSUE DISPLACEMENT (PARATRACHEAL) TECHNIQUE

Description:

The needle is introduced anterior to the body of the 7th cervical vertebra between the trachea and the laterally displaced carotid bundle.

Position:

Supine or semi-recumbent with face directed straight upward. The chin is slightly elevated. Operator stands on the side to be injected.

Landmarks:

    a. Medial border of sternomastoid muscle.
    b. Sternoclavicular articulation.

Materials:

1. $1\frac{1}{2}$ or 2″ 25 G needle with 10 cc. syringe attached.

Procedure:

1. Place the middle and index fingers of the left hand (separated from each other about 1–2 cms.) along medial border or the sternomastoid muscle. Lower finger should be against sternoclavicular articulation.

2. Press finger tips slowly and firmly into the neck so as to displace carotid artery and its accompanying structures laterally. The volar surfaces of fingers lie against the vessel. The trachea and esophagus rest against the dorsal surfaces (Fig. 134A) of the finger. The fingers are between these structures and the carotid bundle (Fig. 134A).

3. Introduce the needle with syringe attached and held in right hand between the two fingers retracting the carotid bundle and sternomastoid. The needle is advanced perpendicular to the skin in the direction

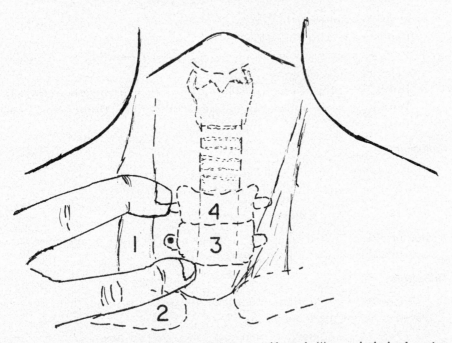

FIG. 134A. Retraction of carotid bundle and sternomastoid muscle (1) to render body of vertebrae (3) more accessible. Trachea (4) remains undisturbed. The index finger is pressed downward at the sternoclavicular joint (2). The needle is introduced perpendicularly between the index and middle finger.

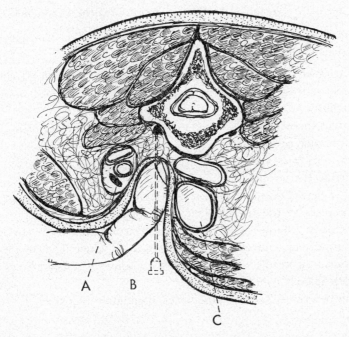

FIG. 134B. Cross section of neck showing method of inducing cervicothoracic sympathetic block by introducing needle between the trachea and anterior border of sternomastoid muscle after carotid sheath is retracted laterally. (A) Carotid bundle. (B) Needle. (C) Trachea.

of the body of the 7th cervical vertebra in region of ganglion until contact is made with bone (Fig. 134B).
4. Remove fingers as soon as bone is encountered. Skin which is depressed slides up shaft of needle.
5. Inject 10 cc. 1% procaine or solution of equivalent strength at this site.
6. Withdraw needle and gently massage area. Wait for Horner's syndrome to appear.

Comment
1. Possibility of piercing pleura avoided.
2. The esophagus may be punctured on the left side.

THORACIC SYMPATHETIC BLOCK

Definition: Block of the sympathetic ganglia of the thoracic chain by paravertebral injection of local anesthetic drugs.

Indications:
  Diagnostic: To differentiate between disease of the sympathetic nervous system and related conditions.
  Therapeutic: To relieve cardiac and other visceral pain.

Anatomy: The thoracic sympathetic ganglia lie along the body of the vertebrae approximately 3 cms. below the transverse processes. They are interconnected by a nervous chain which courses along the anterolateral surface of the vertebral bodies and loops over the heads of the ribs.

Procedure: Preparations and materials are essentially the same as for thoracic paravertebral block.
1. Introduce the 10 cm. needle and establish contact with the rib or transverse process of the desired vertebrae. Start with the bevel pointed medially.
2. Direct the needle in a caudad direction until the inferior border of the transverse process is located.
3. Set marker at 4 cms. on shaft of the needle.
4. Incline the needle at an angle of 20° to median sagittal plane and almost perpendicular to the curvature of the back and advance it until it glances off the lower border of the vertebra.
5. Introduce the needle for a distance of 3 cms. The body of the vertebra is usually encountered at this depth if the angle is correct.
6. Rotate the needle 180° and advance it another centimeter as long as it rests against bone.
7. Inject 5 cc. of 2% procaine for each ganglion blocked.

Comment
1. The ganglia lie 3 cms. below the transverse processes. Incline the

needle more medially if bone is not encountered at this depth and more
vertically if bone is encountered before this depth is attained.

2. Never attach the syringe to the needle in seeking the landmarks and
   ganglia.

ALCOHOL BLOCK OF SYMPATHETIC GANGLIA

Principle: Alcohol is injected into or about nerve tissue to destroy it by its
sclerosing action. The destruction of nerve tissue is similar to that obtained by sectioning a nerve and presents the following features:

1. It is typical of Wallerian degeneration.
2. Nerves regenerate after a variable period of time.
3. Small unsheathed nerves may be permanently destroyed; large heavily
   sheathed nerves are only temporarily impaired.
4. Fibrosis frequently occurs which predisposes to neuritis.

Dose: A single injection of 5 cc. of absolute alcohol causes an area of necrosis
in muscle 1 cm. in diameter.

Procedure:

1. Perform block as described above. Inject 2 cc. of 2% procaine and
   note the extent and distribution of anesthesia.
2. Allow ten minutes to elapse and inject an additional 3 cc. of procaine
   into each needle. This minimizes pain of alcohol injection.
3. Inject 5 cc. of absolute alcohol in half cc. amounts attempting aspiration between each introduction.
4. Introduce 0.25 cc. procaine through each needle as it is withdrawn.
   This washes the alcohol from its lumen.
5. **Maintain patient on his side for an hour to minimize diffusion of the
   alcohol.**

Comment	*Reasons*
1. Do not use excessive quantities of procaine.	The alcohol is diluted and the sclerosing action diminished.
2. Always employ absolute alcohol.	Diluted alcohol is less effective as a sclerosing agent.
3. Inject the alcohol slowly and preferably over a period of several minutes.	The injection is painful, particularly if done rapidly.
4. Attempt aspiration frequently during the injection.	The needle may shift during an injection and a vital structure will be injured.
5. Always wash the alcohol from the hollow of the needle with procaine solution before withdrawing it from the tissues.	A sinus tract may form to the site of injection due to the sclerosing action of alcohol.

BLOCK OF SPLANCHNIC NERVES

Definition:

Block of splanchnic nerves.

Indications:

1. *Diagnostic and therapeutic:* To relieve pain arising from the pancreas, biliary tract and other viscera of the upper abdomen. To relieve spasm of renal vessels and vessels of abdominal viscera.

2. *Anesthetic:* For surgery involving upper abdominal viscera, small intestine, omentum, etc.

Anatomy:

There are three splanchnic nerves (Fig. 134C, 134D):

1. The great splanchnic nerve, formed from roots arising from the 5th or 6th to 9th or 10th thoracic segments, passes downward from the thorax, pierces the crus of the diaphragm and enters the semilunar ganglion on its side (1, Fig. 134C).

2. The lesser or smaller arises from the 10th, 11th or 12th thoracic segments and passes lateral to or with the great splanchnic from the

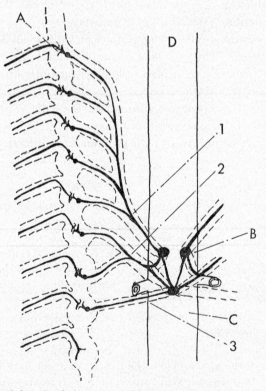

FIG. 134C. Origin of the splanchnic nerves. 1. The great splanchnic nerve. 2. The small or lesser splanchnic nerve. 3. The least splanchnic nerve. (A) Sympathetic ganglia. (B) Coeliac ganglion. (C) Diaphragm. (D) Aorta.

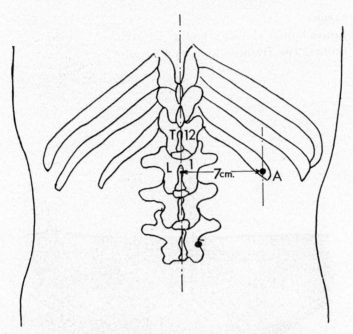

Fig. 134D. Superficial landmarks for performing splanchnic block by the posterior route. (A) point 7 cms. from midline on the 12th rib at which wheal is raised. Needle is introduced perpendicularly to skin until rib is encountered before direction is shifted towards L-1.

thorax to the semilunar ganglion, coeliac and renal plexes (2, Fig. 134C).

3. The least splanchnic nerve arises from the 11th or the 12th thoracic ganglia, passes through the diaphragm, and joins the semilunar ganglia (3—Fig. 134C). The splanchnic nerves are situated in close relation to the first lumbar vertebra. They lie behind the crus of the diaphragm. On the right side the vena cava is anterior and on the left the aorta. The kidneys are lateral on either side.

Types:

The splanchnic nerves may be reached by two routes:
a. The posterior approach through the muscles of the back.
b. The anterior approach through the opened abdominal cavity (used during operation).

Posterior Approach

Materials:

Standard regional set containing a 15 cm. 22 G needle with stylets.

Technique:

1. *Position.* Lateral supine, back arched without distortion of the spine or prone.

2. *Landmarks:*
   a. Lower border of 12th rib (Fig. 134D).
   b. Point 7 cm. from midline on 12th rib.

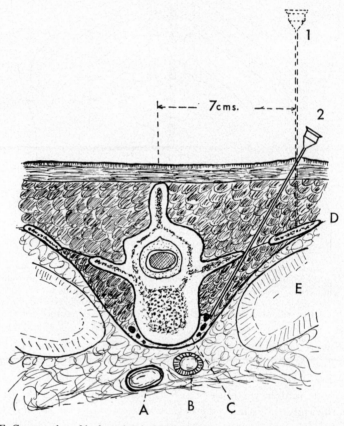

Fɪɢ. 134E. Cross section of body at level of L-1 showing showing method of injecting splanchnic nerve. The needle is introduced perpendicularly to the skin until the first rib (D) is encountered. After sliding off the edge of the rib it is inclined towards the anterolateral edge of the body of the vertebrae. (A) Vena cava. (B) Aorta. (C) Splanchnic nerves. (E) Kidney.

3. *Procedure:*
   a. Palpate lower border of 12th rib.
   b. Mark off a point on the rib 7 cms. from midline and raise wheal at this point (Fig. 31).
   c. Introduce the 15 cm. needle through wheal perpendicular to skin and advance until the rib is encountered.
   d. Partly withdraw needle and then incline it in a caudad direction at an angle that will cause it to slide off lower border of the rib.
   e. Incline the needle towards midline also so that it makes an angle of 30° with median sagittal plane of body.
   f. Advance it at this angle until contact is made with body of verte-

brae (anterolateral face) (E, Fig. 135).

g. Set the marker for 0.5 cm. and rotate needle, attempting to slide off the anterolateral angle for distance of .25 cm. (C, Fig. 135).

h. Inject 20 cc. 1% procaine at this site.

i. Withdraw needle almost to the skin and reintroduce at same angle as in E (30°), but aiming in cephalad direction at point 3 cm. above on body of vertebrae.

j. Inject 10 cc. 1% procaine at this site.

k. Withdraw and reintroduce the needle at the same angle 30° to sagittal plane, aiming caudad at a point 3 cm. below the body of the first lumbar vertebra.

l. Inject 10 cc. 1% procaine at this site.

m. Repeat block on opposite side if it is to be bilateral.

Anesthesia:

1. *Onset.* Approximately five to 10 minutes may be required for the block to become effective if procaine is used. No sensory loss is apparent unless pain is present. Transient fall in blood pressure may be only sign of successful block.

2. *Duration.* One hour to $1\frac{1}{2}$ hours.

3. *Distribution.* Visceroperitoneum is anesthetized. The parietal peritoneum is supplied by the thoracic and upper lumbar nerves and is not anesthetized. The viscera in the upper abdomen, stomach, small intestines, transverse colon, greater and lesser omentum, liver and spleen are under control of the splanchnic nerves and are, therefore, anesthetized. The blood vessels of the viscera, including the kidney, likewise are dilated.

Complications:

1. The needle may pierce the aorta or the vena cava if advanced too far.

2. The drug may be injected into the peritoneal cavity beyond the nerves.

3. The kidney may be pierced.

4. The pancreas, which lies anterior to these nerves, may also be pierced.

5. If the 11th rib is mistaken for the 12th, injection may be made too high and the pleura may be pierced.

Comment:

1. When bilateral block is attempted inject the left side first, so the aorta may be identified, if the needle is advanced too far. Pulsation of the needle makes this structure prominent.

2. Failures are due to variations in the anatomy of the individual. Accurate identification of the first lumbar vertebra depends on the width

of angle between the 12th rib and the vertebral column. The wider the angle the higher the 7 cm. point will be on the vertebral column, the narrower the angle the lower.

3. The 12th rib is identified with difficulty in obese individuals and may be a cause of failure.

4. In certain cases the ganglia occupy a lower level than normal.

5. One injection on each side of the vertebral column is not always followed by complete anesthesia. It is therefore recommended to inject every case at the level above and below, as described.

6. The analgesia resulting from bilateral injection of the splanchnic nerves involves only a relatively small portion of the posterior abdominal wall, especially the area under the direct influence of the maneuvers of the stomach, duodenum, peritoneum and gallbladder. Traction, packing and other manipulation must be gentle.

7. Side effects of a successful block are fall in blood pressure, pallor, cold sweats, nausea and vomiting, slow feeble pulse, due to sympathetic paralysis. In cases when hypotension ensues inject a vasopressor substance intravenously to counteract the fall in blood pressure.

8. Do not use alcohol or sclerosing agents to attempt to secure a prolonged effect. The peritoneal cavity may be entered and vital structures disturbed or injured.

PARAVERTEBRAL BLOCK—LUMBAR REGION

Definition: A block of the spinal nerves of the lumbar region by paravertebral injection of a local anesthetic drug.

Types:

Diagnostic: To determine the presence of vasospastic disease, or diseases of the sympathetic nervous system.

Therapeutic: To produce sympathetic block for diseases characterized by hyperactivity of the autonomic nervous system.

Anesthetic: For abdominal, urological or pelvic operations, used in conjunction with sacral block or paravertebral block of thoracic region.

Anatomy: The anterior primary divisions of the first four lumbar nerves form a series of oblique loops in the substance of the psoas muscle and thus give rise to the lumbar plexus. The 12th thoracic and the 5th lumbar contribute to the plexus. In the lumbar region, the spinal nerve lies cephalad to the transverse process of the corresponding vertebra. The transverse processes of the lumbar vertebrae lie opposite the corresponding spinous processes. A space 1 to 2 cms. in width separates each spine in this region in the midline. The transverse process is located by drawing a transverse line through the tip of the spinous process.

Materials: Standard regional set containing 10 cm. needles.

Technique:

1. *Position:* Arrange the patient lying on the side opposite to the side to be injected.
2. *Landmarks:*
   a. Spine of the lumbar vertebrae.
   b. A line connecting the superior borders of the ilium crosses between the spinous processes of 4th and 5th lumbar vertebrae. Often it may pass across the 4th spinous process.
   c. Transverse process of lumbar vertebrae.
3. *Procedure:*
   a. Raise wheals 4 cms. from the midline opposite the superior borders of the spinous processes of vertebrae selected.
   b. Set the marker at 4–5 cm. on the shaft of a 10 cm. needle.
   c. Introduce the needle perpendicularly through the wheal until the transverse process is encountered. Usually the needle is introduced a depth of 4 to 5 cms. before bone is encountered.
   d. Advance the marker 3 cms. from the skin surface when bone is encountered.
   e. Partly withdraw the needle and reinsert it at an angle of 25° to the medial sagittal plane and at the same angle in a cephalad direction. The needle glances off the edge of the superior border of the transverse process into the substance of the psoas muscle.
   f. Advance it as far as the marker and inject 7–8 cc. of 2% procaine solution after attempting aspiration in two planes.

Anesthesia:

1. *Onset:* Within five minutes if procaine is employed and the needle is in close contact with the lumbar nerves.
2. *Distribution:* Along distribution of the plexus. The ilio hypogastric, ilio inguinal, genitocrural, external femoral cutaneous, and other nerves involved in the lumbar plexus will be affected.
3. *Duration:* Usually one hour if procaine is employed.

Complications:

1. The needle may enter the subarachnoid space if it is inclined at an acute angle.
2. The needle may be advanced too far inward and pierce a major vessel such as the vena cava, aorta, or enter an abdominal organ.

Contra-Indications:

1. Local infections in the lumbar region.

Comment: The fifth lumbar nerve is best blocked by introducing the needle in a caudad and medial direction over the inferior border of the transverse process.

PARAVERTEBRAL BLOCK OF SYMPATHETIC GANGLIA IN LUMBAR REGION

Definition: Block of the sympathetic ganglia of the lumbar region by paravertebral injection of local anesthetic drugs.

Indications:

1. *Diagnostic:* For temporary relief of certain forms of hypertension, vasospastic disturbances of extremities and various diseases of the autonomic nervous system.
2. *Anesthetic:* To permit manipulation of upper abdominal viscera.

Anatomy: The lumbar sympathetic ganglia lie along the anterolateral surfaces of the bodies of 4 lumbar vertebrae 3–4 cms. below the transverse process.

Technique: The technique for sympathetic block in the lumbar region is similar to the paravertebral block except the needles are introduced at a different angle, and deeper into the tissues (Fig. 135).

1. *Landmarks:* Same as for lumbar paravertebral block.
2. *Position:* Same as for lumbar paravertebral block.
3. *Procedure:*
   a. Raise intradermal wheals (over the transverse process) 3 cms. from midline of the desired vertebrae.
   b. Advance needle perpendicularly to skin and establish contact with transverse process of the vertebrae.
   c. Partly withdraw the needle and incline it in a cephalad and medial direction so that it slides off the upper border of transverse process.
   d. Continue to advance the needle in cephalad direction, for 2–3 cms. or until body of vertebra is encountered.
   e. Attempt aspiration and inject 10 to 15 cc. of 1% procaine for each ganglion.

Anesthesia:

1. *Onset:* Almost immediately if the ganglia are encountered directly by the needle.
2. *Distribution:* No sensory anesthesia results unless the lumbar nerves are encountered. Vasodilatation characterized by an increase of warmth, redness, and absence of sweating of the skin over the lower extremity is the most prominent change.
3. *Duration:* Undetermined. The beneficial effects may last from one hour to several days depending upon the condition for which the block is performed.

Complications:

1. The needle may be advanced into the aorta, vena cava, renal vessels, pancreas, and other vital structures.
2. The lumbar nerves may be pierced (these pass between each of the spaces between the transverse processes).

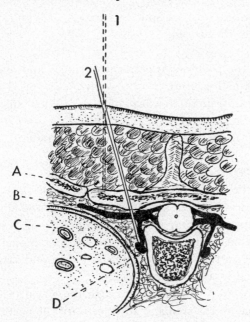

Fig. 135. Method of inducing lumbar sympathetic block.

Comment: Block is preferred if alcohol is to be used as the lumbar nerves are not affected by it.

Transacral Block

Definition: A paravertebral block produced by introducing a local anesthetic solution through the posterior sacral foramina. The sacral nerves are anesthetized as they emerge from the sacral canal.

Uses:

1. *Anesthetic:*
   a. For the same purposes as caudal block. Most frequently employed in cases in which caudal block is not possible because the caudal canal is not accessible.
   b. As an adjunct to caudal block for rectal surgery.
2. *Therapeutic:* For sciatica and other neuralgias involving sacral nerves.

Anatomy: See caudal block for description of sacrum and distribution of caudal nerves.

Materials: Standard regional set containing 10 cm., 8 cm. and 5 cm. needles.

Technique:

1. *Position:* Place the patient in the prone position. Place a pillow beneath the hips to elevate the sacrum.
2. *Landmarks:*
   a. Posterior superior iliac spines.
   b. Cornua of the sacrum.
3. *Procedure:*
   a. Palpate the posterior superior iliac spines and mark their location on the skin (Fig. 136).
   b. Raise an intradermal wheal one cm. medial and caudad to each (Fig. 136).
   c. Palpate the sacral cornua and raise an intradermal wheal over each one (Fig. 136).
   d. Connect both wheals by a line (Fig. 136).
   e. Divide the line into three equal parts and raise a wheal at each point of division. The second, third, fourth, and fifth sacral foramina will lie approximately under these wheals (Fig. 136).
   f. Raise an intradermal wheal 2.5 to 3.0 cms. cephalad to and on the same line as the wheal designating the second sacral foramen. The first sacral foramen is thus located.
   g. Introduce an 8 cm. needle through the wheal (second sacral) perpendicular to the skin and advance until the posterior aspect of the sacrum is encountered.
   h. Incline the needle one way or another, medially, caudad, cephalad, or laterally, until contact with bone is lost and needle enters the foramen.
   i. Advance the needle 1.5 cm. into the foramen (use markers). Inject 5 cc. of 2% procaine at this site.
   j. Repeat procedure for the first sacral foramen advancing the 10 cm. needle 2 cms. after contact with bone is lost. Inject 6 cc. of 2% procaine at this site.
   k. Repeat procedure for 3rd sacral foramen. Advance a 5 cm. needle 1 cm. after contact with bone is lost. Inject 4 cc. solution at this site.
   l. Repeat the procedure for the fourth sacral foramen. Advance a 5 cm. needle 0.5 cm. into the foramen.
   m. Advance a 5 cm. needle laterally to the sacral cornua and inject 2 cc. of 2% procaine. This anesthetizes the fifth sacral nerve as it emerges through the fifth sacral foramen.

Anesthesia:

1. *Onset:* Immediately if procaine is employed.

2. *Duration:* One to two hours or more if procaine is employed.
3. *Distribution:* Approximately the same as for caudal block.

Complications:

1. The needle may pass inward to pelvis if advanced too far.
2. The needle may pass into sacro-iliac joint if directed too far laterally.
3. The solution may be distributed to the posterior aspect of sacrum.

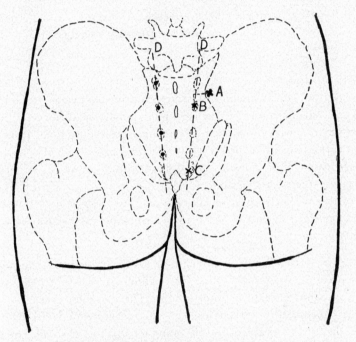

FIG. 136. Landmarks for transacral block. (A) Posterior-superior iliac spines. (B) Sacral foramina. (C) Sacral cornua. (D) 5th lumbar vertebrae.

Comments:

1. Note that the sacrum varies in size and thickness.
2. Note that the needle may advance into the foramen directly without encountering bone.
3. Note that needles may be bent and develop hooklike points if gentleness is not used when bone is encountered.
4. Incline the needles *inward* rather than outward and in the same plane as the wheals.
5. Always begin the block by injecting the second foramen. Then proceed to the others.
6 Block the second and third sacral nerves on both sides if caudal block is associated with transacral block.

NERVE BLOCKS
BLOCK OF CRANIAL NERVES

The cranial nerves which are blocked are the fifth and its branches and, occasionally, the tenth or vagus.

Gasserian Ganglion Block

Definition: Anesthesia obtained by depositing a local anesthetic drug into the area surrounding the Gasserian ganglion (5th cranial nerve).

Types: Although a number of techniques have been described, the one employing the Härtal route through the foramen ovale is the one described here.

Indications:

1. *Diagnostic:* As a means of differentiation between trigeminal and glossopharyngeal neuralgia (the glossopharyngeal nerve supplies the sensory innervation to the posterior third of the tongue). Relief of pain indicates trigeminal neuralgia.

2. *Therapeutic:* For relief of neuralgia (tic-douloureux) if surgery is contraindicated or not desired.

3. *Anesthesia:* For surgery of the face and jaw. Supplemental field blocks, such as cervical plexus block, may also be necessary. Rarely employed for this purpose.

Anatomy: The fifth cranial or trigeminal nerve arises from the pons. It is composed of a sensory dorsal root which gives rise to the Gasserian ganglion and an anterior motor root. The ganglion gives rise to three heads. The motor root passes beneath the ganglion and, after joining with the third expansion of the ganglion, passes through the foramen ovale as the mandibular nerve. The ganglion lies at the posterior extremity of the foramen ovale, which is a canal approximately 1 cm. long. To reach the ganglion, the needle must pass through the foramen ovale. The ganglion extends from the petrous portion of the temporal bone to the foramen ovale and lies on the pterygoid process. The infratemporal plate lies anterior to the foramen. The needle encounters the plate before being diverted towards the foramen.

Materials:

1. Standard regional set containing a 10 cm. needle approximately 1.9 mm. diam.

2. One 2 cc. syringe to aspirate and inject procaine.

Technique:

1. *Position:* Place the patient in the supine position. The operator should stand on side to be injected.

2. *Landmarks:*
   a. Condyloid notch (articulation of condyloid process of mandible).
   b. Midpoint of zygomatic notch on side to be injected.
   c. A point 3 cm. lateral to angle of the mouth, at the level of the 2nd upper molar tooth on side to be injected.
   d. Pupil of eye (as patient looks directly forward) on side to be injected.
3. *Procedure:*
   a. Place the index finger of the left hand in front of the tragus. Palpate the condyloid process and notch as the patient opens and closes his mouth.
   b. Allow the finger to slip anteriorly from the condyloid process along the zygoma until the sigmoid notch of the mandible is palpated.
   c. Hold the finger in the notch, and with finger pointing upward bisect the fingernail, and mark this point on the skin over the zygomatic arch. This point corresponds to the midpoint of the zygoma (A, Fig. 137).
   d. Mark another point on the same level and 1 cm. anterior to the one corresponding to the mid-point of the zygoma (B, Fig. 137).
   e. Locate a point 3 cms. from the angle of the mouth at the level of the 2nd upper molar tooth with the mouth of the patient closed. (C, Fig. 137). Raise an intradermal wheal in the skin at this point.
   f. Project an imaginary line through the pupil of the eye and the skin wheal (X, Fig. 137) and another through the point 1 cm. anterior to the mid-point of the zygomatic arch (point in step d) (Y, Fig. 137) and the skin wheal. This locates two planes one which is almost vertical, one which is inclined at an angle, backwards and upwards.
   g. Introduce the 10 cm. needle through the wheal described in e and advance along a line formed by the intersection of these two planes until the infratemporal plate is encountered, a distance of approximately 5–6 cms. (set recorder at 6 cms.).
   h. Place the recorder 1 cm. from the skin. Withdraw needle to subcutaneous tissue and redirect along a line formed by the intersection of the plane passing through the pupil of the eye and the wheal C and the plane passing through the *mid-point* of the zygomatic arch (point in step a) and the wheal C (Z, Fig. 137). The needle will enter the foramen ovale if guided in this direction. Paresthesias are felt by the patient along the course of the mandibular nerve.
   i. Inject 1 cc. of a 2% procaine solution for anesthesia very slowly so that it literally enters drop by drop. If alcohol is to be employed, inject 5 drops procaine and follow slowly by 1 cc. alcohol.

Anesthesia:

1. *Onset:* Within few minutes after the injection is completed. Rapid in-

jection gives rise to symptoms of increased intracranial pressure.

2. *Distribution:* This corresponds to the distribution of the trigeminal nerve. The cornea, eyelid, face and other structures innervated by this nerve are anesthetized.

3. *Duration:* One or more hours. When alcohol is used, it varies with the individual, but may last from 6 to 12 months.

Complications:

1. Penetration into the brain substance if the needle is advanced more than 1 cm. into the foramen ovale.

2. Arterial puncture. The internal maxillary artery may be encountered and bleeding results.

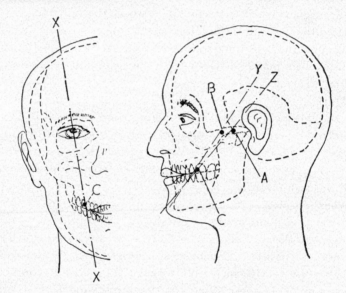

Fig. 137. Landmarks for Gasserian ganglion block (see text).

3. Paralysis and loss of sensation of the conjunctiva and cornea. Causes keratitis.

4. Hemorrhage of the cheek.

5. Herpes about lip—this is usually transient.

6. Paralysis of eye muscles—this is usually transient.

Precautions:

1. **Always inject procaine slowly.**

2. Always employ the supine position and allow the patient to remain in bed for several hours after the procedure.

3. Always attempt aspiration before injection of procaine or alcohol and withdraw needle if spinal fluid is aspirated.

Contra-Indications:

1. Diffuse painful conditions of face.
2. Infections in the site of injection.
3. In cases of neuralgia in which mandibular or maxillary or combined mandibular and maxillary blocks have not been given a trial first.

Remarks:

1. If an alcohol block is desired, perform a procaine block first. Repeat it in several days and follow it by alcohol.
2. **Gasserian ganglion block is a hazardous, difficult procedure. It should not be performed except in extreme cases and only by the initiated.**

Block of Ophthalmic Nerve

Definition: Block of branches of ophthalmic nerve.

Indications:

> *Diagnostic and Therapeutic:* rarely employed for these purposes.
> *Anesthetic:* for enucleation of eyeball or other occular operations and operations on the sinuses.

Anatomy: The ophthalmic nerve is purely a sensory nerve which arises from the Gasserian ganglion. The nerve passes forward, upward and laterally along the lateral wall of the cavernous sinus The nerve passes through the superior orbital fissure and divides into three branches: *lachrymal, frontal* and *nasociliary*. These subdivide into terminal branches.

Types: The ophthalmic nerve may be anesthetized by blocking its branches by two injections, a lateral orbital and medial orbital.

Materials: Standard regional set.

Technique:

1. *Position:* Place the patient in the supine position.
2. *Landmarks:* Margin of the orbit.
3. *Procedure:*

   Lateral orbital block:

   a. Introduce a 5 cm. needle a little above or below outer canthus at margin of orbit (A, Fig. 138).
   b. Allow needle to penetrate along lateral wall for 3.5 cms Retract eyeball either up or down.
   c. Inject 2 3 cc. 2% procaine slowly at this site.

   Medial orbital block:

   a. Introduce 5 cm. needle at point 1 cm. vertically above the caruncle (just below eyebrow).
   b. Insert needle for a distance of 3 cms. along the upper medial angle of orbit close to its wall (A, Fig. 138).
   c. Inject 2 cc. 2% procaine slowly at this site.

Anesthesia:

Onset: immediate if procaine is employed.

Duration: one hour if procaine is employed.

Distribution: The combined lateral and medial blocks produce anesthesia in the following areas: Ethmoidal, sphenoidal and frontal sinuses, as well as nasal cavity, front and tip of nose, upper eyelid and conjunctiva, muscles of eye.

Complications:

1. Protrusion of eyeball.
2. Injury to optic nerve.

Comment: The lower lid is supplied by infra-orbital nerve and is not anesthetized.

Block of Maxillary Nerve

Definition: Block of second or maxillary division of the trigeminal nerve.

Types:

1. Oral route (employed by dentists).
2. Extra oral route:
   a. Orbital route into foramen rotundum (not commonly employed).
   b. Zygomatic or extra oral route—simplest, quickest, safest.

Indications:

1. *Diagnostic:* None.
2. *Therapeutic:* For neuralgia of second division of fifth cranial nerve.
3. *Anesthetic:* Operations on upper lip, antrum, hard and soft palate, upper jaw and tonsils.

Anatomy: The maxillary nerve runs forward from the semi-lunar ganglion between the ophthalmic and mandibular nerves along lower border of the cavernous sinus and passes from the skull through the foramen rotundum, through the pterygopalatine fossa and enters the orbit as the infra-orbital nerve. It divides into the palpebral, nasal, and labial nerves and infra-orbital plexus. En route to the pterygopalatine fossa it gives off the palatine and superior alveolar nerves.

Materials: Standard regional set.

Technique: Zygomatic route:

1. *Position:* Place the patient in the supine position with the head turned to one side and operator standing on the side to be injected.
2. *Landmarks:* The midpoint of the zygomatic notch.
3. *Procedure* (Fig. 139):
   a. Raise an intradermal wheal at the midpoint of the zygomatic notch (Fig. 139).

b. Introduce an 8 cm. needle perpendicularly to the skin surface so that it passes below the zygoma for a distance not to exceed 4.5 cm. to 5 cm. (use marker).

c. Establish contact with the external pterygoid plate which is usually encountered at this depth.

d. Withdraw the marker and set it 1 cm. from skin surface. Reinsert the needle in a direction slightly anterior to the point of contact

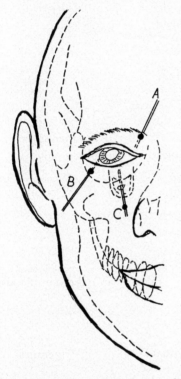

FIG. 138. Landmarks for lateral and medial ophthalmic and infraorbital block.

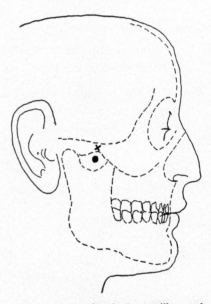

FIG. 139. Landmarks for maxillary and mandibular nerve block. The (X) indicates the midpoint of the notch; the dot, the point of entry of the needle.

with bone. Continue to introduce it until it slips off the anterior portion of the external pterygoid plate and advances as far as the marker.

e. Deposit 2 cc. of 2% procaine solution after carefully attempting aspiration.

Anesthesia:

1. *Onset:* Within five minutes after the injection, if procaine is employed.

2. *Distribution:* The cheek, lower eyelid, side of nose, upper lip, mucous membrane of nose, naso-pharynx, antra and ethmoid cells, soft and hard palate, and tonsils are usually involved.

3. *Duration:* One or more hours if procaine is employed.

Complications:

1. The needle may enter the orbit.
2. The pterygoid plate may be overlooked if the needle is introduced too great a distance posteriorly.
3. The pharynx may be entered if the needle is advanced more than 5 cm.

Precautions: Always use the marker to judge the required depth to advance the needle after the direction is changed.

Contra-Indications:

1. Local infection at the site of injection.
2. Distortions of the landmarks.

Remarks: The procaine block may be followed by an injection of 1 cc. of absolute alcohol if therapeutic block is desired for neuralgia or other conditions necessitating prolonged anesthesia (see page 369).

BLOCK OF MANDIBULAR NERVE

Definition: Block of the third division of the trigeminal nerve.

Types:

1. Oral route.
2. Extra-oral route: This is the more practical and the one usually employed.

Indications:

1. *Diagnostic:* To differentiate glossopharyngeal from trigeminal neuralgia.
2. *Therapeutic:* For relief of trigeminal neuralgia; for relief of masseter spasm in cases of trismus.
3. *Anesthetic:* Operation on lower jaw, lower lip, and for extractions of the lower teeth.

Anatomy: The mandibular or inferior maxillary nerve is the third division of the trigeminal nerve. The nerve is a combined sensory and motor. It runs downward through the foramen ovale and divides into two branches, an anterior branch, which is small and chiefly motor, and a posterior branch which is larger and chiefly sensory. The branches of the mandibular nerve are the auriculotemporal, lingual, buccinator, inferior alveolar and masseteric, anterior, middle and deep temporal, internal and external pterygoid.

Materials: Standard regional set.

Technique: Extra-oral route:

1. *Position:* Place the patient in the supine position. The operator should stand on side to be injected.
2. *Landmarks:* Same as for maxillary block.
3. *Procedure* (Fig. 139):
   a. Follow the same procedure described for the maxillary nerve. The only exception is that the needle is reintroduced to pass posterior to the external pterygoid plate of sphenoid bone for a distance of 0.5 cm. at which point 1 to 2 cc. of 2% procaine solution is injected.

Anesthesia:

1. *Onset:* within 5 to 10 minutes.
2. *Distribution:* Temporal region, dura at base of skull, temporo-mandibular articulation, auricle of ear, external auditory meatus, lower face and eye, mucous membrane of mouth, tongue, salivary glands, muscles of mastication, anterior belly of digastric mylohyoid and tensor palatine and tympanic muscles.
3. *Duration:* One or more hours if procaine is employed.

Complications:

1. The needle may pass into the pharynx if it is introduced a distance greater than 0.5 cm. beyond pterygoid plate.
2. Severe bleeding may result if the internal maxillary artery is encountered.

Precautions:

1. Use a marker to avoid introducing needle too far.
2. Partly withdraw needle after pterygoid plate is encountered and aim approximately 1 cm. behind point of first contact with bone.

Contra-Indications:

1. Infections about the face.
2. Distortion of landmarks.

Remarks: The procaine block may be followed by 1 cc. of absolute alcohol if therapeutic block is desired (see page 369).

BLOCKS OF PERIPHERAL NERVES
Brachial Plexus Block

Definition: Brachial plexus block is a block designed to produce anesthesia of the arm and forearm. It is accomplished by infiltration of the trunks, divisions, or cords of the plexus with a local anesthetic solution.

Indications:

1. *Anesthetic:* For operations on the hand and forearm (particularly tendons).
2. *Therapeutic:* To produce sympathetic block of the hand and forearm.

Types:

1. *Supraclavicular:* This is the most commonly employed approach because it is simplest, most successful, and utilizes the most reliable landmarks.
2. *Infraclavicular:* This approach is less frequently employed because the blood vessels in this region are parallel to the plexus and may be punctured. Often the needle is broken as it is inserted beneath the clavicle.
3. *Axillary:* This approach is not popular because the blood vessels in this region may be punctured. In addition, the plexus fans out at this point and renders infiltration of all component parts difficult.
4. *Paravertebral:* This approach is very difficult to execute technically.

Materials: Standard regional set containing an 8 cm. needle.

The Supraclavicular Approach

Anatomy: The brachial plexus is formed from the anterior primary divisions of the 5th, 6th, 7th cervical and 1st thoracic nerves. These join to form an upper, a middle, and a lower trunk. The trunks give rise to 6 divisions which unite in various ways to form cords which in turn give rise to the nerves of the arm, forearm, and shoulder girdle. The plexus possesses a fan-like arrangement as it runs downward and outward from the vertebrae and converges so that the cords and nerves pass closely together beneath the midpoint of the clavicle over the surface of the first rib.

Technique:

1. *Position:*
   a. Place patient in the supine position. Arrange the arm on the side to be injected in slight abduction, and rotate the head in the opposite direction. The operator should stand on the side to be injected.
2. *Landmarks:*
   a. A point midway and 1 cm. above the superior border of the clavicle. The midpoint of the clavicle is obtained by bisecting the distance between the acromioclavicular and the sternoclavicular joints.
   b. The lateral border of the subclavian artery above the clavicle.
   c. The external jugular vein (rendered prominent by having the patient blow out his cheeks). The vein passes downward and medial to the midpoint of the clavicle.
   d. Tubercle of the 6th cervical vertebra.

3. *Procedure* (Fig. 140):

   a. Raise an intradermal wheal at the point (B, Fig. 140), 1 cm. above the midpoint of clavicle (A, Fig. 140).

   b. Identify, by palpation, the subclavian artery and external jugular vein (C, D, Fig. 140).

   c. Grasp the needle, unattached to the syringe, in the right hand and introduce it through the wheal, exercising care to avoid the artery and vein.

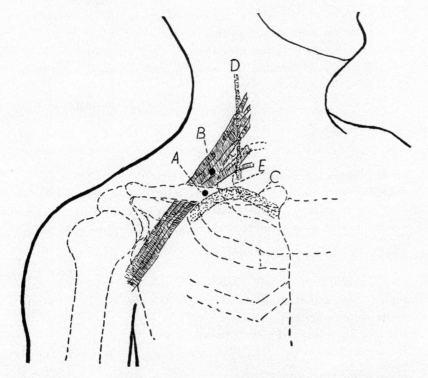

Fig. 140. Landmarks for brachial plexus block by the supraclavicular route. (A) Midpoint of the clavicle. (B) Site of injection. (C) Subclavian artery. (D) External jugular vein. (E) First rib.

   d. Set the marker for 1.5 cms. and advance the needle posteriorly, caudad, and medially until the first rib is encountered. Do not advance the needle any farther than the marker if the rib is not encountered.

   e. Withdraw the needle 2 or 3 mm. after the rib is encountered so that it lies in the same plane as the brachial plexus, i.e., superficial to the deep fascia of the neck.

   f. Place a drop of anesthetic solution on the open end of the hub of needle and ask the patient to take a deep breath. This is to determine whether or not the pleura has been pierced. There should be no movement of the drop.

g. Inject 10 cc. of 2% procaine solution. Perform aspiration frequently during the injection.

h. Palpate and mark the tubercle of the transverse process of the 6th cervical vertebra by placing the left index finger upon it.

i. Withdraw the needle almost to the skin.

j. Push marker all the way back on the shaft of the needle and reinsert the needle deep to the sternocleidomastoid muscle for a distance of approximately 6 cm. towards the tubercle. Allow the index finger of the left hand to remain over the tubercle during the injection.

k. Aspirate to determine the presence of spinal fluid or blood and inject 5 cc. of 2% procaine in this region.

l. Withdraw needle almost to the skin and introduce it again in a lateral caudad direction, inclined to such an angle so as to be directed behind the clavicle and anterior to the first rib.

m. Inject 5 cc. of 2% procaine solution behind clavicle after performing aspiration.

Anesthesia:

1. *Onset:* Ten to fifteen minutes.
2. *Distribution:* Complete in the hands, fingers, and forearm. A zone of hypesthesia exists over the shoulder. No anesthesia exists in the axilla.
3. *Duration:* One hour or more when procaine is employed.

Complications:

1. Piercing of blood vessels. The subclavian artery or vein, external jugular vein and the superficial or deep transverse cervical artery are all liable to puncture.
2. Piercing the pleura. Pneumothorax results.
3. Intraspinal injection. "High" spinal or segmental spinal anesthesia results.

Precautions:

1. Always locate and maintain palpating finger on the subclavian artery while the needle is being introduced.
2. Always contact the first rib with the needle before injecting the drug.
3. Always identify the external jugular vein before making the puncture.
4. Always test for entrance of the needle in the pleural space.
5. Never insert the needle beyond the marker when seeking the first rib.
6. Always perform aspiration to determine whether or not the spinal canal has been entered.
7. Withdraw the needle completely if blood is aspirated in the syringe and make pressure in the supraclavicular fossa before attempting the block again.

Contra-Indications:

1. The presence of infection of the extremity or at the site of the block.
2. The presence of tumor masses which may distort landmarks.
3. In psychically unsuited patients and children.
4. For operations which may last more than one hour.

Comment

1. Withdraw the needle and reinsert it if an artery or other blood vessel is entered.
2. Seek paresthesias when inserting the needle. The patient feels paresthesias radiating up and down the arm.
3. Motor anesthesia is rarely complete in the large muscles. Paresis is usually present, however.

Brachial Plexus Block* (*Alternate Method*)

Procedure:

1. Arrange patient and prepare materials in the same manner for technique described above.
2. Locate junction of middle and inner third of clavicle and mark skin over clavicle.
3. Raise an intradermal wheal 2 cms. above this point.
4. Raise a second intradermal wheal between the first wheal and the clavicle.
5. Raise a third wheal 1 1/2 to 2 cms. above the first wheal.
6. Introduce an 8 cm. needle through the first wheal and establish contact with the first rib.

Brachial Plexus Block (*Axillary Route*)

Definition:

A block of the brachial plexus just as it begins to divide into its branches as it passes into the axilla.

Indications:

Same as branchial plexus block of the supraclavicular route.

Anatomy:

The brachial plexus divides into lateral, medial and posterior cord, which accompanies the axillary artery to the arm at the level of the insertion of the pectoralis major into the humerus. The artery is directly medial to the humerus and rests upon the triceps muscle. The median nerve is medial and superficial to the artery. The musculocutaneous nerve is anterior and lateral. The musculocutaneous nerve may have divided at this site. At the level of

---

* Technique first suggested by Ralph T. Knight.

the insertion of the pectoralis major into the humerus the artery and nerves are superficial and close together and easily palpable.

Technique:

1. *Position:* Supine with the arm adducted at 90°, allowing it to rest on a support in external rotation.

2. *Landmarks:*

   a. Insertion of the pectoralis major anteriorly.
   b. Insertion of the teres major and latissimus dorsi posteriorly.
   c. Axillary artery.

3. *Procedure:*

   a. Locate the insertion of the latissimus dorsi posteriorly and pectoralis major anteriorly. Draw a line between these two points and bisect it (1, Fig. 88). The line lies directly over the brachial artery (2, Fig. 140B).
   b. Raise a wheal at this point and introduce a ¾ inch 25 gauge needle attached to a 10 cc. syringe perpendicularly to the humerus (3, Fig. 140B).
   c. Retract the axillary artery posteriorly with the thumb and index finger of the left hand in order to remove it from the path of the needle.
   d. Continue to advance the needle directly perpendicular to the skin and to the humerus towards the median nerve. Seek paresthesias which radiate to the fingertips (Fig. 140A).
   e. Inject 5 cc. of 2% procaine at this site.
   f. Withdraw the needle almost to the skin and re-introduce it at an angle of 45° anterior to the direction of the first injection toward the insertion of the pectoralis major muscle.
   g. Advance the needle to the musculocutaneous nerve (or its branches, if it has divided) (2, Fig. 140A) and seek paresthesias to the elbow joint. Inject 5 cc. of 2% procaine at this point.
   h. Withdraw the needle almost to the skin and retract the artery towards the upper surface of the arm.
   i. Re-introduce the needle directly posteriorly at an angle of 45° to the line of original injection for the median nerve towards the ulnar nerve (3, Fig. 140A). Seek paresthesias in the fourth and fifth fingers.
   j. Inject 5 cc. of 2% procaine at this site.
   k. Withdraw the needle almost to the skin and re-introduce it with the arm still retracted upward at an angle of almost 90° to the direction of the first injection of the median nerve to reach the radial nerve

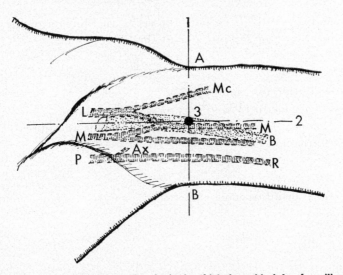

Fig. 140A. View of axilla showing landmarks for brachial plexus block by the axillary route. (1) Line drawn through point of insertion of pectoralis major muscle into humerus (A) and teres major (B). (2) Line drawn through (1) bisected falls directly over brachial artery. (3) Point for raising wheal. (L) lateral cord of plexus (M) medial and (P) posterior. (M₂) Musculocutaneous nerve. (M) medial, ulnar nerve is shown to the medial and (R) radial nerves. Note axillary nerve has been given off before site of block.

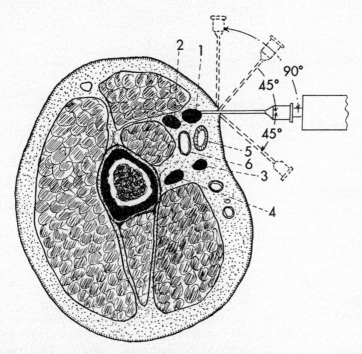

Fig. 140B. Brachial plexus block by the axillary route. Cross section at junction of axilla and arm. (Through Line (1) Fig. 140A). 1. Median nerve. 2. Musculocutaneous nerve. 3. Ulnar nerve. 4. Radial nerve. 5. Brachial artery. 6. Vena comitans.

(4, Fig. 140B). Seek paresthesias to the dorsum of the hand and inject 5 cc. of 2% procaine at this site.

Anesthesia:

1. *Onset:* Within five minutes.
2. *Duration:* One to $1\frac{1}{2}$ hours if procaine is employed.
3. *Distribution:* From the junction of the middle and upper third of the arm to the finger tips.

Complications:

Intra-arterial or intravenous injection if aspiration is not attempted with each injection of drug.

Contra-Indications:

Infections in the axilla.

Comment:

1. Syringe should remain attached to the needle throughout all maneuvers.
2. The needle should be at right angles to the shaft of the humerus at all times and not inclined or pointed upward or downward along the arm.

REFERENCE

Labat, G. Regional Anesthesia. 2nd Ed. Pp. 215–235. W. B. Saunders Co., Philadelphia, 1930.

Block of the Suprascapular Nerve

Definition: Block of the suprascapular nerve as it passes through the suprascapular notch.

Indications:

1. Diagnostic and therapeutic
   (a) For pain affliction of the shoulder joint.
   (b) Subdeltoid bursitis.

2. Anesthetic. None.

Anatomy: The suprascapular nerve arises from the trunk formed by the union of the 5th and 6th cervical nerves. It runs a lateral course beneath the trapezius and it gains access to the infraspinatus fossa by passing through the suprascapular notch below the transverse scapular ligament. The nerve passes beneath the supraspinatus muscle along the lateral border of the scapula to the infraspinatus fossa. It supplies the shoulder joint, infraspinatus and supraspinatus muscles.

Materials: Standard regional set containing 10 cm. needle.

Technique:

1. Position. The patient is placed in the upright sitting position, prefer-ably leaning over a table, resting his elbows on the table.
2. Landmarks.
   (a) The angle of the scapula.
   (b) Scapular spine.
3. Procedure.
   (a) Draw a line along the spine of the scapula.
   (b) Outline lower border of the scapula (Figs. 140C, 140D).
   (c) Bisect the angle formed by the lower border of the scapula and extend it so that it crosses the line overlying that drawn over the spine of the scapula (A, Figs. 140C, 140D).
   (d) Bisect the outer upper angle formed by the intersection of these two lines (3, Figs. 140C, 140D). Raise a wheal 1.5 cm. from the point of intersection along this line (3, Figs. 140C, 140D).
   (e) Introduce a 10 cm. needle through the wheal perpendicular to the skin until the scapula is encountered.
   (f) Set marker for 1.5 cm.
   (g) As soon as bone is encountered partly withdraw the needle and re-introduce towards the midline medially and somewhat caudad until it is felt to slip into the notch.
   (h) As soon as needle slips off into the notch (4, Fig. 140C) advance up to the marker 1.5 cm.
   (i) Inject 10 cc. of 2% procaine at this site.

Anesthesia:

1. Onset. Two to five minutes, if 2% procaine is used.
2. Duration. Approximately an hour and a half.
3. Distribution. The shoulder joint, bursa, and other structures around the shoulder joint completely lose their sensation.

Complications: The needle may be introduced too far and passed into the thorax.

Precautions: Always attempt aspiration.

Contra-indications: Infections about the site of injection.

Remarks:

1. Do not inject alcohol or other long lasting anesthetic substances into the nerve. Prolonged anesthesia of this nerve may cause trophic changes in the shoulder joint.
2. Paresthesias will be felt beneath the scapula or in the shoulder joint as nerve is encountered.

3. Always attempt aspiration. The transverse scapular artery is in close association with this nerve.

4. A small triangular area over the tip of the shoulder may be anesthetic; otherwise no skin anesthesia is encountered.

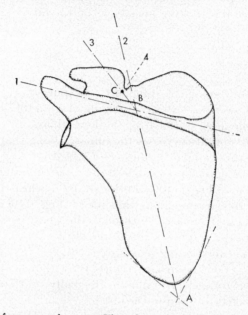

Fig. 140C. Block of suprascapular nerve. View of scapula. (1) Line drawn along spine of scapula. (2) Line drawn to bisect inferior angle of scapula (A). (3) Line bisecting the lateral superior quadrant formed by intersection of (1) and (2). (C) Point 1.5 cm. from intersection at which site wheal is raised through which needle is introducee. (4) Scapular notch.

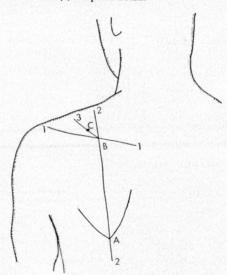

Fig. 140D. Landmarks for block of suprascapular nerve. (1) Line drawn along spine of scapula. (2) Line drawn to bisect inferior angle of scapula. Line bisecting the lateral superior quadrant formed by intersection of (1) and (2). (C) Point 1.5 cm. from intersection at which site wheal is raised through which needle is introduced.

Median Nerve Block

Definition: Anesthesia produced by blocking the median nerve at its most superficial points.

Types:

1. Block at the elbow.
2. Block at the wrist.

Indications:

1. *Anesthetic:* For operations upon the arm and forearm in which brachial plexus block is not feasible.
2. *Therapeutic:* For vasospastic and other diseases involving the autonomic nervous system.

Anatomy: The median nerve arises from the medial cord of the brachial plexus and passes through the axilla along with the brachial artery. It lies lateral to the artery until the elbow is neared. It then crosses over to the inner aspect of the arm. It then passes through the cubital fossa beneath the bicipital fascia and enters the forearm. In the cubital fossa, it lies between the internal condyle of the humerus and the tendon of the biceps muscle. The brachial artery lies between the tendon and the nerve. At the wrist, the nerve becomes superficial and lies beneath the deep fascia, between the palmaris longus and flexor carpi radialis tendons.

Materials: Standard regional set.

Median Block at the Elbow

Technique:

1. *Landmarks:*
   a. Brachial artery.
   b. Tendon of biceps.
   c. Internal condyle of humerus.
2. *Position of patient:* Supine with the arm abducted and forearm extended.
3. *Procedure:*
   a. Place an applicator moistened with iodine or ink in the cubital fossa.
   b. Flex the forearm up on the arm to make an angle of 90° and trace

REFERENCE

Rovenstine, E. A., and Wertheim, H. Cervical Plexus Block. New York State J. Med., *39:* 1311, 1939.*

* This technique originally described by these workers.

or mark junction of skin of arm and forearm with the moistened applicator. A transverse line results (A, Fig. 141).

   c. Locate the tendon of the biceps (felt by flexing and extending forearm with hand in supination) (B, Fig. 141).

   d. Locate the brachial artery (C, Fig. 141) by palpation and raise an intradermal wheal medial to it (D, Fig. 141).

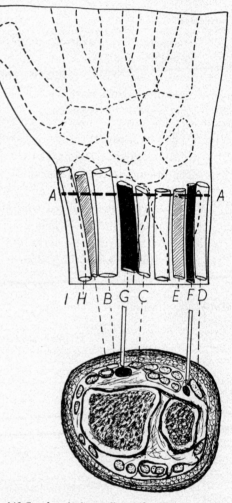

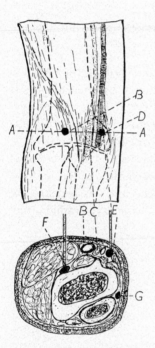

Fig. 141. Landmarks for median and radial nerve block at the elbow: (A) Line above crease of elbow. (B) Tendon of biceps. (C) Brachial artery. (D) Vein. (E) Median nerve. (F) Radial nerve beneath brachioradialis muscle. (G) Ulnar nerve.

Fig. 142. Landmarks for median and radial nerve block at the wrist. (A) Transverse line through ulnar styloid for determining point of injection. (B) Flexor carpi radialis longus tendon. (C) Palmaris longus tendon. (D) Flexor carpi ulnaris tendon. (E) Ulnar artery. (F) Ulnar nerve. (G) Median nerve. (H) Radial artery.

   e. Introduce a 5 cm. needle through the wheal perpendicular to the skin through the superficial and deep fascia and seek paresthesias.

f. Attach the syringe to the needle and inject 3 cc. of 2% procaine at this site.
g. Inject 2 or 3 cc. in fanwise manner over the path of nerve.
h. Circumscribe a "garter" intracutaneously and subcutaneously with 1/2% procaine above the site of injection.

Median Block at the Wrist

Technique:

1. *Landmarks:*
   a. Tendons of palmaris longus and flexor carpi radialis muscles.
   b. Styloid process of the ulna.
2. *Position:* Place the patient in a supine position with the arm on a board and the palm facing upward.
3. *Procedure:*
   a. Locate and mark a cross on the anterior aspect of the wrist through the styloid of the ulna (A, Fig. 142).
   b. Locate and mark the outline of the palmaris longus and flexor carpi radialis tendons (B, C, Fig. 142).
   c. Raise an intradermal wheal between the two tendons on transverse line through the styloid of the ulna.
   d. Introduce a 5 cm. needle perpendicular to the skin through the superficial and deep fascia and advance it 0.5 cm. beyond the deep fascia.
   e. Inject 2 cc. 2% procaine at this site.
   f. Partly withdraw and incline the needle towards the flexor carpi radialis tendon. Introduce needle deep to tendon and inject 2 cc. of 2% procaine at this site.
   g. Massage the area to cause diffusion of solution into the tissues.

Anesthesia:

Onset: Usually within 5 minutes if procaine is employed.
Duration: One hour.

Comment

1. The median nerve lies beneath the flexor carpi radialis tendon in many instances. The needle must be inclined in that direction to seek it.
2. The transverse line marked in the cubital fossa does not correspond to and is above the line drawn through the condyles of the humerus.
3. Median nerve blocks are best employed in conjunction with ulnar and radial nerve blocks.

Note: An intracutaneous and subcutaneous band (garter) of 1% solution of procaine should be infiltrated about the entire arm when a combination of blocks is used to block any overlapping nerve fibres.

Radial Nerve Block

Definition: Anesthesia produced by block of the radial nerve where it is most superficial.

Types:

1. Block at the elbow (lateral).
2. Block at elbow (anterior). This is the most commonly employed type.
3. Block at the wrist.

Block at the Elbow

Indications:

Anesthetic: For surgery of hand or wrist.

Diagnostic and Therapeutic: Same as for median nerve.

Anatomy: The posterior cord of the brachial plexus gives rise to two divisions, one large and one small. The larger gives rise to the radial nerve, the smaller the axillary. The radial nerve passes behind the axillary artery at the anterior surface of the latissimus dorsi muscle across the teres major and proceeds downward posteriorly and laterally into the musculo-spiral groove between the long and medial heads of the triceps muscle. It then passes towards the lateral side of the arm. At approximately 10 cms. above the external condyle it crosses the humerus in an anterior direction between the brachioradialis and brachialis muscles after having pierced the lateral intermuscular septum. As it reaches the external condyle of the humerus, it divides into two branches, the radial and the interosseous.

Materials: Standard regional set.

Technique (Fig. 142):

1. *Landmarks:* Same as for median nerve block.
2. *Position:* Same as for median nerve block.
3. *Procedure:*
   a. Raise an intradermal wheal 1 cm. lateral to the tendon of biceps on a line of bend of elbow as located in the same manner as for the median nerve block.
   b. Introduce a 5 cm. needle through the wheal perpendicular to the skin.
   c. Place the index finger of left hand at the posterior aspect of the lateral condyle of humerus.
   d. Advance needle in the direction of the finger until bone is encountered. Seek paresthesias at this site and inject 5 cc. 2% procaine at this site.

REFERENCE

Labat, G. Regional Anesthesia. 2nd Ed. Pp. 237–246. W. B. Saunders Co., Philadelphia, 1930.

Ulnar Nerve Block

Definition: Anesthesia of the ulnar nerve produced by blocking it at its most superficial points along its course.

Uses:

Anesthetic: Same as for median and radial nerve blocks.
Diagnostic: Same as for median and radial nerve blocks.

Types:

1. Block at the elbow.
2. Block at the wrist.

Anatomy: The ulnar nerve arises from the medial cord of the brachial plexus, passes downward in the arm and becomes superficial between the internal condyle of the humerus and the olecranon process of the ulna. The nerve may be palpated in the groove thus formed. It then courses between the heads of the flexor carpi ulnaris muscle and downward to the wrist where it becomes superficial. It then lies on the outer border of the tendon of the flexor carpi ulnaris before it courses into the hand to supply the skin and muscles there.

Materials: Standard regional set.

Block at the Elbow

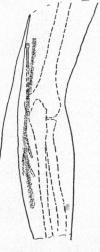

Fig. 143. Landmarks for ulnar block at the elbow (see text).

Technique (Fig. 143):

1. *Landmarks:* The groove between the internal condyle of the humerus and the olecranon process.
2. *Position:*
   a. Place the patient in the lateral prone position on the side opposite the one to be injected.
   b. Allow the arm to rest alongside body.
3. *Procedure:*
   a. Palpate and grasp the nerve above the groove using thumb and index finger of left hand.
   b. Raise an intradermal wheal on the tip of the fold of skin thus grasped. The wheal should be 3 cms. above the bony prominence as shown in Fig. 143.
   c. Introduce a 5 cm. needle in the direction of nerve and nearly parallel to it for a distance of several centimeters.
   d. As soon as paresthesias are felt inject 5 cc. 2% procaine.

Anesthesia:

> *Onset:* Usually within 5 minutes if procaine is employed.
> *Duration:* One hour if procaine is employed.

Block at the Wrist

Technique:

1. *Landmarks:*
   a. Styloid process of ulna (same transverse line as for median block) (A, Fig. 143).
   b. Tendon of the flexor carpi ulnaris muscle.
2. *Position:* Place the patient in the supine position with the hand in supination.
3. *Procedure* (Fig. 143):
   a. Palpate the tendon of the flexor carpi ulnaris at the level of styloid of the ulna (D, Fig. 142, p. 419).
   b. Raise an intradermal wheal on the radial side of the tendon of flexor carpi ulnaris on the line through the ulnar styloid.
   c. Introduce a 5 cm. needle perpendicular to the skin and pierce the deep fascia.
   d. Seek paresthesias and when these are felt inject 3 cc. 2% procaine solution at this site.

Comment: Avoid injection into the tendons, the joint or directly into the nerve.

REFERENCE

Labat, G. Regional Anesthesia. 2nd Ed. Pp. 246–248. W. B. Saunders Co., Philadelphia, 1930.

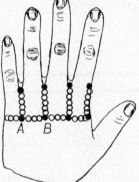

FIG. 144. Block of the digits (see text).

Block at the Thumb and Fingers

Technique:

1. *Landmarks:* Metacarpal bones (Fig. 144).
2. *Position:* Place the patient in the supine position. Dorsum of hand should face upward.
3. *Procedure:*
   a. Raise an intradermal wheal on each side of the midpoint of the metacarpal bone of the digit to be anesthetized or all the digits if desired (A, B, Fig. 144)
   b. Advance a 5 cm. needle towards palm perpendicular to the skin. Inject 1% procaine as the needle is advanced.
   c. Infiltrate along the area from the wheal to web of finger on either side.

Comment: Place a finger on the palm and palpate for the needle so that it does not perforate skin of palm.

Block of Digits

Technique:

1. *Landmarks:* Phalanx proximal to site of operation.
2. *Position:* Dorsum of the finger to be anesthetized should face upward.

Procedure:

1. Raise an intradermal wheal on the dorsum of the digit over the phalanx.
2. Inject 1% procaine through the skin to bone on one side.
3. Almost completely withdraw and insert the needle on the other side in same manner as in step 2.

Comment

1. Do not add vasoconstrictor drugs to the procaine (avoid gangrene).
2. Do not use tourniquet for digital operation when regional anesthesia is induced.
3. Inject drug slowly.

REFERENCES

Adams, R. C. Regional Anesthesia for Operations About the Neck and Upper Extremity. Anesthesiology, *2:* 515, September, 1941.
Labat, G. Regional Anesthesia. 2nd Ed. P. 336. W. B. Saunders Co., Philadelphia, 1930.

Block of Intercostal Nerves

Definition: Block of the intercostal nerves as they course the intercostal grooves.
Uses: Rib section, thoracic and upper abdominal operations.
Anatomy: The intercostal nerve accompanies the intercostal artery and vein in the intercostal groove along the inferior border of the rib. The nerve is inferior to the artery. The vein is superior to both nerve and artery.

Technique (Fig. 145):

1. *Landmarks:*
   a. Midaxillary line.
   b. Inferior border of the rib.
2. *Position:* Sitting upright. The patient's hands should be folded over his head to allow ample exposure of the thorax.
3. *Procedure:*
   a. Raise an intradermal wheal over the lower border of the desired rib in midaxillary line.
   b. Introduce a 5 cm. needle through the wheal until contact is made with the lower border of the rib (A, Fig. 145).

c. Retract the skin and soft tissues in the region of the puncture downward with the thumb of the right hand (B, Fig. 145).

d. Insert the needle 1/4 to 1/2 cms. beyond the lower border of the rib. Paresthesias may result if the needle encounters the nerve.

e. Inject 5 cc. 2% procaine at this site.

f. Infiltrate the skin and subcutaneous tissue in the midaxillary line with 1% procaine to block superficial nerve filaments.

Anesthesia:

1. *Onset:* Within 5 to 10 minutes when procaine is employed.

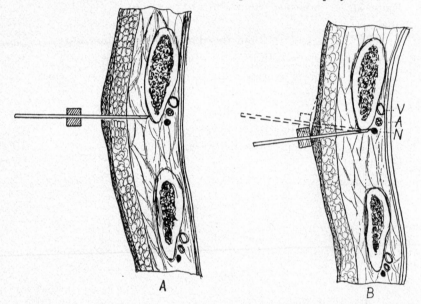

FIG. 145. Block of the intercostal nerves (see text).

2. *Distribution:* Along course of nerve distal to the site of injection.

3. *Duration:* One hour.

Comment: Always attempt aspiration. Vessels or pleura may be entered.

REFERENCE

Bartlett, R. W. Bilateral Intercostal Nerve Block. Surgery, *71:* 194–197, August, 1940.

Femoral Nerve Block

Definition: Block of femoral nerve below the inguinal ligament.

Uses: For operations on the anteromedial aspect of the thigh.

Anatomy: The femoral nerve arises from the lumbar plexus, and emerges beneath the inguinal ligament lateral to the femoral artery and vein to lie beneath the deep fascia of the thigh.

Technique (Fig. 146):

1. *Landmarks:*

a. Inguinal ligament.
b. Femoral artery.
2. *Position:* Supine.
3. *Procedure:*
a. Identify the inguinal ligament (A, Fig. 146).
b. Palpate the femoral artery with left index finger and retract it medially during injection.
c. Raise an intradermal wheal just below the Poupart's ligament lateral to artery (B, Fig. 146).
d. Introduce an 8 cm. needle through the wheal perpendicular to the skin until the iliac fascia has been pierced.
e. Adjust the marker for one centimeter as soon as needle has passed the fascia and insert it 1 cm. beyond the fascia. Attempt to elicit paresthesias.
f. Fix the needle when paresthesias are elicited and inject 5 cc. 2% procaine at this site. If no paresthesias are elicited, inject 25 cc. of the procaine solution in a fanwise direction beneath the fascia and into the muscle.

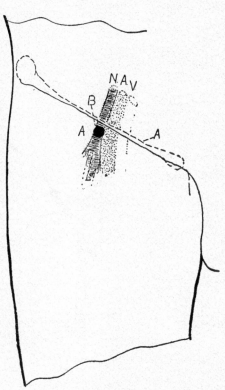

FIG. 146. Landmarks for block of the femoral nerve (see text).

Anesthesia:

Onset: Usually within 5 minutes if procaine is employed.
Distribution: Medial and anterior aspect of thigh.

REFERENCE

Labat, G. Regional Anesthesia. 2nd Ed. P. 480. W. B. Saunders Co., Philadelphia, 1930.

Femoral Cutaneous Nerve Block

Definition: Block of the lateral femoral cutaneous nerve at inguinal region.
Uses: For superficial operations upon the lateral aspect of the thigh (skin grafts, removal of tumors, etc.).
Anatomy: The external femoral cutaneous nerve arises from the lumbar

plexus, traverses the iliac fossa and emerges beneath the inguinal ligament to pass into the thigh.

Technique:

    1. *Landmarks:*
        a. The anterior superior iliac spine.
        b. The inguinal ligament.
    2. *Position:* Supine.

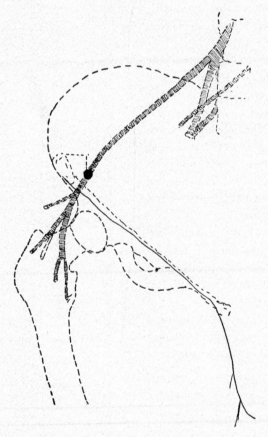

FIG. 147. Landmarks for block of the femoral
cutaneous nerve (see text).

    3. *Procedure:*
        a. Raise an intradermal wheal 1 cm. caudad and medial to the anterior
           superior iliac spine (Fig. 147).
        b. Introduce an 8 cm. needle vertically through the wheal and advance
           it until the iliac bone is encountered.
        c. Inject 1% procaine while needle is advancing and 10 cc. after the
           needle encounters the bone.
        d. Partially withdraw the needle and perform fanlike injections in

lateral and medial direction over an area of 4 or 5 cms. along the spine.

Anesthesia:

1. *Onset:* Usually within 5 minutes if procaine is used.
2. *Distribution:* Anterolateral aspect of the thigh.

REFERENCE

Labat, G. Regional Anesthesia. 2nd Ed. P. 480. W. B. Saunders Co., Philadelphia, 1930.

BLOCK OF THE OBTURATOR NERVE

Definition:

Block of the obturator nerve in the obturator canal before it divides into its terminal branches.

Indications:

Diagnostic and therapeutic; for pain in the hip joint, from arthritis and other causes.

Anesthetic:

For operations about the hip joint in conjunction with sciatic, femoral and lateral femoral cutaneous nerve block.

Anatomy:

The obturator nerve arises from the posterior division of the anterior primary divisions of the second, third and fourth lumbar nerves. It emerges at the medial border of the psoas muscle from which it is separated by the iliolumbar artery. It courses through the pelvis to the obturator canal through which it passes to enter the upper part of the thigh. It divides into an articular and an anterior and a posterior branch, in passing through the obturator foramen. In the obturator foramen it lies above the obturator membrane and below the superior ramus of the pubis. It is sensory to the internal aspect of the thigh and sends off an articular branch to the hip joint, as well as branches to the knee joint (Fig. 147A).

Materials:

Standard regional set.

Technique:

1. *Position:* Supine position with the affected leg partly abducted.
2. *Landmarks.:*
    a. Pubic tubercle medially (a, Fig. 147A).
    b. Pulsation of the femoral artery laterally (B, Fig. 147B).
    c. Superior ramus of the pubis.
    d. Inguinal ligament (C, Fig. 147B).

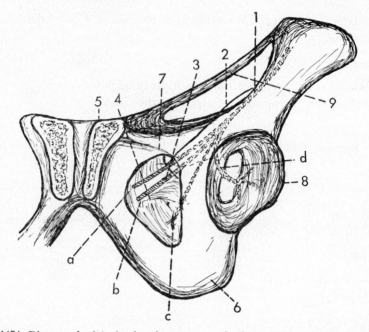

Fig. 147A. Diagram of pelvis showing obturator nerve in obturator foramen. L. Obturator nerve coursing along pelvis into obturator canal dividing into (a) anterior branch, (b) posterior branch, (c) branch to external obturator muscle and (d) articular branch. 2. Accessory obturator nerve. 3. Obturator canal. 4. Obturator foramen and membrane. 5. Pubic tuberosity. 6. Ischial tuberosity. 7. Superior ramus of pubis. 8. Acetabulum. 9. Inguinal ligament.

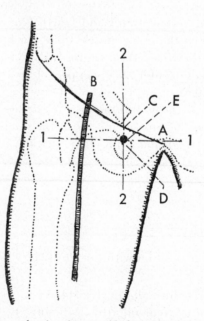

Fig. 147B. Landmarks for performing obturator block. 1. Line drawn through pubic tubercle A and femoral artery B. 2. Line bisecting line (1). E. Point 1.5 cm. below the inguinal ligament (C) on line 2. The wheal is raised at the point. D. The obturator foramen.

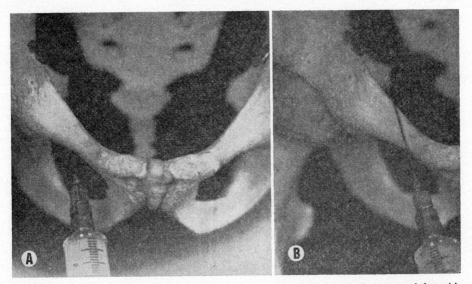

FIG. 147C. (A) The correct position of the needle passing below the superior ramus of the pubis in performing obturator block. (B) The incorrect position. The needle passes over the superior ramus instead of beneath.

3. *Procedure:*
   a. Identify the pubic tubercle and the femoral artery and draw a line connecting these two points (1, Fig. 147B).
   b. Bisect this line and raise a wheal at this midpoint, 1.5 cm. below Poupart's ligament (E, Fig. 147B).
   c. Introduce a 12 cm. needle perpendicularly to the skin and until the superior ramus of the pubis is encountered.
   d. Set marker for an additional 1.5 cm. beyond this depth.
   e. Withdraw the needle almost completely. Tilt it so that it will be directed toward the inferior surface of the ramus of the pubis.
   f. Re-introduce so that it passes beneath the superior ramus of the pubic bone, feeling the way along until needle has been inserted to the marker. The needle is directed cephalad, lateral and posteriorly in this maneuver.
   g. Seek paresthesias and inject 10 cc. of 1% procaine at this site.

Anesthesia:
   1. *Onset:* Requires approximately 15 minutes to be established.
   2. *Duration:* One hour to 1½ hours, if procaine is employed.
   3. *Distribution:* The hip joint, the knee joint and the medial aspect of the thigh are anesthetized. Paresis of the external obturator and of muscles on medial aspect of thigh.

Complications:
   1. Needle may enter the bladder. Patient should empty the bladder before the block is attempted.
   2. The needle may encounter and enter a major blood vessel.

Contra-indications:

Infections at the site of puncture.

Comment:

Failures are due to:

1. If the needle enters the pelvis.
2. If the needle is introduced above the superior ramus rather than at the inferior surface (B, Fig. 147C).
3. The obturator nerve divides and gives off the articular branch before it enters the obturator canal.
4. If the hip joint receives innervation from the nerves of the quadratus femoris muscle. This should be blocked in addition to the obturator nerve.
5. The accessory obturator is present in $\frac{1}{3}$ of the cases. It passes over the ramus of the pubis and joins the branches of the obturator (Fig. 147A).

Sciatic Nerve Block

Definition: Sciatic block is block of the greater sciatic nerve secured by injecting a local anesthetic drug at the point of exit from the pelvis.

Types: The type which employs the lateral approach on thigh is the commonly employed route.

Indication:

1. *Anesthesia:* For fractures and operations on the foot and lateral aspect of the leg.
2. *Therapeutic:* Neuralgias (sciatica).

Anatomy: The sciatic nerve arises from the lumbar plexus (L_4, L_5, S_1, S_2, S_3) and passes from the pelvis between the pyriformis muscle by way of the great sciatic notch. It turns downward between the great trochanter and the tuberosity of the ischium and becomes superficial at the lower border of the gluteus maximus muscle. It then courses down the posterior aspect of the leg to the popliteal fossa where it divides into the tibial and common peroneal nerves. Branches are given off to the muscles of the posterior aspect of the thigh on its descent.

Materials: Standard regional set containing a 10 cm. needle.

Technique:

1. *Position:* Arrange the patient so that he lies on his side with the affected side *upward* and the thigh is flexed to form an angle of 135–150° with the trunk. The operator stands so that *he faces the back* of the patient.
2. *Landmarks:*
   a. Posterior superior iliac spine.
   b. Great trochanter of the femur.

3. *Procedure:*

a. Palpate the greater trochanter and mark a point on the overlying skin.

b. Palpate the posterior superior iliac spine and mark the point on the overlying skin.

c. Draw a line (ilio trochanteric) between the two points (A, B, Fig. 148).

d. Determine the midpoint of the ilio trochanteric line and draw a line perpendicular to it in a caudad direction for a distance of 3 cms. and raise a wheal at its end (C, Fig. 148).

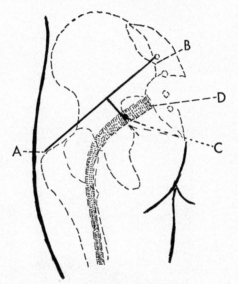

Fig. 148. Landmarks for block of the sciatic nerve (see text).

e. Arrange the marker for 6–7 cms. on the 10 cm. needle and introduce it perpendicularly to the skin through the wheal.

f. Seek paresthesias and inject 10 cc. of 2% procaine slowly.

Anesthesia:

1. *Onset:* Usually appears within 10 minutes if procaine is employed.

2. *Distribution:* Posterior thigh, leg and foot.

3. *Duration:* 1–1 1/2 hours.

Complications: Shock and other circulatory phenomena from trauma to nerve.

Precautions:

1. Do not inject alcohol into the sciatic nerve (motor paralysis may result).

2. Withdraw the needle 1 cm. if bone is encountered and inject the solution.

Contra-Indications: None.

Remarks: This particular block is little employed.

REFERENCE

Labat, G. Regional Anesthesia. 2nd Ed. Pp. 326–332. W. B. Saunders Co., Philadelphia, 1930.

Block of the Great Toe

Uses: For operations involving the large toe if the operative area extends as far as its base.

Technique (Fig. 149):

1. *Landmarks:*
   a. Metatarsal bone of the great toe.
   b. Web between great and second toe.

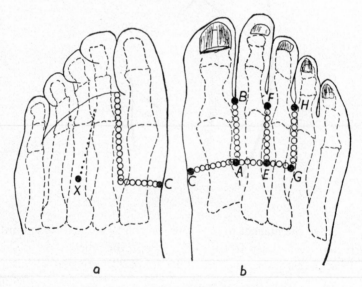

FIG. 149. Landmarks for block of the toes.

2. *Position:* Supine with the sole of the foot in the left hand and dorsum facing upward.
3. *Procedure:*
   a. Raise intradermal wheals at the:
      (1) Dorsomedial border of foot alongside the metatarsal bone (C, Fig. 149).
      (2) Web of the great toe (B, Fig. 149).
      (3) Border of metatarsal of the great toe (A, Fig. 149).

b. Advance an 8 cm. needle attached to a syringe containing 0.5% procaine through the wheal (A) in a direction normal to the skin.

c. Change the direction of needle to an oblique one when the skin has been pierced and inject 0.5% procaine in the interosseous space.

d. Repeat the injection in a fanwise manner along interosseous space (keep the hand beneath the sole to feel the needle as it advances forward).

e. Introduce the needle into wheal over the web (B, Fig. 149) and repeat fanwise injections as above.

f. Introduce the needle through the wheal at the border of the foot and inject in direction beneath the metatarsal and also over it towards the midline of the foot (C, A, Fig. 149).

Comment

1. Do not employ more than 50 cc. of 0.5% procaine to complete the block.

2. Do not add vasoconstrictor drugs to the procaine solution in performing the block (it may cause gangrene).

3. **Do not pierce the sole of the foot with needle at any time.**

REFERENCE

Labat, G. Regional Anesthesia. 2nd Ed. P. 487. W. B. Saunders Co., Philadelphia, 1930.

Block of the Toes

Description: Anesthesia of toes produced by infiltration of the intermetatarsal spaces.

Uses: Amputation and plastic operations of toes.

Technique:

1. *Landmarks:*
   a. Webs adjacent to the selected toe or toes.
   b. Proximal extremities of intermetatarsal space of toe or toes selected.

2. *Position:* Same as for great toe.

3. *Procedure:*
   a. Raise four intradermal wheals, one at each web on either side of the toe (B, F, H, Fig. 149) and one at the extremity of each intertarsal space on either side of the toe (A, E, G, Fig. 149).
   b. Insert the 10 cm. needle through the proximal wheals and perform fanwise injections using 0.5% procaine (same as for great toe).
   c. Incline the needle towards the median sagittal plane of the metatarsal bone and inject 2 or 3 cc. of half per cent procaine on plantar surface of the metatarsal bone (X, Fig. 149). This should be done through both distal wheals.
   d. Repeat injections through the distal wheals in the same manner as the proximal.

Comment

1. Block as many toes as desired, all in the same manner.
2. Inject each interosseous space if more than one toe is blocked.
3. Do not pierce the sole of the foot with the needle. Perform all injections on the dorsum.

REFERENCE

Labat, G. Regional Anesthesia. 2nd Ed. Pp. 485–487. W. B. Saunders Co., Philadelphia, 1930.

FIELD BLOCKS

BLOCK OF SCALP

Definition: Field block of scalp.

Uses: For operations about the head, scalp, or for intra-cranial surgery.

Anatomy: The scalp is innervated by the cervical plexus through the lesser and greater occipital nerves and through the trigeminal by the frontal,

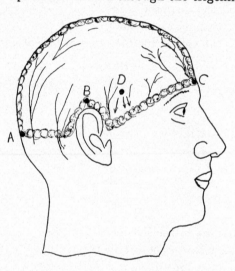

FIG. 150. Landmarks for field block of the scalp.

supratrochlear, supraorbital, auriculotemporal, temporomalar branches.

These nerves pass into the subfascial region at a line which may be described as circling the head above the ear and passing through the glabella and the occiput. Eventually the nerves become subcutaneous at the vertex as they pass through the various layers of the scalp.

Technique:

1. *Landmarks:*
   a. The glabella.
   b. The occiput.

2. *Position:* Place the patient in a sitting or supine position.
3. *Procedure:*
   a. Raise an intradermal wheal at a point over the glabella, and at a point one or two centimeters above the ear. Raise a similar wheal at a point at the occiput (A, B, C, Fig. 150).
   b. Infiltrate intracutaneously, subcutaneously, and subperiosteally through the wheal over the ear and continuing the infiltration in a line to a point anterior to the ear at the level of the meatus (Fig. 150).
   c. Repeat a similar line of infiltration posterior to the ear at the level of the meatus.
   d. Continue the lines of infiltration to the occiput posteriorly and to the glabella anteriorly raising intracutaneous wheals to make a continuous line around the head.
   e. Raise wheals and infiltrate along the midline of the scalp from the glabella to the occiput. Perform the injections in the subcutaneous, intracutaneous, and periosteal layers.
   f At a point anterior to and 3 or 4 cm. above upper border of ear raise a wheal and pass the 8 cm. needle downward toward zygomatic arch into the temporal fossa close to the bone to anesthetize the deep temporal nerves. Deposit 10–25 cc. 1/2% procaine at this site (D, Fig. 150).

Comment

1. Use a fine needle for intracutaneous wheals and 5 or 8 cm. needle for deep injections.
2. Do not use more than 200 cc. of 1/2% procaine for the entire block
3. Use epinephrine to minimize absorption in this highly vascular area

REFERENCE

Mousel, L. H. Anesthesia for Operations About the Head and Neck. Anesthesiology, *2:* 61–73, January, 1941.

LOCAL BLOCK OF PREPUCE

Materials: Standard regional set.
Uses: For operations on foreskin of penis (circumcision).
1. Rinse penis with soap and water, sterilize skin with non-irritating disinfectant and drape field with towels.
2. Raise an intradermal wheal on the dorsum of the penis behind the corona.
3. Establish a line of wheals with 1% procaine behind the corona, to encircle prepuce. Raise each succeeding wheal from the preceding one to make sure the entire procedure is painless (Fig. 151).

4. Retract the foreskin from the corona and raise a line of submucosal wheals in a similar manner as the intradermal wheal.

5. Inject a half cc. of 1% procaine on either side of the frenulum to complete the block. If the block is not satisfactory, it is because this part was not properly injected.

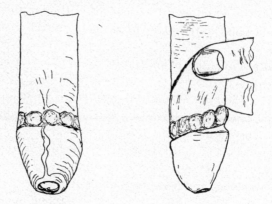

FIG. 151. Landmarks for block of the prepuce.

LOCAL BLOCK OF TONSILS

Uses: To anesthetize peritonsillar tissues for tonsillectomy.

Materials:

1. 1% procaine containing epinephrine 1:10,000.
2. 10% cocaine.
3. One tongue depressor.
4. Light and head mirror.
5. Long curved needle and syringe.
6. Curved grasping forceps.
7. Emesis basin.

Position of Patient: Sitting upright with head cocked backward in a rest.

Landmarks:

1. Upper and lower pole of tonsil (Fig. 152).
2. Border of anterior and posterior pillar.

Procedure:

1. Depress the tongue and paint the fauces with an applicator soaked with 10% cocaine solution squeezed dry.
2. Select three points, one at the upper, one at the middle, and one at the lower border of the anterior pillar and a point at the upper posterior pillar. Inject 1/2 cc. procaine at each one very slowly.
3. Grasp the tonsil with the curved forceps, draw it gently towards the

midline. Inject procaine behind the tonsil to infiltrate its bed and capsule. Use a sufficient quantity to saturate the bed and encircle the tonsil (2 or 3 cc.).

4. Allow several minutes to elapse for establishment of anesthesia.

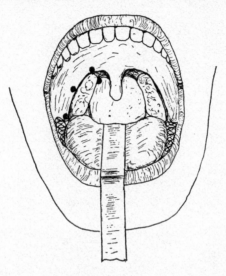

FIG. 152. Block of the tonsil.

REFERENCE

Mousel, L. H. Regional Anesthesia for Operations About the Head and Neck. Anesthesiology, *2:* 61–73, January, 1941.

ABDOMINAL FIELD BLOCK

Definition: Block of ends and branches of thoracic spinal nerves as they pass through the abdominal wall.

Uses: For abdominal operations. Block allows use of median or paramedian incision for either upper or lower abdominal surgery.

Technique:

1. *Landmarks:*
   a. Xyphoid of sternum.
   b. Costal margin.
   c. Lateral border of rectus muscle.
2. *Position:* Place the patient in the supine position.
3. *Procedure* (Fig. 153):
   a. Raise intradermal wheals at the tip of the xyphoid, along the costal margin at 10th costal cartilage and at the lateral border of the rectus at the level of the umbilicus.
   b. Attach a 5 or 8 cm. needle, whichever appears most suitable to the

syringe and commence injection at lowermost wheal by passing needle through the superficial fascia.

c. Incline the needle towards the rectus muscle and pierce the fascia of the muscle. A feeling of break of resistance is noted when the fascia is entered.

d. Advance the needle 0.5 to 1 cm. depending upon whether or not

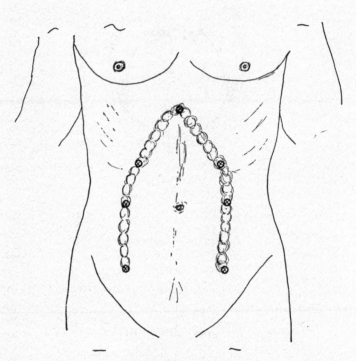

FIG. 153. Abdominal field block.

the patient is lean or obese and inject 2 cc. 0.5% procaine into the area.

e. Withdraw the needle almost to the skin and reintroduce it in a fanwise manner a number of times both in a caudad and a cephalad direction, injecting procaine in a similar amount into the muscle each time (Fig. 153).

f. Withdraw and repeat injections also in a fanwise manner through the remaining wheals along the costal margin.

g. Infiltrate subcutaneous tissues in such a manner that all wheals are connected and make a continuous line from the xyphoid to the last intradermal wheal.

Comment

1. Perform either a unilateral or bilateral block.
2. Prolong the block downward along the entire rectus muscle by raising

other wheals at the lateral border of the rectus below the level of umbilicus as far as the pubis, if lower abdominal surgery is necessary.

FIELD BLOCK OF INGUINAL REGION

Definition: Block of the 11th and 12th thoracic, ilio inguinal, and iliohypogastric nerves as they pass into the inguinal region.

Uses: For inguinal hernioplasty and operations in the inguinal region.

Technique:

1. *Landmarks:*
   a. The anterior superior iliac spine.
   b. The pubic spine.
   c. The inguinal ligament.
   d. The spermatic cord.
   e. The internal and external inguinal rings.
2. *Position:* Supine with operator standing on side to be injected.
3. *Procedure:*
   a. Raise an intradermal wheal 2.5 cms. above and medial to the anterior superior iliac spine (A, Fig. 154).
   b. Introduce a 10 cm. needle (or 8 cm. for thin subjects) connected to 10 cc. syringe filled with 1% procaine and pass through the skin and subcutaneous tissues to transversalis fascia. Inject several cc. of procaine at this site.
   c. Withdraw the needle and perform similar injections in a fanwise manner through the same wheal along a line which extends from the anterior superior iliac spine almost to the umbilicus (A, B, Fig. 154).
   d. Infiltrate subcutaneously along the same line. A total of approximately 50 cc. of solution is required for this part of the block.
   e. Raise an intradermal wheal directly over the pubic spine (C, Fig. 154).
   f. Introduce the 8 cm. needle and inject 8–10 cc. of solution in fanwise direction in the deep tissues along the ramus of the pubis. Inject on each side of the spermatic cord and into edge of the rectus muscle towards the midline (Arrows, Fig. 154).
   g. Infiltrate the subcutaneous tissues along the ramus of the pubis.
   h. Grasp the spermatic cord at the level of the external ring and introduce the needle through the pubic wheal in an upward direction into the cord. Inject 5 cc. 1% procaine at this site.
   i Palpate the internal inguinal ring. Direct the needle with syringe attached through the pubic wheal subcutaneously in a direction medial to the margin of the ring.
   j. Pierce the fascia medially, laterally, and above the ring with a needle and inject 3 cc. each time. This blocks the genitocrural nerve.

k. Raise an intradermal wheal in the skin at the midpoint and immediately below the inguinal ligament and lateral to the femoral artery (D, Fig. 154).

l. Inject 8–10 cc. of 2% procaine into the deep tissues along the upper border of the inguinal ligament in a fanwise manner.

m. Repeat the infiltration into the subcutaneous tissues along inguinal ligament. This blocks the overlapping nerves from the thigh.

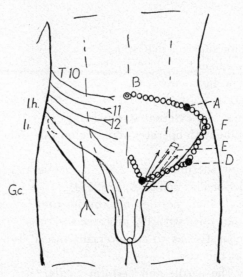

Fig. 154. Inguinal field block. (Ii) Ilio-inguinal nerve. (Ih) Iliohypogastric nerve. (Gc) Genito-crural nerve. Arrows indicate lines of infiltration along the cord E. (See text.)

Comment:

1. Do not inject the internal ring when irreducible hernia is present.
2. Do not cause trauma to the cord by multiple punctures.
3. Avoid piercing the femoral vessels in performing infiltration through the pubic wheal.

REFERENCE

Labat, G. Regional Anesthesia. 2nd Ed. P. 436. W. B. Saunders Co., Philadelphia, 1930.

Field Block of Perineum

Definition: Anesthesia of anterior half of the female perineum by perineal nerve block and infiltration along the vulva.

Uses: For operations on the female perineum

Anatomy: The perineal nerve is the larger and inferior of the two terminal branches of the pudendal nerve. It passes along the lateral wall of the ischio rectal fossa and divides into labial and muscular branches which supply the perineum.

Technique:

1. *Landmarks:* Tuberosity of the ischium (A, Fig. 155).
2. *Position:* Lithotomy.
3. *Procedure:*
   a. Palpate, mark off a point and raise an intradermal wheal over and slightly medial to the tuberosity of the ischium (B, Fig. 155).

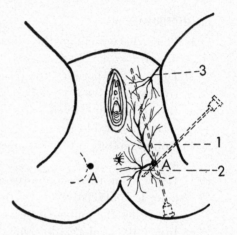

FIG. 155. Field block of the perineum. 1. The skin wheal is raised medial to the ischial tuberosity (A) and the needle is introduced normal to the skin to block the perineal branch of the pudendal (1). 2. Shows the inferior hemorrhoidal branch of the pudendal and the direction of the needle for blocking it. 3. Shows the cutaneous branches of the ilio-inguinal and the direction of the needle for blocking it. All three injections are made through one wheal.

   b. Advance an 8 cm. needle perpendicularly through the skin for a distance of 2.5 cms. and inject 8 cc. of 2% procaine at this site.
   c. Infiltrate both the deep and subcutaneous tissues along the margin of the anterior portion of the vulva. This blocks the ilio inguinal and genito femoral nerve filaments which overlap the perineal nerve in the anterior pubic region (C, Fig. 155).

REFERENCE

Labat, G. Regional Anesthesia. 2nd Ed. Pp. 452–474. W. B. Saunders Co., Philadelphia, 1930.

Pudendal Block (Transvaginal Approach)

I. Landmarks

1. Ischial spines—palpated transvaginally.

II. Position of the Patient

1. Lithotomy

III. Procedure

1. The anesthesiologist is attired with sterile gloves and gown.
2. The right labia is palpated and retracted by the operator's left hand. In the right hand a 10 cc. syringe filled with anesthetic (1% pro-

caine) solution attached to a 20 gauge 8 cm. needle. Tip of needle is held between first and second fingers. Second finger palpates the ischial spine and sacrospinous ligament.

3. Introduce needle point 1 cm. medial to bony tip at ischial spine and 1 cm. below the lower edge of sacrospinous ligament.
4. Perform aspiration and inject 10 cc. of anesthetic solution if no blood appears. If blood appears introduce needle tip slightly inward until no more blood appears.
5. Repeat on left side.

Alternate Route

1. Place the patient in the Sims position with the upper leg sharply flexed.
2. Draw a line between the posterior spine and the tip of the greater trochanter.
3. Bisect this line by a perpendicular similar to technique used for sciatic nerve block.
4. Approximately 6 to 7 cm. downward on the perpendicular line raise a wheal.
5. Insert 8 cm. needle and advance in a slightly outward direction until bone is contacted (bone is the posterior surface of ischial spine on which lies the pudendal nerve).
6. Inject 10 cc. of 1% procaine or solution of equivalent strength.

Comment

1. The spine is missed if the needle is inserted in a perpendicular plane, medially. If introduced at the sacrospinous ligament it is pierced and the needle centers the pelvis.
2. This approach is hazardous for obstetrical use because the needle is too close to infant's head and it may pierce it.
3. Aspirate to identify the pudendal artery and its vein before injecting the solution.

PART VII

SPECIALIZED PROCEDURES

PEDIATRIC ANESTHESIA

The technique of anesthesia for pediatric patients must be modified from that used for adults because of differences in size and physiological development. Some of the factors which make pediatric anesthesia different from adult are as follows:

1. *Nervous System*

   a. Psychic trauma occurs more frequently and is more of a problem.
   b. Effects of analgesic, anesthetic, hypnotic and narcotic drugs upon various centers are more variable.
   c. Convulsions, hyperthermia and other abnormal responses occur more frequently in children.
   d. Temperature control not normal (falls in newborn).

2. *Circulatory System*

   a. The pulse rate is much faster 120–200 first year, 80–150 second year, 70–130 third year.
   b. The blood pressure is more variable, labile and difficult to estimate.
   c. The blood volume is 10% of body weight (same as adult) but blood loss more significant. 0.1 cc. loss = 18 cc. loss in adult, 30 cc. loss = 550 cc. loss in adult.
   d. Cardiac output is greater than in adult. At birth almost 100%.
   e. Sinus arrhythmia may be common and is normal in infants and children.

3. *Respiratory System*

   a. The susceptibility to anoxia and CO_2 excess differs and is probably greater than in the adult.
   b. The respiratory rate is faster, tidal exchange smaller.
   c. Functional residual air volume is smaller in comparison to total lung volume.
   d. Respiratory muscles are not fully developed.
   e. Chest wall is thin and soft and undeveloped.
   f. Air passages are small and easily obstructed.
   g. More lymphoid tissue is present in nasal and oropharynx giving rise to obstruction. Breathing may be entirely through the mouth.
   h. The pressure in the pulmonary artery (newborn) is same as the systemic pressure.

i. Fetal hemoglobin has higher affinity for oxygen than adult.

j. The larynx is placed higher and more anterior and not completely developed.

k. Laryngeal spasm develops more easily and may be quickly followed by cardiac arrest.

l. The pattern of respiration varies considerably. Characterized by gasping, sobbing, inspiratory or expiratory pauses, cog-wheel effect or breath holding.

m. Lungs easily ruptured during positive pressure breathing.

4. *Gastrointestinal System*

a. Secrete saliva easily and obstruct airway.

b. Swallow air causing stomach to dilate and hinder respiratory movements. Use a catheter to deflate.

c. Gastric retention frequent in emergency surgery.

5. *Metabolic Functions*

a. Renal function not fully developed until 6 months of age. Lack concentrating power.

b. Acid base balance fluctuates easily with vomiting, diarrhea or dehydration.

c. Liver function not fully developed.

d. Metabolic rate rises during first year of life to 50 calories per square meter per hour and then gradually declines in later years reaching normal at 15 years.

6. *Skeletal System*

a. Bones not fully developed—easily injured.

b. Soft parts and skin easily traumatized.

7. *Effects of Prematurity*

a. Unable to maintain body temperature at normal limits.

b. Respiratory centers not developed fully. Respiration is irregular—cyanosis may develop periodically. Oxygen restores pattern.

c. Susceptible to infections.

d. Head not calcified and sutures not closed.

e. Response to depressant drugs may be profound.

f. Ventilating surface may not be fully developed and adequate.

UTILITY OF VARIOUS ANESTHETIC DRUGS
FOR PEDIATRIC ANESTHESIA

Drugs: All the drugs ordinarily used for adults may be used for pediatric anesthesia. The following variations are noted in behavior from adults.

A. *Cyclopropane*—behavior is same as in adults.

1. Respiration depressed and apnea results easily.
2. Possibility of overdosage more easily overlooked by novices.
3. Laryngeal spasm may occur, particularly in changing over to ether.
4. An even plane of anesthesia not maintained as easily as in adults.
5. Closed system is necessary and is not always available or practical.

B. *Nitrous Oxide*

1. Resistance to drug varies from child to child. Surgical anesthesia not secured with ease without anoxia.
2. Relaxation poor.
   Uses:
   1. In combination with trichlorethylene or vinyl ether for anesthesia for minor surgical procedures or ethyl ether for major procedures.
   2. In combination with basal narcosis (avertin, or ultra-short-acting barbiturates).

C. *Ethylene*—more potent than nitrous oxide, but used in the same manner and for same purposes.

D. *Ether*—general response is same as in adults with following exceptions. The most widely used and safest of all anesthetic agents for pediatrics.

1. Tachycardia is more frequent due to sympathetic stimulation.
2. Mucous secretion is more prevelant and troublesome.
3. Exaggerated breathing is more pronounced than in adults.
4. Acidosis a greater factor than in adults.

E. *Vinyl Ether*—behavior in general same as adults except that:

1. Convulsions occur more frequently.
2. Secretions may be more abundant and prominent.

F. *Chloroform*—behavior same as in adults. Not used for either adults or children.

G. *Ethyl Chloride*—same objections as for adults—namely it is cardiotoxic.

1. Opisthotonos and muscle spasm common.
2. May cause rapid respiration (vagal effect).

H. *Trichlorethylene*—behavior same for children as for adults.
   Uses:
   1. As an analgesic mixed with air, oxygen or nitrous oxide.
   2. To fortify nitrous oxide in the semi-closed apparatus for minor procedures.

I. *Halothane*—Same advantages and objections as for adults.

J. *Fluoromar*—Same advantages and objections as for adults.

K. *Avertin*—Behavior same as in adults, but response and duration of action more variable:

1. Larger doses required 80–120 mgm./kilo.
2. Readily expelled due to inability to cooperate.
3. More difficult to administer to children. Failures more frequent because of difficulties.

   Uses:

   1. As basal narcotic for *non-painful* diagnostic procedures.
   2. A premedicating agent in unruly subjects followed by ether, cyclopropane, etc.

L. *Ultra-short-acting Barbiturates*

1. Response more variable than in adults.
2. Difficult to administer intravenously because venipuncture not easily performed.
3. Respiratory depression and spasm are vexing and hazardous complications of more serious consequence.

   Uses:

   1. As a basal narcotic for non-painful diagnostic procedures or in conjunction with nitrous oxide, e+her, etc.
   2. To control convulsions.

M. *Muscle Relaxants*—usually not necessary because relaxation is obtained with general anesthesia with ease. Tissues are soft and non-resilient. When used the following objections are noted:

1. Apnea necessitates need for controlled respiration which is undesired.
2. Venipuncture not easily performed.
3. Lethal dose not known—may be given inadvertently.

   Uses: Drug most commonly employed is succinyl choline.

   1. To facilitate intubation.
   2. To relax muscles in large children.

N. *Regional Anesthesia*—children are not psychically suited for regional anesthesia. Only satisfactory in newborns and infants when employed by skillful surgeon and anesthetist.

1. Procaine is the drug of choice because of its low toxicity.
2. Dilute concentrations $\frac{1}{2}\%$ should be employed.
3. Total dose should not exceed 0.1 gram per 15 lbs. of body weight.

Techniques for Pediatric Anesthesia

A. *Open Drop*

Procedure: Same as for adults with following modifications.

1. Use oxygen by nasal catheter under the mask at 1 liter per minute.
2. Do not wrap towels around the mask (Fig. 156).

3. Always use premedication of anticholinergic drug to avoid secretions.

Uses: For ether, vinyl ether, ethyl chloride or chloroform (not advised).

Objections:

1. Oxygen tension in inhaled air not sufficient for adequate oxygenation.
2. Secretions are more prevalent than in adults.
3. Uneven level of anesthesia.
4. Positive pressure and assisted respiration not possible.

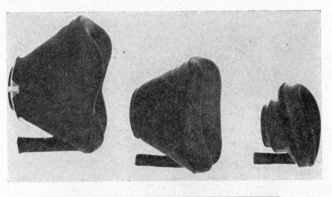

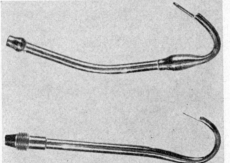

Fig. 156. (A) Infant size mask used for pediatric anesthesia. (B) Ether hooks used for insufflation techniques.

5. Fire hazard exists with flamable agents.
6. Coughing, breathholding and irritation from high concentration of irritating vapors.
7. CO_2 elimination may be inadequate.
8. Cold vapors are inhaled.

Advantages:

1. Simple apparatus.
2. Minimal or no dead space.
3. Permits use of volatile liquids. These are more potent **than** gases.

B. *Insufflation*

Uses: Most often used for ether, but may be used for nitrous oxide, ethylene or cyclopropane.

Procedure: Same as for adults except that Ayre's arrangement intratracheally is most practical, particularly for head and neck or oral surgery (page 196).

1. Anesthetize patient with open drop ether preceded by vinyl ether.
2. Intubate and connect apparatus to insufflator and supply agent in quantity necessary to maintain anesthesia.

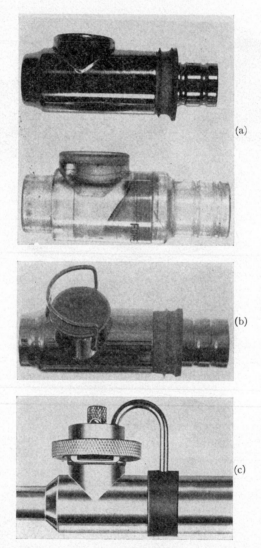

FIG. 157. "Non-rebreathing" valves commonly used for anesthesia for infants and children. (a) Digby Leigh valve (top) and Stephen Slater valve (bottom). (b) Stephen Slater valve with drape guard. (c) Fink valve.

C. *Semi-Closed Method*

Principle: The valves designed by Leigh and modified by Stephen, Slater, Fink and others reduce rebreathing to a minimum. Only the gases contained between the valve and the mask are inhaled. During intratracheal anesthesia the gas in the connector to the valve is inhaled. The minute volume exchange of the patient must be supplied to the apparatus (Fig. 157).

Standard adult type semi-closed inhalers are not suitable because they permit excessive rebreathing.

Procedure (*Leigh valve*):

1. Anesthetize patient with open drop ether and intubate.
2. Connect apparatus to tube (Fig. 158).

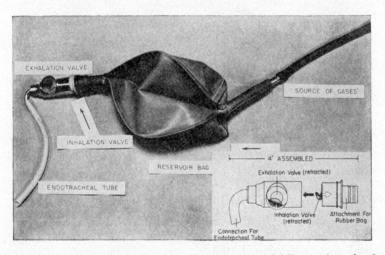

Fig. 158. Non-rebreathing valve assembled to breathing bag and delivery tube and endotracheal catheter. A continuous flow of gases and vapors flow into the inhaler at the minute volume exchange of the patient. Anesthesia is induced by the open mask technique. The patient is intubated and the apparatuses then connected. (Courtesy C. R. Stephen, Elements of Pediatric Anesthesia. Springfield, Thomas, 1954.)

3. Commence flow of nitrous oxide with 20% or more oxygen.
4. Fortify with ether or trichlorethylene or vinyl ether. The gas is bubbled through the liquid.
5. Assist or control respiration by placing thumb over exhalation valve and compressing breathing bag during inspiration and release on expiration.

Advantages:

1. Resistance is minimal.
2. Rebreathing is minimal.
3. Assisted and controlled respiration possible.

Disadvantages:

1. Large volume of gas used
2. Reservoir (bag) deflates readily and gases are lost.
3. Endotracheal tube must be used for successful anesthesia.
4. Positive pressure, controlled respiration and assisted breathing awkward and not easily controlled (require both hands).

Closed Systems

This, as in the case of adults, is the ideal technique if resistance, dead space, and sustained positive pressure can be eliminated.

A. To and Fro (McQuiston) (Fig. 159)

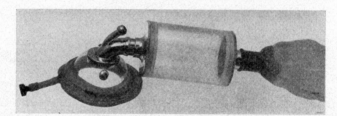

FIG. 159. To and fro absorption unit for anesthesia for infants and children.

Principle: The to and fro inhaler is abbreviated so that the canister is approximately 4×8 cms., the mask is reduced in size and the breathing bag is smaller.

Procedure: Used in exactly same manner as to and fro for adults.

Disadvantages:

1. Dead space excessive. Extends to screen in mask. Tends to extend as canister becomes exhausted.
2. Efficiency of absorber varies as tidal volume varies. Air space in canister must approximate tidal volume for adequate efficiency.
3. Soda lime dust may be inhaled.
4. Excessive warming due to proximity of canister to face.
5. Addition of vapors such as ether not easily controlled.
6. Tight leak proof system difficult to obtain.

Circle Filter

The adult circle filter is unsatisfactory for pediatric use because of the following features.

1. The breathing bag is too large and stiff. Excessive sustained pressure is created in the inhaler. Excursions of bag are too small to be seen or felt by the hand.
2. Dead space in the chimney piece is excessive.

3. Dead space in mask and connectors is often greater than subject's tidal exchange.

4. Valves offer excessive resistance.

5. Total volume of gases in inhaler connectors and tubes excessive—mixing slow

The author's modification of the adult circle filter eliminates these objections. Can be adopted to any standard circle filter (Foregger, Heidbrink, McKesson) (Fig. 160). The apparatus has the following features:

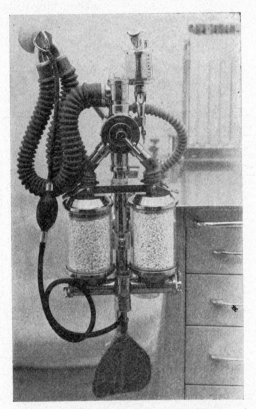

Fig. 160A. Adult anesthetic apparatus modified for use on infants and children. Modification of the Foregger two canister circle filter. The adaptor for the mask has been modified to eliminate all dead space. The bag holder has been modified to accommodate a bag of 500 cc., 1000 cc., or 1500 cc. capacity. The valves are lighter and smaller of the gravity lift type. The bulb interposed between the mask and bag permits flushing the mask and reducing carbon dioxide tension and allows rapid mixing of gases. The canister, ether vaporizer, rubber tubing flow meters are unchanged.

1. Bag holder to accommodate 500 cc. or 1500 cc. thin latex bag.

Bag must be abbreviated and made thin to avoid excessive resistance.

2. Mask holder designed to eliminate dead space completely (Fig. 161).

Dead space in the Y piece is eliminated. Only dead space is in the mask.

3. Light gravity lift valves.

Reduce resistance.

4. Hand bulb interposed between mask holder and bag.

This permits more rapid mixing of gases in mask.

The following remain as they are in the adult machine.

1. Flowmeters

Gases mixed are in same proportion as for adults.

2. Canister.

In circle filter air space in canister may be larger than that of patient without impairing efficiency. Additional soda lime does not increase resistance significantly.

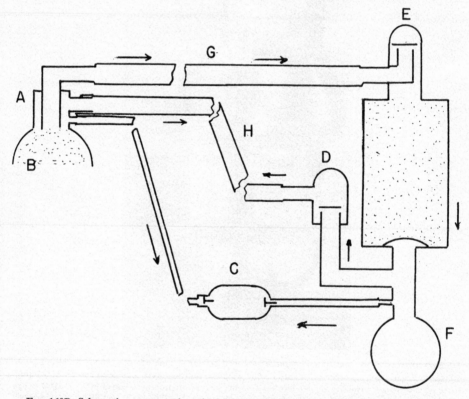

FIG. 160B. Schematic representation of adult circle filter modified for pediatric use. The mask adaptor A is designed to obliterate completely the dead space by conducting one stream of outgoing gases from a tube which is flush with the mouth of the mask. The dead space in the mask (B) cannot be eliminated but is flushed with fresh gases by means of a hand pump C which is interposed between the bag and mask. The valves D and E are abbreviated and are of the gravity lift type. The bag F is made of thin latex and is of 500 cc. capacity. The breathing tubes G & H and Canister I are standard size and not altered.

3. Ether vaporizer.

Dropper or wick type permit addition of ether in desired amount without flooding the apparatus as with bubble type.

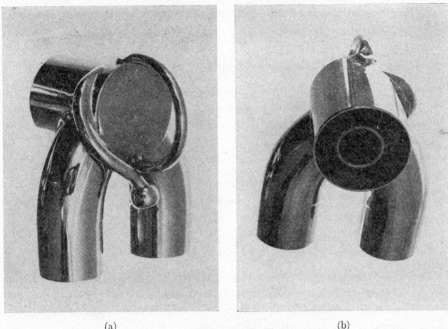

(a)   (b)

Fig. 161. The Y chimney piece has been modified to eliminate all the dead space so that the only gases which are rebreathed are in the mask or connectors to the endotracheal tubes. This is accomplished by having the gases enter the mask through the inner tube and leave in the outer tube. The nipple (a) is used to connect the bypass bulb with the bag.

4. Tubes. — Large size eliminates resistance due to corrugations. Thickness prevents collapse on inspirations and eliminates rebreathing from this source.

5. Exhalation valve. — Permits conversion to a semi-closed inhaler if desired.

6. Size of apperture on chimney piece. — Permits use of standard size masks and intratracheal tube adapters and slip joints.

Advantages:

1. Reduces amount of apparatus required for anesthesia to the interchangeable parts.
2. Permits use of any agent or combination of agents used for adults.
3. Permits use of semi-closed technique without CO_2 accumulation and without supplying volume flow on demand.
4. Permits use of controlled respiration when indicated.
5. Permits rapid induction.

Disadvantages:

1. Tube and chimney piece heavy and awkward.

2. Bag cannot be closed off—gas lost when mask is lifted from face.

3. Awkward for intratracheal use in head and neck surgery.

Use of Modified Adult Circle Filter

Procedure: The basic principles of anesthesia for adults is followed except during induction the hand bulb is used to circulate the gases and ventilate the mask. The absorber is always turned on.

A. *Ethylene or Nitrous Oxide*

1. A flow of nitrous oxide or ethylene 80% oxygen 20% is passed into the inhaler at the minute volume exchange of the subject with the exhalation valve open enough to permit excess to escape.

B. *Ethylene or Nitrous Oxide-Ether Oxygen Sequence*

1. Commence as in (1) above. When patient is in Stage III gradually and slowly add ether using hand pump to facilitate mixing.
2. Gradually reduce flow of nitrous oxide and increase ether as rapidly as possible without coughing or irritation.
3. Reduce oxygen to metabolic flow and close the exhalation valve and shut off ether for several moments.
4. Gradually resume ether again, increase rapidly as tolerated. Use hand pump to circulate gas.

C. *Cyclopropane-Oxygen*

1. Apply mask, and add sufficient oxygen to prevent patients breathing on empty bag.
2. Turn on cyclopropane and oxygen to give a 40%–60% mixture at a rate 200–300 cc. per minute or faster for larger patients.
3. Work hand pump to facilitate rapid mixing.
4. Reduce oxygen to metabolic needs and shut off cyclopropane when bag is filled.
5. Add cyclopropane at 50 to 200 cc. flows at required intervals to meet needs of patient.

D. *Cyclopropane-Ether*

1. Induce anesthesia as in C. When third stage has been attained continue addition of cyclopropane along with ether until patient tolerates ether without aid of cyclopropane.

Comment:

2. Circle filters with abbreviated connectors, bags and valves are avail-

able (Fig. 162) without hand bulb. Principles of use are the same as described above except hand bulb is not used.

Intravenous Anesthesia

The technique is identical to that used for adults. The doses and rate of administration is reduced in proportion. Average for pentothal, surital, evipal is 0.30 gm. per 50 lbs. of body weight.

1. Cannulate vein, if procedure is long.
2. Use small needles for short procedures.

Pentothal Basal Narcosis and Nitrous Oxide

1. Technique same as for adults. Average dose 0.75–1.0 gm. per 50 lbs. of body weight rectally.

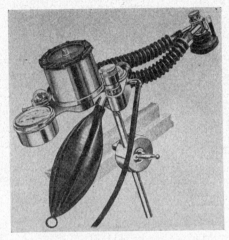

(a)

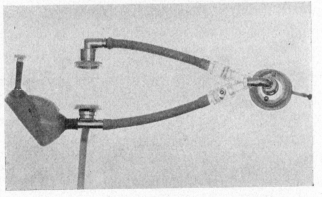

(b)

FIG. 162. (a) Circle filter designed especially for infants and children. The tubing mask, mask holder, valves and canister have been made smaller. Technique and principles underlying its use are similar to those of adult types. (Courtesy Ohio Chemical Company.) (b) Circle filter designed by Leigh for infants and children. (Courtesy Richard Foregger, Ph.D.)

Rectal Anesthesia

Technique is same as described for adults (Part V) with exception of reduction in dosage.

Spinal Anesthesia

Infants and children are not suitable subjects for spinal anesthesia because:
1. They are psychically unsuited for the procedures.
2. The cardiovascular responses are more variable than in adults.
3. Response to physiological alterations more variable and unpredictable.
4. Damage to cord possible because of infancy. It extends further down than in adults.

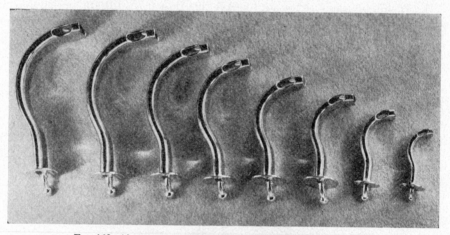

FIG. 163. Airways of various sizes for use for infants and children.
(Courtesy Richard Foregger, Ph.D.)

5. Offers no advantage, as far as relaxation is concerned, to general anesthesia.
6. Extent of anesthesia not easily determined.
7. Status of circulatory system (blood pressure) difficult to follow.
8. Vasopressors not easily administered if hypotension results.

Uses:

1. When general anesthesia is contraindicated in older children.
2. For diagnostic purposes—for autonomic derangements—megacolon.

Procedure: Basic principles and precautions outlined for spinal anesthesia in adults are used with following modifications:

1. Have patient on side or upright to perform block.
2. Premedicate to prevent squirming.
3. Infiltrate skin and interspinous ligament with a local anesthetic.
4. Make puncture below L3.
5. Use shorter needle than used on adults—6–8 cms.—22 or 24 G.

6. Drugs and dosages (average) are as follows:

1 hour or less Procaine 10 mgm. for each year of age in 0.2 cc. 5% dextrose.

2 hours or less Pontocaine 1 mgm. for each year of age in 0.2 cc. 5% dextrose.

3 hours or less Nupercaine 0.75 mgm. for each year of age in 0.2 cc. 5% dextrose.

7. Place in supine position with head flexed sharply by placing folded sheet under neck.

PREPARATION OF PATIENT

Preparations, evaluation, recording etc. are basically the same as for adults.

1. Talk to patient, inspire confidence and avoid instilling fear.
2. Premedicate with an anticholinergic drug, combined with a narcotic or an intramuscular barbiturate or a rectal or intravenous basal narcotic. Use doses in Table VII.
3. Attach stethoscope to chest for continuous auscultation of the heart.
4. Attach blood pressure cuff 2″ wide for infants to right arm or above knee.
5. Restrain patient as soon as consciousness is lost and reflex activity has disappeared.

Premedication

Premedication is administered according to preference of the anesthetist, the status of patient and agent to be used. The following are suggested.

Subcutaneous Route: Narcotics in combination with anticholinergic drugs (Table XVII).

Intravenous Route: Seconal or pentobarbital $\frac{1}{2}$ mgm. per lb. of body weight. Pentothal—fractional doses of $1\frac{1}{2}$–1 cc. at 2–3 minute intervals until narcosis is obtained.

Rectal Route: Avertin—60–80 mgm. per kilo. of body weight (see Part V). Pentothal—1 gm. per 50 lbs. body weight (see Part V Rectal Anesthesia).

COMMENTS AND GENERAL PRINCIPLES ON PEDIATRIC ANESTHESIA

1. Avoid drugs or drug combinations which are spasmogenic—pentothal ether, cyclo-ether. Children are prone to develop severe laryngeal spasm.

2. Have a set of infant size oropharyngeal airways on hand. Oropharynx varies considerably in size from child to child.

3. Do not close mouth tightly when holding mask and supporting Adenoid tissues may prevent free passage of gases through the nose.

TABLE XVII

Age	Weight (lbs.)	Morphine (gr.)	Morphine Dilutions Dose—1 cc.	Scopolamine, Belafoline or Atropine
0– 2 mos.	7–10	1/480	gr. 1/12 in 40 cc. H_2O	1/600
2– 3 mos.	10–12	1/360	gr. 1/12 in 30 cc.	1/600
3– 4 mos.	12–14	1/240	gr. 1/12 in 20 cc.	1/600
4– 7 mos.	14–16	1/144	gr. 1/12 in 12 cc.	1/600
7–11 mos.	16–19	1/120	gr. 1–12 in 10 cc.	1/600
11–18 mos.	19–24	1/108	gr. 1/12 in 9 cc.	1/600
18 mos.–2 yrs.	24–27	1/72	gr. 1/12 in 6 cc.	1/450
2– 3 yrs.	27–30	1/60	gr. 1/12 in 5 cc.	1/450
3– 5 yrs.	30–40	1/48	gr. 1/12 in 4 cc.	1/450
5– 8 yrs.	40–55	1/36	gr. 1/12 in 3 cc.	1/300
8–10 yrs.	55–65	1/24	gr. 1/12 in 2 cc.	1/300
10–12 yrs.	65–80	1/18	gr. 1/12 in 1.5 cc.	1/200
12–14 yrs.	80–90	1/12	gr. 1/12 in 1 cc.	1/150
	over 90	1/8–1/4		1/150

Demerol

12–23 lbs.	5 mgm.		34–45 lbs.	25 mgm.
24–27 lbs.	13 mgm.		45–55 lbs.	37 mgm.
27–30 lbs.	15 mgm.		55–80 lbs.	50 mgm.
30–35 lbs.	18 mgm.		80–90 lbs.	100 mgm.

Seconal

12–15 lbs.	gr. 1/4 to 3/8		30–55 lbs.	gr. 3/4
25–30 lbs.	gr. 3/8 to 1/2		55–90 lbs.	gr. 3/4 to 1 1/2

Nembutal

19–30 lbs.	gr. 1/4		50–80 lbs.	gr. 1
30–50 lbs.	gr. 1/2		80–90 lbs.	gr. 1 1/2

chin, if no airway is in place (Fig. 163).

4. Avoid nasal airways.

Bleeding or obstruction due to adenoid tissue common.

5. Avoid anesthetizing in hot, humid environment.

Hyperpyrexia and convulsions common in summer months.

6. Avoid rebreathing of even the slightest degree.

CO_2 excess may cause convulsions, cardiac arrest, etc.

7. Avoid use of heavy drapes or other objects on chest which inhibit respiratory movements.

Hypoventilation leads to disaster more than any other cause.

8. Measure pressure used to inflate lungs.

Rupture of lungs avoided.

9. Have an assortment of masks for selection and use as small a face piece as possible.

The mask contributes excessive dead space.

10. Take blood pressure on all types of procedures of even the slightest magnitude.

Hypotension occurs as readily in pediatric as in adult cases.

11. Expose chest during induction.	Permits visualization of respiratory movements and detection of obstruction.
12. Do not allow patient to exhale into an overdistended bag.	Continuous positive pressure on airway reduces cardiac output and ultimately leads to circulatory collapse.
13. Administer additional anticholinergic substance if secretions are excessive and persist.	Does not "thicken" secretions as is erroneously claimed.
14. Examine mouth and pharynx for foreign bodies.	Chewing gum, beads, etc. are often concealed by children.
15. Deflate stomach by inserting stomach tube if distended.	Improves respiratory exchange.
16. Do not use "sugar teat" (cotton nipple filled with sugar and soaked with whiskey or brandy) for anesthesia—even during local anesthesia.	Alcohol is not an anesthetic. Secretions form and aspiration occurs frequently.
17. Have all apertures to masks and tubes as wide as possible without being cumbersome.	Obstruction is averted.
18. Watch fluid administration carefully.	Pulmonary edema occurs easily from overloading.
19. Avoid anoxia at all costs.	Asphyxia occurs easily in infants. Anoxia is not tolerated.

PEDIATRIC INTRACHEAL ANESTHESIA

Principle: The differences in position and development and size of the larynx and other parts of the respiratory system in infants and children make intratracheal anesthesia more hazardous and difficult than in the adult. The more pertinent differences are:

1. The infant larynx is placed more cephalad than in the adult.
   a. At birth the lower border of the cricoid cartilage is at the level of the 4th cervical vertebrae.
   b. At the age of 6 it is at the level of the 5th cervical vertebrae.
   c. At the age of 12 it is at the adult level.
2. The epiglottis is longer, stiffer and U shaped.
3. The child's epiglottis is at an angle of 45° with the anterior pharyngeal wall.
4. The infant's hyoid bone is closely attached to the thyroid cartilage.
5. The cricoid ring is the narrowest point of the larynx. In the adult the rima glottidis is the narrowest.
6. The transverse diameter of the trachea is greater than the anteroposterior.

7. The angle between trachea and bronchi is more obtuse (120°) and same on both sides. The angle changes with age.

8. The trachea is short and intubation of a bronchus occurs easily.

9. The nasopharynx contains an abundance of lymphoid tissue and nasal intubation is difficult or impossible.

10. The mouth is small and does not accommodate the laryngoscope unless abbreviated for pediatric use.

11. The trachea moves up and down (tugs) particularly in diaphragmatic breathers.

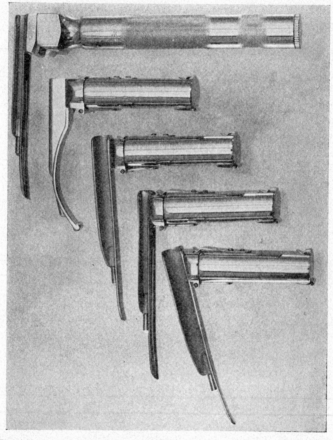

Fig. 164. Laryngoscopes of various designs for use for infants and children.
(Courtesy Richard Foregger, Ph.D.)

Technique: The details, procedures, and materials needed are similar to those employed for endotracheal intubation in adults with modifications to conform to above anatomic and functional differences.

Materials:

1. Infant laryngoscopes with small, medium and large blade of Miller and Mcintosh type (Fig. 164).

2. Intratracheal catheters embodying following features (Fig. 165):

    a. As thin a wall as possible without losing its rigidity.

    b. The length from tip of nose to lobe of ear plus approximately 1/2 cm. for each year of age of subject.

3. Bite block constructed from partly used roll of small size bandage.

4. An assortment of slip joints and connectors to fit the catheters.

5. Non-drying, non-oily local anesthetic lubricant.

6. Support for head—folded sheet or doughnut shaped pillow.

7. A plastic catheter for suctioning to fit into lumen of intratracheal catheter.

8. Sawed off needle of proper size. This should be inserted at one end to connect to the suction tube.

Procedure:

A. *Oral Intubation*

1. Anesthetize patient to point of relaxation with cyclopropane, ether or pentothal—succinyl choline or other agent of choice.

2. Place "doughnut" under the head and extend head.

3. Remove mask and airway as soon as all details are readied.

4. Introduce laryngoscope with left hand, in same manner as described for adults, at right side of mouth and work it over to midline.

5. Pick up the epiglottis, remove secretions if necessary by suction and introduce the endotracheal tube.

6. Introduce the bite block and remove laryngoscope.

7. Connect tube to anesthetic apparatus and anchor.

8. Pack pharynx lightly.

B. *Nasal Intubation*

1. Anesthetize as for oral intubation.

2. Introduce well lubricated Magill tube along into nostril until posterior pharyngeal wall is encountered (an obstruction results due to the adenoids).

3. Hyperextend the head and gently wiggle tube past this obstruction.

4. Expose larynx and pass tube into the trachea, using forceps if necessary.

5. Connect catheter and proceed as above.

Comments

1. Cleanliness is of utmost importance. Sterilize tubes and suction catheters and instruments used for intubation with alcohol or by boiling.

    Laryngeal edema and tracheitis may be caused by unsterile unclean instruments or chemical sterilizing agents.

2. Inspect thorax and auscultate both sides after intubation.

    Labored breathing, lag, absent breath sounds or expiratory

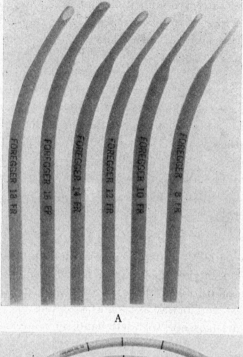

A

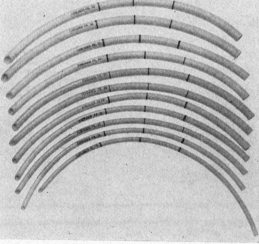

B

FIG. 165. Endotracheal catheters for use for infants and children. A. Cole tubes for infant anesthesia. B. Plastic Magill tubes. C (*at top of facing page*).

3. Inspect teeth before intubation. Note status and missing ones.

4. An oversize catheter may pass the vocal cords, but not into the trachea.

wheeze may indicate catheter is in a bronchus or obstructed.

Deciduous teeth may be dislodged and lost particularly after age of 5 or 6.

The rim of the glottis is larger than the cricothyroid ring in infants.

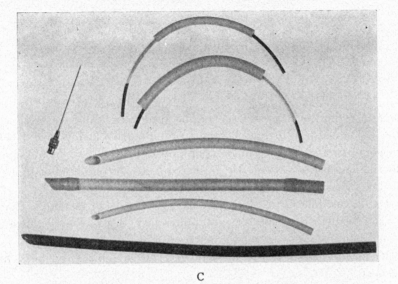

C

Top: Plastic (polyethylene tubing) reinforced with rubber to prevent kinking with stylets. *Center:* Magill rubber catheter and wire woven latex tube. *Bottom:* Plastic dipped catheter.

5. Avoid the use of muscle relaxants.	Not needed. Tissues of infants and children are easily relaxed. Muscles are not fully developed.
6. A catheter large enough for oral use usually passes through the nares.	Undersized nasal catheters are often selected.
7. Have an assortment of tubes of 3 or 4 different lengths for a particular diameter.	Variations in distance from teeth to carina much more frequent than in adults for a given height and weight.
8. Always use connectors of same internal diameter as internal diameter of tube.	Obstruction results if fittings are smaller.
9. Nasal catheter should be longer than oral.	The distance is several centimeters greater for infants and 4–5 cms. greater for adults.
10. Do not attempt to use cuffs.	Trauma, and encroachment upon lumen result.
11. Use as thin walled, pliable and firm a tube as possible.	In a 3 mm. bore tube a 1 mm. wall occludes cross sectional area 33%.
12. Do not make repeated attempts to intubate.	Edema invariably results from trauma.
13. Extubate on expiration.	Spasm occurs less frequently because the vocal cords relax on expiration.

REFERENCES

Leigh, D. and Belton, K. Pediatric Anesthesia. New York, 1949.
Stephen, C. R. Pediatric Anesthesia. Charles C Thomas, Springfield, Ill., 1955.
Adriani, John, and Griggs, T. Rebreathing in Pediatric Anesthesia. Anesthesiology, *14:* 337, 1953.

ANESTHESIA IN AGED (GERIATRIC) PATIENTS

Principle: Technique of anesthesia for the aged is basically the same as for any adult subject to modifications prompted by factors listed below. Selection of anesthesia is made upon physical status rather than chronological age. Factors which are most frequently encountered or should be looked for which are due to sensescence are as follows:

1. Cardiovascular status. Influence of degenerative or metabolic changes (arteriosclerosis, hypertension, pulmonary disease) may cause abnormalities.
2. Respiratory system may be deranged (emphysema, bronchitis, fibrosis etc.).
3. Renal function may be decreased. Power of concentration diminished.
4. Nutrition may be poor. Diseases of digestive system may have interfered with proper assimilation resulting in weight loss, emaciation, anemia, avitaminosis, neuritis, etc.
5. Liver function may be impaired due to fibrosis and other causes; ability to metabolize drugs is impaired.
6. Metabolic rate lower. It gradually decreases from fourth decade on.
7. Metabolic diseases and degenerative diseases such as diabetes, nephritis, etc. may be present.
8. Blood volume may be contracted. Anemia may be present.
9. Mental disturbances, functional and organic may be present.
10. Muscular system altered. Atrophy, tremors, spasticity may be present.
11. Skeletal system may be altered—fixation of joints due to arthritis.
12. May have generalized tissue waste with atrophy of skin, mucous membranes and other structures.
13. May be edentulate.
14. Power of repair and ability to resist infections, shock, trauma diminished.
15. Reflex activity diminished. Cough, laryngeal, pharyngeal, corneal or pupillary reflexes may be decreased in activity.

Principles to Observe:

1. Avoid or use minimal doses of narcotics, hypnotics, basal narcotics for medication or pain relief. Use 1/3 to 1/2 the ordinary adult dose. Suggested dose of morphine for premedication is:

40–60 yrs.	morphine gr. 1/6
60–70 yrs.	morphine gr. 1/8
70–80 yrs.	morphine gr. 1/12
80–90 yrs.	morphine gr. 1/16

2. Correct blood volume, anemia, disturbances in electrolytes, deficiency of serum protein, nitrogen balance, etc. before operation.
3. Digitalize patients who are in cardiac failure or borderline failure.
4. Select agent or combination of agents which permit most rapid recovery, and early ambulation.
5. Avoid agents or methods which cause variations in blood pressure or depress the cardiovascular system.
6. Perform long procedures in two stages if possible.

EVALUATION OF DRUGS AND METHODS

Local and Nerve Blocks

Most desirable choice where feasible.

Advantages:

1. Causes least disturbances in metabolism, respiration or vascular system.
2. Permit early ambulation.

Disadvantages:

1. Cannot be used in all situations.
2. Operation may outlast block.
3. Systemic reactions occur from absorption of excess amounts of drug.
4. Epinephrine used in conjunction with local anesthetic may cause gangrene in extremities.
5. Psychic makeup of patient may preclude its use.

Spinal

Suitable only if the extent is low or if cardiovascular and respiratory systems are adequate.

Advantages:

1. Postoperative somnolence reduced to minimum allowing early ambulation.
2. Nausea and vomiting reduced to minimum.
3. Metabolic disturbances minimal.

Disadvantages:

1. Lumbar puncture may be difficult to perform.
2. Hypotension occurs frequently; may be severe and uncontrollable.

Ether

Avoid wherever possible.

Advantages:

1. Wide margin of safety.
2. Is not cardiotoxic.
3. Does not depress respiration.

Disadvantages:

1. Slow recovery. Ambulation delayed.
2. Nausea, vomiting, dehydration, acidosis are frequent following its use.
3. Disturbs metabolic functions—liver—kidney.

Cyclopropane

Suitable when cardiovascular system is not diseased.

Advantages:

1. Rapid, pleasant induction and recovery.
2. Labile. Yields light or deep anesthesia at will.
3. Permits adequate oxygenation at all times.

Disadvantages:

1. May cause cardiac irregularities.
2. May elevate blood pressure.
3. May cause laryngeal and bronchospasm.
4. Depresses respiration.

Ethylene

Very useful in aged.

Advantages:

1. Characterized by rapid induction and recovery.
2. Disturbs metabolism little or not at all.
3. Nausea minimal.
4. Aged subjects less resistant to the drug. Second and even top third plane anesthesia possible.

Disadvantages:

1. Flammable.
2. May not yield desired relaxation at all times.

Pentothal-Nitrous Oxide and Other Thiobarbiturates

This is one of the few choices when fire hazard exists and general anesthesia is needed.

Advantages:

1. Nitrous oxide permits reduction of total pentothal needed.
2. Nausea and vomiting minimal.

Disadvantages:

1. Prolonged somnolence and depression may occur due to slow detoxification of pentothal.
2. Relaxation not adequate at all times (use succinyl choline).
3. Anoxia a possibility.

Avertin

Avoid. Respiratory depression, hypotension and prolonged somnolence common.

Trichlorethylene

Suitable for analgesia only.

Halothane

Suitable for anesthesia. nonspasmogenic.

REFERENCES

Adriani, John. Selection of Anesthesia. Charles C Thomas, Springfield, Ill., 1955.
Lorhan, P. Geriatric Anesthesia. Charles C Thomas, Springfield, Ill., 1955.

THORACIC SURGERY

Types

Thoracic surgery is of the following types:

1. On the pleura and chest wall—decortications, drainage of empyema, thoracoplasty.
2. On the lung proper—pneumonectomy, partial or complete.
3. In the mediastinum—on the heart, great vessels, thymus or oesophagus.

Problems Encountered

1. Diminished pulmonary reserve from pulmonary or cardiac disease giving rise to:
   a. Cyanosis, anoxia or CO_2 retention.
   b. Orthopnea and dyspnea.
2. Diminished ventilation from lateral position required for operation and from the pneumothorax.
3. Secretions, particularly when suppurative disease is present.
4. Obstruction due to:
   a. Mass in chest compressing trachea or bronchi.
   b. Cord paralysis.
   c. Secretions.

5. Hyperactive reflexes.
   a. Cough.
   b. Tracheobronchial.
   c. Vagal.
6. Circulatory strain due to:
   a. Respiratory difficulty, anoxia, CO_2 excess.
   b. Existing cardiac disease.
   c. Fluid loss and shock.
7. May be long and tedious and accompanied by blood loss.

*Management of Cases for
Pulmonary Surgery*

Comment	*Reason*
1. Delay operation to latter part of morning to institute postural drainage.	Purulent material is evacuated from the lung before arrival in operating room.
2. Intubate all patients especially if suppurative disease exists.	Prevents build up of high intrapulmonary pressure (cough).
3. Bronchoscope patient preoperatively if suppurative disease is present and secretions are excessive.	Provide clear airway.
4. Aspirate frequently during operation if secretions are present.	Secretions may accumulate without causing noisy breathing.
5. Avoid non-volatile drugs particularly narcotics.	Cause depression of respiration which carries over to postoperative period.
6. Use controlled respiration or assisted respiration.	Ventilation with open chest is not adequate unassisted.
7. Premedicate with anticholinergic drug.	Vagal reflexes minimized. Secretions reduced.
8. Use inclined position by breaking table in V shape and tilt head down.	Effects of gravity are utilized for drainage of secretions into trachea.
9. Use endobronchial tube in suppurative diseases.	Isolates one lung from the other.
10. Introduce suction catheter quickly, aspirate once, oxygenate.	Severe anoxia may be instituted by occluding the lumen of the catheter and application of suction.
11. Infiltrate hilum with procaine when respiratory disturbances, bradycardia, cardiac irregularities or "bucking" occurs.	Troublesome vagal reflexes may be blocked.
12. Replace fluid as it is lost.	Avoid overloading the circulation. Pulmonary edema follows.

13. Use supine position as often as possible.	Lateral position undesirable because patient is on healthy lung. Diminished ventilation and contamination result.
14. Periodically (about every 20 minutes) inflate lung.	Oxygenates blood in the collapsed lung.
15. Apply blood pressure cuff to upper arm if patient is on side.	Weight of body occludes vessel partly and sounds are inaudible if the lower arm is used.
16. Pad shoulder and arm in prone or lateral position.	Palsies due to nerve injury from traction and pressure may occur.
17. Cocainize larynx prior to intubation and after.	Abolish cough reflex which is often hyperactive in patient with chronic pulmonary disease.
18. Use cyclopropane as agent of first choice and ether second choice.	Assures quiet operative field. Ether causes exaggerated breathing.
19. Do not permit sustained positive pressure on the airway.	Causes a decrease in cardiac output.

Management of Cardiac Surgery

Comment	Reason
1. Sedate with basal narcotic.	Apprehension causes increase in cardiac activity which is detrimental.
2. Monitor rhythm with electrocardiogram.	Irregularities common when heart is manipulated.
3. Use hypothermia in congenital lesions.	Reduces metabolic activity of patient.
4. Use drugs which do not increase cardiac irritability.	Ether causes least irritability.
5. Control respiration particularly if depression or hypoventilation is present.	Carbon dioxide excess increases cardiac irritability.
6. Be prepared for cardiac massage or to defibrilate heart.	Sudden stoppage or fibrillation readily occurs without warning when heart is manipulated.
7. Have available cardiac drugs— pronestyl, quinidine, procaine, calcium chloride.	May be needed for reducing cardiac irritability.
8. Avoid excessive amounts of antichlorinergic drugs.	Increases pulse rate unduly.
9. Use supine position whenever possible.	Ventilation is more adequate.

10. Limit fluids to blood lost.

Overloading readily occurs resulting in cardiac failure.

11. Block vagus if signs of hyperactivity appear.

Procaine block may be performed directly.

REFERENCES

Adriani, J. Selection of Anesthesia. Charles C Thomas, Springfield, Ill., 1955.

Beecher, H. K. Principles and Practices of Anesthesia for Thoracic Surgery. Charles C Thomas, Springfield, Ill., 1955.

OBSTETRIC ANALGESIA AND ANESTHESIA

Obstetric analgesia and anesthesia differs from other forms of surgical anesthesia, in the following respects.

1. Two physiologically and somatically different individuals are to be considered.
2. The patients are young and vigorous.
3. Patients are unprepared. They may have eaten, or may be exhausted physically from long labor and may be emotionally upset.
4. Toxemia, hypertension, anemia, dehydration and other complications may be present.
5. Labor may be premature in which case the fetus may be adversely affected by drugs and the obstetric procedure.

Analgesic Methods

1. A barbiturate (gr. $1\frac{1}{2}$) meperidine (100 mgm.) and scopolamine (gr. 1/100) in early stages. Thorazine 25 mgm. may be used combined with half the barbiturate or meperidine.
2. a. Analgesia with nitrous oxide with each contraction until full dilatation occurs and the head is in position on perineum (Fig. 161).
   b. Analgesia with trichlorethylene by self-administration or with nitrous oxide.
   c. Analgesia with ethylene.
   d. Continuous caudal block.

Anesthetic Methods for Uncomplicated Cases at Time of Application of Forceps

1. Cyclopropane for all types of vaginal deliveries.
2. Ethylene reinforced by ether.
3. Pentothal or nitrous oxide for short procedures.
4. Saddle block.
5. Caudal block.
6. Pudendal block.

HYPOTHERMIA DURING ANESTHESIA

Definition: The lowering of body temperature during anesthesia to reduce cardiac irritability and the total oxygen consumption. The body temperature is reduced by depressing the thermoregulatory center with a central nervous system depressant and then placing the patient in a cold environment.

Indications:

1. Cardiac or extra-cardiac operations on the great vessels of cyanotic infants and children.

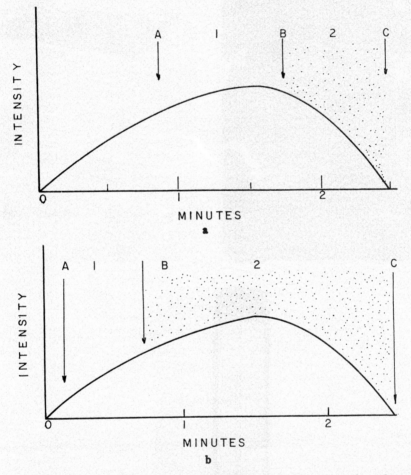

Fig. 166. Nitrous oxide used for analgesia must be administered at the moment the patient senses the onset of an impending contraction, so that analgesia will be established as soon as the peak of the contraction has been attained (A). When the administration is begun while the contraction is in progress analgesia may not be established until the pain begins to recede (B).

2. Operations which require complete interruption of the circulation for brief periods of time—resections of major vessels.
3. Major surgery of any type in debilitated infants and children.
4. To deliberately stop the heart using the heat exchanger and reaching temperatures of 10°C.
5. To reduce fever.

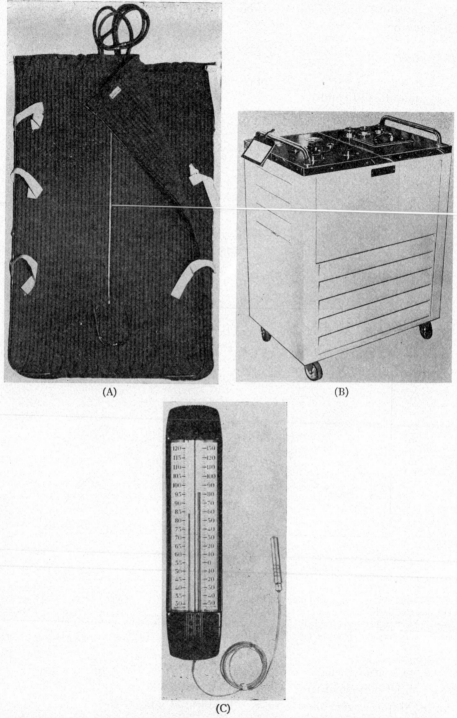

(A)

(B)

(C)

FIG. 167. A. Blanket for inducing hypothermia, composed of multiple coils through which ice water circulates. It may also be used for controlling hyperthermia during and after operation. B. Refrigerating and warming unit (Thermorite) which operates electrically and automatically controls temperature of liquid circulating through the blanket. C. Indoor-outdoor thermometer used for recording rectal temperature. Outdoor portion is inserted into rectum.

6. To reduce brain volume for neurosurgery.
7. To prevent brain damage from anoxia after cardiac arrest.

Methods of Cooling:

1. Placing ice packs around patient on table (very slow).
2. Placing subject in a deep freezing unit and cooling with cold air (frost bite).
3. Immersion in tub of ice water (most rapid).
4. Placing on a specially devised ice blanket through which cold alcohol circulates.
5. Using extracorporeal circulation through coils surrounded by coolant (heat exchanger.) This is complicated and tedious.

Materials:

1. Direct writing electrocardiograph.
2. The usual anesthetic apparatus, endotracheal equipment for closed technique (cuff).
3. Cooling blanket, refrigerating unit, (Thermorite), numerous ice bags or tub for submerging patient (Fig. 167).
4. Ice, unless mechanical coolers are used.
5. Water.
6. At the conclusion of anesthesia, warm water at 42–44° C. or diathermy machine. Not required if Thermorite is used.
7. A thermocouple or recording thermometer equipped with bulbs which can be introduced into the patient's rectum and into the esophagus (Outdoor portion of outdoor-indoor thermometer may be used).
8. Intravenous procaine (.2% in 5% glucose in distilled water) optional. To reduce cardiac irritability.

Technique (Blanket):

1. Premedicate with a narcotic and an anticholinergic drug 1 hour prior to induction of anesthesia.
2. Anesthetize with cyclopropane, pentothal or other desired agent.
3. Intubate with a cuffed tube using a muscle relaxant if necessary to augment anesthesia and set up closed system with carbon dioxide absorption.
4. Cannulate a vein with polyethylene tubing and commence 0.2% procaine (optional) in 5% glucose distilled water at a rate of 30 to 60 drops per minute.
5. Introduce bulb of a thermocouple or thermometer into the patient's rectum and esophagus and set recording mechanism in operation or record temperatures on chart every 5 minutes.
6. Attach electrocardiographic leads to limbs.

7. Place the patient on the cooling blanket and commence the flow of cold water through the blanket (Fig. 168).
8. Cool to 26° C.—Prepare in advance. Allow minimum of one hour for cooling period.
9. Perform operation.
10. Run warm (40° C.) water or warm coolant if Thermorite is used through blanket.

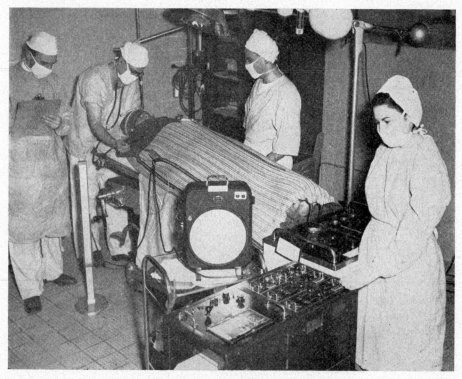

Fig. 168A. Inducing hypothermia in the operating room.

Technique (Tub):

1. Induce anesthesia with desired agent, intubate as described above.
2. Connect rectal thermometers as described above.
3. Immerse patient in tub filled with sufficient ice and water to submerge entire body except the head.
4. Cool to 95° F or 15 minutes whichever is soonest; remove from tub.
5. Place on table and attach electrocardiograph and other monitering devices.
6. Perform operation.
7. Remove to tub containing water at 40° C. and warm to 28° C. quickly. (See page 549)

Technique (Ice Bags):

1. Induce anesthesia and make preparations as above.
2. Place ice bags in axilla, over groin, under back, along thighs and cover body with rubber sheet or blanket.

Signs of Anesthesia and Appearance During Hypothermia

1. The skin has cherry red color where in contact with cold water.
2. Lungs slow to deflate after artificial inflation.
3. Pupils dilated, particularly during ether anesthesia and also during recovery.
4. Planes and stages of anesthesia are nullified as patient is cooled. Use electroencephalogram.
5. Spasticity of muscles may occur. Use relaxant to overcome it.
6. Nerve conduction, reflexes and respiratory activity decreased as 28°C is approached and cease below this temperature.

Complications:

1. Ventricular fibrillation may develop if cooled below 26° C.
2. Frost bite may occur (usually in deep freeze technique).
3. Subcutaneous fat necrosis.
4. Respiratory acidosis.
5. Rewarming shock.

Contra-Indications:

1. The presence of acquired heart disease for non cardiac operations.
2. Surgery of the heart in non-cyanotic infants and children (left sided lesions).
3. For operations not requiring interruption of the circulation.

Comment	*Reason*
1. Monitor the heart rhythm by continuous electrocardiography.	(a) Electrocardiograms show changes, usually prolonged PR and ST intervals.
	(b) Sinus rhythm predominates in temperatures above 23.3 C.
	(c) Ventricular fibrillation occurs easily. Once it occurs it is difficult to reverse.
	(d) Pulse rate is accelerated initially then becomes slower at lower temperatures.
2. Prevent shivering by adding intermittent doses of pentothal or deepening anesthesia.	Shivering may precipitate ventricular fibrillation or exhaustion. Cooling ceases when shivering be-

3. Be prepared to do controlled respiration.

4. Hyperventilate throughout operation.

gins. O_2 consumption markedly increased.

Apnea occurs when body temperature falls below 28°C.

CO_2 excess occurs readily and causes ventricular fibrillation as well as acidosis.

5. Do not have full weight of blanket on thorax.

Water is heavy and respiratory movements may be inhibited.

6. Cool to above 5° (about 60%) of desired temperature. Allow ample time for cooling.

Temperature may continue to drop another 5° after cooling is stopped.

7. 60 to 90 minutes are required for cooling for the blanket technique, several hours with ice bags, 20 minutes with tub.

Use bath tub on wheels for adults or small wash tub for infants or plastic tub which fits on operating table.

8. Use thermometer to test temperature of warming water.

Testing by hand has led to use of too hot water and burns have resulted.

9. Warm by artificial means at conclusion of operation.

Natural warming may require 10 hours.

10. Hyperventilate to raise pH to 7.5 when circulation is occluded.

May prevent accumulation of CO_2 to point of ventricular fibrillation.

11. Discontinue addition of agent below 28°C.

The cold acts as anesthesia, No additional drug is required.

12. Inject 0.25 to 0.5 mgm, prostigmine intravenously when desired temperature is attained 3/5 of maximal cooling.

Prophylaxis for ventricular fibrillation.

13. Warm rapidly at conclusion of operation (use blanket with warm water at 104–110° F or Thermorite unit with warm chemical or diathermy—Virtue's technique).

Audible blood pressure is obtained before wound closure.

14. Allow rectal thermometer to remain in situ several hours after warming.

Rectal temperature may raise above normal. Cool with ice bags or on ice blanket.

15. Monitor heart with electrocardiogram for several hours postoperative.

Cardiac irregularities may develop.

16. Warm if fibrillation develops.

More easily reversed at near normal temperature.

17. Avoid tight fastenings of cuff, E.K.G. leads, etc.

Necrosis develops easily.

18. Be prepared to do a thoracotomy during period of cooling.

Ventricular fibrillation may develop from deep anesthesia and cold.

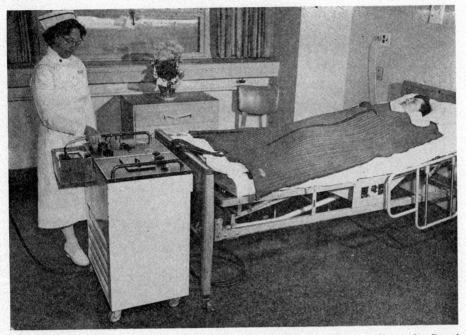

Fig. 168B. Thermorite unit used for rewarming after hypothermia. (Courtesy Thermorite Corp.)

19. Avoid arm or nerve traction.	Injury and necrosis may result.
20. Replace blood as needed.	Blood volume must be maintained at adequate levels.

REWARMING AFTER HYPOTHERMIA

Methods

a. By running warm water (104°F) through blanket.
b. By immersing in warm water in tub.
c. By use of diathermy coils (method of Virtue).
d. By use of mechanical cooler-warmer (Thermorite). (Fig. 168B)

Procedure Using
Diathermy:

1. Wrap 1″ felt around abdomen and hips.
2. Wrap coils around felt.
3. Allow patient and wrappings to rest on wood strip, the ends of which are supported 2″ above operating table.
4. Support legs and upper part of body with short mattresses.
5. Use diathermy at 2 minutes on and 1 minute off.

Comment	*Reason*
1. Do not allow body to rest on coils.	Burns may result.
2. Watch circulatory system as 32° is approached.	Pallor, circulatory collapse may develop.

3. Use 50% nitrous oxide if patient is restless during warming.

Awakening and reflex activity reappear at 34°. May be unruly.

4. Consciousness returns at 32° (lower rectal temperature) with surface warming.

Heat is applied to entire surface of body. With diathermy it is localized.

5. Do not rely upon packs and hot water bags for rewarming.

This method is not efficient.

6. Always measure temperature of warm water with thermometer.

Burns may result if this is not done.

REFERENCE

Virtue, Robert. Hypothermia. Charles C Thomas, Springfield, Ill., 1955.

REFRIGERATION ANESTHESIA

Definition: Anesthesia obtained by the application of ice or iced water to tissues until insensibility to pain is obtained.

Uses:

1. For producing insensibility for amputation of limbs, for gangrene, devitalization of tissues, etc.
2. To arrest hemorrhage, relieve pain, or to minimize devitalization of tissue in extremities in crushing injuries. Metabolism of the cells is decreased.

Materials:

1. Cracked ice (1″ to 2″ pieces).
2. One large pail of several gallons capacity.
3. Rubber sheet approximately 3′×4′.
4. One medium sized pillow.
5. Tourniquet composed of gum rubber tubing half inch in diameter.
6. Large clamp or sponge holder for tourniquet.
7. Six ice bags.
8. Roll of bandage (2″ wide).

Premedication: Morphine and scopolamine one hour prior to the operation.

Procedure:

1. Place the rubber sheet under the extremity so that it may be wrapped completely about it to form a gutter and so that the roll projects 8″ to 10″ over the end of the bed over the bucket.
2. Elevate the extremity upon the pillow to allow blood to drain from the vessels.
3. Surround the region of the' proposed site of the tourniquet with ice bags for half an hour to minimize pain.
4. Apply one turn of the tourniquet about the extremity. This first wrapping should occlude the circulation.

5. Apply a second wrapping over first and fasten the ends securely with the clamp to prevent slipping.
6. Place a layer of ice upon the sheet and place extremity upon this layer of ice.
7. Surround the entire extremity with ice beginning one or two inches proximal (above) to the tourniquet and extending to the end of the limb.

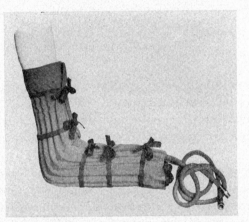

FIG. 168C. Leg wrapper for use with Thermorite unit to cool extremities for refrigeration anesthesia. (Courtesy Thermorite Corp.)

8. Encircle the rubber sheet about the extremity and secure it with several turns of bandage.
9. Allow the end of the roll of the rubber sheet to project over the edge of the bed so that the water from the melting ice drips into the bucket.
10. Allow the limb to cool as follows:
    Foot—1 hour   Upper third of leg—2 hours
    Lower leg—1 1/2 hours   Midthigh—2 1/2 hours
11. Remove the patient to the operating room, place on the table, unwrap the extremity as soon as all preparations for surgery are made and the surgical team is ready.
12. Dry the extremity without rubbing, drape and prepare quickly in the desired manner (leave tourniquet in place).
13. Arrange to follow blood pressure and pulse, etc., as for other types of anesthesia.

Alternate Method: Use Thermorite unit with special wrapper for extremities. (Fig. 168C).

Duration of Anesthesia: Approximately 30 minutes.

Advantages:
1. No inhalation or other type of anesthesia by drugs is necessary.
2. Shock during surgery is minimal.

3. Lowered temperature reduces oxygen and other metabolic requirements of the extremity.
4. Low temperature reduces metabolism of cells.
5. May be used postoperatively to reduce pain.

Disadvantages:

1. Period of insensitivity to pain may not outlast operation.
2. Cumbersome in its execution.
3. Reduced temperature interferes with healing (postoperative use).

Contra-Indications: None.

Comments

1. Do not remove tourniquet until all blood vessels are tied and apparently satisfactory hemostasis is obtained.
2. Observe blood pressure, pulse, and respiration closely during surgery.
3. Administer a barbiturate or other sedative prior to initiation of cooling process.
4. Use sufficient ice and keep limb well covered to insure success.
5. Use cold solutions for irrigations, sponges, etc., during the operation. This prevents extremity from becoming warm too quickly.
6. Always use a tourniquet. It prevents chilling of the remainder of the body but allows thorough chilling of limb.
7. Employ a pure elastic narrow tubing for tourniquets.

REFERENCE

Allen, F. M., Crossman, L. W., et al. Refrigeration Anesthesia. Anesth. & Analg., *21:* 241, October, 1942.

INTENTIONAL HYPOTENSION (HYPOTENSIVE ANESTHESIA)

Description: The deliberate lowering of blood pressure during anesthesia to reduce blood loss in procedures in which excessive bleeding or acute hemorrhage is anticipated.

Rationale: Subjects whose autonomic nervous system is denervated withstand periods of hypotension due to hemorrhage for longer periods of time that those whose vasomotor systems are intact.

Methods of Induction:

1. By use of central depressants (narcotics, basal hypnotics and hypotensive agents) which depress the medullary centers.
2. By use of high spinal block by inducing spinal anesthesia with a dilute solution of procaine.
3. By use of ganglionic blocking agents (hexamethonium, arfonad or pendiomide).
4. By use of sympatholytic agents (priscol, regetine, thorazine).
5. By use of smooth muscle depressants (nitrites).

6. By reducing blood volume by use of arteriotomy (does not denervate blood vessels).

Situations in Which it is of Value:

1. Resection of malignant or highly vascular neoplasms about head, face, neck, pelvis or other areas.
2. Resection of highly vascular intracranial tumors or aneurysms.
3. Resections of major vessels, fenestration operations, or other operations in which hemorrhage nullifies results.
4. Pelvic eviscerectomies and other radical resections for carcinoma which are accompanied by bleeding.
5. Hemisection of the kidney for removal of calculi, neoplasms, etc.
6. Unavailability of rare types of blood or inability to match incompatable subjects for transfusion.

Present Technique Using Ganglionic Blocking Agents:

A. *Arfonad*

1. Anesthetize patient with desired anesthetic such as pentothal-nitrous oxide or cyclopropane. Intubate using topical anesthesia and succinyl choline if desired.
2. Canulate a vein to be prepared for infusion and transfusion.
3. At approximately 10 minutes before anticipated time for need for the hypotension commence drip of drug (arfonad 0.1% solution in 5% dextrose—1 mgm. per cc.) and quickly reduce blood pressure to 80 or less; 75–150 mgm. may be required.
4. Maintain infusion at a rate to keep blood pressure at hypotensive level 1–1.5 mgm. per min. Dose varies for each patient.
5. Tilt head down or feet down to raise or lower blood pressure as required.

B. *Hexamethonium*

Same technique as above except 20–25 mgm. of drug are given into infusion tubing in single injection. Dose varies from 5–35 or 40 mgm. May have to be repeated several times before effective blockade occurs.

Advantages of Arfonad over Hexamethonium:

1. Arfonad is more rapid acting and its action is of shorter duration and therefore permits greater control.

Technique Using Spinal Anesthesia (see Spinal Anesthesia Section for details):

1. Induce spinal anesthesia using 150–200 mgm. procaine and steep Trendelenburg position to have level above T4.
2. Use continuous spinal technique.

Advantages of Ganglionic Blockade over Other Methods:

1. Greater degree of controllability.
2. Sensitivity to epinephrine and vasoconstriction remains.
3. May be interrupted or reversed with greater ease.
4. Vasoconstrictor effects are absent.

Comment	*Reason*
1. Elevate blood pressure by tilting head down during blockade.	Autonomic denervation inhibits centers for vasomotor control and the blood shifts to dependent areas.
2. Replace blood as lost to avoid irreversible shock.	Sympathectomized subjects do not stand severe blood loss.
3. Lower blood pressure below 80, but not below 60 mm. systolic.	Renal and cerebral damage result from impaired blood flow if below 60. Bleeding not overcome if above 80.
4. Do not allow hypotension to persist for more than one hour.	Cerebral damage or anuria may result.
5. Lighten anesthesia during period of hypotension.	The amount of agent necessary to maintain anesthesia is reduced during period of decreased pressure.
6. Watch body temperature.	May fall during hypotension. Vasodilatation causes heat loss and heat regulating center is depressed also.
7. Reduce blood pressure quickly and maintain it at desired level. Do not permit it to rise.	Tachyphylaxis develops after repeated administration in some subjects and patient becomes refractory to drug.
8. Watch patient closely until blockade has worn off.	Blood pressure may continue to fall after procedure is completed.
9. Use vasopressors cautiously.	Patients may be more sensitive to these drugs while blockade is in progress.
10. Keep head as much as possible at level of or below level of heart.	In the head-up position the blood pressure in the head is lower than in the rest of the body because the blood shifts to dependent portion due to vascular atony.
11. Use electroencephalogram if available.	Cortical potential becomes flat when cerebral perfusion is inadequate.

Complications:

1. Reactionary hemorrhage due to inadequate hemostasis.
2. Prolonged depression in postoperative period.
3. Thrombosis of cerebral and coronary arteries.
4. Oliguria or anuria postoperatively.
5. Cerebral damage due to impaired nutrition of cells.
6. Unexplained cardiac arrest.

Contra-Indications:

1. Arteriosclerosis with well defined changes in most vessels.
2. Essential hypotension and hypotension due to other causes.
3. Impaired renal function.
4. Anemias of all types (uncorrected).
5 Heart disease, particularly advanced coronary artery disease.
6. Liver dysfunction.

REFERENCES

Hale, D. E. Controlled Hypotension. Anesthesiology, *16:* 1, 1955.
Little D. Hypotensive Anesthesia. Charles C Thomas, Springfield, Ill., 1956.

"CONTROLLED" RESPIRATION

Definition: The continuance of pulmonary ventilation by artificial methods during a deliberately induced apnea produced by inhibiting the stimulus to respiration.

Uses:

1. To provide an intermittently motionless field in thoracic and abdominal surgery.
2. To provide adequate saturation of tissues with gaseous and volatile anesthetic drugs in the face of respiratory depression.

Principle: The apnea in controlled respiration is the result of one or a combination of these four factors:

1. The removal of enough carbon dioxide from the alveoli and blood by hyperventilation so that the normal stimulus no longer exists.
2. A decrease in sensitivity of the respiratory center by depressant drugs so that its threshold to carbon dioxide is raised.
3. Stimulation of the Hering-Breuer reflex by overdistension of the alveoli so that the inspiration is inhibited.
4 The patient may be completely paralyzed by use of a muscle relaxant.

Procedure:

1. Anesthetize the patient with cyclopropane or ether by the carbon dioxide absorption technique and attain the desired depth of anesthe-

sia. The patient should be heavily premedicated if no relaxants are to be used.

2. Intubate patient and secure an entirely leakproof system (use either the open or closed intra-tracheal techniques).

3. Augment the volume of respiration by compressing the breathing bag during inspiration. Inspiration should be rapid and not occupy more than one third of the cycle (Fig. 168D).

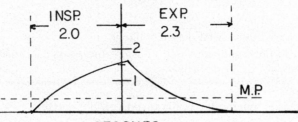

FIG. 168D. Cournand Type III curve. The pressure falls to ambient pressure during expiration. Expiration is of sufficient duration to permit least disturbance in cardiac output.

4. Allow the lungs to empty quickly by releasing bag promptly during expiration. Expiration and the interrespiratory pause occupies two thirds of the cycle.

5. Omit pressure after eight or ten inspirations, and note if voluntary respiratory movement occurs when inflation is halted

6. Continue ventilation by manual pressure on the bag at the rate and volume of exchange comparable to rate during normal sleep. Add anesthetic agent and oxygen as required.

7. Judge depth of anesthesia by observing the reflexes in the eyes and muscle tone or by using the electroencephalograph.

Comment

1. Observe circulation closely throughout the entire period of artificial ventilation.

2. **Always establish an absolutely clear airway. An endotracheal airway is desirable but not imperative for short periods. It is mandatory for long periods.**

3. Do not attempt controlled respiration during the period when the tracheal reflex is active.

4. Secure a leakproof system for optimum results.

Reasons

The circulation is impaired by the positive pressure which decreases the venous return to the heart and reduces cardiac output.

The stomach is often inflated when pharyngeal airways are employed.

Lungs are difficult to inflate during active coughing stage and a high degree of positive pressure is established in the inhaler.

Loss of anesthestic mixture results in uneven depth of anesthesia.

5. Do not exceed a pressure of 20 cms. of water to inflate lungs. Use a manometer.

Excessive pressure may be dangerous and cause trauma to the alveoli.

6. Use muscle relaxant if voluntary respiratory efforts cannot be abolished.

Inflation of lung is easier if patient does not oppose it.

REFERENCES

Guedel, A. E., and Treweek, O. N. Ether Apneas. Anesth. & Analg., 7: 238, 1928.

Waters, R. M. Absorption of Carbon Dioxide from Anesthetic Atmospheres. Proc. Roy. Soc. Med., 34: 11, 1936.

CONTROLLED RESPIRATION USING THE MECHANICAL (JEFFERSON) RESPIRATOR

Description: Various insufflators are available for artificially respiring patients with mixtures of anesthetic gases or vapors and oxygen. The Jefferson ventilator (Fig. 169) inflates the lungs with a stream of gases under positive pressure. Varying degrees of negative pressure may be applied on expiration. The gases circulate through the circle filter in the same manner that the patient circulates them using voluntary breathing. The apparatus is used as follows:

1. Induce apnea by hyperventilation or by use of muscle relaxant.
2. Remove rebreathing bag from anesthetic apparatus and attach flexible hose from ventilator.
3. Attach rebreathing bag from anesthesia apparatus to vertical leg of T-valve.
4. Turn T-valve to manual position.
5. Turn negative and positive pressure controls counterclockwise to their limit.
6. Connect pressure hose to any standard oxygen flowmeter or regulator. Set flow high enough to maintain 12 pounds pressure on gauge just below timer.
7. *Partially* inflate rebreathing bag in glass control by turning T-valve to automatic, and adding oxygen to respiratory circuit.
8. Make desired control settings (see below), then turn T-valve to automatic position.

SETTINGS FOR CONTROLS

Phase

Equal duration of inflation (positive pressure) phase and deflation (negative pressure) phase appear to be satisfactory with both open and closed thorax.

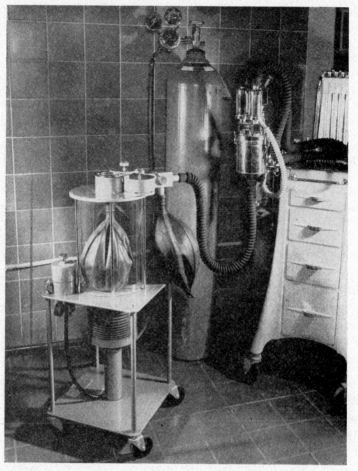

FIG. 169. Automatic "breathing machine" for controlled respiration (Jefferson). The apparatus utilizes compressed air as source of energy. Positive pressure is made by raising the pressure on the exterior of the bag. Negative pressure may also be applied during expiration. A lever permits instant shift from mechanical to manual controlled respiration or normal breathing. (Courtesy Air-Shields Company.)

Pressure

Open Thorax: 15 cm. H_2O positive and 5 cm. H_2O negative with equal phasing.

Closed Thorax: 10 cm. H_2O positive and 10 cm. H_2O negative with equal phasing.

Rate

Respiratory rates in the order of 18 to 20 per minute appear to provide adequate ventilation for most patients.

Disadvantages of Mechanical Methods of Controlled Respiration

1. Depth of anesthesia not easily estimated during artificial ventilation.
2. Volume of gas delivered not known with most devices.

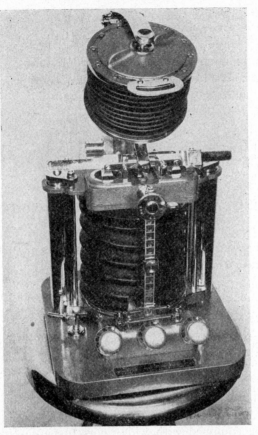

Fig. 169a. The Stephenson mechanical ventilator (designed by Goodner) utilizes a bellows to assure delivery of a fixed volume of gas for controlled respiration. The desired tidal volume can be set by adjusting the sliding vertical scale. The apparatus is connected by means of a corrugated tube to a standard anesthetic apparatus of either the circle or to and fro design in place of the breathing bag. The mechanism operates by compressed gas or oxygen. Respiratory rate, duration of inspiration, duration of expiration and length of inter-respiratory pause are adjusted by means of dials at the base. The sliding weights on the beams are adjusted to deliver the desired positive pressure and the pressure necessary to overcome any resistance in the airway or apparatus. Varying degrees of negative pressure during the expiratory phase of respiration may be applied by adjusting the sliding weight along the beam on the right. An auxiliary (safety) bellow is provided at the top to act as the breathing bag before the mechanism commences to operate or when obstruction or mechanical failure causes interference with delivery of the set volume of gas.

3. Machines may continue to appear to operate if obstruction occurs and lungs are not being inflated.

4. Effects on circulation difficult to predict; usually adverse particularly if pressure does not return to zero or subatmospheric on expiration.

Comment

1. To clean or replace internal rebreathing bag, lift entire gauge and T-valve assembly straight up.

2. Flowmeter settings of 12–14 liters per minute are required to maintain proper operating pressure. However actual consumption is 6–8 l.p.m.

3. Use compressed air instead of oxygen as a source of pressure to operate

machine if desired.

4. Change soda lime canister frequently because of the greater ventilation provided.

5. Switch to "manual" when aspirating the trachea, or when a bronchus is open to avoid loss of anesthesia gases. Do not turn off ventilator when on "manual." It continues to operate.

6. Make suitable adjustment of pressure settings to insure maintenance of safe and effective mean lung pressure if relative duration of inflation phase is changed from two to one.

7. *Always* keep rebreathing bag inside control *partially* inflated.

POSTANESTHETIC RECOVERY ROOM

Definition: The postanesthetic recovery room is a special room for observing and attending patients recovering from anesthesia. It should possess the following features.

A. 1. Should be on the same floor as and close to operating room.

2. Should be properly warmed (winter) and air conditioned (summer) and free from drafts.

3. Should be a well lighted single open square or oblong space so that patients can be seen from any part of room.

4. Should lead into a corridor not traversed by visitors and non-medical personnel. Corridor should be wide enough to permit turning of a bed or roller.

5. Should be equipped with wide doors to permit passage of rollers, portable x-ray equipment, oxygen tents, etc.

6. Should be large enough to accommodate desired number of rollers or special recovery room beds so that they are at least 3 feet apart.

7. Should have outlets for piped oxygen, double electric plugs and wall suction at each bed or roller station.

8. Should have terrazzo asphalt tile or other easily cleaned floor (need not be conductive).

9. Should be adjacent to laboratory for doing urine, blood counts and hematocrit.

10. Should have ample closet, storage and cabinet space for supplies.

B. *Beds*

Recovery room beds or rollers (Fig. 169b) should be sturdily constructed preferably of stainless steel and have the following features:

1. Wide enough to permit patient to be rolled on side with comfort and safety.

2. Large casters equipped with conductive rubber type or grounded by chains.

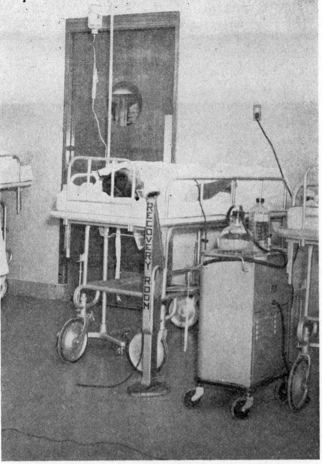

FIG. 169b. Recovery room combination roller and bed.

3. At least 3 feet from floor—to permit easy care and removal from operating table and to ward bed.
4. Tiltable at head and foot end to permit head down or head up position.
5. Locking mechanism for wheels.
6. Side boards and head and foot ends which are removable for bronchoscopy, venipuncture and other treatment, etc.
7. Infusion stand placeable at foot, head or side of bed.
8. Arm board which can be placed at either side.
9. Straps for restraining and anchors for them on bed.
10. Shelf beneath for placing suction bottles and other equipment.
11. Hooks for hanging suction bottles, catheter draining bottles, etc.
12. Comfortable washable rubber covered matress pad.

C. *Materials—Resuscitative for Ventilation*

1. Tracheotomy set.

2. Suction apparatus for aspiration of respiratory tract (catheter and tonsil suction).
3. Set of airways, oral and nasal.
4. Set of endotracheal catheters (plastic).
5. Laryngoscopes with assortment of blades.
6. Aspirating bronchoscope (Davis).
7. Mechanical insufflator for resuscitation—Stanton, Kriselman; AMBU, to and fro etc.
8. Pneumothorax set and water trap.
9. Availability of Iron Lung (for respiratory paralysis—head injury, brain injury etc.).

D. *Materials—Resuscitative for Circulation*
1. Cardiac arrest set (scalpel, rib spreader, hemostats) sterile and ready to use.
2. Defibrillator and pacemaker.
3. Arterial transfusion set.
4. Ordinary transfusion sets.
5. Sternal puncture needle for infusion into bone marrow.
6. Blood pressure apparatus (cuff and stethoscope).
7. Phlebotomy set.

E. *Oxygen Therapy Unit*
1. Tent (adult), O.E.M. mask and catheter equipment.
2. Tent (infant), Croupette or similar type with nebulizer for water.
3. Bennet, Bird or other positive pressure device for treating pulmonary edema.
4. Coughlator or similar exsufflator.
5. Carbon dioxide, 5% oxygen with semi-closed mask and flow meter.
6. Nebulizers for aerosol therapy.

F. *Surgical Supplies*
1. Syringes and needles of various sizes for medications and aspiration.
2. Emesis basins.
3. Gastric tubes.
4. Rectal tubes and suction.
5. Urinary catheterization set.
6. Ice bags.
7. Hot water bags.
8. Ice cooling mattress for hyperthermic patients
9. Thermometers—oral-rectal.
10. Bed pans.
11. Urinals.
12. Ice box for storage of perishable drugs, blood, etc.
13. Goose neck lamps for bedside therapy (venipuncture, etc.).

G. *Drugs*

    a. Respiratory—stimulants
        1. Nallorphine
        2. Metrazole
        3. Picrotoxin
        4. Coramine
        5. Bemegrid (Megimide)
    b. Narcotics—for pain
        1. Morphine
        2. Demerol
        3. Dilaudid
        4. Nisentil
        5. Methadon and other synthetic narcotics the physicians desire.
    c. Barbiturates
        1. Pentobarbital or Secobarbital for injection (drug reaction).
        2. Phenobarbital
        3. Pentothal or other ultra short-acting barbiturates.
    d. Anti-curare Drugs
        1. Edrophonium (Tensilon)
        2. Prostigmine
    e. Anti-cholinergic Drugs
        1. Atropine
        2. Hyoscyamine
        3. Scopolamine
    f. Cardiac Drugs
        1. Pronestyl
        2. Quinidine
        3. Aminophylline
        4. Procaine—5 cc. ampules (20%) for I.V. use
        5. Digitalis preparations
    g. Antihistaminic Drugs
        1. Benadryl
        2. Chlortrimeton
        3. Pyribenzamine
    h. Vasopressor Drugs
        1. Arfonad
        2. Hexamethonium
    i. Anti-nausea Drugs
        1. Marezine
        2. Dramamine, Tigan
        3. Thorazine
    j. Fluids
        1. Blood

    2. Plasma or plasmanate
    3. Serum albumin
    4. Fibrinogen
    5. Dextran
    6. Normal saline
  k. Antibiotics and Chemotherapeutic Agents
    1. Streptomycin
    2. Penicillin
    3. Tetracycline
    4. Sulfa drugs

H. *Personnel*

1. Graduate nurses trained in management of airways, intravenous therapy, inhalation therapy and surgical nursing should be in attendance constantly (one nurse per 2 or 3 patients).
2. Resident physician anesthetist or staff anesthesiologist should make rounds at frequent intervals and be available on call.
3. Surgical residents available for surgical complications.
4. Orderlies, maids and ward aids.

I. *Duties of Recovery Room Personnel*

1. Maintain adequate airway.
2. Watch respiration of patient—color, rate, depth.
3. Restrain to prevent injury.
4. Administer drugs required for sedation and supportive therapy.
5. Watch circulatory system—pulse, blood pressure, etc.
6. Prevent aspiration and pulmonary complications.
7. Watch for bleeding.
8. Watch fluid intake and output.
9. General nursing care—catheterizing, changing gowns, administration of narcotics and other drugs.
10. Initiate or continue specialized therapy once it has been instituted by physician or technician.

J. *Hours of Operation of Recovery Room*

1. Varies with size of hospital.
    Large institution—24 hours 7 days a week.
    Small—day time operation only. Closed nights and holidays.

K. *Supervision*

The recovery room may be supervised in a number of ways. Method depends upon local situation.

1. Anesthesiologist only.

2. Jointly by anesthesiologist and surgeon.

3. By nursing service with assistance and advice of anesthesiologists and surgeon.

L. *Duration of Stay of Patients in Recovery*

1. Remain until all reflexes have returned and patient is rational and no artificial airway is needed.

2. Remain until blood pressure has stabilized and possibility of shock is over.

3. Remain until vomiting and nausea are over.

4. Remain until possibility that movement and shifting will cause no circulatory depression.

M. *Records*

The following data should be recorded on a special recovery room chart or on the patient's regular chart.

1. Time of arrival and discharge and condition upon arrival and discharge.

2. Name of physicians visiting and treatments performed by them.

3. Blood pressure, pulse, temperature, respiration, color, etc.

4. Fluids and medication given from time of arrival.

5. Therapy instituted and time of administration.

6. Laboratory tests done or ordered.

7. Time of recovery from anesthesia.

8. Unusual episodes, and method of treatment.

N. *Prevention of Pulmonary Complications*

1. Turn patient from side to side frequently.

2. Use narcotics sparingly.

3. Encourage patient to breathe deeply.

4. Induce coughing by endotracheal suction or aspirate in comatose patients.

5. Ambulate as soon as possible.

O. *Maintaining Airway*

1. Hold chin (Fig. 75).

2. Turn patient on side.

3. Aspirate saliva.

4. Use airway if reflexes have not returned.

5. Administer anticholinergic drug if secretions are excessive.

6. Perform tracheotomy if supralaryngeal obstruction is present.

P. *Prevention of Aspiration*

1. Remove airways as soon as reflexes return to avoid gagging.

2. Maintain in supine head down position.
3. Connect stomach tubes to suction.

Q. *Prevention of Urinary Retention*

1. Catheterize every six hours or use retention catheter to prevent dilatation of bladder.

R. *Treatment of Nausea*

1. Hydrate (if ketosis or acidosis is present).
2. Discontinue narcotics or change to different type.
3. Introduce Levine tube and lavage stomach.
4. Use phenobarbital, dramamine, or thorazine.

Comment

1. Do not allow visitors in recovery room.
2. Place nurse's station so that all patients can be seen from her position.
3. Have direct communication system by phone or speaker system to surgeon and anesthesiologist.
4. Do not remove patients from recovery until fully reacted and danger of hypotension has passed.
5. Remain with patient until vomiting is over.
6. Instruct nurses never to leave patients alone at any time.

POST ANESTHETIC COMPLICATIONS
ATELECTASIS

A clinical syndrome occasionally occurring during anesthesia but more often afterwards, characterized by collapse of the parenchyma of the lung due to obstruction of a bronchus and resulting in non-aeration of the segment and pneumonitis.

A. Types

1. Lobular—involves a single lobule.
2. Partial or patchy—involves a number of lobules completely or partially.
3. Lobar—involves one or more lobes completely.
4. Total—one or both lungs are involved.

B. Pathogenesis

1. Obstruction
   (a) Reflex bronchospasm of neurogenic origin.
   (b) Swelling of the mucosa due to edema.
   (c) Plugs of mucous occluding bronchi.
   (d) Endotracheal catheter down too far during anesthesia or in postoperative period if necessary to retain it.

2. Hypoventilation
   (a) Drugs which depress respiration.
   (b) Restriction of ventilatory movements due to obesity
   (c) Poor posture which favors hypoventilation.
   (d) Use of tight binders.
3. Incidence
   (a) More common in males than females.
   (b) Occurs more frequently in debilitated patients.
   (c) Greater in upper abdominal than lower or other operations.
   (d) Influenced little if at all by types of anesthetic agents.
   (e) Greater with "high" spinal anesthesia in upper abdominal surgery.
   (f) Greater in operations performed under deep anesthesia.
   (g) Greater in lung and other intrathoracic operations.
   (h) Influenced by reduced vital capacity by splinting of upper ab-abdomen.
   (i) It is the most common major postoperative pulmonary complication.

C. Predisposing Factors

1. Pre-existing pulmonary disease or acute upper respiratory infections.
2. Hyper-secretions of saliva and mucous.
3. Aspiration of vomitus.
4. Awkward positions which restrict ventilation, particularly lateral or prone.
5. Ineffective cough, particularly in debilitated acutely-ill patients. Secretions accumulate.

D. Characteristics

1. Usually occurs within 48 hours postoperatively.
2. Occurs more often on the right side than left.
3. Sudden onset as a rule.

E. Symptoms

1. Abrupt onset of dyspnea and orthopnea and other manifestations of respiratory distress.
2. Cough.
3. Tachypnea.
4. Pain in affected side of chest aggravated by respiratory movements.
5. Elevation in temperature up to 103° or 104°F.
6. Abrupt onset of tachycardia.

F. Physical Signs

1. Cyanosis
2. Lag of chest on affected side.

3. Hyper-resonance to percussion on the sound side—dullness on affected side.
4. Shifting of point of maximum impulse of the heart to affected side.
5. Elevated diaphragm.
6. Rales on affected side.
7. Bronchial breathing.

G. Laboratory Findings

1. X-ray shows emphysema on the sound side and dense shadow on the affected side.
2. Leukocytosis.

H. Treatment

1. Attempt re-expansion of the lungs by removing secretions by intratracheal suction. Tracheobronchial "toilet" (see below).
2. Perform bronchoscopy or use Cofflator if steps in 1 are ineffective.
3. Administer antibiotics or chemotherapeutic agents to prevent pneumonitis.
4. Inhalation of oxygen to relieve respiratory distress.

I. Sequelae

1. Re-expansion of the lung and relief of symptoms if treatment is applied immediately.
2. Pneumonitis in debilitated patients or if treatment is delayed.
3. Possibility of lung abscess, particularly in cases caused by aspiration.

J. Prevention

1. Avoid long operations, deep anesthesia, formation of secretions.
2. Avoid hypoventilation postoperatively.
3. Remove secretions. Use atropine or other anticholinergic agent intravenously to inhibit formation of more.
4. Perform "breathing exercises" during recovery period.
5. Change position hourly.
6. Ambulate early whenever feasible.
7. Block upper abdominal wall (lower six intercostal nerves) to relieve pain in order to permit patient to expand lungs by breathing deeply.

K. Differential Diagnosis. Most common entities with which atelectasis might be confused are:

1. Coronary Thrombosis. Points helpful in differentiation are:
   (a) Hypotension, feeble, pulse, irregularities, etc.
   (b) Pain substernally and in left arm.
   (c) Electrocardiographic changes characteristic of ischemia.
   (d) Signs of heart failure.
   (e) Absence of finding in chest x-ray.

2. Pulmonary Embolus.
    (a) Bloody sputum.
    (b) Hypotension, tachycardia and other manifestations of shock.
    (c) Sharp pleuritic type of pain often related to respiration.
    (d) Findings by x-ray are negative (early).
3. Pneumothorax
    (a) Pleuritic type of pain. Site shifts with positional changes.
    (b) Physical examination reveals resonance on affected side, mediastinal shift to opposite side, depressed diaphragm, absent breath sounds, etc.
    (c) X-ray reveals air in pleural space.
4. Pneumonia
    (a) Cough with bloody sputum.
    (b) Dullness, absent breath sounds over affected side, rales over affected side.
    (c) Signs of consolitation in x-ray examination.

PNEUMOTHORAX

Definition

Collapse of lung due to admission of air into pleural space due to opening or puncture of visceral or parietal pleura.

Causes

1. Excessive positive pressure on airway during controlled breathing.
2. Spontaneous rupture of an emphysematous bleb.
3. Needle puncture of lung in attempting brachial plexus, stellate or thoracic paravertebral block.
4. Inadvertent opening of the pleural space during nephrectomy and other operations in the area of the diaphragm.
5. Blast injury.

Symptoms

1. Dyspnea, cyanosis and other signs of respiratory distress.
2. Lag of chest on affected side.
3. Pleuritic pain associated with respiration.
4. Sucking sound with respiratory movements (open).

Signs

1. Tympanitic areas on percussion over the affected lung.
2. Absent breath sounds on the affected side.
3. Mediastinal shift of the lung to opposite side.

Treatment

1. Aspirate the air using a suction or attach a water trap for large collection of air.
2. No treatment for small collection without symptoms.

RESPIRATORY DEPRESSION OR APNEA

Definition

Inadequate gaseous exchange due to diminished ventilation or cessation of ventilating movements.

Causes

1. Excess of or intolerance to narcotics, barbiturates and other central nervous system depressants.
2. Excess of or intolerance to muscle relaxants, such as succinyl choline, d-tubocurarine, etc. used during operation.
3. Shock due to hypovolemia or trauma.
4. Restriction of thoracic movements by dressings, binders, position, etc.
5. Obstruction of airway (see Part III).
6. High spinal anesthesia or other factors causing paralysis of the muscles.
7. Hypothermia (intentional or inadvertent). After prolonged procedures in a cool operating room.
8. Intraperitoneal instillation or intravenous use of antibiotic, such as Neomycin.
9. Intracranial bleeding or expanding lesions.

Treatment

1. Establish airway and assist or control breathing using intermittent insufflation with a bag or mask.
2. Use anti-narcotics (Nalline) if due to narcotic (see Part).

POST-INTUBATION LARYNGEAL EDEMA

Definition

Edema involving the larynx and trachea following intratracheal anesthesia.

Causes

1. Trauma from forceful introduction of intratracheal catheters.
2. Friction from manipulation of the trachea (during neck surgery) so that the trachea is mobile and rubs over the catheter which is made stationary in its lumen by anchoring it at the lips. This also occurs when patient is in the prone position, particularly in children (cerebellar position).
3. Use of unsterile, unclean catheters.

4. Allergic manifestation to substances of which the catheter is composed or to the substance used as a lubricant for the tube.

Symptoms

1. Hoarseness, phonation, stridor.
2. Dysnpea and obstruction to breathing.
3. Retraction of the chest (in infants).
4. Cyanosis, tachycardia and elevation in blood pressure.

Treatment

1. Inhalations of moist air (water).
2. Antihistamines such as Benadryl and a steroid.
3 Tracheotomy.
4 Antibiotics, if infection is present.

Comment

1. In children the antihistamine ($\frac{1}{4}$–$\frac{1}{2}$ mgm. per lb.), (Benadryl I.V.) and steroid (introduced by Demming) afford rapid relief by reducing the swelling within several hours. Decadron 4 mgm. I.V. for patients one year or less and 8 mgm. over 1 year are used.
2. One millimeter thickness of edema may obliterate the cross sectional area of the trachea as much as 60%.

HYPERTENSION IN THE IMMEDIATE POSTOPERATIVE PERIOD

Description

Elevation in blood pressure in the postoperative period in patients previously normotensive is uncommon. When it occurs it is usually a carryover from hypertension developing during anesthesia. Usually, hypertension, developing during anesthesia reverts to normal at the discontinuance of anesthesia.

Causes

1. Persistence of hypertension arising during maintenance phase of anesthesia.
2. Misuse of vasopressors. Absorption of unabsorbed vasopressors administered during hypotensive state during anesthesia.
3. Respiratory obstruction causing carbon dioxide retention and anoxia.
4. Water absorption syndrome. May occur after transurethral resection.
5. Increased intracranial pressure (neurosurgical procedures, head injuries).
6. Use of oxytoxics after spinal anesthesia for obstetrical purposes.

7. Unrecognized pheochromocytoma.
8. Thyroid crisis after thyroidectomy.
9. Emergence delirium, excitement, struggling.

Treatment

1. Determine and eliminate the cause if possible.
2. Vasodepressor drugs are best omitted unless the hypertension is of severe proportions and a cerebrovascular accident is feared. If required use:
   (a) Thiophanium (Arfonad) in slow infusion.
   (b) Phentolamine (Regitine) 20 mgm. diluted in 500 cc. saline given slowly by intravenous drip.

HYPOTENSION IN THE IMMEDIATE POSTOPERATIVE PERIOD

Description

A decrease in blood pressure may occur at the conclusion of anesthesia. Blood pressure readings should be taken immediately upon transferral of patient from the operating table to the recovery room bed or roller and at frequent intervals during the first hour in the recovery room.

Causes of Hypotension

1. Postural due to changes in position from roller to bed.
2. Motion during transport on rollers and in elevators.
3. Surgical shock.
4. Unrecognized blood loss or inadequately treated hypovolemia during operation.
5. Reactionary hemorrhage from slipped ligatures, oozing after hypothermia, controlled hypotension.
6. Narcotics administered for pain, particularly if quantities are excessive or are administered rapidly intravenously or to patients in borderline shock.
7. Transfusion reaction in an "unreacted" patient.
8. Reflex from rapid recovery from general anesthesia (halothane, cyclopropane) and stimulation from pain.
9. Respiratory acidosis during anesthesia followed by a rapid decrease in carbon dioxide tension.
10. Withdrawal of high oxygen concentration when mask is removed.
11. Drugs added to blood which have vasodilator effect (antihistamines, procaine).
12. Emboli—pulmonary, fat, air, or amniotic fluid.

Treatment

1. Determine cause and:
   (a) when due to hypovolemia, administer blood or plasma volume expanders.

(b) when due to neurogenic and reflex factors, administer vasopressors—ephedrine 10–15 mgm. increments or phenylephrine in 0.25 mgm. increments.

CONVULSIONS

Description

Convulsions during anesthesia are described in Part III. The etiology of convulsions occurring postoperatively usually differ from those occurring during anesthesia. In general they are due to:

1. Pre-existing neurologic disease—brain tumors, brain abscesses, head injury, etc.
2. Inadvertent use of an excess respiratory stimulant of the non-specific type, such as bemegride, metrazol, picrotoxin, etc. in attempting to overcome respiratory depression due to anesthetic or other causes mistaken for those due to anesthesia.
3. Hyperthermia (heat retention) particularly in infants and children.
4. As an event of progressive damage to the brain due to anoxia following cardiac arrest. Preceded by or accompanied by spasticity, coma, etc.
5. Tetany from parathyroid deficiency or hyperventilation.
6. Idiosyncrasy to drugs, such as atropine, intravenous contrast media, etc.
7. As part of the train of symptoms of toxemia of pregnancy.
8. Pentothal or other barbiturates inadvertently given to patients who have porphyria.

Treatment

1. Attempt to ascertain etiology and remove cause.
2. Establish and maintain a patent airway with a pharyngeal, nasal or intratracheal tube.
3. Administer oxygen using a non-return (non-rebreathing) technique.
4. Relax using a muscle relaxant or control with secobarbital or pentothal if cause is undetermined.
5. Reduce body temperature by immersion in tepid water or by use of Thermorite blanket.

Comment

1. Severe shivering from chill could possibly be mistaken for convulsions. Take rectal temperature.
2. Local anesthetics produce convulsions shortly after injection. Convulsions do not persist into the postoperative period. Look for other cause if they develop after a local is used.
3. Convulsions commencing spontaneously after anesthesia has been discontinued and consciousness has been partially regained are seldom due to direct effect of the anesthetic drugs.

HYPERTHERMIA—POST-ANESTHESIA

Causes

1. Aggravation of pre-existing fever due to the patient's disease.
2. Pyrogenic reaction from contaminated intravenous solution.
3. Rebound after hypothermia.
4. Hot external environment causing heat retention.
5. Belladonna alkaloids may inhibit sweating in fever prone patient.
6. Damage to the central nervous system from anoxia after cardiac arrest, shock, etc.
7. Thyroid crisis after thyroidectomy.
8. Dehydration.

Treatment

1. Cool with hypothermic unit employing ice-blanket.
2. Sponge with alcohol.
3. Use antipyretics if due to aggravation of pre-existing fever.
4. Hydrate and correct electrolyte deficiencies.

COMA OR FAILURE OF AROUSAL

Causes

1. Excess of non-volatile drugs such as thiopental, narcotics, etc. administered during anesthesia.
2. Prolonged anesthesia using ether, Penthrane (methoxyflurane) or other slowly eliminated volatile drugs.
3. Anoxia damaging the brain after cardiac arrest or prolonged severe hypotension.
4. Shock from trauma, hemorrhage or "toxemia," etc.
5. Prolonged apnea resulting after use of muscle relaxant, such as succinyl choline.
6. Liver failure precipitated by operation and anesthetic drugs in patients with hepatic insufficiency.
7. Acidosis from renal shutdown, diabetes, or other metabolic disturbances.
8. "Cerebral vascular accident."
9. Administration of anti-nausea drugs which are central depressants (phenothiazines).

Comment

1. Determine the cause and institute appropriate treatment:
   (a) administer bemegride in 50 mgm. increments I.V. if believed due to barbiturates or other hypnotics.
   (b) use nalorphine (Nalline) in 5 mgm. increments or levallorphan (Lorfan) if due to narcotics (see Sec. VII).
   (c) administer fluids or vasopressors if due to hypotension.
   (d) correct acidosis and electrolyte imbalance if this is the cause.

2. Prolonged somnolence with return of reflex activity requires no treatment.

3. Often seen after ether anesthesia, Penthrane, chloroform and the use of drugs with high air-blood ratios administered over long period of time at a deep level of anesthesia.

NERVE INJURIES

Nerve injuries manifesting themselves in the postoperative period are usually the result of injury during operation. They are characterized by sensory changes, paresthesias (pins and needles), weakness of muscle groups, paralysis, fasciculations or tremors. They are caused by:

(1) Pre-existing central nervous system disease, brain tumor, cerebral hemorrhage, multiple sclerosis, etc.

(2) Systemic toxicity of exogenous or endogenous agents. Anesthesia of the face caused by the impurities in Trilene is an example.

(3) Pre-existing vitamin deficiencies.

(4) Local injury.

Those caused by local injury are of the most interest in Anesthesiology and are due to:

(1) Trauma from needles. This occurs most often in attempting venepuncture or arterial puncture.

(2) Accidental severance during operation (facial, recurrent laryngeal).

(3) Pressure from straps, posture, retractors, etc.

(4) Impaired blood supply to a given area.

(5) Toxic manifestations of local anesthetics.

The nerves most commonly injured, the causes of injury and usual manifestations are as follows:

(1) Supratrochlear. Manifested by numbness over the forehead. May result from pressure by the mask.

(2) Branches of the mental nerve. Manifested by numbness over the chin. May be caused by pressure.

(3) Trigeminal nerve. Characterized by anesthesia of the face. May be diffuse, unilateral or bilateral. Caused by toxic agents. Usually follows the use of trichlorethylene which has deteriorated to dichloracetylene or phosgene, particularly after being in contact with soda lime. Onset may be delayed days or weeks. May develop in patients not receiving trichlorethylene but who followed patients who had trichlorethylene and the charge of absorbent not discarded.

(4) Sixth cranial nerve (external rectus). Associated with spinal anesthesia. Caused by traction made on a nerve as it passes through the cavernous sinus following low spinal pressure fluid syndrome. Chief symptom is diplopia. Appears several days after spinal anesthetic. Treatment consists of applying eye patch. Usually lasts approximately six weeks.

(5) Facial nerve. May be caused by hyper-extension of the head in cases

in which the distribution of nerve is atypical and is superficial or subject to traction. May also be caused by severance during mastoidectomy or may occur without apparent cause (Bell's palsy).

(6) Laryngeal nerves. Usually injured after thyroidectomy. Bears no relationship to anesthesia or endotracheal intubation.

(7) Brachial plexus palsy. This is usually due to traction on the arm, hyper-extension and manifested by sensory and motor effects of the ulnar, median and radial nerves. Manifestations are usually mixed.

(8) Median nerve. Usually injured by direct needling in attempting venepuncture or brachial plexus block.

(9) Ulnar nerve. Usually injured by needling, occasionally by pressure, paresthesias in the fifth finger and half of the fourth. Inability to spread fingers apart.

(10) Radial nerve. Usually injured by allowing arm to hang over side of operating table, due to direct pressure manifested by wrist drop.

(11) Lateral femoral cutaneous nerve. Symptoms consist of loss of sensation on lateral aspect of thigh. Caused by injury to the nerve by retractors and intra-abdominal manipulations. Possible pre-existence from meralgia paraesthetica.

(12) Common perineal nerve. Caused by pressure on the common perineal nerve by straps or stirrups during lithotomy position. Characterized by anesthesia on lateral aspect of the leg and motor weakness of lateral leg muscles. Differentiated from cauda equina syndrome or central lesions in cord by peripheral localization, unilateral distribution and confinement of neurologic deficit to area supplied by the nerve.

(13) Cauda equina syndrome. Manifested by paraplegia in the lower extremities. May follow spinal anesthesia. Possibly caused by arachnoiditis, myelitis due to detergents used for cleansing spinal anesthesia equipment, caustic agents used for sterilization.

OTITIS MEDIA

Causes

1. Extension of unrecognized pharyngitis into Eustachian tube.
2. Passage of contaminated blood into Eustachian tube following nasal intubation.

Treatment

1. Myringotomy if purulent.

WOUND DISRUPTION

Causes

1. Failure of the wound to heal with subsequent disruption after removal of sutures.
2. Straining and coughing in immediate postoperative period or during emergence from anesthesia.

3. Improper suturing.

Treatment

1. Resuture.

CONJUNCTIVITIS AND CORNEAL IRRITATION

Causes

1. Chemicals inadvertently instilled into the eye, such as ether, vinyl ether, etc., or rancid castor oil or unsterile mineral oil or vaseline.
2. Inadvertent passage of vomitus and blood into the eye.
3. Abrasions from masks, eye shields and other instruments during anesthesia.
4. Contamination from masks, towels and other devices used by anesthetists or by unclean hands.
5. Allergic manifestations to drugs, rubber or inhalants.

Treatment

1. Irrigate eye with saline to remove foreign bodies, vomitus, chemicals, etc. (except in cases due to allergy).
2. Use ophthalmic ointment with antiseptic properties (infection).
3. Seek advice of ophthalmologist.

VASOSPASM AND THROMBOSIS FROM INTRAVASCULAR INJECTION

Causes

Mistaking artery for a vein and injecting an irritating solution inadvertently. Usually occurs in antecubital fossae while administering pentothal and other ultra short acting barbiturates. May also occur in other areas with other drugs. Due to direct injury on the endothelium and vessel wall.

Symptoms

1. Bright red blood pulsates into syringe.
2. Intense pain and blanching due to intense vasospasm and damage to the intima.

Sequelae

Not predictable. Nothing may occur or gangrene of area supplied by vessel may result.

Treatment

1. Promote vasodilatation by using:
   (a) 10 cc. 1% procaine slowly in artery. Leave needle in after accident to use for injection.
   (b) Inject heparin through needle. Use anti-coagulants afterward, such as Dicomourol.
   (c) Stellate ganglion block.

SLOUGH

Causes

1. Extravasation of alkaline, acidic, or otherwise irritating solutions during intravenous therapy (Thiopental).
2. Infusion of vasopressors (Norepinephrine).
3. External pressure from straps, parts of the operating table, retractors, blood pressure cuffs especially during prolonged bouts of hypotension or during hypothermia.
4. Injection of irritating drugs and inadvertent injection of necrotizing drugs into the tissues (local anesthetics in oil, drugs, etc.).
5. Frostbite. Most frequently encountered after hypothermia.
6. Burns. Misuse of hot water bottles, inadvertent contact of skin with caustic chemicals (phenols). May occur during rewarming following hypothermia.

Treatment

Prevention is better than cure. Once injury has occurred and death of tissue is apparent steps should be taken to prevent infection. Immediately after an accident has occurred steps to promote vasodilatation are indicated when vasospasm is present. The following are recommended:

1. For extravasation of thiopental and related drugs. Infiltrate area with 5–10 cc. 1% procaine. Promote vasodilatation with warmth (immersion in water bath at 105°–108°F.) or by stellate ganglion block.
2. For extravasation of norepinephrine. Phentolamine (Regetine) 5 mgm. diluted and infiltrated in area.

SUBCUTANEOUS EMPHYSEMA

Causes

1. Trauma to the mucosa of the pharynx, trachea, bronchi or alveoli from:
   (a) faulty intubation.
   (b) excessive manual pressure on breathing bag.
   (c) excessive positive pressure in system due to inadvertent direct connection from "straight-over oxygen" to the inhaler.
   (d) tears or cuts in lung or bronchi occurring during pulmonary surgery.
   (e) explosion in anesthetic apparatus.

Treatment

1. Remove source of leak.
2. Tracheotomy if emphysema in neck is severe and encroaches on the airway.
3. Incision of the skin to relieve tension and prevent necrosis (see comment).
4. Inhalation of 100% oxygen by mask to help eliminate nitrogen from tissues (of questionable value).

Comment

1. The incision should be made in skin crease if in the neck. It should be approximately 1 cm. long.
2. The air should be milked towards incision. Wound does not require suturing.

SKIN RASHES

Causes

1. Exposure to excessive heat.
2. Exposure to excessive cold.
3. Inadvertent direct contact with chemical irritants, such as adhesive, sterilizers, plastic substances, drugs, etc.
4. Systemic injection of drugs such as bromides, barbiturates, narcotics, etc.
5. Vasodilatation following hypothermia.
6. Allergic responses due to drugs, blood, proteins, etc.

Treatment

1. Determine etiology if possible and remove cause. Discontinue drugs.
2. Cleanse skin by irrigation if due to contact with chemical irritants.
3. Administer an antihistaminic if the response is of an allergic nature. Benedryl (25–50 mgm. I.V.) may be used.

TRACHEOBRONCHIAL ASPIRATION WITH CATHETER

Purpose: To induce patient to cough in order to aspirate mucoid secretions from tracheobronchial tree. Used for treating atelectasis and other pulmonary infections.

Material:

1. Magill catheter—29 F. approximately, depending on size of patient.
2. Jelly type lubricant containing local anesthetic (xylocaine, metycaine, Americaine, etc.).
3. Suction or urethral catheter about 10 F. which will pass through endotracheal tube.

Procedure:

1 Lubricate gently, introduce the Magill tube into one nostril which has no obstruction until larynx is reached.
2. Have patient inspire deeply and at height of inspiration direct Magill tube into trachea.
3. Pass suction catheter into Magill tube and remove secretions.
4. Keep Magill tube in as long as patient tolerates until no further secretions are removed.

Comments

1. In cases of atelectasis if lung fails to expand due to inability to remove secretions because they are too far down, perform bronchoscopy.
2. In cases of excessive gagging or coughing anesthetize nasopharynx with local anesthetic spray

PART VIII

RESUSCITATION

Definition: Resuscitation is *Restoration to life of the apparent dead (Webster).* **It might be added that the dead cannot be revived.**

Subjects requiring resuscitation fall into three categories, according to the symptoms they present:

1. Those with no signs of circulatory or respiratory activity. *This is the most common picture encountered.*
2. Those in whom *respiration* has failed, but *circulation* is still active. This state is usually caused by depressant drugs, anesthesia, intra-cranial and other nervous system lesions. Circulation soon fails unless *treatment* is instituted.
3. Those in whom respiration is active, but circulation is depressed—shock, spinal anesthesia, etc. Respiratory depression or failure soon follows if the circulatory depression is not corrected.

Treatment:

1. If a patient is not breathing or respiratory movements are inadequate, institute artificial respiration *immediately.*
2. Institute cardiac resuscitation.

Comment: Do not neglect artificial respiration and waste time administering stimulating drugs. The oxygen the patient needs in such circumstances cannot be administered with a syringe from an ampule! ! !

ARTIFICIAL RESPIRATION

Definition: The process of maintaining as near as possible physiological oxygen and carbon dioxide tensions in alveoli by artificial methods when voluntary respiratory movements are absent.

Methods: There are numerous methods of artificial respiration. All fall into one of these two following groups:

1. *Manual* or *non-mechanical.* These are methods in which no apparatus is required.
2. *Mechanical.* These are methods which require some form of apparatus or machinery.
   Methods of artificial respiration are based upon one of these two principles:
1. The principle in which an intermittent negative or positive pressure in the pleural space is produced by a force applied to the exterior of the

581

thorax or by causing the diaphragm to move. The following embody this principle:

    a. Nielsen's arm lift back pressure method (manual).
    b. Silvester's method (manual).
    c. Drinker's method (using the "iron lung," mechanical).
    d. Eve's method (using the tilt table).

2. The principle in which expansion of the thorax is produced by insufflating gases under pressure into the alveoli.

    The following methods embody this principle:

    a. Insufflation by mouth to mouth breathing (non-mechanical).
    b. Insufflation by an inhaler composed of mask, breathing bag and an oxygen supply (mechanical). The inflated bag is compressed manually.
    c. Insufflation by an automatic mechanism. The E & J, Emerson, McKesson and such insufflators are purely automatic mechanical devices.

REFERENCE

Waters, R. M. Methods of Resuscitation. Jour. Lab. & Clin. Med., *26:* 272–278, October, 1940.

Nielsen's Method (Arm Lift—Back Pressure Technique)

Definition: The establishment of respiratory movements by compression and relaxation of the thorax using the arm lift back pressure technique.

Principle:

1. *Inspiration*—Obtained by having the operator grasp the elbows and elevate them to create active inspiration.
2. *Expiration*—Obtained by releasing the elbows and applying pressure over the scapulae.
3. Oxygen tension—this is the same as that of the atmosphere.
4. Carbon dioxide—this is the same as that of the atmosphere.

Technique:

1. Place the subject in the prone position with hands under the forehead.
2. Kneel at the head and face the feet of the patient. (Fig. 170)
3. Grasp the patient's arms and raise them until the upper thorax is off the floor.
4. Release the arms and allow the thorax to go back to the floor.
5. Make pressure over the scapulae with both hands by leaning forward. (Fig. 170)
6. Repeat this maneuver rhythmically sixteen times per minute. All movements should be gradual.

Advantages:

1. May be instituted immediately by one operator.
2. May be instituted by having the patient in the prone position.
3. The tidal exchange is approximately 500–600 cc. per minute, greater than any other manual method.

Disadvantages:

1. The airway may become obstructed because the patient is in the prone position and the airway is not under direct control of the operator.
2. The method is not suitable for long periods because it is tiring to the operator.

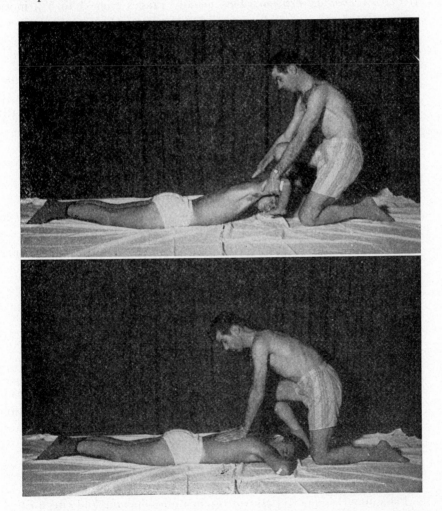

Fig. 170. Maneuvers in performing Nielsen's method of artificial respiration. (Courtesy Meyer Saklad. Inhalation Therapy and Resuscitation. Thomas, Springfield, 1953.)

INSUFFLATION BY MOUTH TO MOUTH BREATHING

Definition: The establishment of respiratory movements by inflating the patient's lung by breathing into the patient's mouth.

Principle:

1. *Inspiration:* This is obtained by forcing the operator's exhalation into the alveoli.
2. *Expiration:* This is obtained by the elastic recoil of lungs and tissues of the chest wall.
3. *Oxygen Tension:* This is usually subatmospheric, 12%–15%, in the insufflated gas.
4. *Carbon Dioxide Tension:* This usually ranges from 3 to 5% in the insufflated gas.

Technique:

1. Stand on left side of subject and extend head as far backward as possible to establish airway by placing palm of left hand on the back of the neck and palm of right hand on forehead lifting head so that it tilts backward.
2. Open subject's mouth if it does not open automatically.
3. Take deep breath and open (operator's) mouth.
4. Place mouth (operator's) over subject's making a tight seal.
5. Blow forcefully (adult) and gently (children) into subject's mouth.
6. Press (operator's) right cheek against nostrils (subject's) to prevent leakage through nose.
7. Be aware of movement of thorax. When inflation and elevation of thorax ceases remove mouth (operator's) to allow subject to exhale.
8. Repeat every 3 to 5 seconds (adult); 2 to 3 seconds (child).

MOUTH TO NOSE BREATHING

1. Close subject's mouth by extending chin upward with left hand.
2. Place mouth (operator's) opened widely over nostrils in such a manner as not to pinch them and obstruct airway.
3. Inflate chest as described in mouth to mouth technique above.
4. Open subject's mouth to allow deflation of lungs after each insufflation.

MOUTH TO TRACHEOTOMY TUBE BREATHING

1. Pinch nose and close mouth.
2. Take deep breath and open mouth.
3. Place mouth (operator's) over tracheotomy opening and effect a tight seal.
4. All exhalations to come out of tracheotomy cannula.

Mouth to Mask Breathing

1. Insert pharyngeal airway.
2. Adjust mask over face in same manner as for inhalation anesthesia with
   (a) Last three fingers supporting chin.
   (b) Thumb and index finger supporting and adjusting mask to make tight fit.
3. Extend head to obtain patent airway.
4. Take deep breath and blow into opening of mask as in mouth to mouth breathing.
5. Remove mouth and allow exhalations to escape.

Mouth to Airway Breathing

1. Introduce S shaped ("Safar" Resuscitube) airway in same manner as ordinary pharyngeal airway.
2. Blow into airway in same manner as described for mouth to mouth breathing.

Mouth to Endotracheal Tube Breathing

1. Intubate after patient has been oxygenated several times by mouth to mouth breathing.
2. Blow into tube using same procedure and precautions outlined for mouth to mouth.

Comment

1. No method of insufflation is successful unless tight seal of operator's and subject's lips is made and no leaks occur.
2. Rhythm is not important but regularity is desirable if attainable.
3. Use mouth to nose breathing when patent airway is difficult to establish by mouth to mouth technique.
4. Remember that exhalation is passive and allowance must be made for it.
5. Blowing into nose provides adequate insufflation, but may not permit adequate exhalation.
6. In small children hold mouth (operator's) over both mouth and nose.
7. In infants use only puffs from the mouth and not air from lungs to prevent rupture of alveoli.
8. Air may pass into stomach. Can be overcome by placing hand over epigastrium.
9. Introduce pharyngeal airway (or Resuscitube) if available and if:
   (a) person is limp and has no reflexes
10. Adults require forceful blowing particularly if leakage is present.
11. In operating room or recovery ward mouth to mask method more effective than mouth to mouth.

Advantages of mouth insufflation techniques

1. The method is immediately available. It requires no special apparatus.
2. It may be executed by anyone or delegated to assistants if necessary after a moment's instruction.

Disadvantages:

1. The oxygen tension of the insufflated air is below that of the atmosphere.
2. The carbon dioxide from operator's exhalation introduced into an asphyxiated patient is not desirable.
3. The excessive force exerted by adults may rupture alveoli of infants.
4. Tiring to the operator.
5. Is ineffective when spastic muscles prevent opening of the mouth.
6. May be a source of infection to the operator.

SILVESTER'S METHOD

Definition: Establishment of respiratory movements by compression and relaxation of lower portion of the thorax with the patient's elbows.

Principle:

1. *Inspiration:* This is obtained by expansion of the thoracic cage, by extending patient's arms over his head.
2. *Expiration:* This is obtained by compression of lower ribs and thorax with the patient's elbows.
3. *Oxygen Tension:* This is the same as that of the atmosphere.
4. *Carbon Dioxide Tension:* This is the same as that of the atmosphere.

Technique (Fig. 171):

1. Place the patient in the supine position and lower his head and shoulders.
2. Grasp patient's hands at the wrist. Extend the patient's arms without flexing at the elbow joint backward and upward over beyond head. This expands ribs for inspiration.
3. Return the patient's arms so that his elbows are flexed almost at a right angle with the humeri. The elbows are placed along lower anterior chest wall. Pressure is made on forearms so that the humeri compress the ribs and force air out of the chest.
4. Repeat this maneuver rhythmically 16 times per minute. All movements should be gradual.

Advantages: This method is useful when the patient must be maintained in a supine position (surgical cases).

Disadvantages:
1. The airway becomes obstructed because the patient is in the supine position. The tongue rolls back easily.
2. The method is not suitable for long periods because it is tiring for the operator.

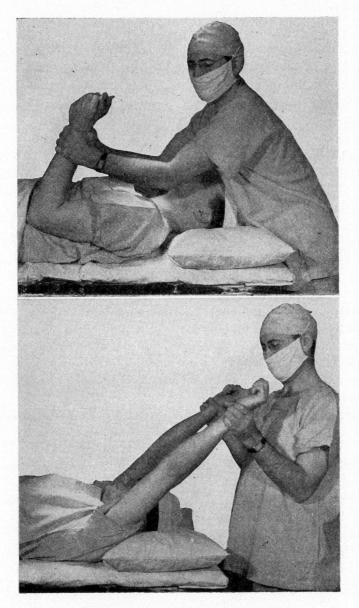

Fig. 171. Silvester's method of artificial respiration.

REFERENCE

Silvester, H. Restoring Persons Apparently Drowned or Dead. British M. J., p. 575, 1858.

"Iron Lung" or Drinker Respirator

Principle: An intermittent negative pressure is produced in an airtight steel chamber by the alternate compression and relaxation of a large diaphragm. The chamber encloses all of a patient's body but his head. Atmospheric air is drawn into the lungs during the phase of negative pressure (Fig. 172).

Apparatus: A cylindrical chamber constructed to enclose an adult human being. The chamber has the following features:
1. A cot which slides out at head end of the chamber. This is attached to the cover which is quickly clamped to body of the chamber.
2. A sponge-like collar fitting about the patient's neck to insure an airtight fit.
3. A motor to operate the diaphragm to produce variations in pressure within the chamber.
4. A manometer to record changes in pressure within the chamber.
5. A regulator for varying pressure changes within the chamber.
6. A rheostat to control the motor to vary the rate of respiration.
7. A lever for hand operation of the diaphragm in event the power fails.
8. Windows and port holes for administering treatments and examinations of patients.

Principle:
1. *Inspiration:* This is produced by creating a negative pressure in pleural space by creating a subatmospheric tension about the thorax.
2. *Expiration:* This is produced by the elastic recoil of lung tissue (or by positive pressure device on machine if desired).
3. *Oxygen Tension:* This is the same as the atmosphere, unless oxygen is supplied by mask or catheter.
4. *Carbon Dioxide Tension:* This is the same as that of atmosphere.

Technique:
1. Unclamp the front, pull out the cot, adjust patient comfortably upon it and replace in chamber. Lock clamps securely. (Fig. 173)
2. Turn on the switch which starts the respirator. Regulate the rate to 14–18 times per minute (rate may be increased by adjusting rheostat which controls the motor).
3. Adjust collar so that it fits snugly and comfortably. Pad with cotton if necessary. Place the head upon the head rest.
4. Regulate depth of respiration by adjusting negative pressure to ap-

proximately 18 cms. water pressure. Determine the threshold of the negative pressure to be employed by asking the patient to count out loud. Increase the pressure to the point at which speech disappears. This is the optimum pressure.

Precautions:

1. Be positive the airway is patent and air passes in and out of mouth (place hand over mouth to be certain). Insert a pharyngeal airway if it is tolerated by the patient or if the patient is unconscious.

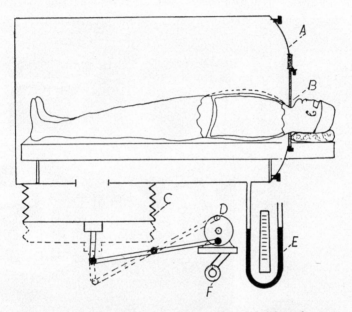

FIG. 172. Schematic diagram of iron lung. (A) Steel airtight enclosure. (B) Rubber collar. (C) Movable diaphragm and bellows. (D) Motor for operating the diaphragm. (E) Manometer for gauging changes in the pressure. (F) Rheostat for controlling the rate of ventilation.

2. Synchronize mechanical breathing with ineffective natural breathing if respiratory depression is present.
3. Do not use positive pressure for expiration. Natural passive expiration is sufficient and satisfactory.
4. Do not waste time adjusting the collar if the patient is in serious condition. Start respirator and adjust collar later. Slight leaks do not render machine entirely ineffective.
5. Tilt body so that head is low if secretions are present. Use pharyngeal suction if necessary.
6. Operate apparatus at the lowest possible speed required to maintain effective respiration and circulation.

REFERENCES

Drinker, P., and Shaw, L. A. An Apparatus for Prolonged Administration of Artificial Respiration. J. Clin. Investigation, 7: 229, 1929.
Schmidt, G. F., and Seldon, T. H. Practical Management of Patients in the Respirator. Proc. Staff Meeting Mayo Clinic, 16: 456, July, 1941.

AUTOMATIC MECHANICAL INSUFFLATORS

A number of different designs are available. They derive energy from cylinders of compressed oxygen and inflate the lungs by an intermittent stream of oxygen. The high pressure also operates a suction mechanism used

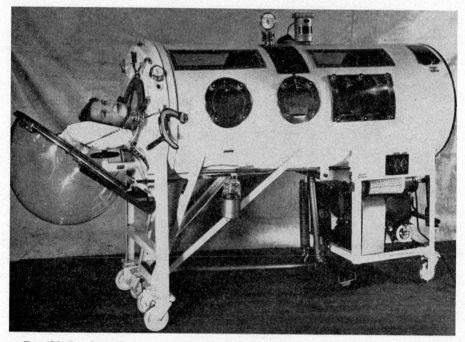

FIG. 173. Iron lung (Tank respirator). The dome permits the use of intermittent positive pressure for insufflation for maintaining respiration when patient is out of tank. (Courtesy J. H. Emerson Company.)

to assist in deflating of the lungs. Although they differ in many ways, all have some or all of the following features:

1. They inflate the lungs by supplying a stream of oxygen to a mask. As soon as a pressure of 14 to 18 cms. of water is attained, the stream is automatically interrupted.
2. They attempt to deflate the lungs by negative pressure induced by suction (9–12 cms. of water).
3. They have a suction mechanism operated by the compressed gas to remove secretions.
4. They are equipped with a valve which allows the apparatus to be

converted to an inhaler to allow patients pure oxygen or oxygen and carbon dioxide.

5. They are equipped with an automatic release which shuts off the stream of gases when calibrated pressure is attained in the mask.

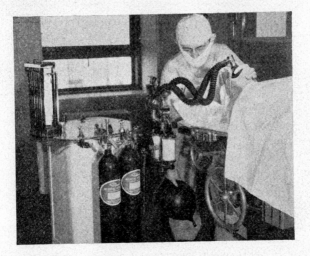

FIG. 174. Artificial respiration by insufflation. Use of circle filter for manual ventilation of lungs.

6. They are equipped with a valve which institutes negative pressure when positive insufflation pressure is interrupted.
7. They have a valve for varying the rate of inflation.

Note Numerous models of this type introduced by different manufacturers are available. For each model the instructions provided by the manufacturer should be followed. The E&J is the better known and its use is described below.

Use of E&J Resuscitator (Fig. 176)

1 Turn oxygen cylinder valve on completely.
2. Turn operating lever to "resuscitator" side if on "suction" or inhaler.
3. Turn oxygen control valve until gas is heard to flow.
4. Apply mask snugly to face using right hand and extend chin to support airway.
5. Adjust gas flow to desired respiratory rate.

Comment

1. A series of rapid clicks indicates obstruction of respiratory passages. Adjust airway.
2. Remember the respiratory rate depends upon volume flow. The larger

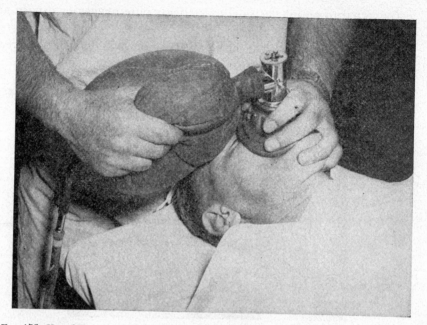

FIG. 175. Use of To and Fro inhaler for artificial respiration. Insufflation is accomplished by intermittently compressing the breathing bag. Expiration is passive. (Courtesy Meyer Saklad, Inhalation Therapy and Resuscitation. Springfield, Thomas, 1953.)

the patient's tidal exchange the slower the rate which the machine delivers. For large subjects the rate cannot exceed a fixed limit.

3. A flow of gas but absence of respiratory movements indicates improper application of mask.

4. Mask is held and airway maintained in same manner described for inhalation anesthesia.

5. May fail to operate in face of slight respiratory obstruction which requires pressure greater than calibrated pressure to be overcome.

Kreiselman Resuscitator

Description: A simple apparatus, uses air or oxygen when available, composed of an accordian type bellows and mask. Valves permit escape of exhaled gases to outside atmosphere while bellows is being loaded with fresh gas. (Fig. 177)

Principle:

1. *Inspiration.* This is obtained by manually compressing the breathing bag filled with oxygen and forcing the gas into the alveoli.

2. *Expiration.* This is obtained by recoil of chest wall and elastic tissue of lungs when pressure is reduced by extending the bellows. Exhaled air escapes at side.

3. *Oxygen tension.* Air is used. A nipple at the top permits attachment

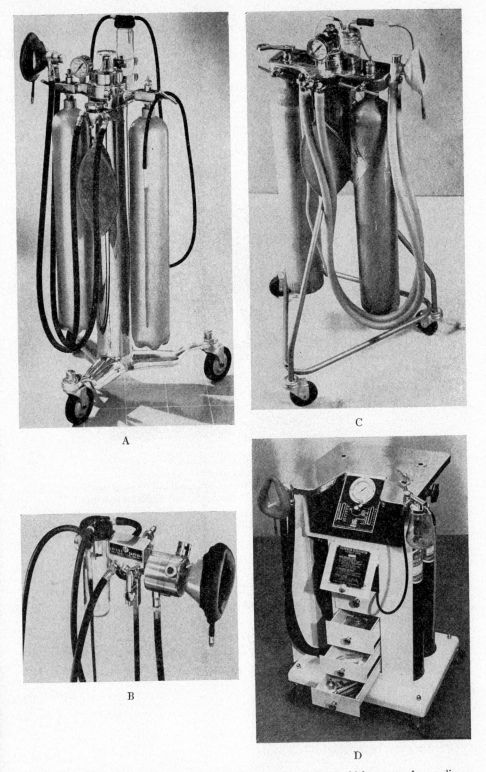

FIG. 176. Positive-negative ("blow and suck") respirators. A. E & J which operates from ordinary oxygen cylinders. B. Portable E & J model which operates from oxygen piping system. C. Emerson. D. Stephenson.

to hose from ordinary oxygen regulator at 4–5 liters per minute to enrich the mixture.

4. *Carbon dioxide tension.* Only that which is in air in mask.

Procedure:

1. Position of patient, insertion of airway, holding mask and rate of manipulation are as described above for insufflation technique.

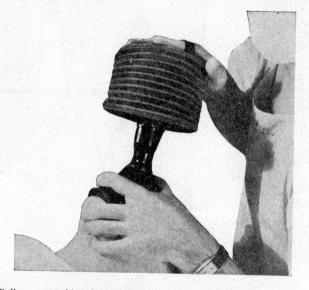

FIG. 177A. Bellows type of insufflator devised by Dr. Joseph Kreiselman. Inspiration is actively performed by graded amounts of positive pressure. Expiration is passive and due entirely to the elastic recoil of the lungs without suction, because an outlet valve opens to allow exhalations to escape while bellows are being extended. Air is used but a nipple attachment for oxygen is provided.

2. Insufflate lungs by compressing the bellows downward and allow lungs to deflate while replenishing.

Advantages:

1. Simple and instantly readied for use.
2. Easily demonstrated to novices.
3. Inexpensive.
4. Mechanical difficulties easily detected and corrected.
5. Allows gradation of pressure up to 25 cms. H_2O.
6. Excess pressure not possible. Is provided with safety escape valve to prevent rupture of lungs.

Disadvantages:

1. Prolonged use may interfere with venous return to heart.
2. Air may be pushed into stomach if respiratory obstruction is present.

Ambu Resuscitator

Operates on same principle as Kreiselman resuscitator except that bag contains sponge rubber. Utilizes air or oxygen which is admitted at the tail of the bag (Fig. 177B).

MANUAL INSUFFLATION

Definition: The establishment of respiratory movements by insufflating oxygen into the alveoli by alternately compressing and releasing the breathing bag. (Fig. 174, 175)

Apparatus: Any inhaler used for anesthesia composed of a mask, bag and canister and oxygen supply may be employed. The to and fro or circle filter inhaler is satisfactory and this is the equipment usually employed.

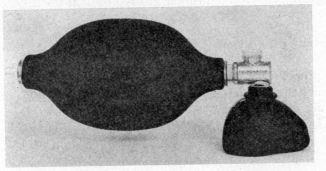

FIG. 177B. The Ambu resuscitator. (Courtesy Air Shields Co.)

Principle:
1. *Inspiration:* This is obtained by manually compressing the breathing bag filled with oxygen and forcing the gas into the alveoli.
2. *Expiration:* This is obtained by recoil of chest wall and elastic tissue of lungs when the pressure is reduced by releasing the bag.
3. *Oxygen Tension:* Concentrations as great as 100% may be used.
4. *Carbon Dioxide Tension:* Slight or none.

Procedure:
1. Place patient in the supine position.
2. Insert a pharyngeal airway or, if available, an intra-tracheal airway.
3. Apply mask to face and secure a snug fit. Hold mask tightly to the face.
4. Fill the breathing bag with pure oxygen. Compress the bag rhythmically 12–18 times per minute to inflate the thorax.
5. Release the pressure. The bag inflates as the thorax deflates.
6. Repeat this maneuver 12–18 times per minute. Replace oxygen which leaks out.

Advantages:
1. It is instantly available in the operating room during surgery.
2. Expiration is not accomplished by negative pressure but by the elastic recoil of the lungs.
3. Insufflation pressure, rate of manipulation and oxygen tensions may

be graded according to needs of patient and the wishes of the operator.

4. It may be used over long periods of time.

Disadvantages:

1. The insufflation pressure, if excessive, may rupture the alveoli.
2. Gases other than oxygen may be erroneously employed (when anesthesia machines are used).
3. The thoracic negative pressure necessary to facilitate the venous return to the heart is not maintained and circulatory disturbances may follow.
4. Oxygen is often forced into the gastrointestinal tract.

Comment

1. **Be positive the airway is free at all times and that the thorax expands and recoils easily.**
2. Use pure oxygen for insufflation.
3. **Discard the mixture and fill the bag with pure oxygen at frequent intervals when treating overdosage of volatile drugs.**
4. Connect the intra-tracheal catheters if they are used to the inhaler with slip joints.
5. Attach a manometer to the inhaler and do not exceed 20 cms. water pressure when inflating the thorax of infants and children.

REFERENCES

Waters, R. M. Artificial Respiration by Means of Intermittent High Pressure Inflation of the Chest with Oxygen. Anesth. & Analg., *15:* p. 10, October, 1921.

Saklad, M. Inhalation Therapy and Resuscitation. Charles C Thomas, Springfield, Ill., 1953.

DISADVANTAGES OF MECHANICAL DEVICES

1. The machines are not always instantly available.
2. **Their use requires knowledge and skill for proper management.**
3. They do not necessarily employ sound physiological principles for ventilation of lungs.
4. They are subject to mechanical defects and uncertainty in proper function of automatic adjustments.
5. The negative pressure which some utilize for deflation is unnecessary and may predispose to pulmonary edema if used over long periods of time.
6. They may inflate the gastro-intestinal tract and cause trauma to vital organs.
7. They may develop leaks in masks and other parts which render the apparatus ineffective.
8. They are difficult to synchronize with natural but shallow ineffective breathing in instances in which respiration is depressed but has not failed.

Summary

1. The "mouth to mouth" method is the accepted method for general purposes, particularly in urgent cases when apparatus is not available.
2. The "Drinker Respirator" is the most desirable for protracted periods of artificial respiration.
3. Insufflation with the inhaler of the anesthesia apparatus is the most desirable and convenient for anesthesia and surgery.

Remember:

1. Initiate artificial respiration immediately. Order assistants to carry out treatments or diagnostic procedures or ask a particularly competent assistant to maintain artificial respiration while the operator attends to other details.
2. Maintain a patent airway. The object of the manipulation is to remove carbon dioxide from alveoli and introduce oxygen in to them.
3. **Be gentle, slow, and deliberate in manipulations.** Gradual and rhythmic movements are the most desirable and effective.
   a. If manipulations are executed too rapidly, carbon dioxide will be removed by hyperventilation and the apnea may continue from the resulting acarbia.
   b. If movements are too forceful, alveoli may be overdistended and apnea may result from stimulation of the Hering-Breur reflex.
   c. If insufflation is forceful, it may rupture the alveoli.
   d. If movements are too slow, inadequate ventilation results.
4. Always use pure oxygen whenever available. **Air is satisfactory if no oxygen is available.**
5. After artificial respiration has been instituted, supply:
   a. Warmth.
   b. Fluids, if necessary.
   c. Analeptic drugs and other treatments as desired.
6. Although the muscles of patients suffering from acute anoxemia may be spastic in the early phase, they are relaxed after prolonged asphyxia and do not have same resilience as normal tissues.
7. **Do not add carbon dioxide to the oxygen mixture. The use of carbon dioxide for respiratory failure is a controversial subject. Do not worry if it is not available. Oxygen is the gas which must be introduced into the alveoli.**
8. Do not be too generous in the use of analeptic drugs. Patients may recover unexpectedly and develop convulsions, or depression may follow stimulation by the drug.
9. **Always remain with a patient being treated with a mechanical device for maintaining artificial respiration until effective natural breathing is restored.**
10. When a protracted period of artificial respiration is required and the

use of a mechanical method is contemplated, maintain the manual method until the apparatus is available and the transfer can be accomplished without interruption of ventilation.

11. **Do not hesitate to perform a tracheotomy in irremediable obstruction of the upper respiratory tract.** *One more often regrets not having done a tracheotomy than having done one.*

ANALEPTIC DRUGS

Definition: An analeptic drug is a stimulating drug used as a restorative for depressed respiratory and circulatory mechanisms.

Available Drugs: The following drugs are the currently employed respiratory stimulants:

> Metrazol
> Nikethamide (Coramine)
> Picrotoxin
> Nalorphine (Nalline)
> Bemegride (Megimide)
> Methyl Phenidate (Ritalin)
> Ethemivan (Vandid)

Mode of Action: Analeptic drugs exert their action by one or a combination of several of the following mechanisms:

1. By stimulation of medullary and other vital centers: Metrazol, coramine, picrotoxin, and carbon dioxide act in this manner.
2. By stimulation of the carotid body, which, in turn, reflexly stimulates the respiratory center. Lobeline, coramine, and cyanide derivatives act in this manner.
3. By stimulation of sympathetic receptors in the arterioles to elevate blood pressure and improve general and cerebral circulation: Epinephrine, ephedrine, and other sympathomimetic drugs act in this manner.
4. By stimulation of the smooth muscle of the blood vessels to elevate blood pressure and improve general and cerebral circulation: Pitressin, pituitrin, and ephedrine act in this manner.
5. By stimulating the heart muscle and improving the cardiac output: Digitalis (perhaps some of the above act in this manner).
6. By influencing capillary permeability and preventing fluid loss: Adrenal cortical hormone acts in this manner.

Uses:

1. *Respiratory Failure:* Administer metrazol 100 milligrams (10% solution) intravenously as the initial dose and repeat, or coramine 250 milligrams (25% solution) intravenously. Use these drugs as adjuncts to artificial respiration only.

2. *Circulatory Failure:*
   a. Cardiac arrest. Cardiac massage, and intracardiac injection of epinephrine.
   b. Peripheral circulatory failure (primary). Vasopressor drugs.
   c. Peripheral circulatory failure (secondary). Fluids and cortical extract or cortisone.
3. *Overdosage of Depressant Drugs:*
   a. Inhalation anesthesia: Metrazol as described under respiratory failure.
   b. Barbiturate overdosage: Bemegrid for massive overdosage. Bemegrid for ultra short acting barbiturates.
   c. Other non-volatile drugs: Bemegrid or methyl phenidate (Ritalin).

Objection to Analeptic Drugs:

1. They stimulate cells of the nervous system in the face of acute oxygen lack.
2. They produce depression after the initial stimulation. The depression may persist after the "emergency" is over.
3. The period of stimulation may persist after the disturbance is relieved resulting in elevated blood pressure, convulsions, and hyperpnea.
4. They antagonize the narcotic action of depressant drugs, but do not hasten the destruction of the drug. The summation of the depression (which follows the stimulation) with the action of the narcotic produces even a greater depression.

MANAGEMENT OF COMA DUE TO DEPRESSANT DRUGS (NON-VOLATILE)

The manifestations of overdosage of sedative drugs are: loss of reflexes, respiratory depression, coma, and, in certain instances, circulatory depression. The following measures should be instituted for all cases of drug poisoning of this type:

1. *Institute Adequate Ventilation:*
   a. Provide a satisfactory airway. Support the chin, introduce a pharyngeal airway or intubate the patient, if necessary, to obtain unimpeded ventilation.
   b. Augment respiratory movements, if they are inadequate, with artificial respiration. Insufflation with inhaler of the anesthesia apparatus is satisfactory for short periods. Place patient in Drinker respirator for protracted periods of respiratory failure.
   c. Oxygen (100%) by nasal catheter or mask.
2. *Remove Drug from Stomach:*
   a. Introduce a stomach tube through the nose, aspirate the entire

contents, and **send a specimen to the laboratory for immediate analysis.**

   b. **Lavage the stomach with warm dilute sodium bicarbonate solution if drug is suspected of being acid (barbiturates).** Use dilute vinegar if drug is alkaline, or potassium permanganate ($\frac{1}{4}\%$) if drug is an alkaloid.

   c. **Introduce saline cathartic into stomach through tube.** Do not use magnesium salts as they may further enhance the depression.

3. *Support Circulation if Depression Is Present:*

   a. Administer 1000 cc. glucose in distilled water (5%) intravenously. Fasten arm on board **(particularly if the patient is restless).**

   b. Administer plasma if hemocentration is present.

   c. Administer a vasopressor substance, such as ephedrine or neosynephrine cautiously. These are indicated when hypotension is present.

4. *Promote Diuresis:*

   a. Catheterize and measure the urinary output. Send specimen to laboratory for analysis.

   b. Administer glucose in distilled water (5%).

5. *Lavage the Colon with Physiological Saline Solution:* This step is imperative, particularly if the drug is known to be excreted into colon (morphine).

6. *Administer an Analeptic Drug* to antagonize the depression. The type depends upon the drug causing the depression. Metrazol, coramine, or Bemegrid are the most commonly employed (see analeptics).

7. *Institute General Nursing Care:*

Comment	*Reasons*
1. Remove secretions by suction if they appear. Atropine gr. 1/150 may be employed.	Secretions become inspissated and obstruct airway.
2. Chart intake and output of all fluids administered.	Pulmonary edema may result if an excess of fluid (over 3500 cc. in 24 hours) is administered.
3. Turn patient from one side to his back to other side at least every hour.	This procedure may assist in prevention of bronchopneumonia which frequently complicates these cases.
4. Use antibiotics in long cases.	Pulmonary infection may occur from hypoventilation.

TREATMENT OF DEPRESSION DUE TO NARCOTICS WITH NALORPHINE (NALLINE)

Uses: To overcome depression due to opium alkaloids (morphine, codeine) their derivatives—dilaudid, heroin, dicodid, metapon and synthetic narcotics, demerol (meperidine), dromoran, nisentil.

Procedure:

1. Administer 5 mgm. nalorphine intravenously over period of 1/2 to 1 minute and note response.
2. Allow several minutes to elapse and administer an additional 5 milligrams if there is a response.
3. If no response occurs administer an additional 5 milligrams.

Comment

1. If no response has occurred after 15 milligram's use no more drug. Depression is probably not due to narcotic.
2. If response has occurred with first dose but not second, administer no additional drug.
3. If second dose causes a response or augments response of first, administer additional 5 milligrams.

Precautions:

1. Large doses cause depression. Do not exceed 15 mgm in ordinary circumstances.
2. The drug is not suitable for ether, barbiturates, chloral, avertin and central nervous system depressants other than narcotics.

Use of Levallorphan (Lorfan) as Antinarcotic

Levallorphan is approximately 5 times more potent than nalorphine. Use 1 mgm. doses for each 5 of nalorphine in same manner as nalorphine.

Use of Picrotoxin for Overdosage of Barbiturate

1. Follow routine described above for management of coma.
2. Administer picrotoxin intravenously as a constant infusion at the rate of one milligram each sixty seconds until a lightening of narcosis appears. The following manifestations are significant:
   a. Stirring, opening the eyes, movement of hands and feet, etc.
   b. Return of reflexes such as laryngeal, pharyngeal, superficial skin.
   c. Increased amplitude of respiration.
3. Repeat half the intravenous dose required to obtain this effect subcutaneously within 30 minutes and each succeeding 30 minutes if the patient continues in the restored level of depression.

Comment	*Reasons*
1. Administer picrotoxin until the desired therapeutic effect is obtained.	In severe depressions, large initial doses are required to rouse the subject (10 milligrams or more).
2. Observe the patient closely for twitchings of small muscles, retching, vomiting or convulsions. Ad-	These are toxic manifestations of overdosage of picrotoxin, due to too rapid administration.

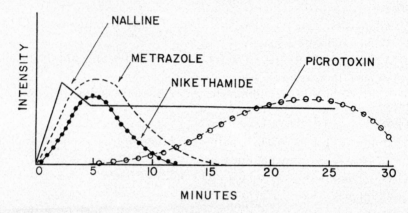

FIG. 178. The relationship of onset and intensity of action to time manifested by metrazole, nikethamide, picrotoxin and N-allyl nor-morphine when used as analeptics during narcosis. Note that the peak effect is reached within several minutes when metrazole is used. Minute volume exchange is the criterion used to designate intensity of stimulation. A latent period of 30 or more seconds precedes the onset of stimulation. There is a gradual recession of respiratory activity after three or four minutes with a return to the pre-injection state. The latent period with nikethamide is somewhat longer, the peak of action is not quite as intense and the duration of action is briefer, compared to metrazole. Picrotoxin manifests a long latent period with a gradual rise in intensity to a plateau which may be sustained as long as 25 or 30 minutes. The intensity is greatest with the substance. The response depicted by these three drugs is by the intravenous route in a subject narcotized with barbiturate. The N-allyl nor-morphine is used to reverse overdosage from morphine. Note that the effect is sustained, in contradistinction to the other analeptics.

minister pentothal in event convulsions occur and decrease succeeding doses of picrotoxin.

3. Lengthen the time interval for successive doses during the treatment to 45 minutes—or to one hour if signs of hyperirritability appear.

The barbiturate is being detoxified by the tissues and the level of narcosis is being elevated because of the detoxification.

4. Resort to intravenous injection of the picrotoxin in event the patient relapses into depression during the treatment.

The subcutaneous dose may not always be sufficient to maintain the patient at the roused level.

5. Remember that a latent period exists between the moment of injection and the onset of stimulation. (Fig. 178).

Overdosage may result if the drug is injected too rapidly because of this delayed effect.

6. Remember that picrotoxin merely antagonizes the effect of the barbiturate and does not accelerate its destruction.

Both picrotoxin and the barbiturate must be detoxified or eliminated from the body.

Use of Bemegride (Megimide) for Drug Induced Coma

Follow directions above described for picrotoxin but instead
(1) inject bemegride (Megimide) at 50 mgm. increments at 3–4 minute intervals intravenously until signs of reflex activity appear.

Comment

1. Fractionate drug as needed. As many as 600 mgms. may be required before arousal occurs.
2. Watch for signs of twitchings and convulsive movements. Discontinue drug if these appear and subject has not showed signs of increased activity.
3. Give drug slowly allowing sufficient time to lapse between doses (3–4 minutes).
4. Watch for signs of relapse particularly in case of long lasting drug.

Evaluation and Management of Newborn Infant (Apgar Score)

Definition:

In most cases the newborn makes his transition from uterine life to the neonatal period without difficulty. The condition of the infant and the need for resuscitation may be judged by observing the following five signs:

1. Heart rate. Should not be below 100 per minute. Use stethoscope to auscultate.
2. Respiratory effort. Should be spontaneous and established within one minute.
3. Muscle tone. Active motion of the extremities should be in evidence. Flaccidity and poor muscle tone may be a sign of shock.
4. Reflex irritability Should have an active cough or sneeze reflex when the mucosa of these parts is stimulated by a catheter.
5. Color. Should be completely pink over the head, torso and extremities.

Scoring:

Within *one minute* after delivery the above factors should be evaluated and rated and given a score of 2, 1 or 0 depending upon the infant's status, as described below:

Score	2	1	0
Heart rate.	Over 100.	Slow, less than 100.	Absent.
Respiratory effort.	Active with crying.	Slow, irregular.	Absent.
Muscle tone.	Active.	Some flexion of arms and legs.	Limp.
Reflex irritability.	Sneezing and coughing.	Grimace when stimulated.	No response.
Color.	Pink over entire body.	Body pink; extremities cyanotic.	Blue or pale.

Score of: 10 to 5— No treatment is indicated except routine care described below.
4 to 0— Resuscitation or other treatment which appears to be indicated from pre senting symptoms.

Comment

1. Over 90% of newborns have score of 7 or more.

Materials for Infant Resuscitation:

1. Inhaler composed of infant sized mask and holder, breathing bag of 500 to 1000 capacity with bag holder, and nipple or tail for attachment of delivery tube, delivery tube, oxygen supply, and flow meter.
2. Aneroid or water manometer attached to right angled tube which is connected at some convenient point to the delivery tube.
3. Infant size airways (plastic or metal).
4. DeLee glass suction trap.
5. Two holed suction catheters (Raush).
6. Pencil handled laryngoscope with a premature blade.
7. Cole endotracheal catheters size 10, 12, 14 with stylets.
8. Sterile lubricant for endotracheal tube.

Procedure for Routine Care of the Newborn at Birth:

1. Hold with head down to prevent aspiration of mucous, amniotic fluid, blood, etc.
2. Gently aspirate mouth, throat and nose by applying gentle suction with mouth on the catheter and DeLee trap.
3. Wrap to prevent chilling to assure and maintain a normal body temperature.

For Infants with Score of 4 or Less:

Technique same as for adults.

1. Ventilate using controlled intermittent positive pressure (of 15–20 cms. water pressure) with mask and bag.
2. Relieve obstruction due to secretions by using a suction. Insert an airway if needed. An endotracheal tube should be used last if necessary.
3. Administer blood of shock is present. Indications are pallor, or history of blood loss.

Comment

1. Omit analeptics. Non-speicfic stimulants (metrazole, coramine, bemegride, etc.) are of no benefit and even may be harmful. Bemegride may be of service if apnea is due to barbiturates. Administer in 5 mgm. increments intravenously into umbilical cord at 2–3 minute intervals. Do not exceed 25 mgm. if no response is obtained.
2. Use anti-narcotics, such as nalorphine (Nalline) in 0.5 mgm. increments up to 2 mgm. or levallorphan (Lorfan) if depression is known to be due to a narcotic. Should be administered intravenously into umbilical

vein. Do not exceed doses suggested, particularly if no effect is observed.

3. In absence of mechanical apparatus, mouth to mouth breathing or mouth to airway or mouth to endotracheal tube may be used. Blow in only air from mouth. Blow none from lung otherwise pressure will be excessive and lungs will be ruptured.

REFERENCES

Adriani, J. Pharmacology of Anesthetic Drugs. 4th Ed. Charles C Thomas, Springfield, Ill., 1960.

Dille, J. M. Picrotoxin. Northwest Med., *38:* 80, March, 1939.

Volpitto, P. P. The Treatment of Acute Barbiturate Poisoning. Anesth. & Analg., *18:* 205, 1939.

PART IX

INHALATION THERAPY

OXYGEN THERAPY

Definition: The administration of oxygen enriched atmospheres by inhalation for therapeutic reasons.

Purpose:

1. To attempt to relieve anoxia by raising the alveolar oxygen tension.
2. To increase oxygen in tissues above the normal concentration. This is accomplished by increasing the dissolved gas by inhalation of nearly 100% oxygen.
3. To facilitate the removal of gases, such as nitrogen or helium, from hollow viscera, body cavities, blood and other tissues.

Methods of Administration:

1. *By catheters* or inhalers placed in the nostril or nasopharynx. **This method is simplest and most practical for ordinary routine use.**
2. *By mask:* This method is necessary to secure high alveolar concentrations of oxygen and for the successful desaturation of tissues of such gases as nitrogen or helium.
3. *In a tent* or canopy equipped with a conditioner. This method is suitable for children and patients who cannot tolerate masks or catheters.
4. *In an oxygen room:* This method is ideal but the least practical from economic standpoint.

Source of Oxygen for Clinical Use

Use: Oxygen is delivered to the bedside in one of 2 ways. (1) In individual cylinders; (2) piped from a central source where it is stored in bulk. Oxygen used for medicinal purposes has the following features.

1. Is 99%–100% pure. The contaminent is nitrogen.
2. Is tasteless, colorless and odorless.
3. Exists as a compressed gas in the cylinder at room temperature (not liquid).
4. Is made from liquid air.
5. Differs in no way from chemically pure commercial oxygen.
6. Is anhydrous.

Features of Cylinders:

1. Usually contain 244 cubic feet of gas expressed at room temperature and atmosphere pressure.

2. Usually is at 2000 lbs. per square inch.
3. Are usually painted green.
4. Are made of drawn steel.
5. Have single valve protected by removable caps when not in use.

OXYGEN THERAPY USING PIPING SYSTEM

Principle: Oxygen in bulk is delivered to a central storage unit in the hospital and distributed to outlets located at the patient's bedside by a system of copper pipes.

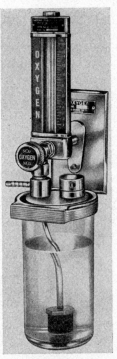

FIG. 179. Wall unit consisting of humidifier and flowmeter. (Courtesy National Cylinder Co.)

Features:

1. The gas is piped at a low pressure (60–100 lbs.) from the high pressure (2000 lbs.) storage unit.
2. Only the flowmeter is required. The pressure gauge is not necessary. These are quickly detachable and replaceable to the wall unit (Fig. 179).
3. Details of therapy after regulator is connected same as outlined for cylinder oxygen. The wall unit takes the place of the cylinder and regulator described in the following procedures.

Advantages:

1. Reduces cost and labor.
2. Eliminates cylinder handling and its inconveniences and hazards.
3. Convenient and instantly available.
4. Assures uninterrupted therapy.

NASAL CATHETER TECHNIQUE

Principle: The concentration of oxygen in the alveoli is raised by flowing pure oxygen through a nasopharyngeal catheter.

Materials:

1. One cylinder of oxygen. The size usually employed contains 244 cu. ft. at 2200 lbs. per square inch pressure.
2. A suitable regulator consisting of a reducing valve, a flow meter calibrated in liters, a humidifier, and a pressure gauge (Fig. 180).

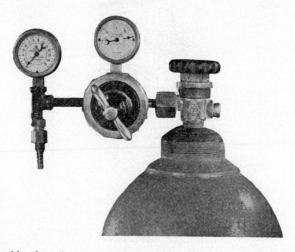

FIG. 180. Assembly of regulator and pressure gauge for oxygen therapy. A humidifing bottle is attached to the outlet when the catheter technique is employed. (Courtesy of The Linde Air Products Company.)

3. A catheter #12F which has four or five perforations at the tip (for children #10, or #8 in some cases).
4. A cotton or canvas wrapper or cover for the cylinder.
5. A strap for securing the cylinder to the bed post.
6. A cork or rubber mat 12″ × 12″ to place beneath the cylinder to protect floor.
7. Adhesive cut in strips 4″ long × 1/2″ wide.
8. Petrolatum for lubricating the catheter.
9. A rubber delivery tube from humidifier to catheter (5 feet long, 1/4″ inside diameter).

10. Stainless steel or plastic connector for catheter (5/16"×3").
11. Wrench for tightening regulator.

Procedure:

1. Attach gauge and flowmeter to cylinder and tighten joints.
2. Fill humidifier jar with water to designated line.
3. Arrange cylinder on the mat at the right hand side of the head end of the bed. Fasten securely with strap to the bed post.

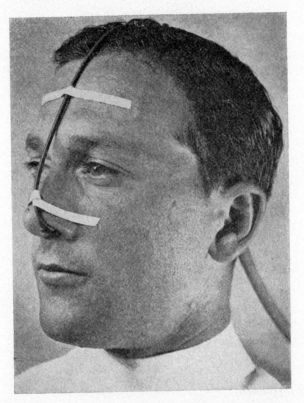

Fig. 181. Administration of oxygen by nasal catheter. (Courtesy of The Linde Air Products Company.)

4. **Explain the contemplated procedure to the patient.**
5. Mark off a distance on the catheter equivalent to the distance from tip of nose to the tragus of ear of the patient.
6. Attach connecting rubber tubing to regulator and connect catheter to glass tip.
7. Lubricate the catheter half its length from the tip with petrolatum.
8. Commence the flow of oxygen at 5 liters per minute.
9. Insert catheter as far as the designated mark gently into either nostril. Use no force whatsoever in placing it. The nostril through which the

catheter passes easiest and is most comfortable is the one to be selected.

10. Immobilize the catheter over the forehead and bridge of the nose with several strips of adhesive so that it remains securely anchored (Fig. 181).

Precautions:

1. **Always inspect the tubing leading from regulator to the catheter for perforations or kinks and be positive all of the oxygen is flowing to the patient.**

2. Be positive catheters are not kinked or obstructed by plugs of mucus in perforations.

3. Be positive the catheter is not doubled upon itself in the nostril and that it is placed correctly in the nasopharynx (Fig. 182).

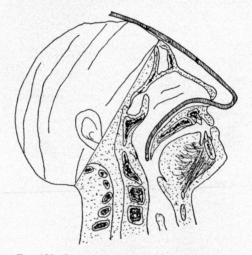

Fig. 182. Correct placement of the catheter in the nasopharynx for oxygen therapy.

Discontinuing Treatment:

1. Loosen adhesive from head and nose and gently wiggle catheter. Be certain that it is loose before withdrawing it from the nose.
2. Turn off oxygen at regulator valve.
3. Turn off main cylinder valve (turn anti-clockwise).
4. Return all equipment to the supply room for cleaning and storing.

Advantages of Catheter Technique:

1. It is simple, easily installed, and serviced.
2. It is relatively inexpensive.
3. It is comfortable for the patient.
4. It supplies a high tension of oxygen in the alveoli (approximately three times the normal alveolar oxygen tension).

5. It does not interfere with the elimination of carbon dioxide.
6. The catheter is tolerated and easily managed in comatose patients.
7. It requires little care, once treatment is initiated.
8. The flow of gas need not be discontinued during treatments, meals, or examinations.

Disadvantages:

1. Uncooperative subjects do not always tolerate the catheter (children, delirious subjects).
2. It cannot be employed when high oxygen tension or when desaturation of other gases from tissues is desired.

Comment

1. Be certain catheters are provided with several perforations. This prevents the stream of gas from impinging on one area and irritating the mucous membranes.
2. **Be sure the oxygen is humidified.** The gas is anhydrous as it issues from the cylinder and irritates the mucous membranes.
3. **Vary the flow of oxygen according to the needs of the patient.** A flow of 5 liters per minute usually provides 35 to 40% oxygen in the inspired air. Pulse and respiratory rate should be guide to efficiency of treatment.
4. Do not insert the catheter beyond the measured distance into the pharynx. If it rests in the oropharynx, oxygen is swallowed.
5. Do not insert the catheter too short a distance into the nasopharynx. The oxygen tension falls below 35% and the therapy is not satisfactory.
6. **Do not fail to strap the cylinder to the bed post.**
7. Do not use oil or grease to lubricate oxygen therapy equipment.
8. Replace the catheter every 8 to 12 hours with a clean one.
9. Maintain a record of the treatment upon a special form designed to indicate the following data:
   a. Date.
   b. Hour treatment was instituted.
   c. Temperature curve.
   d. Pulse rate.
   e. Respiratory rate.
   f. Color of skin.
   g. Flow of oxygen.
   h. Type of treatment.

REFERENCES

Boothby, W. M. Oxygen Therapy. J.A.M.A., *99:* 2026, 1932.
Evans, J. H. Oxygen Therapy in Pneumonia. Anesth. & Analg., *6:* 57, 1927.
Waters, R. M., and Buerki, R. C. Oxygen Therapy at the Wisconsin General Hospital Hospitals, March, 1936.

Waters, R. M., Buerki, R. C., and Hathaway, H. R. Oxygen Therapy at the Wisconsin General Hospital. Hospitals, March, 1936.
Wineland, A. J., and Waters, R. M. Oxygen Therapy. Archives Surg., *22:* 67, 1930.

Oxygen by the Mask Technique

Principle: The alveolar oxygen concentration is raised by allowing the patient to breathe from a semi-open, semi-closed, or closed inhaler.

Types of Inhalers:

1. *Semi-open:* The semi-open inhaler consists of loosely fitting celluloid, rubber, or plastic face pieces into which oxygen is conducted. No valves or bags are employed (Fig. 183).
2. *Semi-closed:* The semi-closed inhaler designed for inhalation anesthesia may be employed for oxygen therapy. The semi-closed system is necessary for the administration of 100% oxygen and the desaturation of nitrogen from tissues. Various simpler forms than those for anesthesia have been devised to be used for inhalation therapy. The following are some of the most popular:
   a. B.L.B.: This is composed of a mask, a rebreathing bag of one liter capacity and an exhalation valve composed of sponge rubber.
   b. Barach-Eckman: This is composed of a bag, mask, and exhalation valve. A calibrated injector is attached to the regulator for aspiration of air to dilute oxygen when concentrations less than 100% are desired. Also known as the O.E.M. mask.
3. *Closed:* The circle or to and fro inhaler designed for inhalation anesthesia may likewise be used to administer oxygen by the closed system.

Note: Follow the instructions provided by the manufacturer for each type of mask.

REFERENCE

Barach, A. L., and Eckman, Morris. A Mask Apparatus for High Oxygen Concentrations J. Aviation M., March, 1941.

B.L.B. Mask Technique

Materials:

1. Assemble the same material for the nasal catheter technique.
2. Select the type mask desired.
   Two types of masks are available: *Oronasal and nasal.* The nasal type is suitable for conscious subjects who can breathe through the nose. Two sizes of B.L.B. masks are available, a small and large.

Procedure:

1. Arrange the cylinder, flowmeter, tubing, etc., in the same manner described for the catheter technique.

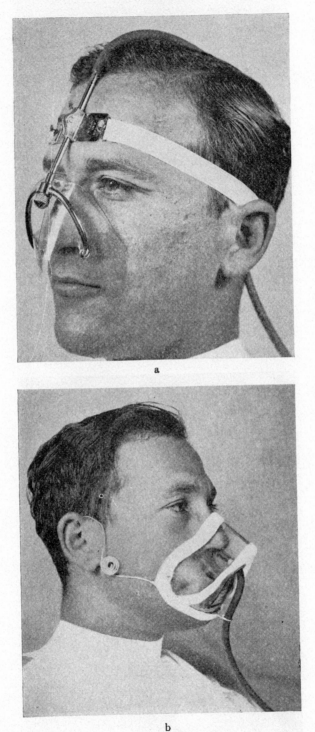

a

b

FIG. 183a and b. Lombard face shield for oxygen therapy. (Courtesy of The Linde Air Products Company.)

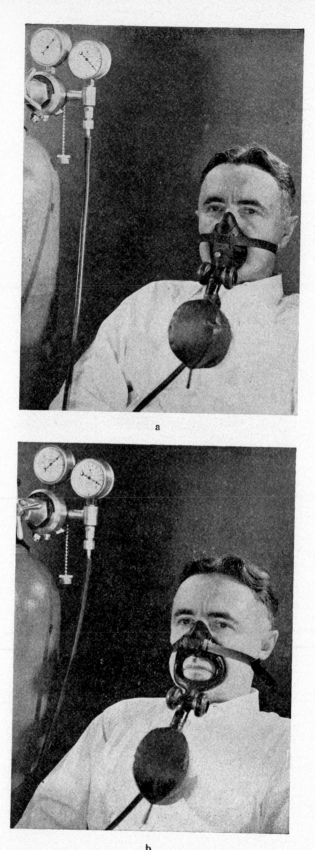

a

b

FIG. 184 (a) B.L.B. oronasal mask in use. (b) Nasal B.L.B. mask in use.
(Courtesy of The Linde Air Products Company.)

2. Connect the mask to the delivery tube in place of the catheter.
3. Commence the oxygen flowing at approximately 8 liters per minute.
4. Apply the mask so that it fits snugly to face. Pack leaks with cotton to insure a comfortable and snug fit (Fig. 184).
5. Fasten the head strap to maintain this fit.
6. Readjust the flow of gas to suit the needs of the patient.

Precautions:

1. Be certain the mask fits properly and the flow of oxygen is sufficient to allow the rebreathing bag to remain inflated at all times.
2. Restrain delirious patients.
3. Be positive the exhalation valve is in satisfactory working order and that it allows the excess oxygen and carbon dioxide to escape without resistance.

Discontinuing Treatment:

1. Loosen the strap and remove the mask.
2. Turn off oxygen at regulator valve and then at the main valve.

Advantages of Mask:

1. It allows the use of high oxygen tensions (100% if necessary).
2. It allows desaturation of tissues from other gases.
3. It is portable and simple to service.
4. It is inexpensive.

Disadvantages:

1. It allows some rebreathing. Carbon dioxide may accumulate in the mask and bag if valves are not patent.
2. The oxygen must be discontinued to administer medication and other treatments.
3. The expiratory valve, particularly the sponge type, creates resistance to respiration.
4. The mask is not comfortable and does not fit the face of all patients snugly.

Comment

1. Remember that the B.L.B. mask allows some rebreathing. The first third of the expiration passes into the bag, the remainder passes through the sponge exhalation valve.
2. Use a rapid flow of oxygen (7–10 liters per minute) to eliminate inspiratory resistance and to avoid carbon dioxide in the inspiratory air.
3. Remember that the oxygen concentration is controlled by the flow of gas as follows: 50–60%—4 liters per minute and allow bag to collapse. 95–100%—8 liters and allow bag to remain distended.

4. Omit the humidifier if rebreathing is employed.
5. Pass stomach tubes through the nipple provided for the purpose to insure a snug fit.
6. Remove the plug at the end of the bag from time to time to drain off condensed vapor.

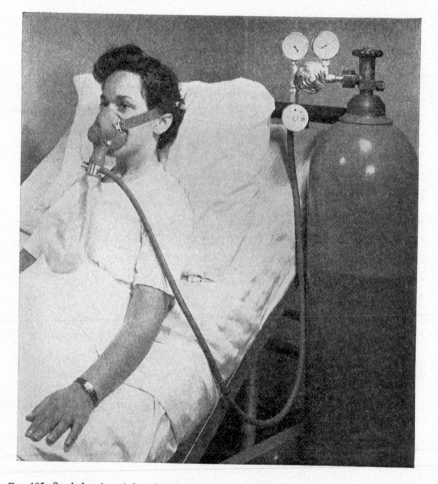

Fig. 185. Semi-closed mask for administering oxygen. Rebreathing is minimized by an inspiratory valve at the neck of the bag and an expiratory valve at the top. A calibrated resistance may be placed at the top at the exhalation port for expiratory positive pressure. The O.E.M. mask operates on this principle. (Courtesy Meyer Saklad, Inhalation Therapy and Resuscitation. Springfield, Thomas, 1953.)

BARACH ECKMAN METER MASK TECHNIQUE (O.E.M.)

1. Assemble same material used for nasal catheter technique plus air injector.
2. Semi-closed mask with valves at inlet and outlet (Fig. 185).

Procedure:

1. Arrange cylinder, flowmeter, tubing in the same manner described for B.L.B. technique.
2. Attach mixing meter at outlet of regulator (instead of humidifier).
3. Adjust mixing valve to supply desired percentage of oxygen and air. The figure indicates percent oxygen delivered.
4. Turn on oxygen at rate sufficient to maintain a full bag.

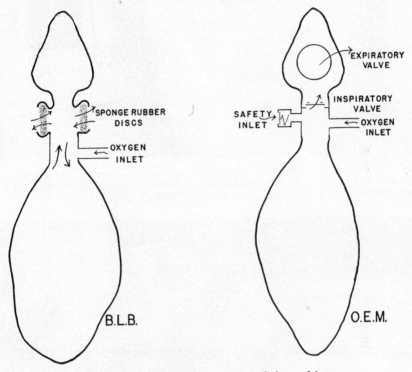

Fig. 186. Schematic diagram of semi-closed inhaler used for oxygen therapy. (Courtesy Meyer Saklad.)

Advantages:

1. Eliminates rebreathing (except air in mask) (Fig. 186).
2. Permits proportion of oxygen and air to be accurately fixed and maintained.
3. Permits use of expiratory positive pressure to be applied.
4. System is entirely semi-closed.

Disadvantages: Same as those outlined for mask therapy with B.L.B.

REFERENCE

Boothby, W. M., Lovelace, W. R., and Bulbulian, A. H. Proc. Staff Meeting Mayo Clinic, *15:* 194, 1940.

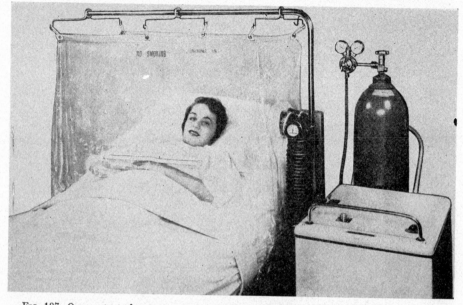

FIG. 187. Oxygen tent of canopy type operated by mechanical refrigeration. The mechanical unit recirculates the gases from the tent through the conditioning unit which removes moisture and carbon dioxide and cools the gas. (Courtesy National Cylinder Company.)

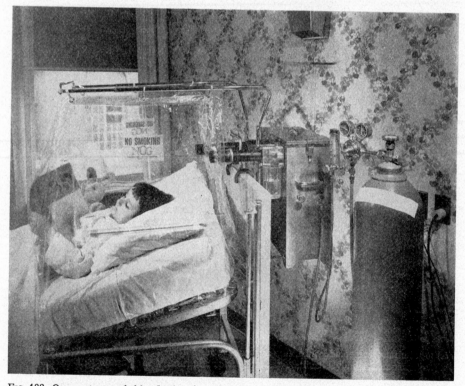

FIG. 188. Oxygen tent cooled by flowing the gas through crushed ice. Some recirculation is obtained by a jet utilizing the Venturi principle. (Courtesy National Cylinder Company.)

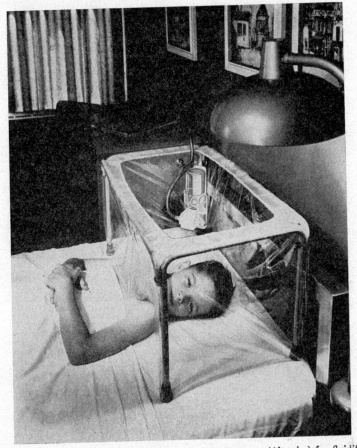

Fig. 189. Open top tent with nebulizer for water and detergent (Alevaire) for fluidifying secretions. The stream of oxygen is passed through the nebulizer creating a fine mist. Antibiotics and other therapeutic agents may be administered by inhalation. (Courtesy National Cylinder Company.)

OXYGEN BY TENT

Definition of a Tent: A tent consists of a gas-proof canopy or hood which encloses the head or upper portion of the patient's body. Connected to this canopy is a source of oxygen, a unit composed of a dehumidifier, a cooler, and a carbon dioxide absorber.

Types: Many types of tents are manufactured and available for clinical use. These may be resolved into two types:

1. Canopies which fit over the bed over the upper half of the patient's body (Fig. 187).
2. Open box tent or canopies. These are for infants and small children because the entire body is enclosed (Fig. 191).

Procedure for Use of Tents: Each type tent must be manipulated according

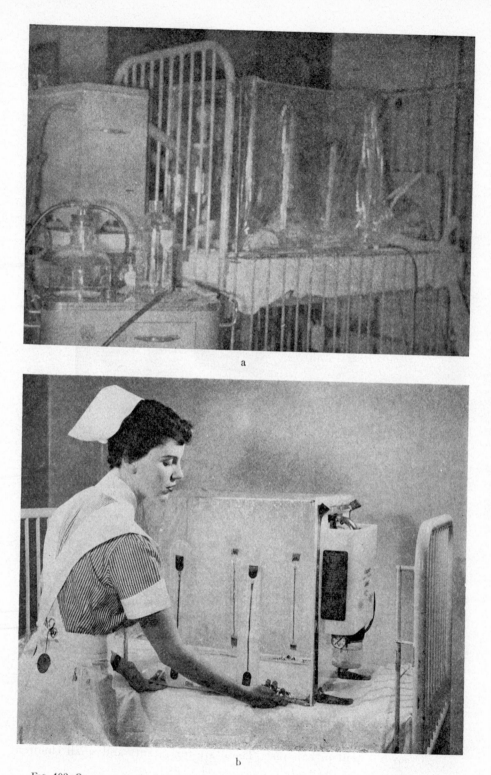

a

b

FIG. 190. Oxygen tents for infants. (a) Canopy type. (b) Canopy type tent which supplies nebulized water in fine mist for humidification as well as oxygen.

to the instructions and recommendations of the manufacturer. However, these general remarks apply to all tents:

1. Analyze the concentration of oxygen at least every three hours.
2. Watch the temperature and humidity in the tent closely. Maintain at patient's comfort.
3. Increase the flow of oxygen temporarily each time the tent is opened for treatments or examinations (15 liters for 15 minutes).
4. Inspect the canopy for leaks and see that skirts of the tent canopy are tucked in tightly beneath the bed covers.
5. Use a rubber sheet over the mattress with the canopy type of tent.

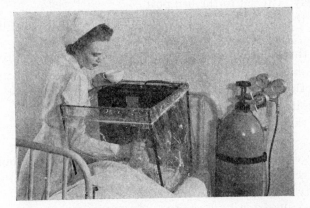

FIG. 191. Open box tent permits ready access to patient for treatments and general care. (Courtesy of The Linde Air Products Company.)

Advantages of Tents:

1. They allow a greater degree of comfort to the patient than catheters or masks. They provide air conditioning in warm climates.
2. They permit use of vaporized drugs.

Disadvantages:

1. The initial cost of the equipment prohibits its use in many institutions.
2. They are more difficult to service than catheters or masks and require constant attention by trained attendants.
3. The enclosure by the canopy psychically disturbs some patients.
4. They are a fire hazard. Permit no smoking at any time in or around tents.
5. They interfere with treatments, medical examinations, and general care.

REFERENCES

Barach, A. L., A New Oxygen Tent. J.A.M.A., *87:* 1213, 1926.
Campbell, J. A., A Box for the Administration of Oxygen. Brit. M. J., *1:* 1245, 1936.
Saklad, M. Inhalation Therapy. Charles C Thomas, Springfield, Ill., 1953.

MAKING ROUNDS ON PATIENTS RECEIVING INHALATION THERAPY

The inhalation therapist on duty should make rounds every three hours or as often as possible and do or note the following:

1. Be certain that proper pressure exists in cylinders and flow of gases is adequate.
2. Change all cylinders whose pressure is 100 lbs. or less. Such cylinders are near exhaustion.
3. Remove and return equipment to the storage room on discontinued cases.
4. Note whether or not the cylinder is properly placed on the mat and is securely fastened to the bed post.
5. Note that the water is at proper water level in the humidifier bottle (3″).
6. Note that no leaks exist in the line from the flowmeter to the catheter or mask.
7. Note that catheter has not been displaced, kinked, or coated with inspissated mucus.
8. Note that all masks are properly applied, leak proof, and in working order.
9. Analyze the oxygen concentration in all tents every 3 hours.
10. Observe that no smoking or other source of ignition is in the immediate vicinity of oxygen therapy apparatus.
11. Change all catheters every 12 hours.

PRACTICAL HINTS

1. Maintain a record or chart for each patient. Include the following items: Date, hour, patient's temperature, pulse, respiration, color, type of treatment, duration.
2. Open the cylinder valve slightly and then turn it on slowly at first when initiating a fresh cylinder.
3. Store cylinders in a cool room away from all combustible materials.
4. Mark used cylinders "empty" and arrange in an orderly fashion in a part of the store room away from full cylinders.
5. Never attempt to administer oxygen or other compressed gases without a regulator.
6. Transport cylinders on trucks designed for the purpose.
7. Remove all oil and grease from the hands when handling cylinders.
8. Always crack the cylinder valve (open slightly, and close quickly) to remove dust before applying the regulator.
9. Never use any heating or electrical device in any oxygen tent.
10. Commence treatment with an excess flow of oxygen and reduce according to respiration and pulse of patient.

11. Do not use water soluble lubricants for catheters as they dissolve in the nasal discharge.
12. Always fasten the catheter over the bridge of the nose and over center of forehead for comfort and for correct placement of tip of catheter in nasopharynx.

CLEANING CATHETERS AND INHALERS

1. Scrub catheters with soap and warm water and rinse. Remove adhesive with ether.
2. Soak in bichloride of mercury 1 to 1000 or Wescodyne Solution for 30 minutes and rinse (do not use creosol or phenol).
3. Rinse, dry, and coat lightly with talcum if they are to be stored.

CARE OF MASKS

1. Wash with hot soap and water.
2. Rinse with 70% alcohol and wipe with clean towel.
3. Dry and powder with talcum to absorb moisture.
4. Place in cool cabinet to prevent drying.

CARBON DIOXIDE-OXYGEN THERAPY

Purposes: Inhalation of carbon dioxide in air or oxygen is employed for respiratory stimulation in the following conditions:

1. Depressed states resulting from morphine, barbiturates or other drugs.
2. To attempt to relieve persistent hiccoughs.
3. To induce hyperventilation in the postoperative period to prevent respiratory complications by the forced expansion of the thorax.
4. To hasten the dissociation of the carbon monoxide hemoglobin complex in carbon monoxide poisoning.

Methods of Administration:

1. By allowing a patient to rebreathe from a paper bag or a closed inhaler.
2. By supplying a continuous flow of a preformed mixture to a semiclosed inhaler from a storage cylinder.

Concentration: Five per cent carbon dioxide in oxygen or air is usually employed.

TECHNIQUE BY REBREATHING

Materials:

1. The closed inhaler of an anesthesia machine.
2. A cylinder of pure oxygen.

Procedure:

1. Fill inhaler with oxygen and strap mask snugly to the face of the subject. Turn on metabolic flow of oxygen.
2. Close the soda lime absorber and allow patient to rebreathe his exhaled carbon dioxide until a hyperpnea is well established.

TECHNIQUE USING PREFORMED MIXTURES

Materials:

1. One cylinder of carbon dioxide (5%) oxygen (95%) mixture.
2. A reducing valve, pressure gauge, and flowmeter.
3. A semi-closed inhaler consisting of rebreathing bag, mask, and exhalation valve.

Procedure:

1. Fill the bag of inhaler by closing the exhalation valve and obturator.
2. Apply the mask to the face, open obturator and allow patient to breathe from filled inhaler.
3. Allow gas to flow at the rate of 2 or 3 liters per minute, or fast enough to allow bag of inhaler to remain distended.
4. Open exhalation valve sufficiently to allow the expired and excess gas to pass from the mask.
5. Allow the hyperpnea to become well established.

Note: If pure carbon dioxide is available, the flowmeter of anesthesia apparatus may be used to form the desired mixture as follows: 4 3/4 liters of oxygen to 250 cc. of carbon dioxide for 95:5% mixture, or 4 1/2 liters to 500 cc. for 90:10% mixture.

Contra-Indications to Inhalation of Carbon Dioxide:

1. The presence of cardiac disease.
2. The presence of hypertension.
3. Dyspnea, hyperpnea, obstruction, and other types of respiratory difficulty.
4. Acidosis from any cause.
5. Emphysema, asthma, or pneumonia.

HELIUM-OXYGEN THERAPY

Definition: Helium is an extremely light, inert inorganic gas. It is the second lightest gas; also one of the least soluble gases known.

Uses: Mixtures of helium and oxygen are administered by inhalation to reduce the respiratory effort. This is accomplished by one or a combination of the two following factors:

1. By decreasing the respiratory load (80% helium and 20% oxygen equals 1/3 the weight of an equivalent volume of air).
2. By increasing the rate of diffusion of the mixture. The lightness of the helium molecule is responsible for this property.
   The mixture, therefore, appears to be of benefit to patients with dyspnea due to respiratory obstruction, bronchiolar constriction, stenosis of the trachea, etc.

Methods of Administration: Helium may be administered by:

1. The semi-closed technique (B.L.B.). The cost is prohibitive because a continuous flow is required.
2. The closed system by the rebreathing technique. The circle filter, the to and fro filter, or the hood type of tent (page 523) may be employed.

Technique Using B.L.B. Mask

Materials:

1. A cylinder of pure oxygen (type G—220 cu. ft.).
2. A cylinder of helium-oxygen mixture 80%–20% (type G).
3. One regulator for each type gas without humidifier.
4. One Y connecting piece to fit connecting tube.
5. One section of delivery tube 4 feet long, 1/4" inside diameter.
6. B.L.B. mask—oronasal or nasal.
7. Two sections of delivery tubes 18" long.

Procedure:

1. Connect one short section of delivery tubing to the regulator on the oxygen cylinder, the other to the regulator on the helium cylinder.
2. Connect the long tubing to the mask and to the stem of the Y piece.
3. Connect the Y to the oxygen and helium.
4. Allow the helium mixture to flow into inhaler so that the rebreathing bag is not quite emptied with each inspiration.
5. Pad the mask well to occlude all leaks. Decrease the flow of helium-oxygen mixture and gradually turn on pure oxygen until the patient is able to tolerate 100% oxygen.
6. Continue the flow of gas mixture until the symptoms disappear.

Techniques Using Closed Inhalers

Materials:

1. A circle filter or a to and fro inhaler equipped with an exhalation valve.
2. One cylinder of pure oxygen.
3. One cylinder of helium-oxygen mixture (80%–20% or 75%–25%).
4. Flowmeter with yokes for oxygen, and helium-oxygen mixture.

Procedure:

1. Arrange patient in comfortable position.
2. Fill the breathing bag or inhaler with oxygen and apply mask to the patient's face so that a snug fit is secured.
3. Open the exhalation valve, deflate rebreathing bag almost completely, and fill with oxygen-helium mixture.
4. Turn on oxygen at the rate of 500 cc. per minute or in a quantity to satisfy the metabolic requirement of the patient.
5. Allow patient to rebreathe the mixture for 3 to 5 minutes.
6. Open exhalation valve, deflate bag and fill with oxygen-helium mixture once again (this removes nitrogen).
7. Repeat several times after 3 or 4 minutes.

Comment	*Reasons*
1. Eliminate nitrogen in the alveoli and inhaler by emptying the bag to obtain effective treatment.	Nitrogen has a higher molecular weight than helium (7 times greater). It lacks the physical properties which render helium effective.
2. Do not use pure helium for inhalation therapy.	The gas is inert and causes asphyxia if oxygen is not added.
3. Always supply oxygen when the rebreathing technique is employed.	The oxygen in the mixture is gradually consumed by the tissues.
4. Do not be alarmed if the patient's voice assumes a nasal tone.	The speed of sound is decreased in the lighter medium and changes the quality of the voice.

REFERENCES

Barach, A. L. Recent Advances in Oxygen and Helium Therapy. Med. Clinics North America, *24:* 261, 1940.

Lovelace, W. R. Technique of Treatment With Helium and Oxygen Using B.L.B. Inhalation Apparatus. Proc. Staff Meeting Mayo Clinic, *13:* 786, 1938.

POSITIVE PRESSURE OXYGEN THERAPY

Methods:

1. Continuous. Positive pressure is applied during inspiration and expiration.
2. Inspiratory. Positive pressure is applied during the inspiratory phase of respiration. Expiration is without resistance.
3. Expiratory. Positive pressure is applied during expiration. Inspiration is unimpeded or unaided.

Uses:

1. For treatment of pulmonary edema.

2. For treatment of obstructive dyspnea.

3. For treatment of emphysematous states.

CONTINUOUS POSITIVE PRESSURE

Material:

1. Closed inhaler. To and fro or circle filter used for anesthesia equipped with water or aneroid manometer.

2. Oxygen supply.

Procedure:

1. Fill inhaler with oxygen and distend bag to 8–10 cms. H_2O pressure.

2. Adjust flow into inhaler to maintain desired pressure on inspiration and expiration (10–4 cms. H_2O).

Caution: Prolonged use has deleterious effects on the circulation.

POSITIVE PRESSURE ON INSPIRATION

Material: Inhaler with demand valve activated by negative pressure (flow sensitive type of Bennett, Fig. 192).

1. Select proper size mask.

2. Open the oxygen supply by turning shut off lever down.

3. Set control pressure gauge to read desired pressure.

4. Apply mask and ask patient to breathe in normal manner.

5. Adjust pressure to patient's comfort.

POSITIVE PRESSURE ON EXPIRATION

A. *Using Semi-closed inhaler with expiratory resistance (Barach Eckman, O.E.M. mask)*

Procedure: Adjust mask in same manner outlined for ordinary oxygen therapy and set resistance on expiratory valve at desired pressure (4 cms.)

B. *Using Anesthesia Apparatus*

Material:

1. Closed to and fro or circle inhaler.

2. Water manometer (Fig. 14) or calibrated expiratory valve.

Procedure: Allow gas to flow into inhaler at rate to maintain a zero pressure at inspiration and to allow excess to escape through valve or the stem of the water manometer at desired positive pressure on expiration (4 cms.).

ETHYL ALCOHOL INHALATIONS

Description: Inhalation of vaporized ethyl alcohol as an anti-foaming agent.

Uses: For the treatment of pulmonary edema.

Materials:

1. Standard oxygen therapy regulator and humidifier.
2. Ethyl alcohol—95%.
3. Semi-closed inhaler or oronasal catheter set-up used for oxygen therapy.

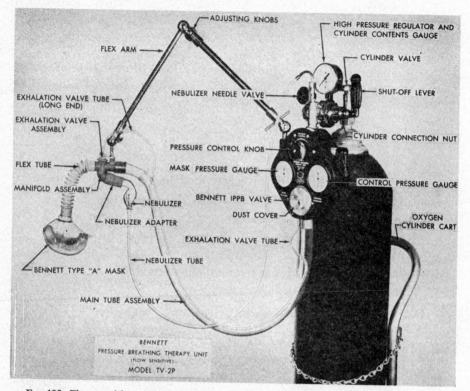

Fig. 192. Flow sensitive pressure breathing therapy unit (Bennett) for administering positive pressure on inspiration. The Bennett valve is activated by negative pressure caused by the patient's inspiration. Flow ceases at initiation of expiratory phase of the cycle. The device permits administration of nebulized agents for therapeutic purpose. Automatic cycling for intermittent positive pressure breathing in apneic states may also be induced.

Procedure:

1. Place 2 cc. alcohol for each 8 cc. water (total 10 cc.) in vaporizer jar almost to "full level."
2. Commence flow of oxygen at 5 liters into semi-closed inhaler (O.E.M. or B.L.B. mask) or lubricated catheter placed into oropharynx.
3. Continue treatment for 5 minutes. If there is no sign of improvement increase alcohol adding 2 cc additional for each 8 cc of water originally used. If still additional alcohol is needed add 2 cc. more for each 8 cc. water used

Precautions:

1. The mixture is highly inflammable.
2. Do not leave alcohol in apparatus after use.
3. Do not smear alcohol on regulator—it may pass into the device and cause a flash fire or an explosion.
4. Do not nebulize alcohol in tents, or hoods. Explosions may result.

Comment

1. Ethyl hexanol may be used with same effect instead of alcohol to reduce fire hazard.
2. Do not use more than a total of 6 cc. of alcohol for each 8 cc. water.

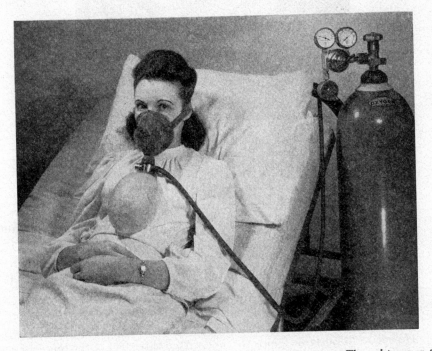

FIG. 193. The O.E.M. mask being used for expiratory positive pressure. The resistance on the valve is calibrated to 4 cms. H_2O pressure. (Courtesy Meyer Saklad, Inhalation Therapy and Resuscitation. Springfield, Thomas, 1953.)

RULES FOR SAFETY USING OXYGEN TENT

1. Do not use alcohol, oil or other flammable material for back rubs on a patient receiving oxygen in a tent.
2. Do not place an E.K.G. cardiac Pacemaker or monitoring device within three feet of an oxygen tent canopy.
3. Switch the nasal oxygen or mask or roll canopy up around neck of patient. Do not use flashlight inside oxygen tent.
4. Do not place electric suction pump within three feet of an oxygen tent.

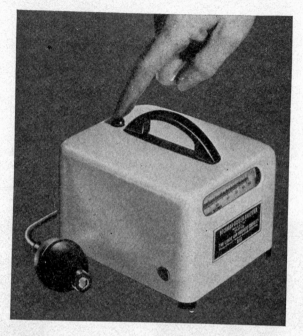

Fig. 194. Oxygen analyzer (Beckman) based upon the principle that oxygen is paramagnetic. (Courtesy Meyer Saklad, Inhalation Therapy and Resuscitation. Springfield, Thomas, 1953.)

5. Do not use oxygen tents on electrically operated bed unless electrical operating mechanism carries Underwriter's label.
6. Do not place an electric fan, radio, television or other electrical appliance within three feet of an oxygen tent.
7. Do not allow a patient to use a hearing aid, electric heating pad, telephone, transistor remote control unit, electric razor or electrical call bell inside the oxygen canopy.
8. Remove electric lamps, radios attached to the headboard of beds during oxygen tent therapy.
9. Do not allow portable lamps to come within three feet of the tent.
10. Do not permit the use of mechanical toys operating by revolving drum inside oxygen tent.

Analyzing for Oxygen Using Beckman Analyzer

Description: The Beckman oxygen analyzer employs the Pauling principle which takes advantage of the fact that oxygen is paramagnetic and affects the lines of force in a magnetic field (Fig. 194).

Uses:

1. Place free end of rubber tube which connects with sampling bulb at point from which sample is to be taken.

2. Slowly squeeze and release aspirator bulb 4 or 5 times to insure complete removal of previous sample and take in new sample.
3. Press light with switch on top of instrument.
4. Read oxygen concentration on top of scale.

Comment

1. Glass tube on back containing silica absorbs moisture so that dry gases are led into apparatus.
2. Readings are affected by temperature. Device should be used in temperature range between 65 and 85°F.
3. Failure to obtain image on scale is due to:
   a. Burned out lamp in apparatus.
   b. Exhausted dry cells.
   c. Quartz string which suspends mirror inside is broken.
4. Pink color in quartz indicates drying power is gone. May be regenerated to blue by heating to 300°F.

APPENDIX

TABLE I (APPENDIX)

URINE ANALYSIS

Volume in 24 hours..750–2,000 cc.
pH..4.8–7.5
Specific Gravity...1.015–1.020
Total Nitrogen...12–18 gm. in 24 hrs.
Urea Nitrogen...10–40 gm. in 24 hrs.
Creatinine...1,000–1,500 mgm. 24 hrs.
Ammonia Nitrogen...600 mgm. in 24 hrs.
Uric Acid..400–1,000 mgm. 24 hrs.
Chloride (as Sodium Chloride)..10–15 gm. in 24 hrs.
Phosphates...1–2 gm. in 24 hrs.
Sulfates..1.5–3.5 gm. in 24 hrs.
Urobilinogen (Watson)..0–4.0 mgm.
Urinary Diastase (Amylase)..8–32 units
17-ketosteroids..12–15 mgm. in 24 hrs.

KIDNEY FUNCTUON

Phenosulfonephthalein test.............................75% excretion of dye in 2 hrs.
Urea clearance...75–130%

BLOOD CHEMISTRY

Constituent	Test Material	mgm./100 cc.
Total solids	whole blood	10.23
Total protein	plasma	6.5–8.2
Albumin	plasma	3.8–6.7
Globulin	plasma	1.2–3.5
Fibrinogen	plasma	0.3–0.6
Total nitrogen	whole blood	3.0–3.7
Non-protein nitrogen	whole blood	25–35
Ammonia nitrogen	whole blood	0.1–0.2
Undetermined nitrogen	whole blood	4–18
Hemoglobin		
(men)	whole blood	14–17 (gms. per 100 cc.)
(women)	whole blood	13–16 (gms. per 100 cc.)
Glucose	whole blood	80–120
Total Lipoids	plasma	450–550
Total Fatty Acids	plasma	190–450
Neutral Fat	plasma	0–370
Cholesterol	plasma	130–230
Lecithin (Phospholipids)	plasma	60–350
Bilirubin	serum	0.1–0.8
Chlorides (as Sodium Chloride)	whole blood	450–500
Chlorides (as Sodium Chloride)	plasma	570–620
Sulfates (inorganic as S)	whole blood	1.04±0.05
Phosphorus, inorganic	plasma	570–620
Calcium	serum	9.3–11.0
Magnesium	serum	1–3
Sodium	serum	330
	whole blood	310–345
Potassium	serum	16–22
Diastase (Amylase)	plasma or serum	80–150 units (Somogyi)
Vitamin C (Ascorbic acid)	plasma	0.8–2.4
Iodine (Protein bound)	serum	3.5–8.5 gamma
Lipase	plasma or serum	Less than 1.5 cc. of N/20 NaOH
Alkaline Phosphatase-Adult	serum	1.5–4.0 Bodansky units
Alkaline Phosphatase-Children	serum	5–12 Bodansky units
CO2 combining Power	plasma	50–80 vol. per cent
Hydrogen ion conc.	whole blood serum	pH 7.4
	serum	pH 7.6–7.9

632

TABLE I (APPENDIX)—*(continued)*

CEREBROSPINAL FLUID

Amount	60–150 cc.
Specific Gravity	1.001–1.010
Reaction	alkaline
Total solids	0.8–1.2 gm./100 cc.
Calcium	2.5–11.2 mgm./100 cc.
Chlorides	740 mgm./100 cc.
Sugar	45–85 mgm./100 cc.
Total protein	15–40 mgm./100 cc.

LIVER FUNCTION TESTS

Normal Values

Serum Bilirubin-less than	1.0 mgm./100 of serum
Cephalin-cholesterol Flocculation (Hanger)-less than	4 units
Urobilinogen in urine-less than (Watson)	1.2 Ehrlich units
Bromsulphalein Excretion	No retention of dye after 45 min.
Icterus Index (Bilirubin content)	4–6
Hippuric Acid Excretion	
Oral test	3.0 gm. of Sodium Benzoate as Benzoic acid
Intravenous test	0.7 gm. of Sodium Benzoate as Benzoic acid
Galactose Tolerance	Less than 3.0 gms. of sugar excreted in 5 hr. test period
Levulose Tolerance	Blood sugar not to rise above 130 mgm./100 cc. of blood
Thymol Turbidity	0–4 units
Cholesterol—cholesterol ester ratio	60–90% of total cholesterol
Iso-Iodeikon Test	10% retention in serum 1/2 hr.
	5% or less retention in serum 1 hr.

(greater the retention, the greater the impaired liver function)

HEMATOLOGY

Coagulation time (Lee-White)	5–8 minutes
Bleeding time	1–2 minutes
Contraction of clot	1–2 hours
Prothrombin time (Quick)	22–25 seconds
Prothrombin time	
(Shapiro)—whole blood	15.5 seconds ± 1.5
diluted blood	39.5 seconds ± 2.5
Erythrocyte Sedimentation Rate	
Westergren—men	1–5 mm./hr.
women	2–0 mm./hr.
Linzenmeier—men	350–600 minutes
women	300–600 minutes
Wintrobe—men	0–9 mm./hr.
women	0–30 mm./hr.
Blood Volume (Plasma)	49–55 cc. Kgm.
Blood Volume (Whole)	72–100 cc. Kgm.

CARDIAC HEMODYNAMICS (CARDIAC CATHETERIZATION)

Right auricular mean pressure	−2 to +3 mm. Hg.
Right ventricular pressure	25 systolic
	2 diastolic
	mean 13
Pulmonary artery	25/8 mean 15
Brachial artery	120/70 mean 90
Cardiac index (cc./mm./m²)	3.1 ± 0.4
A-V O_2 difference	4.2–4.7
Stroke volume—cc.	80
O_2 consumption (cc./min./m²)	150
Peripheral resistance (dynes/sec./cm.²)	1138–1216

Blood Enzyme Studies

(S.G.OT

Serum Glutamic Oxalacetic Transaminase...10–40 units
Serum Glutamic Pyruvic Transaminase...8–25 units
Lactic Dehydrogenase..250–500 units
Isocitric Dehydrogenase...250–500 units

TABLE II (APPENDIX)

CONVERSION FACTORS FOR METRIC SYSTEM

	Exact	*Approximate*
1 cubic centimeter	16.23 minims	15 minims
1 liter (1000 cc.)	33.8 fl. oz.	1 qt.
1 milligram	0.0154 grain	1/60 gr.
1 gram	15.423 grains	15 gr.
1 grain	64.8 milligrams	60 mgm.
1 dram	3.89 grams	4 gm. or 4 cc.
1 ounce	28.35 grams	30 gm. or 30 cc.
1 millimeter	—	1/25 inch
1 inch	2.54 cm.	2.5 cm.
1 pint (16 oz.)	475.00 cc.	500 cc.

TABLE III (APPENDIX)

TEMPERATURE CONVERSION FACTORS

Fahrenheit to Centigrade—Subtract 32 from F.° reading and multiply by 5/9.
Centigrade to Fahrenheit—Multiply C.° by 9/5 and add 32 to the result.

INDEX

635